Retinal Pigment Epithelium in Health and Disease

Alexa Karina Klettner • Stefan Dithmar
Editors

Retinal Pigment Epithelium in Health and Disease

Springer

Editors
Alexa Karina Klettner
Department of Ophthalmology
University of Kiel
University Medical Center
Kiel
Schleswig-Holstein
Germany

Stefan Dithmar
Department of Ophthalmology
HSK Wiesbaden
University of Mainz
Wiesbaden
Germany

ISBN 978-3-030-28383-4 ISBN 978-3-030-28384-1 (eBook)
https://doi.org/10.1007/978-3-030-28384-1

This Springer imprint is published by the registered company Springer Nature Switzerland AG
The registered company address is: Gewerbestrasse 11, 6330 Cham, Switzerland

Preface

When studying the eye, one cannot help to be fascinated by its complexity, its functionality, and its beauty. When working on the retina, the most fascinated cell, at least in our humble opinion, is the retinal pigment epithelium (though we do acknowledge that opinions might differ here, researchers tend to find their own field to be the most interesting subject in the world). The retinal pigment epithelium (RPE) has many functions, many aspects, and many ways to be elucidated. When this introduction was written, the term "retinal pigment epithelium" had 14,142 hits in PubMed. We are aware that neither we nor any other book could possibly do justice to the knowledge about this cell type, nor do we make any claim to be complete. However, the last comprehensive book on the retinal pigment epithelium was published more than 20 years ago, and we felt the urge and the need to present a compendium on the modern RPE, as it is studied in the twenty-first century.

We have divided the book in five different aspects: (1) physiological RPE function, (2) RPE in disease, (3) RPE in diagnostics, (4) RPE in therapy, and (5) RPE models to portray the different aspects of RPE research.

In the first chapter, "**RPE Histopathology and Morphometry**," *Szalai*, *Nickerson*, and *Grossniklaus* introduce the histology, morphology, distribution, and topography of these cells, comparing the physiological appearance with changes seen in age and furthermore in pathological conditions such as age-related macular degeneration, retinal dystrophies, proliferative retinopathies, mitochondrial disease, and tumors.

A major characteristic of the RPE is its polarity, and the functions associated with it. *Rizzolo* gives an overview on "**RPE Polarity and Barrier Function**," describing the unique polarity of the RPE (considered to be "upside down" or rather "right side up" due to reversed membrane polarity), explaining the blood-retinal-barrier and its maturation and the structure and composition of tight junctions, stressing the claudins, and introducing reader into the ways of analyzing barrier function. Finally, the breakdown of the barrier in pathological situation, such as edema, is covered.

A major function of the polarized RPE cells is the phagocytosis of shed photoreceptor outer segment fragments, which is covered in this volume by *Müller and Finnemann* in their chapter "**RPE Phagocytosis**." The authors introduce the reader to the experimental approaches to study phagocytosis in RPE cells and give insights into the molecular mechanisms of phagocytosis, including the recognition and binding by the RPE cells, consequent signaling pathways, as well as processing and degradation of the phagocytosed material.

Finally, they cover defects in the process and its relevance to retinal diseases.

In order to fulfill its functions, ion channels play an important part in RPE cells. In their chapter "**Ion Channels of the Retinal Pigment Epithelium**," *Reichhart* and *Strauss* introduce the reader into the profile, function, and pathological role of ion channels. Both apical and epithelial transports are covered, as well as their role of ion buffering in the subretinal space. Also, a major topic is the role of Ca^{2+} signaling in RPE function.

Vascular endothelial growth factor (VEGF) is a major cytokine in health and disease in the retina, with the RPE being an important source, as described in this volume by *Klettner*. The chapter "**RPE and the Vascular Endothelial Growth Factor**" introduces VEGF and its regulatory mechanisms; gives an overview on its roles in development, adult, and diseased retina; and elaborates on regulatory mechanisms under various conditions, such as hypoxia, oxidative stress, inflammation, and hyperthermia.

The chapter "**The RPE cell and the Immune System**" by *Detrick* and *Hooks* covers the important role of the RPE in the innate immunity of the retina. Components of the innate immunity, such as toll-like receptors, cytokines, and complement, are introduced, and the role of the RPE in their interaction with microglia, in immune regulation, and in adaptive immune responses is described.

The RPE is involved in the development of different ocular diseases. In their chapter "**The RPE in Myopia Development**," *Zhang* and *Wildsoet* describe the role of the RPE in eye growth and refractive development, covering the changes of the RPE in high myopia and their part in regulation of eye size, elucidating on the role of different cytokines, neurotransmitters, and ion channels.

Dik, *Bastiaans*, and *van Meurs* address "**Retinal Pigment Epithelium in Proliferative Disorders**," with the focus on the molecular regulation of the RPE's contribution to proliferative disease. In their chapter, after an introduction into the mechanisms of fibrosis in the retina, they elaborate on the epithelial mesenchymal transition and contributions of the RPE to inflammation as well as to angiogenesis.

In the chapter "**Retinal Pigment Epithelium in Health and Disease: Maturation, Aging and Age-Related Macular Degeneration**," *Ach*, *Tarau*, and *Curcio* elaborate on the development, differentiation, and transdifferentiation of the RPE, stressing on alterations in adolescence and age as they present in the RPE, leading up to the changes seen in age-related macular degeneration (AMD).

Taking the topic of AMD further, *Kaarniranta*, *Salminen*, and *Kauppinen* shed more light on the role of the RPE in the pathology of AMD in chapter "**Retinal Pigment Epithelium in Age-Related Macular Degeneration**," stressing the role of proteasomes and lysosomal autophagy, organelle cross-talk, and inflammation in the development of this disease.

A different aspect is covered by *Schnabolk*, *Obert*, and *Rohrer* in their chapter "**Sex Related Differences in Retinal Pigment Epithelium and Retinal Disease**." The authors discuss the importance of sex hormones and the sex (and gender) differences within the eye, in RPE function, and in retinal disease, with a special focus on autoimmune diseases.

The role of the RPE in diagnostics is covered in two chapters. *Hassenstein* and *Grohmann* describe the role of the **RPE in Optical Coherence Tomography**, where they introduce the different techniques of OCT used and elaborate on the appearances of the RPE in several diseases.

Dithmar and *Celik* cover **RPE Autofluorescence** in their chapter, introducing the fluorophores responsible and the imaging devices making RPE autofluorescence visible. They further elaborate on the fluorescent signals in health and disease, which may help to understand disease progression and pathophysiology.

In the next step, RPE cells can be part of the therapy of retinal diseases. An exciting new field is the **RPE and Stem Cell Therapy**, which is covered by *Skottman*. The reader is introduced into cell-based RPE therapy and educated on the differences of human pluripotent and human embryonic stem cells. Major topics are the differentiation and characterization of the stem-cell-derived RPE and the current status of transplantation studies, both in preclinical and in clinical trials.

Another exciting field is **RPE and Gene Therapy**, in which *Stieger* and *Lorenz* summarize the current state and further direction of RPE-based gene therapy, introducing the different approaches of gene therapy and gene transfer and describing the different gene therapies for inherited retinal diseases as well as acquired retinal disorders.

The role of the RPE in laser therapy is covered by *von der Burchard* and *Roider* in their chapter "**RPE and Laser**." The authors introduce the physics of laser-tissue interactions and elaborate on the different concepts of RPE laser treatment, with a major topic being selective RPE treatment.

In the final part of this volume, we focus on the experimental potential of the retinal pigment epithelium in the different model systems. *Klettner* introduces the reader in **RPE Cell Culture**, starting with a brief historical overview on different model species and describing the challenges of RPE cell culture. An overview on different RPE cell lines, stressing their usage and limits, is given, and the features of primary fetal and adult RPE cells in culture are discussed. Finally, an outlook is given on current co-culture and 3D techniques.

In the chapter "**Retinal Pigment Epithelium Organ Culture**," *Miura* takes us to the next level of complexity. After an introduction into the history and donor species of RPE organ culture, reader is presented the different types of explants and culture systems as well as the morphological changes during the different culturing methods. Finally, different applications of RPE organ culture in research are described.

In their chapter, *Fletcher* and *co-workers* present **Animal Models of Diseases of the Retinal Pigment Epithelium**. After an introduction into the function and structure of the RPE, the authors described several models for retinal disease, such as retinitis pigmentosa, Leber's congenital amaurosis, inherited macular degenerations, melanin-associated disorders, and age-related macular degeneration. In addition, they cover pharmacological as well as transgenic models of RPE dysfunction.

We wish to thank all authors for their contribution to this volume and to the highly active and versatile field of RPE research. While being aware of the limitation of a printed volume of limited space in this time of online publications and rapid new findings, we believe that this book can become any RPE researcher's compendium to refer to anytime. We hope that the reader will enjoy reading the book at least as much as we enjoyed putting it together! We would also like to thank our young research, PhD students, postdocs, and technicians for the constant contribution to research as well as our families for their support for us.

Kiel, Germany — Alexa Karina Klettner
Wiesbaden, Germany — Stefan Dithmar

Contents

About the Editors

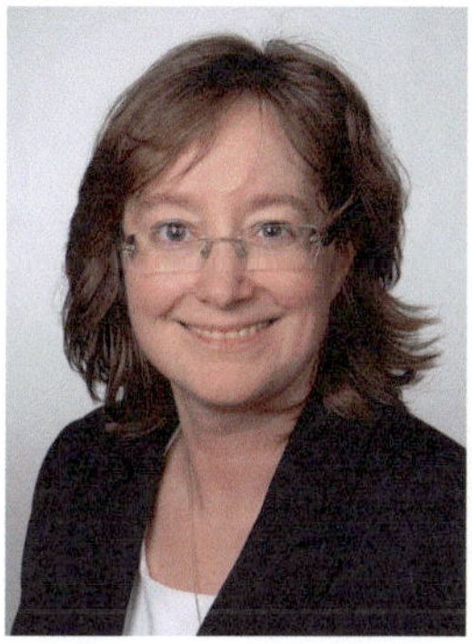

Alexa Karina Klettner studied biology at the Christian-Albrechts-University in Kiel and did her diploma thesis at the Research Center Borstel. She did her PhD in pharmacology, working on neuroprotection, and habilitated in experimental ophthalmology, studying antagonists of the vascular endothelial growth factor (VEGF). Since 2013, she is professor for experimental retinology at Kiel University, Germany, and since 2017 adjunct professor at the University of Cairo, Egpyt. Her main research interests are the cellular aspects of pathogenesis and therapy of age-related macular degeneration (AMD), with a strong focus on the retinal pigment epithelium (RPE), investigating VEGF regulation, long-term consequence of retinal therapy, interaction of the RPE with the innate immune system, and development of new therapeutics for AMD.

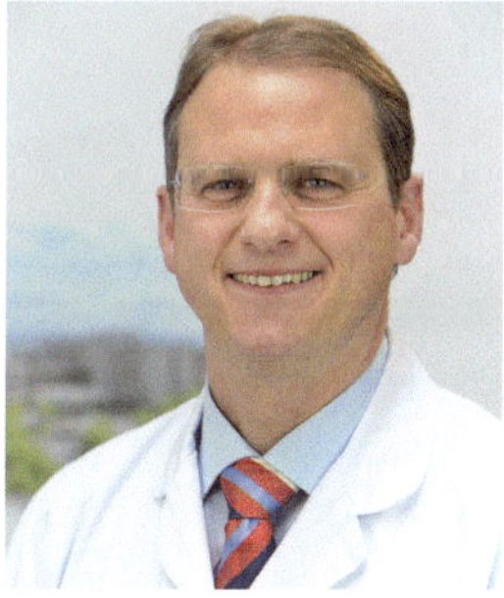

Stefan Dithmar, MD, PhD is professor of ophthalmology. He studied medicine at the Universities of Göttingen (Germany), and Heidelberg (Germany), in Great Britain and the USA (Harvard Medical School, Boston MA). He completed his specialist training in ophthalmology at Heidelberg University. He then worked as a research fellow with Professor H.E. Grossniklaus at the Emory Eye Clinic, Emory University (Atlanta, USA), and worked on numerous projects in the posterior segment of the eye. He became professor at the University of Heidelberg and head of the Retina Department at the University Eye Clinic. His research activities include the establishment of an interdisciplinary working group with Prof. Dr. C. Cremer, Kirchhoff Institute for Physics, University of Heidelberg, and the further development of the methodology of structured illumination microscopy applied to the retinal pigment epithelium. He has been director and chairman of the Department of Ophthalmology, HSK-Wiesbaden, University of Mainz (Germany), since 2014.

Part I

Physiological RPE Function

RPE Histopathology and Morphometry

1

Eszter Szalai, John M. Nickerson, and Hans E. Grossniklaus

Introduction

Retinal pigment epithelium (RPE) is a single layer of hexagonal/cuboidal epithelial cells which separates the neuroretina from the underlying choroid. These cells are arranged in a mosaic-like pattern. Regular hexagon cell pattern is thought to be the most stable and energetically the most favorable cell arrangement [1–3]. Embryologically, RPE is a neuroepithelial derivative. In the early development, RPE differentiates from the neuroectoderm of the optic vesicle and later becomes highly specialized [4]. The apical membrane faces the photoreceptor outer segments and interphotoreceptor matrix [5], the RPE basal lamina is in close contact with the inner collagenous layer of the Bruch's membrane. This special polarized structure is required for the proper development of the photoreceptors and choroid and this allows for multiple functions of the RPE cells such as adsorbing scattered light to improve spatial resolution, recycling visual pigments to ensure light sensitivity of photoreceptors, and transporting nutrients and metabolites between the choriocapillaris and the neurosensory retina [6]. The impact of RPE in the regulation of eye growth has also been implicated by transmitting signals between the retina and the adjacent choroid and sclera [7]. Tight junctions between neighboring RPE cells constitute the outer blood-retinal barrier, i.e. barrier between the subretinal space and the choriocapillaris. The highly dynamic cytoskeletal elements of the plasma membrane and cytoplasm provide membrane motility, intracellular transport and mechanical strength of the cells. RPE cells show topographic differences, and they also vary within one particular region based on their melanin pigment granule content [3].

Improperly functioning RPE cells can have primary or secondary contribution to several disease processes including dry and wet age-related macular degeneration (AMD), proliferative vitreoretinopathy (PVR), central and peripheral retinal dystrophies, mitochondrial diseases, and RPE neoplasias. Progressive RPE dysfunction and cell loss may lead to a secondary degeneration of photoreceptor rods and cones due to the close relationship between the RPE and photoreceptor cells and due to the loss of barrier functions.

Normal Histology

Normal human RPE is a monolayer of cuboidal cells in which the cytoplasm is filled with melanin pigment granules (also known as melanosomes). The thickness of this layer varies according to the location and age, RPE cells are about 14 μm in height in the macular region whereas toward the periphery they become

E. Szalai (✉) · J. M. Nickerson · H. E. Grossniklaus
Department of Ophthalmology, Emory University, Atlanta, GA, USA
e-mail: eszalai@emory.edu; litjn@emory.edu; ophtheg@emory.edu

A. K. Klettner, S. Dithmar (eds.), *Retinal Pigment Epithelium in Health and Disease*,
https://doi.org/10.1007/978-3-030-28384-1_1

significantly shorter [8]. Numerous microvilli of the apical membrane extend to the photoreceptor outer segments. The morphology of the polarized RPE layer is visible by transmission electron microscopy (TEM), in which tight junctions, apical microvilli, basal infoldings, shed photoreceptor outer segment disks, melanin pigments, lipofuscin and melanolipofuscin granules can be observed (Fig. 1.1). Melanins are complex pigment structures in the skin, retina and uveal tract which are synthesized within melanosomes. There are two types of cells in the eye which produce melanin: (1) melanocytes in the uveal tract and (2) neuroepithelial cells, such as pigment epithelial cells in the iris, ciliary body and retina. There are substantial differences in the phenotype of melanosomes between the skin, uveal tract and retina. The RPE melanosomes are more elongated or bullet shaped whereas skin and choroidal melanosomes are more spherical [9, 10]. The basal surface of an RPE cell faces the Bruch's membrane, a five-layer complex structure with multiple functions which lies between the retina and choroid. The RPE basement membrane (basal lamina) is the innermost layer of the Bruch's membrane with an average thickness of 0.15 μm in young individuals [11]. The structure of this basement membrane is not unique, it consists of type IV collagens, fibronectin, laminin, heparan, chondroitin and dermatan sulfate [12]. The basal plasma membrane of the RPE cells is separated from the basement membrane and it contains several infoldings in order to increase its membrane surface for needed ion transport. Anteriorly there are less infoldings, and they are more pronounced on the posterior pole except adjacent to the optic nerve head where they tend to be less marked. Desmosome and hemidesmosome-like structures are present in the basal plasma membrane resulting in a tight connection between the RPE and Bruch's membrane [13]. In the lateral surface, zonula occludens, zonula adherens, gap junctions, and occasional desmosomes are present to maintain paracellular permeability, cellular integrity, and cell-cell contact. Zonula occludens or tight junctions are present in the apical half of the cell and are responsible for maintaining the outer blood-retinal barrier. Na,K-ATPase function has been shown to be involved in the normal tight junction structure and permeability in human RPE cells [14]. Zonula adherens or adherens junctions are associated with a rich network of actin filaments. They have multiple functions by supporting cellular motility but also by providing mechanical strength in response to various intracellular signals [15]. The apical microvilli provide increased surface area and play role in special functions, such as phagocytosis of the

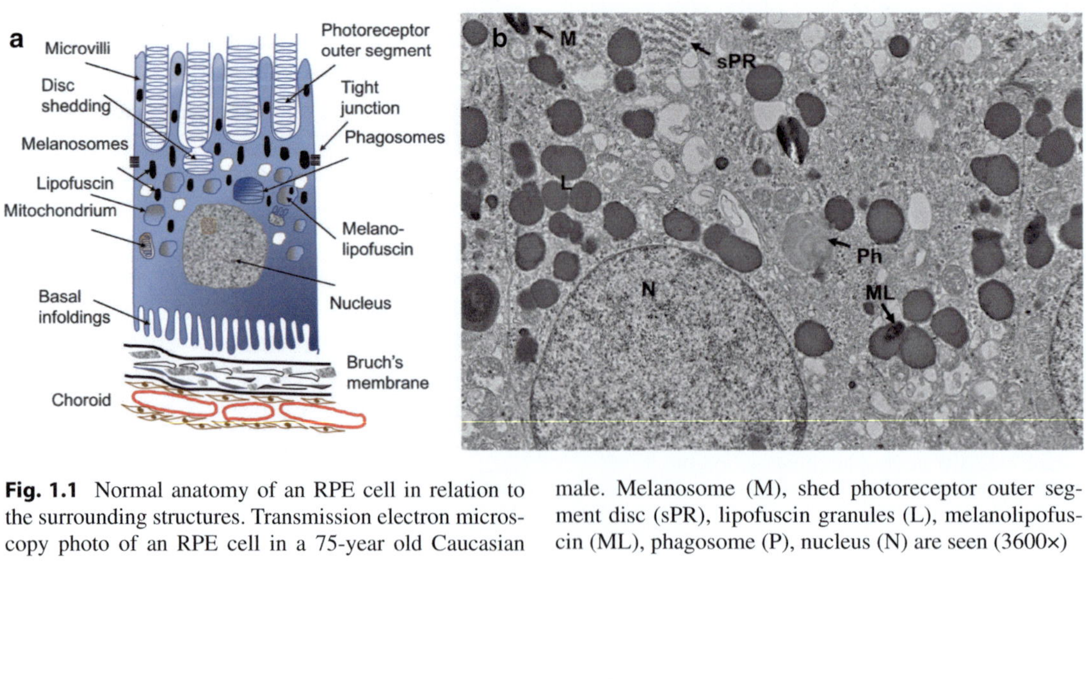

Fig. 1.1 Normal anatomy of an RPE cell in relation to the surrounding structures. Transmission electron microscopy photo of an RPE cell in a 75-year old Caucasian male. Melanosome (M), shed photoreceptor outer segment disc (sPR), lipofuscin granules (L), melanolipofuscin (ML), phagosome (P), nucleus (N) are seen (3600×)

shed photoreceptor outer segment disks, movements of melanin granules due to light exposure and adhesion to the neurosensory retina. The apical surface faces the subretinal space, the microvilli connect and interdigitate with the photoreceptor outer segments. Light exposure causes the pigment granules migrate into the microvilli in order to decrease the light amount that reaches the rods and cones [16–20]. On the contrary, in scotopic conditions the pigments migrate back to the cell body to allow more light to reach the photoreceptors [16–20].

RPE cells also contain lipofuscin granules, which increase in amount throughout life due to outer segment phagocytosis. The RPE cells are known to show large degrees of heterogeneity in melanin and lipofuscin granule content [3]. It has been proposed that higher melanin content of RPE cells might be protective against the formation of lipofuscin granules [21, 22]. One of the major metabolic roles of RPE cells is to degrade phagocytosed photoreceptor outer segment disk membranes, which are very densely packed structures. Young and Bok observed that approximately 10% of the outer segment disks are generated each day [23], and the same fraction of outer segment dics are phagocytosed by the RPE daily. This is on a circadian rhythm, with rod outer segments consumed at daybreak, and cone outer segments at dusk. Thus, it takes about 10 days for an outer segment disc to traverse from its proximal site of biosynthesis to the distal tip of the outer segment, where it is consumed by the RPE.

Qualitative, morphological analysis of the RPE cells has traditionally been performed during routine histopathologic examination in vitro (Fig. 1.2). More recently, non-invasive imaging modalities are capable of automatic segmentation of the human RPE layer in vivo [24–27]. Polarization-sensitive optical coherence tomog-

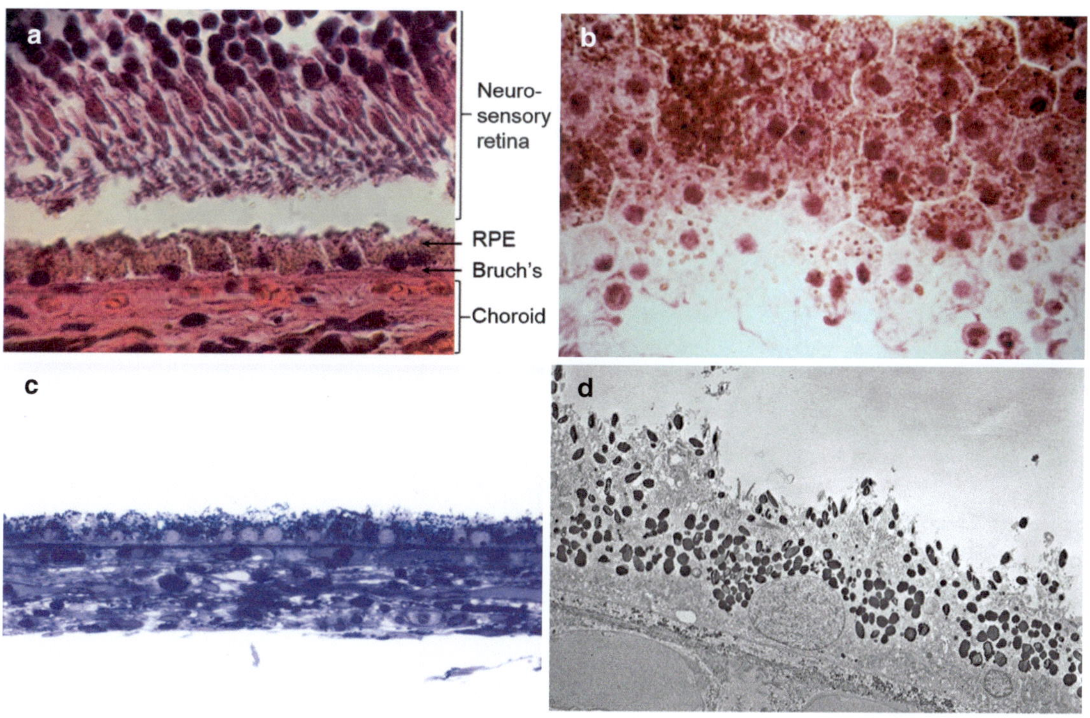

Fig. 1.2 Normal histological appearance of the human RPE in relation to the neurosensory retinal layers and Bruch's membrane (hematoxylin and eosin, 100×) (**a**). En face (flat mount) light micrograph of the hexagonal RPE cells (hematoxylin & eosin, 250×) (**b**). Toluidine blue stain of the normal RPE layer highlighting the intracellular pigment granules (150×) (**c**). Transmission electron microscopy of the RPE cells with normal cell organelles (1900×) (**d**)

raphy (OCT) reveals RPE cell bodies specifically in optical biopsy of the retina [27]. Adaptive optics scanning laser ophthalmoscope combined with lipofuscin autofluorescence, dual wavelength imaging and registration is an applicable tool to measure and quantify RPE cell morphometry in vivo [28].

Cell Morphometry

Pleomorphism, Polymegathism

The total number of RPE cells has been reported to vary between 3.6 and 6.1 million in a healthy human eye [29, 30]. Qualitatively, both aging and degenerative retinal disorders are associated with not only a decline of the relative number of regular hexagonal RPE cells and an increase in the variability of the shape of the RPE cell and increased variability in the number of sides of a cell (pleomorphism), but also with an increase in the variability of cell area (polymegethism).

Hexagonal cells are most frequently (>50–60%) located in the fovea, and the proportion of six-sided RPE cells decreases from the fovea towards the peripheral retina [28, 31]. Cell areas are more variable in older eyes (>80 year old) than in younger ones (≤51 year old) [31]. A previous study confirmed a predominance of hexagonal cells only in the younger adult fovea, where almost 60% of cells had six neighbors [31]. However, RPE cells show continuous remodeling and rearrangement during lifetime, which is thought to reflect a propensity of RPE cells to remain tightly attached to each other so that the outer blood retina barrier remains intact at all costs.

An inter-RPE cell variability (mosaicism) has been described in animal and human studies affecting different cell properties both in macroscopic and molecular level [3]. The pigment granule content varies highly between RPE cells and the expression level of certain proteins. This heterogeneity is thought be due to both genetic and epigenetic processes and contribute to the functional diversity of the RPE layer [3].

Spatial Distribution, Topography

RPE cells extend from the edge of the optic disc to the ora serrata. Anterior to the ora serrata the RPE continues to the pars plana pigment epithelium of the ciliary body. Certain fundamental differences have been shown between RPE cell density (Fig. 1.3) and morphometry in distinct topographical locations (Fig. 1.4) and in different age groups [32]. Cell density at the posterior pole was about four times greater than at the far

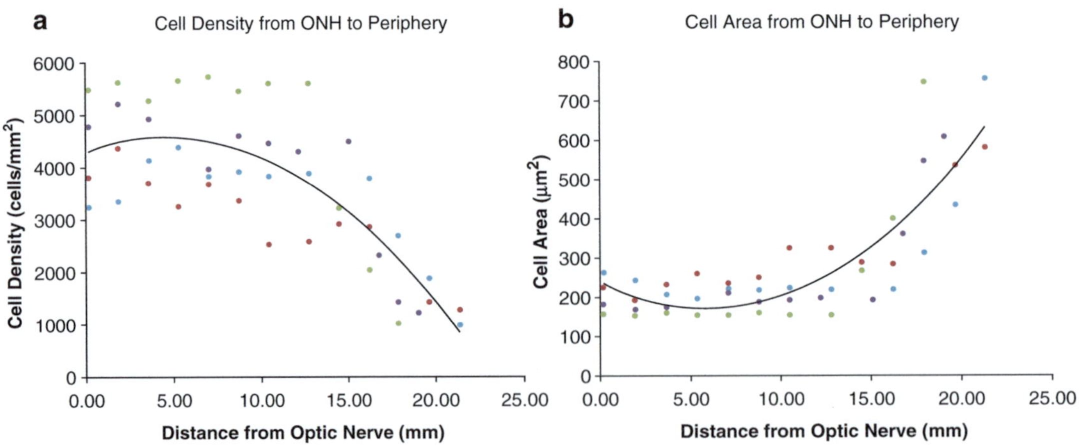

Fig. 1.3 RPE cell density (**a**) and area (**b**) from the optic nerve head (ONH) to the far peripheral retina. (With permission of the authors: Bhatia SK, Rashid A, Chrenek MA, Zhang Q, Bruce BB, Klein M, et al. Analysis of RPE morphometry in human eyes. Mol Vis. 2016;22:898–916)

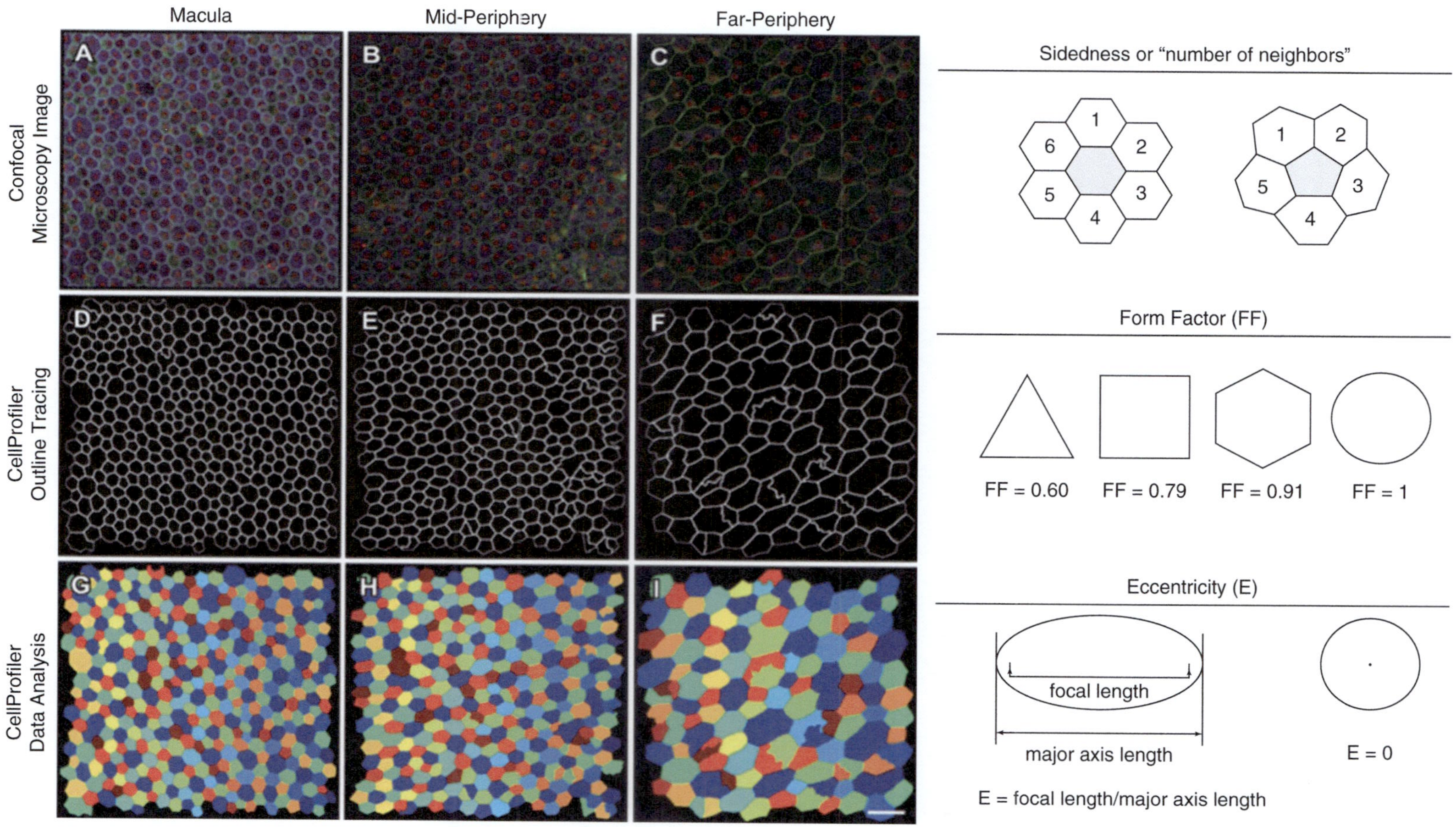

Fig. 1.4 Differences in RPE morphometry in the macula, mid-periphery and far-periphery demonstrated by image analysis techniques. (With permission of the authors: Bhatia SK, Rashid A, Chrenek MA, Zhang Q, Bruce BB, Klein M, et al. Analysis of RPE morphometry in human eyes. Mol Vis. 2016;22:898–916)

periphery with inverse correlation to cell area (Fig. 1.3) [32]. The literature shows large ranges of RPE cell density with high variability across age, retinal location and between individuals [3, 28, 30, 33–37]. The RPE cell density has been shown to decrease from the fovea (4220 cells/mm^2) to the midperiphery (3002 cells/mm^2) and to the peripheral retina (1600 cells/mm^2) in normal human eyes [30]. Another investigation described the highest density of 7500 RPE cells/mm^2 at the fovea in both younger (≤51 year old) and older subjects (>80 year old) [31]. RPE cell density decreases gradually towards the equator (it measures approximately 5000 cells/mm^2 at the edge of the macula) [31]. Also foveal RPE cells are found to be significantly smaller in size than the peripheral cells [2, 31, 38].

There is a physiologic variation in RPE cell shape between different locations, i.e. cells are flat and wider anteriorly, whereas they are elongated and narrow posterior to the equator. Salzmann reported the height of RPE cells to be 11–14 μm in the macular region and 8 μm in the other parts of the fundus [8]. The cells also contain more melanin pigment granules within the macular area.

Pathology

Extensive research of the cellular and subcellular pathogenesis of retinal disorders has identified RPE dysfunction as having either a primary role or a secondary role. RPE cells might interact with the neurosensory retina, Bruch's membrane, and choriocapillary network in different diseases such as age-related macular degeneration (AMD), proliferative retinopathies, central and peripheral retinal dystrophies, mitochondrial diseases and tumors of the RPE.

Age-Related Changes

Normal human RPE cells are mitotically quiescent. Age-related decline of RPE density and the corresponding morphology changes (Fig. 1.5) have been extensively studied [30, 31, 34, 38–41]. In a previous investigation, the RPE cell density in the fovea decreased significantly ($p < 0.001$) by about 0.3% per year with increasing age [30]. Such a continuous age-related decline of RPE cell count is commonly found in the literature but the quantification of the magnitude of the decline is not well understood [31, 34, 38–41]. With age, the number of hexagonal RPE cells decreases in the fovea and parafoveal areas [31]. Ach et al. indicated that the density of five-sided RPE cells increased significantly in the fovea, whereas in the parafovea the proportion of five and seven-sided cells tends to dominate as a result of an age-related remodeling [31].

Lipofuscin granules are known to localize close to the RPE cell borders when low lipofuscin granule density is present which is expected for young, healthy individuals [42]. RPE cells are responsible for the phagocytosis of diurnally shed photoreceptor outer segments [43]. Lipofuscin arises in the RPE from incomplete digestion of the outer-segment fragments within the lysosomes [44]. Lipofuscin accumulation in RPE cells has been proved to lead to a range of retinal disorders (Fig. 1.6).

The major fluorophores of lipofuscin are the bis-retinoid, *N*-retinylidene-*N*-retinylethanolamine (A2E), closely related A2E phosphatidyl esters, and retinyl dimers [45]. In clinical setting, fundus autofluorescence (FAF) is informative for monitoring RPE health and metabolism by enabling detection of autofluorescence (AF) attributable to lipofuscin and melanolipofuscin, long-lasting intracellular residual bodies rich in bisretinoid derivatives of vitamin A. The loss of fundus autofluorescence (detected as black patches in FAF) thus represents the loss of RPE cells that contain these highly fluorescent molecules (Fig. 1.7). In 2005, eight phenotypic FAF patterns have been defined to be associated with non-exudative AMD, such as normal, minimal change, focal increase, patchy, linear, lacelike, reticular and speckled pattern [46]. Diffuse and banded phenotypes are associated with a higher risk for disease progression [47].

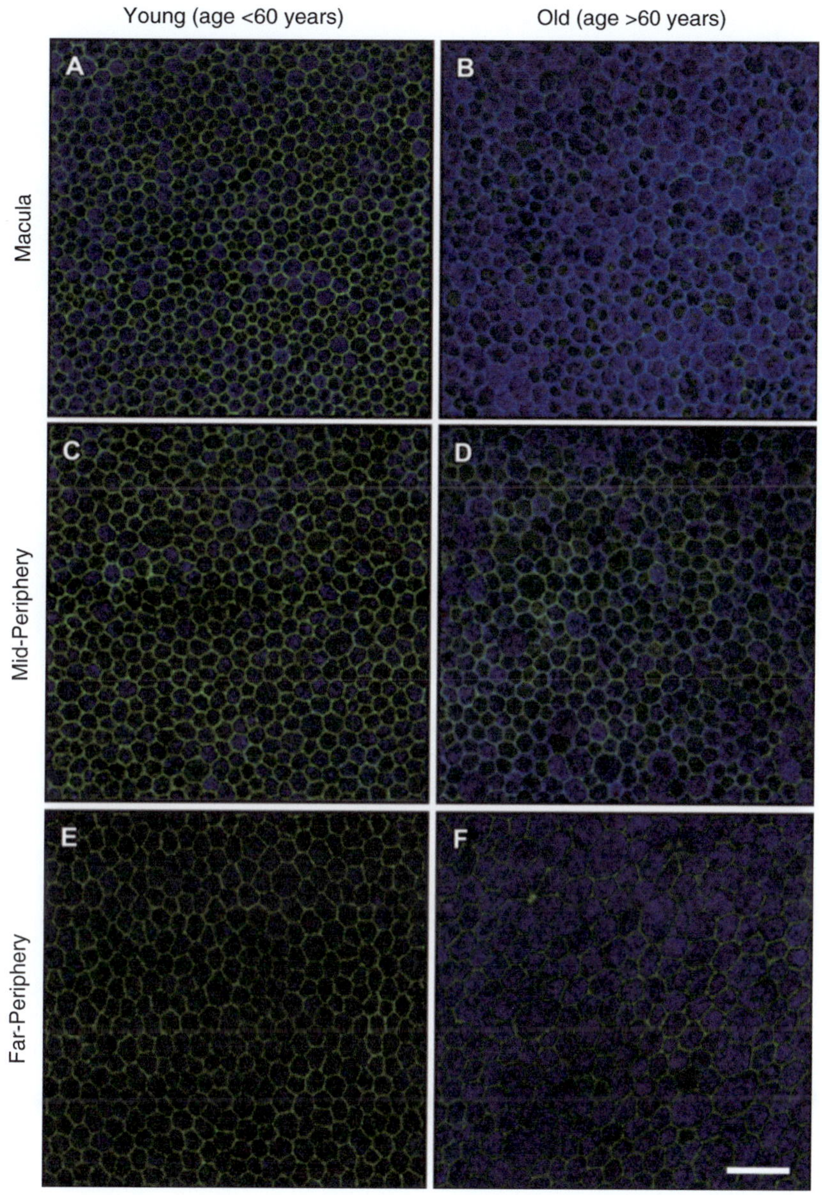

Fig. 1.5 RPE cell morphology of a "young" individual (37-year-old; **a**, **c**, and **e**) and an "old" individual (75-year-old; **b**, **d**, and **f**). (With permission of the authors: Bhatia SK, Rashid A, Chrenek MA, Zhang Q, Bruce BB, Klein M, et al. Analysis of RPE morphometry in human eyes. Mol Vis. 2016;22:898–916.) Note the increase in the bluish autofluorescence in the "old" sample in comparing the right and left images. This signal is thought to reflect an increase in autofluorescent lipofuscin with age

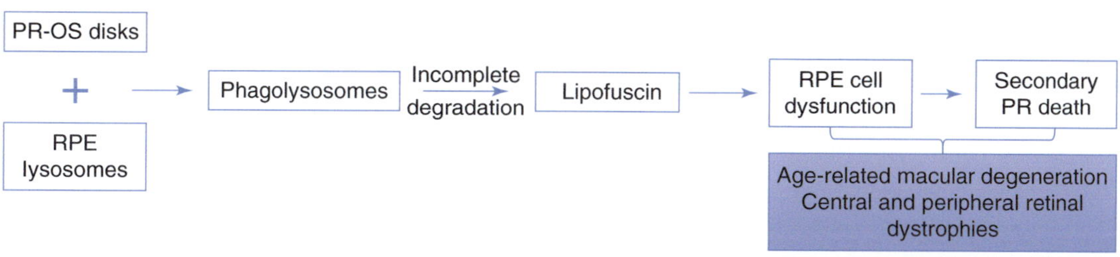

Fig. 1.6 Photoreceptor outer segment (PR-OS) degradation and lipofuscin formation in the RPE cells

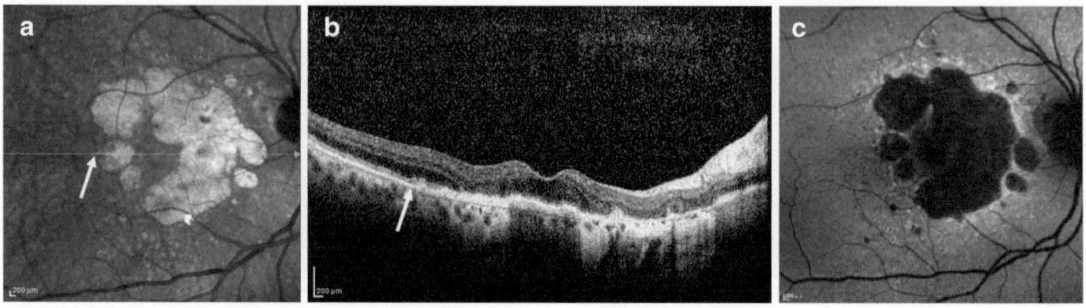

Fig. 1.7 Infrared reflectance (**a**) and spectral domain optical coherence tomography (**b**) image of the fovea in geographic RPE atrophy. Note the junction (arrow) between the normal RPE layer and the atrophic lesion (**b**). On fundus autofluorescence image (**c**), the hypo-autofluorescent areas correspond to RPE atrophy and they are surrounded by diffuse reticular hyper-autofluorescence in the junctional zone, which represent areas of current RPE cell dysfunction. This is a 76-year-old female patient with 20/25 best corrected visual acuity due to foveal sparing of geographic atrophy

Degenerations

Biometry-Related Changes

RPE has been shown to play a critical role in ocular growth regulation by controlling ion/fluid transport and signal transduction between the retina, choroid and sclera [7]. A profound decrease in the RPE cell density was reported in the equatorial to retro-equatorial region in association with longer axial length and a lower degree of decline at the midpoint between equator/posterior pole [41]. RPE cell density at the posterior pole was not significantly associated with axial length in a previous study [41].

Age-Related Macular Degeneration

With aging RPE cells gradually decrease in density and enlarge in size associated with intracellular lipofuscin accumulation [48]. Lipofuscin was found to be photocytotoxic to RPE cells in a wavelength dependent manner (390–550 nm), it reduced significantly the RPE cell viability by at least 41% 2 days after 390–550 nm exposure when compared to lipofuscin-free cells [49]. Its accumulation is associated with photooxidation, RPE cell damage, and inflammation. These alterations with age-related changes of the Bruch's membrane (calcification and fragmentation) may lead to age-related macular degeneration [50]. However, the heterogeneous clinical picture of RPE dysfunction could be explained by the susceptibility of RPE cells in vivo due to the balance between the amount of lipofuscin granules and the antioxidant potential of the cell [49]. Moreover, RPE cell pattern has been shown to have a much reduced regularity in AMD [40].

AMD starts with the formation of basal laminar deposits and drusen and hypertrophy and loss of the RPE cells (Fig. 1.8). In more advance stages, these processes may lead to geographic atrophy (Fig. 1.7) and choroidal neovascularization. It has also been proposed that RPE cells might undergo transdifferentiation [51, 52]. Drusen are deposits of amorphous extracellular material lying between the RPE and the inner collagenous zone of Bruch's membrane [53]. The transformation theory [54], deposition theory [55] and the vascular theory [56] have been proposed to explain the exact origin of drusen. Hard drusen may progress into atrophic AMD, whereas soft drusen may precede choroidal neovascularization. Softening of drusen is associated with accumulation of membranous debris external to the RPE basement membrane which may arise from the photoreceptors [57]. Large drusen are associated with diffuse thickening of Bruch's membrane with basal linear deposit, whereas confluent soft drusen resemble an exudative RPE detachment [57]. Basal laminar deposit is a diffuse accumulation of hyalinized material between the RPE basal plasma membrane and its basement membrane. It is composed of widely spaced type IV collagen and other fibrillar mate-

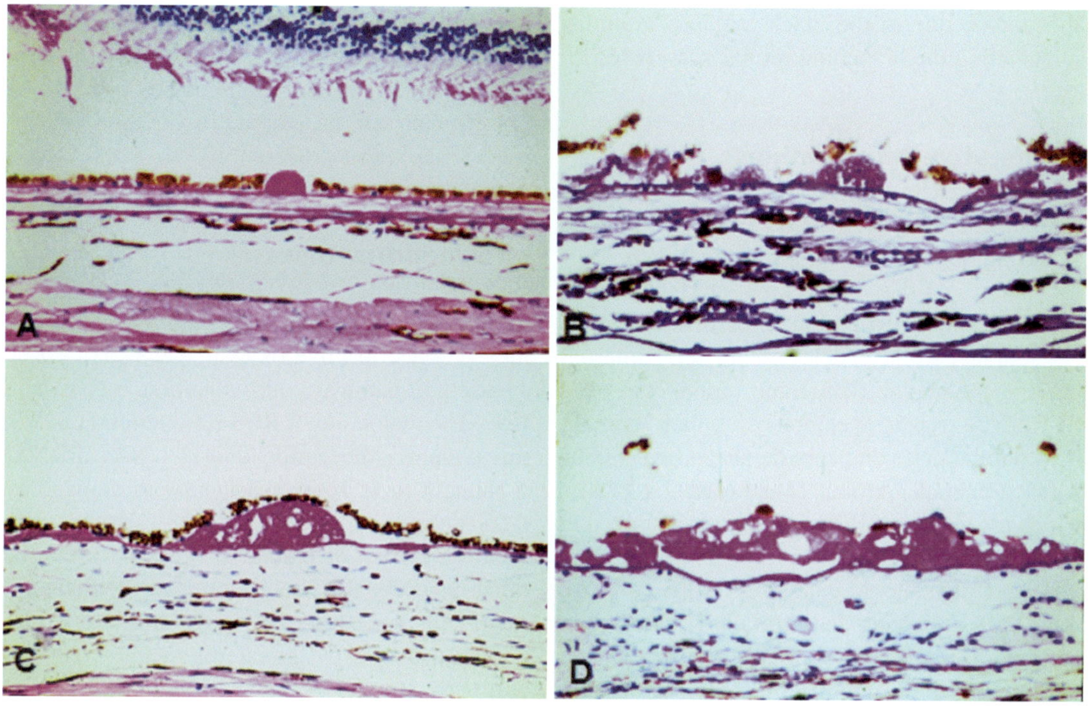

Fig. 1.8 Light microscopy of hard drusen (hematoxylin and eosin, 160×) (**a**), soft drusen (periodic acid-Schiff, 160×) (**b**), large drusen (hematoxylin and eosin, 160×) (**c**) and confluent drusen (hematoxylin and eosin, 160×) (**d**). (Reproduced with permission from Spraul CW, Grossniklaus HE. Characteristics of drusen and Bruch's membrane in postmortem eyes with age-related macular degeneration. Arch Ophthalmol. 1997;115:267–273)

rials [58]. They can be either the cause or consequence of compromised RPE cell functions [59]. Multiple studies concluded that there is a significant risk of progression to exudative AMD if there is a large drusen size, drusen confluence or focal macular hyperpigmentation on initial presentation [57]. Spraul et al. postulated that choroidal neovascular membranes represent a nonspecific wound-repair mechanism since their composition (i.e. RPE cells, vascular endothelial cells, fibrocytes, macrophages, photoreceptors, erythrocytes, lymphocytes, myofibroblasts, collagen, fibrin and basal laminar deposit) is not characteristic of a specific disease process [59].

Retinal Dystrophies

Retinal dystrophy refers to a heterogeneous group of inherited central and peripheral retinal diseases associated with various mutations in the human retina affecting the retinal pigment epithelium and the photoreceptor layer [60]. These mutations may impact a number of molecular cascades by interfering with intra- and intercellular interactions in different layers of the retina. Those processes may compromise the integrity of the RPE plasma membranes (bestrophinopathies, e.g. Best vitelliform macular dystrophy) [61] and/or photoreceptor membranes (pattern dystrophies, e.g. butterfly-shaped pattern dystrophy) [62]. Histopathologically, pattern dystrophies are associated with accumulation of excessive lipofuscin in the RPE, whereas in later stages these changes are replaced by extensive atrophic depigmented areas of the RPE and degeneration of photoreceptor cells [62–64]. In retinitis pigmentosa, the initial degenerative changes occur in the rod photoreceptors followed by secondary changes in the cones, RPE, retinal glia and ganglion cells [65]. The RPE cells migrate to perivascular sites in the inner retina after extensive photoreceptor damage, producing the characteristic bone-spicule appearance due to the black melanin granules surrounding the branching retinal vessels [65].

Proliferative Retinopathies

Epiretinal membrane (ERM) formation can be occurring secondary to a number of pathological changes on the vitreoretinal interface. Snead et al. classified ERMs into three distinct types: (1) simple ERMs, which contain only internal limiting membrane (ILM) and laminocytes; (2) PVR/tissue repair membranes, which contain ILM, laminocytes and spindle-shaped RPE cells with extracellular stroma; (3) neovascular ERMs, which are devoid of ILM and contain vessels and hyaline stroma [66].

Under physiologic conditions, RPE cells are mitotically quiescent and virtually stationary. In various disease processes such as proliferative vitreoretinopathy, retinitis pigmentosa, or choroidal neovascularization, the RPE cells detach from the basement membrane and exhibit migratory potential [65, 67, 68]. The term PVR refers to various conditions characterized by cell proliferation and matrix deposition within the retina (Fig. 1.9). Essentially in PVR cases, the ERM is usually complicated by the presence of RPE cells [66]. Besides RPE cells, occasional macrophages, fibrocytes and lymphocytes can also be present with various amount of collagen indicating a tissue repair process [66].

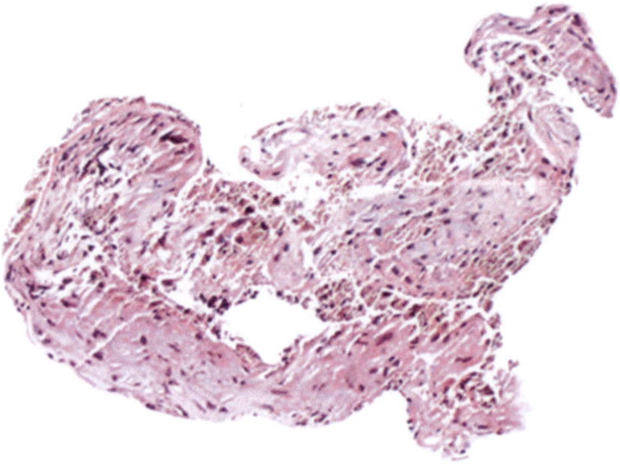

Fig. 1.9 Light microscopy of subretinal PVR showing fibrocellular tissue composed of RPE (pigmented cells), collagen, fibrocytes and macrophages (hematoxylin and eosin, 25×). This is a 10-year-old highly myopic male with a history of prematurity and long standing retinal detachment. During pars plana vitrectomy, a "napkin ring" band of PVR was removed from the subretinal space through a small retinotomy site

Mitochondrial Diseases

RPE cells are metabolically highly active and they produce reactive oxygen species (ROS) by a variety of pathways during aerobic metabolism [69]. The major site of ROS production is within mitochondria, thus mitochondrial DNA (mtDNA) is thought to be more susceptible to damage by ROS than nuclear DNA. mtDNA damage is a good biomarker of oxidative stress [70]. On the other hand, the RPE cells along with retinal ganglion cells are particularly susceptible to oxidative damage [71]. Retinal pigmentary changes and optic atrophy both are common ophthalmic manifestations of mitochondrial disorders [72]. Histopathological studies showed a primary RPE degeneration followed by secondary changes of the photoreceptors and choriocapillaris, and proved abnormally enlarged mitochondria in the RPE cells [73]. The same ROS-mediated mtDNA damage and RPE cell death mechanisms are thought to play key roles in the pathogenesis of AMD in susceptible eyes [70].

RPE Tumors

The retinal pigment epithelium often undergoes reactive hyperplasia secondary to intraocular inflammation or trauma (Fig. 1.10). Although less common, it can produce a variety of tumors and related lesions [74]. The main tumors of the RPE include congenital hypertrophy of the RPE (CHRPE), congenital simple (solitary or grouped) hamartoma, combined hamartoma, adenoma, and adenocarcinoma.

Histopathologically, both solitary and grouped CHRPE lesions consist of a single layer of hypertrophied RPE cells (Fig. 1.11) which are densely packed with round macromelanosomes [75]. A hypopigmented halo is often seen around the

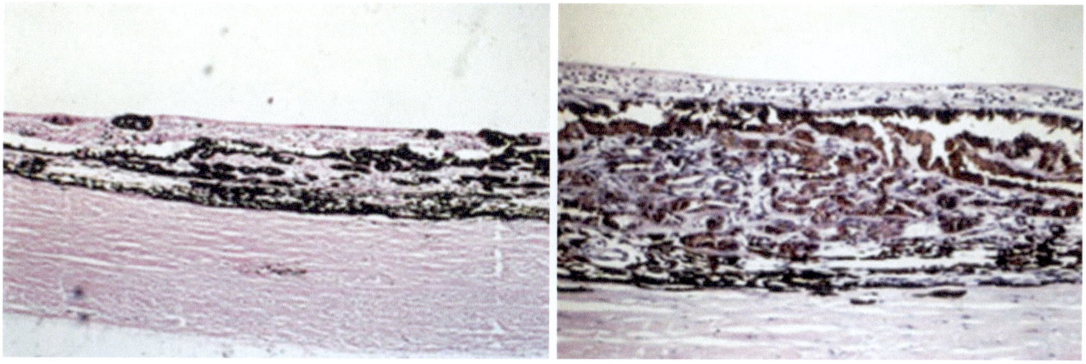

Fig. 1.10 Light microscopy of RPE hyperplasia showing multiple layers of RPE cells (hematoxylin and eosin left 25×, right 100×)

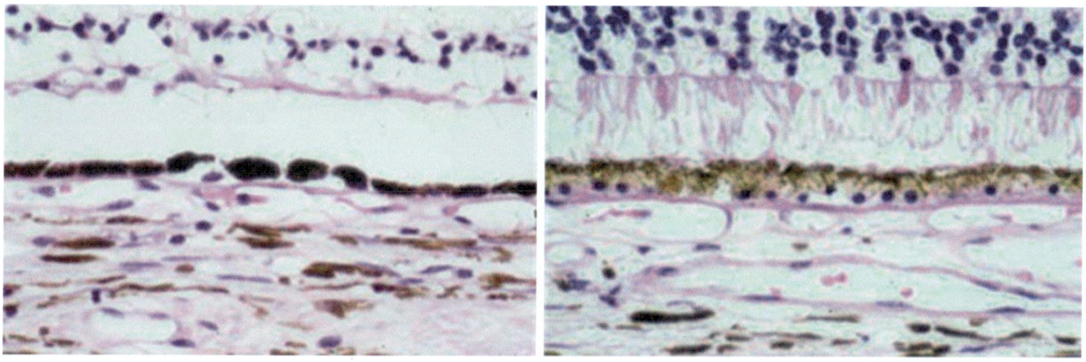

Fig. 1.11 Light microscopy of RPE hypertrophy indicating a single layer of enlarged RPE cells in volume. The left figure shows RPE hypertrophy associated with the dark part of a congenital hypertrophy of the RPE (CHRPE) lesion and the right shows depigmented RPE in the lacunae in CHRPE (hematoxylin and eosin 100×)

lesion representing taller RPE cells with less and smaller melanosomes. The Bruch's membrane is thickened, but the neurosensory retina remains unaffected [76]. Multilayered (hyperplastic) lesions with hypertrophic RPE cells are often referred to as hamartomas, i.e. abnormal amount of mature tissue in the normal anatomic location [75]. There is a distinct autosomal dominant disorder when the RPE hamartomas are associated with familial adenomatous polyposis. This disease entity was recently termed as "RPE hamartomas associated with familial adenomatous polyposis" by Shields and Shields to avoid the confusion because neither simple nor grouped hamartomas possess a higher risk of colon carcinoma [77]. Combined hamartoma of the retina and RPE has been described in juxtapapillary location when the RPE proliferation extended into the optic disc [78]. Proliferation of glial elements on the retinal surface and intraretinally was also observed [79]. The RPE cells proliferate in the neurosensory retinal layers as sheets and cords [76].

Adenoma of the RPE usually shows tubules and cords of proliferating RPE cells, separated by basement membrane and fibrous stroma histopathologically [80]. They usually arise from the peripheral retina but can occasionally be observed juxtapapillary masquerading melanocytoma of the optic disc or peripapillary uveal melanoma [81]. Adenocarcinoma of the RPE is composed of cords and tubular proliferations of cells with pleomorphic, hyperchromatic nuclei and variable amounts of cytoplasm (Fig. 1.12). There can be focal desmoplastic reaction to the tumor and bone formation (osseous metaplasia) in some

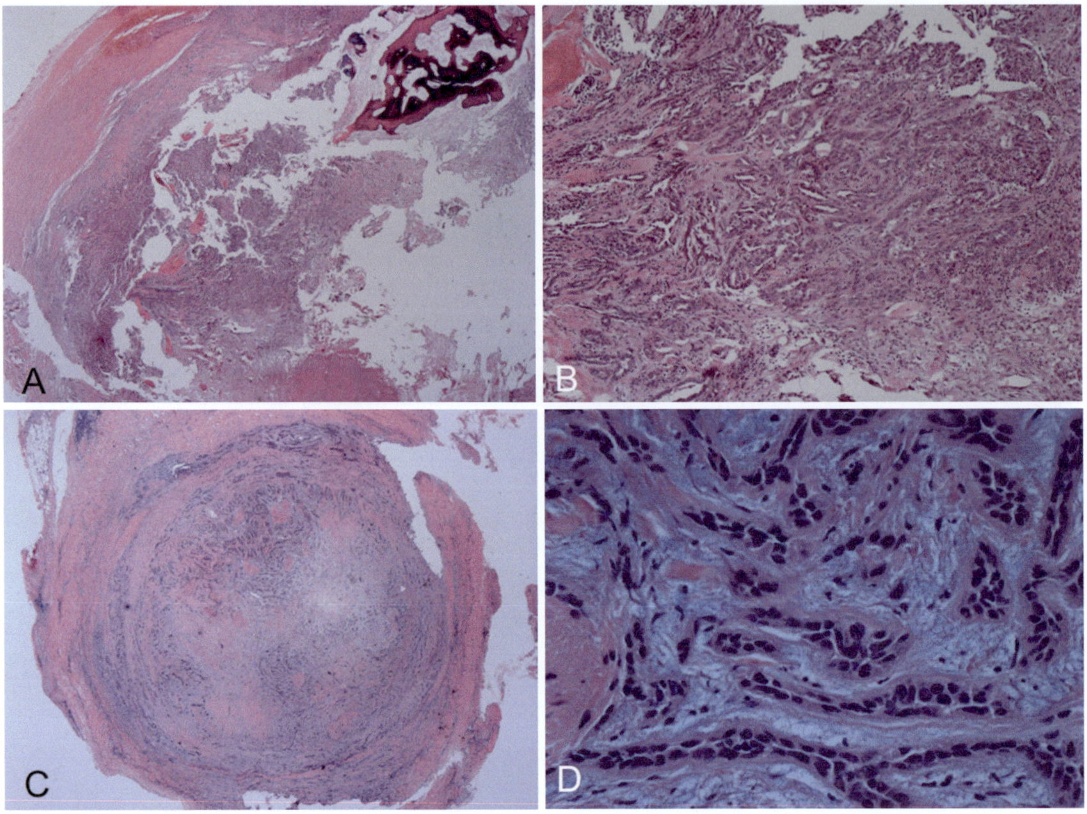

Fig. 1.12 Light microscopy of RPE adenocarcinoma. The tumor is composed of tubular and chord-like proliferations of cells with associated osseous metaplasia (**a**, **b**). The tumor has also invaded the optic nerve (**c**, **d**) (hematoxylin and eosin 5×, 25×, 5×, 100×, respectively)

areas. RPE adenocarcinoma can be highly invasive with extensive intraocular invasion, including lens, choroidal, scleral and optic nerve invasion, extension through emissary canals to the epibulbar surface with conjunctival and orbital invasion. However, tumors of the RPE seem to have no potential to metastasize [82]. Malignant transformation of a preexisting CHRPE into an adenocarcinoma has also been reported [83].

Pigmented RPE lesions can clinically simulate choroidal melanoma, thus they often referred to as pseudomelanoma [84]. Most commonly, CHRPE may appear similar to choroidal melanoma on routine clinical examination. However, differentiating between a benign RPE hypertrophy and malignant choroidal melanoma is crucial. CHRPE is typically a sharply demarcated dark pigmented lesion and usually flat or slightly elevated. A pigmented or non-pigmented halo can often be seen surrounding the lesion and intralesional lacunae are present in 43% of cases [85]. The diagnosis of RPE tumors is usually made on the basis of ophthalmoscopic findings and diagnostic imaging.

Acknowledgements The authors thank Nancy L'Hernault for the assistance in transmission electron microscopy. We are grateful for support provided by NIH R01EY021592, R01EY016470, P30EY006360, and an unrestricted grant to the Department of Ophthalmology at Emory University from Research to Prevent Blindness, Inc.

References

1. Yamashita M, Gotoh M. Impact behavior of honeycomb structures with various cell specifications—numerical simulation and experiment. Int J Impact Eng. 2005;32:618–30.
2. Streeten BW. Development of the human retinal pigment epithelium and the posterior segment. Arch Ophthalmol. 1969;81:383–94.
3. Burke JM, Hjelmeland LM. Mosaicism of the retinal pigment epithelium: seeing the small picture. Mol Interv. 2005;5:241–9.
4. Fuhrmann S, Zou C, Levine EM. Retinal pigment epithelium development, plasticity, and tissue homeostasis. Exp Eye Res. 2014;123:141–50.
5. Röhlich P. The interphotoreceptor matrix: electron microscopic and histochemical observations on the vertebrate retina. Exp Eye Res. 1970;10:80–6.
6. Strauss O. The retinal pigment epithelium in visual function. Physiol Rev. 2005;85:845–81.
7. Rymer J, Wildsoet CF. The role of the retinal pigment epithelium in eye growth regulation and myopia: a review. Vis Neurosci. 2005;22:251–61.
8. Salzmann M. Anatomie und Histologie des menschlichen Augapfels. Leipzig: F. Deuticke; 1912.
9. Liu Y, Hong L, Wakamatsu K, Ito S, Adhyaru BB, Cheng CY, et al. Comparisons of the structural and chemical properties of melanosomes isolated from retinal pigment epithelium, iris and choroid of newborn and mature bovine eyes. Photochem Photobiol. 2005;81:510–6.
10. Nakagawa H, Imokawa G. Characterization of melanogenesis in normal human epidermal melanocytes by chemical and ultrastructural analysis. Pigment Cell Res. 1996;9:175–8.
11. Guymer R, Bird A. Bruch's membrane, drusen, and age-related macular degeneration. In: Marmor M, Wolfensberger T, editors. The retinal pigment epithelium. New York: Oxford University Press; 1998. p. 693–705.
12. Booij JC, Baas DC, Beisekeeva J, Gorgels TG, Bergen AA. The dynamic nature of Bruch's membrane. Prog Retin Eye Res. 2010;29:1–18.
13. Miki H, Bellhorn MB, Henkind P. Specializations of the retinochoroidal juncture. Invest Ophthalmol. 1975;14:701–7.
14. Rajasekaran SA, Hu J, Gopal J, Gallemore R, Ryazantsev S, Bok D, Rajasekaran AK, et al. Am J Physiol Cell Physiol. 2003;284:C1497–507.
15. Pollard TD, Cooper JA. Actin and actin-binding proteins. A critical evaluation of mechanisms and functions. Annu Rev Biochem. 1986;55:987–1035.
16. Bruenner U, Burnside B. Pigment granule migration in isolated cells of the teleost retinal pigment epithelium. Invest Ophthalmol Vis Sci. 1986;27:1634–43.
17. Burnside B, Adler R, O'Connor P. Retinomotor pigment migration in the teleost retinal pigment epithelium. I. Roles for actin and microtubules in pigment granule transport and cone movement. Invest Ophthalmol Vis Sci. 1983;24:1–15.
18. Mondragón R, Frixione E. Retinomotor movements in the frog retinal pigment epithelium: dependence of pigment migration on Na+ and Ca2+. Exp Eye Res. 1989;48:589–603.
19. Lythgoe JN, Shand J. Endogenous circadian retinomotor movements in the neon tetra (Paracheirodon innesi). Invest Ophthalmol Vis Sci. 1983;24:1203–10.
20. Zhang QX, Lu RW, Messinger JD, Curcio CA, Guarcello V, Yao XC. In vivo optical coherence tomography of light-driven melanosome translocation in retinal pigment epithelium. Sci Rep. 2013;3:2644.
21. Sundelin SP, Nilsson SE, Brunk UT. Lipofuscin-formation in cultured retinal pigment epithelial cells is related to their melanin content. Free Radic Biol Med. 2001;30:74–81.
22. Schraermeyer U, Heimann K. Current understanding on the role of retinal pigment epithelium and its pigmentation. Pigment Cell Res. 1999;12:219–36.
23. Young RW, Bok D. Participation of the retinal pigment epithelium in the rod outer segment renewal process. J Cell Biol. 1969;42:392–403.
24. Rangel-Fonseca P, Gómez-Vieyra A, Malacara-Hernández D, Wilson MC, Williams DR, Rossi EA. Automated segmentation of retinal pigment epithelium cells in fluorescence adaptive optics images. J Opt Soc Am A Opt Image Sci Vis. 2013;30:2595–604.
25. Rossi EA, Rangel-Fonseca P, Parkins K, Fischer W, Latchney LR, Folwell MA, et al. In vivo imaging of retinal pigment epithelium cells in age related macular degeneration. Biomed Opt Express. 2013;4:2527–39.
26. Rossi EA, Chung M, Dubra A, Hunter JJ, Merigan WH, Williams DR. Imaging retinal mosaics in the living eye. Eye (Lond). 2011;25:301–8.
27. Schütze C, Wedl M, Baumann B, Pircher M, Hitzenberger CK, Schmidt-Erfurth U. Progression of retinal pigment epithelial atrophy in antiangiogenic therapy of neo-vascular age-related macular degeneration. Am J Ophthalmol. 2015;159:1100–4e1.
28. Morgan JIW, Dubra A, Wolfe R, Merigan WH, Williams DR. In vivo autofluorescence imaging of the human and macaque retinal pigment epithelial cell mosaic. Invest Ophthalmol Vis Sci. 2009;50:1350–9.
29. Hogan MJ, Alvaraso JA, Weddell JE. Chapter 9. In: Hogan MJ, Alvaraso JA, Weddell JE, editors. Histology of the human eye. Philadelphia: W. B. Saunders; 1971. p. 393–522.
30. Panda-Jonas S, Jonas JB, Jakobczyk-Zmija M. Retinal pigment epithelial cell count, distribution, and correlations in normal human eyes. Am J Ophthalmol. 1996;121:181–9.

31. Ach T, Huisingh C, McGwin G Jr, Messinger JD, Zhang T, Bentley MJ, et al. Quantitative autofluorescence and cell density maps of the human retinal pigment epithelium. Invest Ophthalmol Vis Sci. 2014;55:4832–41.
32. Bhatia SK, Rashid A, Chrenek MA, Zhang Q, Bruce BB, Klein M, et al. Analysis of RPE morphometry in human eyes. Mol Vis. 2016;22:898–916.
33. Gao H, Hollyfield JG. Aging of the human retina: differential loss of neurons and retinal pigment epithelial cells. Invest Ophthalmol Vis Sci. 1992;33:1–17.
34. Watzke RC, Soldevilla JD, Trune DR. Morphometric analysis of human retinal pigment epithelium: correlation with age and location. Curr Eye Res. 1993;12:133–42.
35. Harman AM, Fleming PA, Hoskins RV, Moore SR. Development and aging of cell topography in the human retinal pigment epithelium. Invest Ophthalmol Vis Sci. 1997;38:2016–26.
36. Del Priore LV, Kuo Y-H, Tazel TH. Age-related changes in human RPE cell density and apoptosis proportion in situ. Invest Ophthalmol Vis Sci. 2002;43:3312–8.
37. Leung IY, Sandstrom MM, Zucker CL, Neuringer M, Snodderly DM. Nutritional manipulation of primate retinas, II: effects of age, n-3 fatty acids, lutein, and zeaxanthin on retinal pigment epithelium. Invest Ophthalmol Vis Sci. 2004;45:3244–56.
38. Ts'o MO, Friedman E. The retinal pigment epithelium. 3. Growth and development. Arch Ophthalmol. 1968;80:214–6.
39. Dorey CK, Wu G, Ebenstein D, Garsd A, Weiter JJ. Cell loss in the aging retina. Relationship to lipofuscin accumulation and macular degeneration. Invest Ophthalmol Vis Sci. 1989;30:1691–9.
40. Rashid A, Bhatia SK, Mazzitello KI, Chrenek MA, Zhang Q, Boatright JH, et al. RPE cell and sheet properties in normal and diseased eyes. Adv Exp Med Biol. 2016;854:757–63.
41. Jonas JB, Ohno-Matsui K, Holbach L, Panda-Jonas S. Retinal pigment epithelium cell density in relationship to axial length in human eyes. Acta Ophthalmol. 2017;95:e22–8.
42. Cabral L, Unger W, Boulton M, Lightfoot R, McKechnie N, Grierson I, et al. Regional distribution of lysosomal enzymes in the canine retinal pigment epithelium. Invest Ophthalmol Vis Sci. 1990;31:670–6.
43. Bok D. The retinal pigment epithelium: a versatile partner in vision. J Cell Sci Suppl. 1993;17:189–95.
44. Kennedy CJ, Rakoczy PE, Constable IJ. Lipofuscin of the retinal pigment epithelium: a review. Eye (Lond). 1995;9:763–71.
45. Eldred GE, Lasky MR. Retinal age pigments generated by self-assembling lysosomotropic detergents. Nature. 1993;361:724–6.
46. Bindewald A, Bird AC, Dandekar SS, Dolar-Szczasny J, Dreyhaupt J, Fitzke FW, et al. Classification of fundus autofluorescence patterns in early age-related macular disease. Invest Ophthalmol Vis Sci. 2005;46:3309–14.
47. Holz FG, Bindewald-Wittich A, Fleckenstein M, Dreyhaupt J, Scholl HP, Schmitz-Valckenberg S. Progression of geographic atrophy and impact of fundus autofluorescence patterns in age-related macular degeneration. Am J Ophthalmol. 2007;143:463–72.
48. Hogan MJ. Role of the retinal pigment epithelium in macular disease. Trans Am Acad Ophthalmol Otolaryngol. 1972;76:64–80.
49. Davies S, Elliott MH, Floor E, Truscott TG, Zareba M, Sarna T, et al. Photocytotoxicity of lipofuscin in human retinal pigment epithelial cells. Free Radic Biol Med. 2001;31:256–65.
50. Spraul CW, Grossniklaus HE. Characteristics of Drusen and Bruch's membrane in postmortem eyes with age-related macular degeneration. Arch Ophthalmol. 1997;115:267–73.
51. Grisanti S, Guidry C. Transdifferentiation of retinal pigment epithelial cells from epithelial to mesenchymal phenotype. Invest Ophthalmol Vis Sci. 1995;36:391–405.
52. Lopez PF, Sippy BD, Lambert HM, Thach AB, Hinton DR. Transdifferentiated retinal pigment epithelial cells are immunoreactive for vascular endothelial growth factor in surgically excised age-related macular degeneration-related choroidal neovascular membranes. Invest Ophthalmol Vis Sci. 1996;37:855–68.
53. Farkas TG, Syvlester V, Archer D. The ultrastructure of drusen. Am J Ophthalmol. 1971;71:1196–205.
54. Donders FC. Beitrage zur pathologischen Anatomie des Auges. Arch Ophthalmol. 1854;1:106.
55. Muller H. Untersuchungen uber die gladuates des Auges, insbesondere die Glaslamelle der Choroidea und ihr senilen Veranderungen. Arch Ophthalmol. 1856;2:1.
56. Friedman E, Smith T, Kuwabara T. Senile choroidal vascular patterns and drusen. Arch Ophthalmol. 1963;69:114.
57. Abdelsalam A, Del Priore L, Zarbin MA. Drusen in age-related macular degeneration: pathogenesis, natural course, and laser photocoagulation-induced regression. Surv Ophthalmol. 1999;44:1–29.
58. Löffler KU, Lee WR. Basal linear deposit in the human macula. Graefes Arch Clin Exp Ophthalmol. 1986;224:493–501.
59. Spraul CW, Lang GE, Grossniklaus HE, Lang GK. Histologic and morphometric analysis of the choroid, Bruch's membrane, and retinal pigment epithelium in postmortem eyes with age-related macular degeneration and histologic examination of surgically excised choroidal neovascular membranes. Surv Ophthalmol. 1999;44:S10–32.
60. Broadgate S, Yu J, Downes SM, Halford S. Unravelling the genetics of inherited retinal dystrophies: past, present and future. Prog Retin Eye Res. 2017;59:53–96. https://doi.org/10.1016/j.preteyeres.2017.03.003.
61. Guziewicz KE, Sinha D, Gómez NM, Zorych K, Dutrow EV, Dhingra A, et al. Bestrophinopathy: an RPE-photoreceptor interface disease. Prog Retin Eye Res. 2017;58:70–88.

62. Zhang K, Garibaldi DC, Li Y, Green WR, Zack DJ. Butterfly-shaped pattern dystrophy: a genetic, clinical, and histopathological report. Ophthalmic Mol Genet. 2002;120:485–90.
63. Gass JMD. Stereoscopic atlas of macular disease. Philadelphia: Elsevier; 1997.
64. Birnbach CD, Jarvelainen M, Possin DE, Milam AH. Histopathology and immunocytochemistry of the neurosensory retina in fundus flavimaculatus. Ophthalmology. 1994;101:1211–9.
65. Li ZY, Possin DE, Milam AH. Histopathology of bone spicule pigmentation in retinitis pigmentosa. Ophthalmology. 1995;102:805–16.
66. Snead DR, James S, Snead MP. Pathological changes in the vitreoretinal junction 1: epiretinal membrane formation. Eye (Lond). 2008;22:1310–7.
67. Machemer R, Laqua H. Pigment epithelial proliferation in retinal detachment (massive periretinal proliferation). Am J Ophthalmol. 1975;80:1–23.
68. Miller H, Miller B, Ryan SJ. The role of retinal pigment epithelium in the involution of subretinal neovascularization. Invest Ophthalmol Vis Sci. 1986;27:1644–52.
69. Jin GF, Hurst JS, Godley BF. Rod outer segments mediate mitochondrial DNA damage and apoptosis in human retinal pigment epithelium. Curr Eye Res. 2001;23:11–9.
70. Liang FQ, Godley BF. Oxidative stress-induced mitochondrial DNA damage in human retinal pigment epithelial cells: a possible mechanism for RPE aging and age-related macular degeneration. Exp Eye Res. 2003;76:397–403.
71. Newman NJ. Mitochondrial diseases and the eye. Ophthalmol Clin North Am. 1992;5:405–24.
72. Fraser JA, Biousse V, Newman NJ. The neuro-ophthalmology of mitochondrial disease. Surv Ophthalmol. 2010;55:299–334.
73. McKechnie NM, King M, Lee WR. Retinal pathology in Kearns-Sayre syndrome. Br J Ophthalmol. 1985;69:63–75.
74. Shields JA, Shields CL. Tumors and related lesions of the pigment epithelium. In: Shields JA, Shields CL, editors. Atlas of intraocular tumors. Philadelphia: Lippincott, Williams and Wilkins; 1999. p. 287–307.
75. Lloyd WC 3rd, Eagle RC Jr, Shields JA, Kwa DM, Arbizo VV. Congenital hypertrophy of the retinal pigment epithelium. Electron microscopic and morphometric observations. Ophthalmology. 1990;97:1052–60.
76. Meyer CH, Gerding H. Congenital hypertrophy of the retinal pigment epithelium. In: Ryan SJ, editor. Retina. 5th ed. St. Louis: Elsevier; 2013. p. 2209–13.
77. Shields JA, Shields CL. Tumors and related lesions of the pigmented epithelium. Asia Pac J Ophthalmol (Phila). 2017;6:215–23.
78. Theobald GD, Floyd G, Kirk HQ. Hyperplasia of the retinal pigment epithelium simulating a neoplasm: report of two cases. Am J Ophthalmol. 1958;45(4 Pt 2):235–40.
79. Vogel MH, Zimmerman LE, Gass JD. Proliferation of the juxtapapillary retinal pigment epithelium simulating malignant melanoma. Doc Ophthalmol. 1969;26:461–81.
80. Shields JA, Eagle RC Jr, Dutton J, Ehya H, Shields CL. Adenocarcinoma of the retinal pigment epithelium: clinicopathologic correlation with paradoxical immunohistochemical findings. JAMA Ophthalmol. 2014;132:1249–52.
81. Shields JA, Melki T, Shields CL, Eagle RC Jr, Singh AD. Epipapillary adenoma of retinal pigment epithelium. Retina. 2001;21:76–8.
82. Shields JA, Shields CL. Tumors and related lesions of the pigment epithelium. In: Shields JA, Shields CL, editors. Intraocular tumors: an atlas and textbook. 2nd ed. Philadelphia: Lippincott, Williams & Wilkins; 2008. p. 432–83.
83. Shields JA, Eagle RC Jr, Shields CL, Brown GC, Lally SE. Malignant transformation of congenital hypertrophy of the retinal pigment epithelium. Ophthalmology. 2009;116:2213–6.
84. Shields CL, Manalac J, Das C, Ferguson K, Shields JA. Choroidal melanoma: clinical features, classification, and top 10 pseudomelanomas. Curr Opin Ophthalmol. 2014;25:177–85.
85. Shields CL, Mashayekhi A, Ho T, Cater J, Shields JA. Solitary congenital hypertrophy of the retinal pigment epithelium: clinical features and frequency of enlargement in 330 patients. Ophthalmology. 2003;110:1968–76.

2 RPE Polarity and Barrier Function

Lawrence J. Rizzolo

Introduction

The RPE separates the developing neurosensory retina from its blood supply in the choroid. Because choroidal capillaries are fenestrated, RPE functions as the outer blood-retinal barrier (BRB). This dynamic barrier regulates the extracellular milieu of the developing retina, and later the mature photoreceptors. Because the retina lacks lymphatics, it relies in part on the RPE to recover fluid extravasated from retinal capillaries by pumping fluid out of the subretinal space. RPE also removes fluid from the vitreous that is driven into the retina by ocular pressure. The RPE maintains the ionic composition of the subretinal space that is optimal for photoreceptor activity. RPE participates in the visual cycle whereby 11-*cis* retinal that was converted to all-trans-retinal upon capturing a photon of light was transported from photoreceptors to the RPE, re-isomerized, and returned to the photoreceptors. RPE phagocytizes the spent disc membranes that are shed daily by the photoreceptors. Each of these processes is related to barrier function and depends upon epithelial polarity and a structure called the tight junction.

L. J. Rizzolo (✉)
Department of Surgery, Yale University School of Medicine, New Haven, CT, USA

Department of Ophthalmology and Visual Science, Yale University School of Medicine, New Haven, CT, USA
e-mail: Lawrence.rizzolo@yale.edu

Epithelial polarity refers to the asymmetric distribution of proteins between the apical and basolateral membranes of an epithelial cell and is known as cell polarity. RPE was thought to be an "upside down" epithelium with reversed membrane polarity. The reason was that a plasma membrane pump protein, the Na,K-ATPase, that drives fluid transport across epithelia is located in the apical plasma membrane [1, 2]. The Na,K-ATPase is in the basolateral plasma membrane of most epithelium. In general, cell polarity refers to the asymmetric distribution of any protein, mRNA, or organelle within a cell. Polarity may be transient, as in a migrating cell with its leading and trailing ends. Polarity may be an enduring feature as in ciliated cells or neurons with dendrites at one pole and an axon at the other. The mechanisms that underlie polarity are largely conserved and have been adapted and retooled during evolution to polarize specialized cells that function in asymmetric environments [3–5].

Compared with the polarity of other epithelia, the RPE is actually "right side up" with variations on a basic theme [1, 2, 6–8]. Generally, simple, transporting epithelia are monolayers with an apical pole that faces a lumen and a basolateral pole that faces a solid tissue. Interactions between the basolateral membrane and the underlying tissue induce epithelial polarity. RPE uses these same basolateral mechanisms for house-keeping proteins, and shares a polarity in common with many epithelia [7, 9–13].

A. K. Klettner, S. Dithmar (eds.), *Retinal Pigment Epithelium in Health and Disease*,
https://doi.org/10.1007/978-3-030-28384-1_2

To understand how the variations in RPE polarity arise and affect barrier function, it will be instructive to compare RPE with other epithelia derived from the same embryonic primordium, the neuroepithelium. These include the epithelium of the choroid plexus, the ciliary body of the eye, and the iris. The apical membrane of these epithelia faces the lumen of the brain's ventricular system. The epithelium of the choroid plexus also has an apical Na,K-ATPase, and secretes cerebral spinal fluid into this lumen. The other epithelia are found in the eye, where the lumen of the ventricular system is reduced to a potential space. Accordingly, the apical membranes of these epithelia face a solid tissue. Despite its apical Na,K-ATPase, RPE absorbs fluid from the potential (subretinal) space to prevent serous retinal detachment. Rather than secrete fluid into the potential space, the functional unit of ciliary body expresses a non-polarized Na,K-ATPase to secrete fluid into the aqueous chamber. This chapter explores how RPE's apical interactions with the neurosensory retina underlie the differences in barrier function between RPE and the epithelia of the choroid plexus and ciliary body.

There is an intimate relationship between cell polarity and tight junctions (Fig. 2.1). Tight junctions form a partially occluding seal between the neighbors of an epithelial monolayer. They

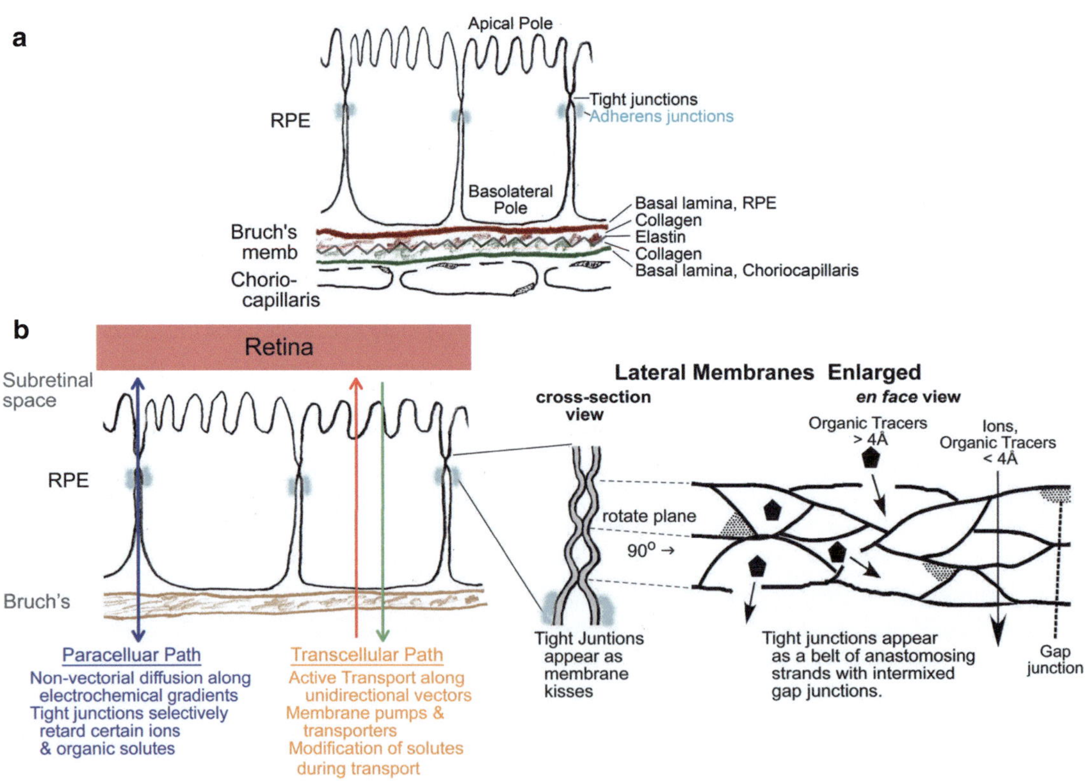

Fig. 2.1 Schema of RPE and tight junctions. (**a**) Microvilli at the apical pole of RPE extend into the subretinal space. At the basal pole, five-layered Bruch's membrane separates RPE from the choriocapillaris. Fenestra in the walls of the choriocapillaris lie next to Bruch's membrane. Tight and adherens junctions lie at the apical end of the lateral membranes. (**b**) The properties of the paracellular and transcellular pathways are indicated. The enlarged views schematize the appearance of tight junctions by transmission (cross-section) and freeze-fracture electron (enface) microscopy. The enface schematic illustrates two pathways for solutes. The pathway for small solutes (<4 Å) is often called the "pore" pathway. The pathway for large and small solutes is called the "leak" pathway. Modified with permission from Rizzolo (Histol Histopathol. 1997;12:1057–67) and Rizzolo et al., (Reference Module in Neuroscience and Biobehavioral Psychology, Elsevier, 2017)

are part of the apical junctional complex, which includes adherens and gap junctions. The complex separates the apical from the basolateral plasma membranes. Together, these junctions regulate cell shape, proliferation, and polarity. By locating different pump, transport and channel proteins on either side of the apical junctional complex, cells can use the energy of ATP to pump solutes against a concentration gradient from one side of the monolayer to the other. Tight junctions prevent this gradient from dissipating. The pumps and transporters of the apical membrane are electrically coupled to those of the basolateral membrane intracellularly and via tight junctions. Accordingly, the functional composition of tight junctions and membrane transporters are interconnected and tailored to the unique functions of a given epithelium.

This chapter relates cell polarity to the function of tight junctions in the RPE. To fully appreciate the unique features of this region of the BRB, RPE is discussed in the context of other tissue barriers and in particular other epithelia derived from the neuroepithelium.

The Blood-Retinal Barrier (BRB) Is a Division of the Blood-Brain Barrier (BBB)

Properties of a Blood-Tissue Barrier

Ehrlich and Goldman provided the first description of a blood-tissue barrier. Intravenous injections of dye permeated most tissues, but were excluded from the brain, testes, and placenta [14, 15]. This initial conception of the barrier has been expanded to include the five pathways that are illustrated in Fig. 2.2, using RPE as an example.

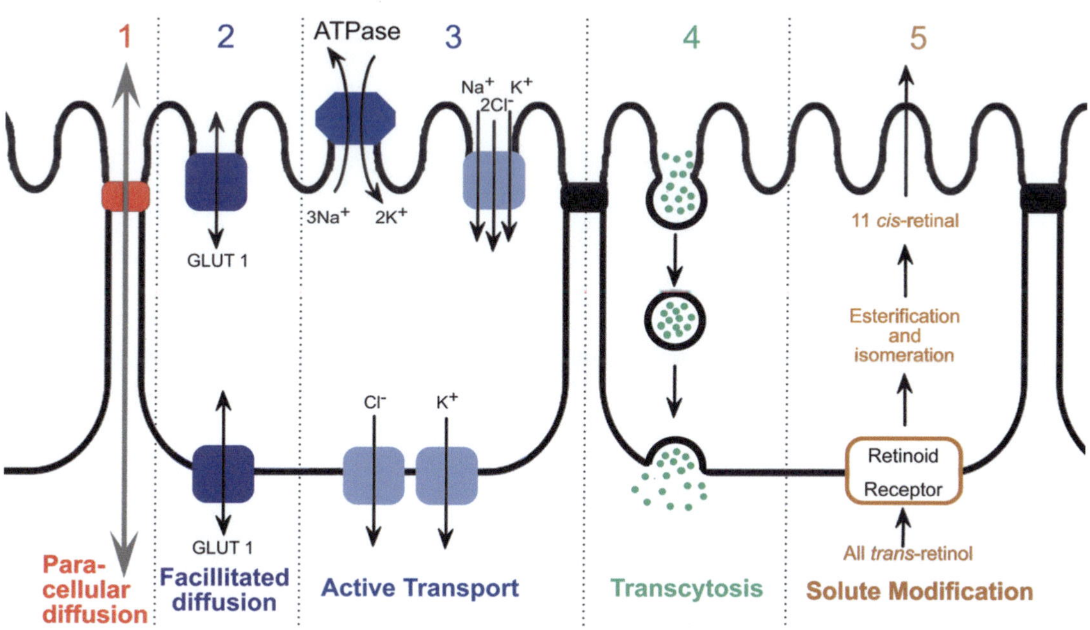

Fig. 2.2 Five pathways for the transepithelial transport in RPE. The apical membrane appears at the top. (1) Small solutes can diffuse across tight junctions, but the junctions allow some solutes to diffuse more readily than others. (2) Channels allow diffusion in either direction, but are specific for certain solutes. (3) Active transport: The Na/KATPase uses the energy of ATP to pump ions vectorially across the plasma membrane. The electrochemical gradients that are established drive other solutes vectorially through channels, symporters, and antiporters. (4) Transcytosis: Bulk phase transcytosis is illustrated. Receptor-mediated transcytosis may also occur. (5) Solute modification: Solutes, e.g., all trans-retinol enters the cell by receptor-mediated endocytosis. The solute is modified as it crosses the monolayer. From Xia and Rizzolo (Vision Res. 2017;139:72–81) with permission

1. Tight junctions were thought to block transepithelial diffusion through the paracellular spaces, but physiologists demonstrated that tight junctions were semi-permeable, semi-selective, and tissue specific [16–19]. They will be detailed in sections "The Structure of Tight Junctions and Pathways for Solutes to Traverse Them", "Analysis of Paracellular Barrier Function", and "The Interplay of Tight Junctions and Membrane Transporters".

   The remaining pathways are transcellular and more finely regulated than tight junctions. Nonetheless, RPE tight junctions affect proteins involved in these pathways
2. Facilitated diffusion relies on bidirectional channels in the plasma membrane. Their selectivity is orders of magnitude greater than that of the semi-selective tight junctions. Solutes only move down their transepithelial electrochemical gradient. RPE glucose transporters are examples [20]. They are often incorporated into active transport mechanisms.
3. Active transport moves solutes against an electrochemical gradient. The energy of ATP is used by pump proteins to (a) move solutes against a concentration gradient or (b) establish the electrochemical gradients that are used by symporters and antiporters. The second application couples the transport of one solute to another. The first solute travels down its electrochemical gradient, while the second solute comes with it or is moved in the opposite direction. The second application does not necessarily require a polarized ATPase, but does require that the various channels, symporters and antiporters be distributed to either the apical or basolateral membrane, as illustrated in Fig. 2.3.
4. Transcytosis uses receptor-mediated or bulk-phase (fluid-phase) endocytosis to encapsulate solutes. The endocytic vesicles that are formed traverse the cell to fuse with the opposite plasma membrane, and release their contents to the other side of the cell. Transcytosis is a typical feature of systemic capillaries, but not capillaries of the BBB. In the RPE, there is evidence of a bulk-phase, apical-to-basal pathway that partially recovers VEGF that is secreted from the apical membrane [21, 22].
5. Solute modification alters solutes as they traverse the cell. Rod outer segments are an extreme example. They are endocytosed by the apical membrane, degraded, and in aged individuals the degradation products are extruded from the basal membrane and contribute to drusen. More conventional examples are vitamin A and CO_2. Vitamin A crosses the basolateral membrane of RPE by receptor mediated endocytosis, is transformed in microsomes to 11-*cis*-retinal, and is exocytosed from the apical membrane into the subretinal space for use by photoreceptors. CO_2 that crosses the apical membrane of RPE is converted to HCO_3, which leaves the cell though the basolateral membrane [23, 24].

Epithelial Contributions to the Blood Retinal Barrier (BRB)

Transport across capillary walls of the inner BRB, and of the BBB in general, is tightly regulated [25–27]. In contrast, very leaky capillaries are found in the outer BRB (choriocapillaris), choroid plexus, and ciliary body. In these locations, the transport across the barrier is tightly regulated by epithelia derived from neuroepithelium (Fig. 2.3) [28, 29]. Despite their different barrier properties, their common origin sets these epithelia apart from other epithelia. To understand the RPE barrier, it is instructive to compare and contrast the differentiation of RPE to its cousins.

During embryogenesis, the neuroectoderm forms the neuroepithelium of the neural tube (Fig. 2.3). In the adult, the lumen of this tube becomes the central spinal canal and ventricular system of the brain. The cerebral spinal fluid that will eventually fill this lumen will be secreted by the epithelium of the choroid plexus (Fig. 2.3b). The lumen and the apical surface of the epithelium are continuous with the subretinal space and RPE. The subretinal space is a potential space, because the RPE continuously pumps fluid out of it. To envision this, recall that the optic vesicle is a diverticulum of the neurotube (Fig. 2.3a). Imagine the optic vesicle is a balloon. Punch your fist into the balloon to form a double-walled cup. Your fist will become the

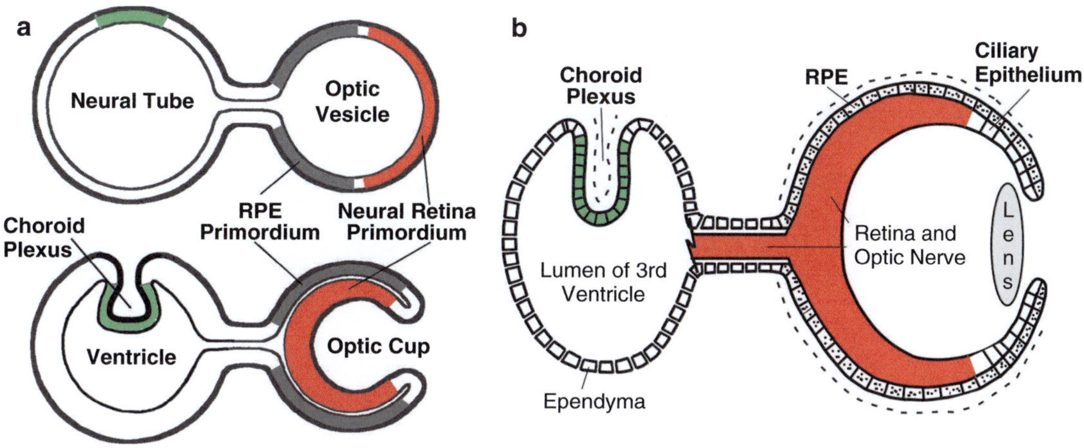

Fig. 2.3 Development of the epithelial regions of the blood-brain barrier. (**a**) The basal aspect of the neuroepithelium (thick line) faces the mesoderm, and the apical aspect with apical junctional complexes (thin line) faces a central lumen. The optic vesicle is a diverticulum of this tube that invaginates to form a two-layered optic cup with the apical surfaces apposed. The potential space between the layers is the subretinal space and remains continuous with the lumen of the ventricle. The outer layer becomes pigmented (RPE). A portion of the ventricular wall invaginates to house a tuft of fenestrated capillaries. (**b**) The linings of the ventricular system and subretinal space. Although adherens junctions encircle ependymal cells, the width of the lateral spaces is exaggerated to emphasize the lack of tight junctions [94]. Not shown are the similar junctions that form the outer limiting membrane, which link photoreceptors and Müller cells at the apical surface of the neural retina. Tight junctions are present in the RPE and epithelium of the choroid plexus. Dashed lines represent fenestrated capillaries. Modified with permission of Routledge/Taylor & Francis Group, LLC [29]

vitreous, your wrist represents the pupil, and the lens would be found at the base of the hand. The space between the two walls of the optic cup is reduced to a potential space, the subretinal space. The outer wall of the cup becomes a monolayer, the RPE. Anteriorly, the RPE is continuous with the pigment epithelium of the ciliary body and iris. In the iris, the pigment epithelium folds back on itself to form the inner wall of the cup. Continuing posteriorly, the inner wall courses over the pigment epithelium of the ciliary body and remains a monolayer but loses its pigment. The apical membranes of the non-pigment and pigment epithelium contact each other and are electrically coupled by gap junctions. This region of the blood-ocular barrier secretes aqueous humor. Where the non-pigment epithelium transitions into the neurosensory retina, the tissue thickens to give rise to all the non-vascular cell types of the neurosensory retina. The apical surface of the neurosensory retina is lined by photoreceptors whose outer segments interdigitate with the apical microvilli of the RPE.

RPE organizes the outer BRB. RPE induces the formation of fenestra in the choriocapillaris, which are distributed to the side of the capillary that faces the RPE. The RPE and choriocapillaris collaborate to form the five layers of Bruch's membrane, which lies between them (Fig. 2.1) [30–32]. RPE pumps fluid out of the subretinal space to prevent serous retinal detachment and retinal edema. Fluids continuously enter the retina from two sources: First, a portion of the fluid that retinal capillaries extravasate at the arteriole end is not normally resorbed by the capillaries at the venous end. Second, fluid from the vitreous humor is driven towards the choroid by intraocular pressure [33, 34]. RPE helps remove this fluid.

In general, the driving force for unidirectional transport of fluid and selected solutes is the Na,K-ATPase. Since this pump is in the apical membrane of RPE and the epithelium of the choroid plexus [1, 2, 6, 13, 35–40], why does one absorb fluid while the other secretes it? The answer lies in the polarized distribution of channels, symporters and antiporters, which differs between the RPE and epithelium of the choroid plexus (Fig. 2.4a, b) [41, 42]. The Na,K-ATPase does not need to be polarized to provide energy for the process, and is less polarized

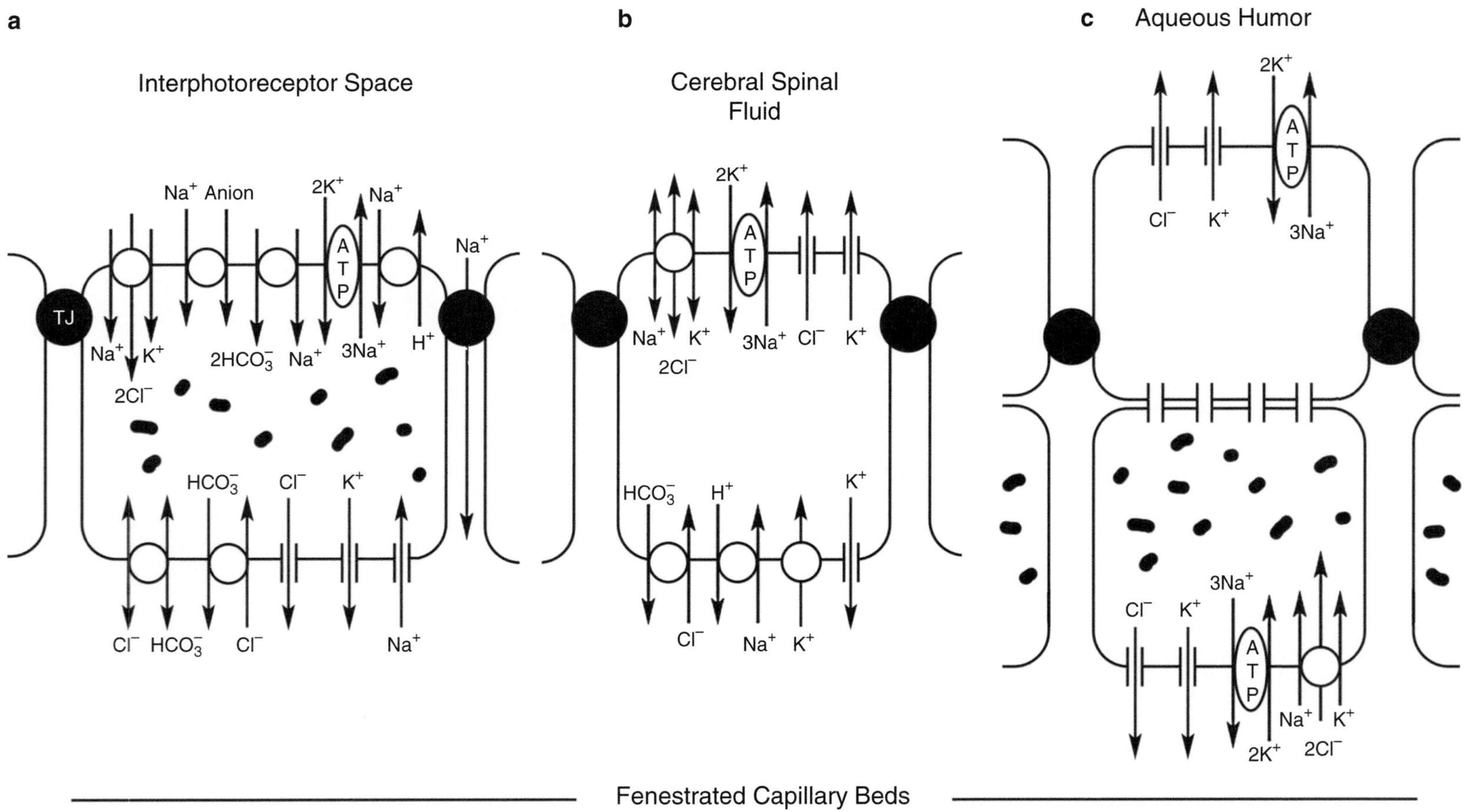

Fig. 2.4 Ion transport in derivatives of the neuroepithelium. (**a**) RPE (modified from Gallemore et al. 1997). (**b**) Choroid plexus (modified from Keep et al. Am J Physiol. 1994;267:C1616–C22). (**c**) Ciliary epithelium (modified from Edelman et al. 1994). With permission of Elsevier [6]

than the other transporters [43–45]. In fact the Na,K-ATPase is not polarized in the epithelium of the ciliary body, in which a pigmented and non-pigmented cell combine to function as a single cell (Fig. 2.4c). The two cells are coupled along their apical membranes by gap junctions that link the cytoplasms of the two cells. Tight junctions are only found in the non-pigment layer, and the Na,K-ATPase is in the basolateral membranes of each epithelium [46–50]. In other words, the Na,K-ATPase is non-polarized in this functional unit and is still able to drive the secretion of aqueous humor. The details of fluid absorption by the RPE will be revisited in section "The Interplay of Tight Junctions and Membrane Transporters".

Differentiation vs Maturation *In Vivo* and in Culture

Originally, the RPE was viewed as an uninteresting epithelium from the viewpoint of development. It was the first retinal cell to differentiate and changed little after it was established, morphological changes notwithstanding [51]. However, dynamic, fundamental changes underlie the increase in the number of melanin granules, elongation of apical microvilli, and infolding of the basal and lateral plasma membranes. The RPE works cooperatively with the fenestrated choriocapillaris and with the retina to serve the retina's changing needs as retinal differentiation proceeds. Accordingly, the functions of RPE mature with the differentiation and maturation of its neighboring tissues. Given the absence of choroidal capillaries and a neural retina, how does cultured RPE compare with native RPE? To approach this question, consider that RPE with the best barrier properties were isolated during embryonic, fetal, or newborn animals [52]. To some extent, the barrier properties of these cultures reflect the molecular and functional properties of the developmental stage from which the RPE was isolated. The following sections discuss the development and maturation of RPE relative to neighboring tissues.

What Is an RPE Cell?

Epithelia in the iris and ciliary body aside, cells of the optic vesicle that express melanin granules are committed to become mature RPE, but what is meant by maturity? It takes 6–8 weeks in culture for an RPE monolayer to "mature". Mature in this context means that: gene and protein expression becomes stable, barrier function becomes stable, and filamentous actin redistributes from stress fibers to cortical rings. The latter marks the end of the gradual remodeling that tight and adherens junctions undergo throughout this period [52, 53]. In another sense, "mature" means "become more like an adult RPE cell *in vivo*". This type of maturation does not happen unless the culture environment replicates aspects of the *in vivo* environment. Because of the difficulties of procuring human globes close to the time of death, cultures of 15–17 WG hfRPE have become the gold standard for authenticating cultures of human RPE [54–56].

Traditionally, investigators defined RPE by the expression or polarized distribution of a handful of RPE specific or enriched markers, supplemented by functional tests related to barrier function e.g., phagocytosis (a combination of barrier pathways 4 and 5, Fig. 2.2), retinoid processing pathway (5), paracellular resistance (pathway 1), and transcellular transport (pathways 2 and 3). To develop a more complete fingerprint of an RPE cell, the Miller laboratory identified a set of 154 "signature genes" by comparing the transcriptome of hfRPE with a panel of other tissues [57]. The rationale was that some cellular processes may be common to many cells, but are hyperactive in RPE. The phagocytic and lysosomal pathways would be examples. The list was narrowed to 87 genes, by eliminating genes that were highly expressed in human embryonic stem cell (hESC) and induced pluripotent cell (hiPSC) lines, before they were differentiated into RPE [58]. These are quantitative assays. Expression levels are of interest, because the proteins expressed by these genes function in a network of signaling and functional pathways. A protein that is expressed out of balance with its functional partners could have diverse effects on cell behavior. Surprisingly, the tight junction protein, claudin-19, is not included in this panel. Further study revealed that claudin-19 is not only an important determinant of RPE-specific properties of barrier pathway (1), claudin-19 regulates the expression of other RPE-specific, barrier-related pathways [59, 60].

To authenticate cultures of RPE, several strategies have been described that combine gene and protein expression with functional assays [52, 56, 61]. A complete assessment helps investigators evaluate the relative maturity of the cultures and integrate data from multiple laboratories. Many studies are difficult to compare, because they are performed in subconfluent or newly confluent cultures, which may be relevant to wound-repair or proliferative disease. Unfortunately, this practice makes it difficult to standardize experiments or compare data from different laboratories. Stem cell-derived and primary cultures of RPE derived from fetuses or young individuals are considered the best, but many studies rely on the convenience of established cell lines [52, 53]. Of the several human cell lines, ARPE-19 has been favored, because it replicates more of the native RPE phenotype [62]. Early passage cells, grown in specialized media under strict protocols, are the most RPE-like [63]. Most studies with ARPE-19 fail to meet these criteria. They are difficult to interpret, because the investigators used subconfluent cultures maintained in a media that does not allow ARPE-19 to mature. With time, the cell line has become heterogeneous, and more difficult to re-differentiate [59, 64]. ARPE-19 fails to express claudin-19. Exogenous expression of claudin-19 restores some of these lost properties [59]. Increasingly, leading eye journals currently require ARPE-19 studies be corroborated with animal studies, other cultures, or provide extensive documentation of cell phenotype.

One difficulty in developing a molecular/functional definition of an RPE cell is that the molecular fingerprint and barrier function change with time in development. Without environmental cues, maturation likely does not continue in culture as it does *in vivo*. For example, the epigenetic modifications of chromosomes that regulate gene expression are remodeled in response to changes in the environment. One could hypothesize that the epigenetics of RPE isolated from one stage of development would differ from those of RPE isolated from a later stage or from an adult. This hypothesis would explain the differences in gene expression and barrier function that are observed when chick RPE is isolated from different stages of development. It would also explain why the properties of primary cell cultures change as the cells are passaged. Barrier function as a function of development is explored in the following subsections.

Maturation of RPE Barrier Function in Chick Embryos and Small Mammals

Regardless of the length of gestation, developmental milestones for the choroid and RPE can be tied to the appearance of photoreceptor inner segments and outer segments [28, 65, 66]. These milestones of photoreceptor development divide ocular development into early, middle and late stages. For example, the ability of RPE to process retinoids appears in rodents when outer segments are made and *cis*-retinal is needed [67]. The process has been most thoroughly studied in chick. Between the early and late stages, 40% of the chick RPE transcriptome will turn on, turn off, or change its level of expression [66].

All epithelia sit on a basal lamina that contains tissue-specific isoforms of laminin, collagen IV, and associated proteins. Each provides signals that induce the epithelial phenotype and define the apical and basal surfaces of the cell [68–70]. For RPE, Bruch's membrane is composed of five layers (Fig. 2.1a). The basal lamina of the RPE and the endothelial cells each have an adjacent collagenous layer. An elastin fiber layer separates the two collagenous layers. Different layers appear gradually during development, beginning with the basal lamina and ending with the elastin layer [28]. RPE isolated from early-stage chick embryos could be cultured on a wide variety of matrixes. RPE isolated from the end of the middle stage adhered to fewer substrates, and only some substrates allowed the RPE to respond to physiologic stimuli from the neurosensory retina [71, 72]. The data are consistent with normal chick development. The RPE secretes different isoforms of extracellular matrix proteins as embryogenesis proceeds. Early embryonic forms of laminin and collagen IV (laminin $\alpha1\beta1\gamma1$ and collagen IV $\alpha2$ chains) are replaced with more mature forms (laminins $\alpha3\beta2\gamma1$, $\alpha1\beta2\gamma1$, and $\alpha5\beta2\gamma1$ and collagen IV $\alpha4$ chains) [66]. These results suggest that receptors for the extracellular matrix and associated signaling pathways are remodeled as development progresses.

During the late stage of development, construction of Bruch's membrane, elaboration of basal plasma membrane infoldings, and the fenestration of the choriocapillaris is completed [65]. In chick, this corresponds with the completion of RPE's barrier mechanisms. Like studies of the chick RPE transcriptome [66], studies of the mouse choriocapillaris transcriptome revealed potential remodeling of Bruch's membrane [73]. These authors used endothelial cell-RPE co-culture and endothelial cell conditioned medium to explore the mechanism of remodeling. The matrix remodeling by endothelial cells was sensed by integrin receptors in the RPE that triggered Rho GTPase signaling. The result was an increase in barrier function of the RPE.

Concurrent with the gradual remodeling of basal interactions, gradual remodeling of lateral membranes occurs at the apical junctional complex. The claudins (tight junctions) and cadherins (adherens junctions) are families of transmembrane proteins that reach across the paracellular space to form homotypic dimers. The family members that are expressed change throughout chick development [66, 74–76]. Because these proteins activate signaling pathways it is likely that cell-cell signaling is remodeled during development [77]. Section "Analysis of Paracellular Barrier Function" will describe how claudin expression affects barrier function directly via pathway (1) (Fig. 2.2), and indirectly by affecting the expression of genes related to the transcellular pathways of barrier function.

Concurrent with basal and lateral remodeling, signaling across the apical membrane also changes during chick development, as the neurosensory retina differentiates and matures. These signaling pathways are mediated by secretions of the neurosensory retina and direct contact of the RPE apical membrane with it [28]. Direct contact caused certain integrins and the Na^+/K^+-ATPase to concentrate in the apical membrane [7, 29]. Retinal secretions were studied using a conditioned medium that was prepared by organ culture of retinas isolated from different embryonic ages. Retinal conditioned medium increased the expression of many RPE related genes, including those for: melanogenesis, the visual cycle, lysosomes, phagocytosis, adherens junctions, tight junctions, gap junctions, plasma membrane transporters, cytoskeletal elements and their regulators, and proteins of the extracellular matrix and their receptors [28, 77]. Retinal conditioned medium converted rudimentary, discontinuous tight junctions into a continuous network of tight junctional strands [72, 78]. Although all of the components required to make a tight junction were present, retinal signaling was required to trigger assembly into a functional tight junction [79, 80].

Maturation of RPE Barrier Function in Humans

Differentiation and maturation appears to be different in humans. The first indicator is that the choriocapillaris becomes fenestrated near the beginning of the middle stage (as defined by photoreceptor morphology, section "Epithelial Contributions to the Blood Retinal Barrier (BRB)"), 21–22 weeks gestation (WG), much earlier than in non-primate vertebrates [52, 81]. However, RPE tight junctions are well formed by 12–13 WG. RPE isolated at this age forms a robust barrier [82]. Retinoid processing appears to be completely established in RPE isolated from 16 to 22 WG fetuses, before outer segments are made [81, 83]. Although RPE cells isolated from the early stage can phagocytize outer segment disc membranes, the machinery for digesting disc membranes may not be upregulated until late development. This hypothesis is based on a comparison of RPE-derived from stem cells with cultured hfRPE and adult RPE. Flux through the degradative pathway followed the order: hiPSC-RPE < hfRPE (16 week gestation) ≪ adult RPE (K. Davis and L. Rizzolo, unpublished data).

To ascertain which principals gleaned from the study of non-primate vertebrates might apply to human development, researchers have turned to hESC and hiPSC. Though highly differentiated, hESC—derived RPE are not as mature as 15–16 WG human fetal RPE (hfRPE), as judged by RNA sequencing [61]. The relative immaturity provides an assay to screen for agents that promote maturation. A second indication of the immaturity of stem cell-derived RPE is the affinity for extracellular matrix. The best matrix to culture highly differentiated hfRPE is derived from human placenta, which expresses mature family members of laminin and collagen IV [54]. Stem cell-derived RPE will not form monolayers on this matrix, but will do so on matrixes that contain embryonic forms of laminin and collagen IV [61, 84, 85].

Similarly, stem cell-derived RPE cells were less able than hfRPE to populate native Bruch's membrane that was isolated from cadaveric eyes [86]. RPE was unable to form monolayers on Bruch's membrane from aged eyes with macular disease [87]. The importance of basal signaling pathways is illustrated by modifying Bruch's membrane from cadaveric eyes. The lamina of Bruch's membrane can be removed sequentially. RPE is unable to form a monolayer on the collagen and elastin lamina, or on a chemically modified basal lamina. Cell attachment and proliferation increases, allowing patches of monolayers to form if the surface is recoated with laminin or collagen IV [87–90]. The electron micrographs suggest that an apical junctional complex reformed, but the experimental protocol did not investigate whether functional tight junctions are formed. Gene expression was not examined in any of these studies.

To explore RPE-neurosensory retina interactions of human RPE, cultures of planar retinal organoids are needed to place the RPE and neurosensory retina in their normal morphological relationship. When the apical membrane of RPE contacts the photoreceptor layer, tissue-tissue interactions are potentially enhanced two ways: (1) cell-cell contact allows for receptor-mediated signaling, and (2) a subretinal space is recreated that allows secreted factors to attain effective concentrations without being diluted by the bulk medium. Stem cell-derived retinal organoids can be made from hESC and hiPSC [91]. The maturation of retinal organoids approximates normal retinal development in vivo, but the essential morphological relationship of the RPE and neurosensory retina was not re-established. The native RPE-neurosensory retina relationship was retained if the retinal cup-like structures were established in two-dimensional culture [92]. Retinal lamina did not form, but the maturation of photoreceptors was enhanced. The method illustrates a role for RPE in promoting an aspect of retinal development, but the method is limited by the experimenter's lack of independent access to the RPE and retinal tissue. By constructing a scaffold that emulates the extracellular matrix of the retina, a planar retinal tissue can be established [93]. Coating the scaffold with components of the inner limiting membrane resulted in a laminated retinal organoid (Rizzolo, manuscript in preparation). Co-culture of this organoid with RPE promoted the maturation of both tissues, analogous to the co-dependence of RPE and neurosensory retina in chick development [66, 77]. Besides effects on gene expression in the RPE and developing neurosensory retina, barrier function (pathway 1) of the RPE was enhanced. The method allows independent access to both sides of the organoid using the device illustrated in Fig. 2.5a, which enables the assays of barrier function discussed in section "Analysis of Paracellular Barrier Function".

The Structure of Tight Junctions and Pathways for Solutes to Traverse Them

Epithelia can be classified as leaky or tight based on how readily ions pass through the paracellular space. At one extreme, the paracellular path of the urinary bladder is virtually blocked by tight junc-

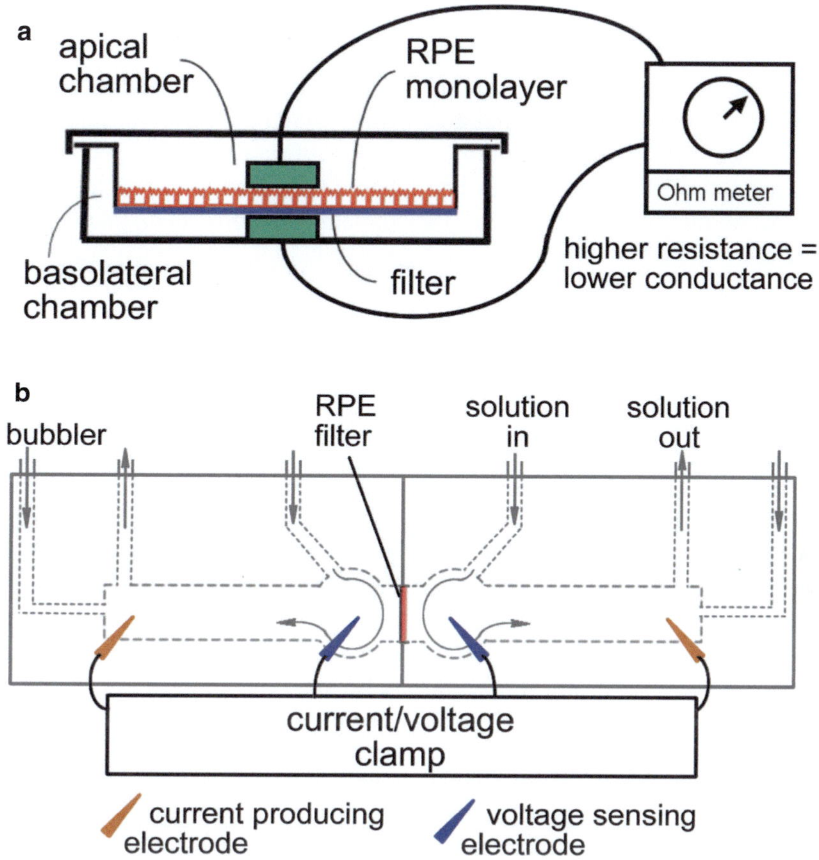

Fig. 2.5 Culture of RPE on filters and measurement of barrier properties. (**a**) The monolayers separate the media into apical and basal compartments. Barrier function can be assessed by placing solutes on one side of the monolayer and measuring the rate by which it travels to the opposite side. Alternatively, electrodes can be placed on either side to estimate the TER during culture. (**b**) For more rigorous assessment of barrier properties, the filters can be placed in an Ussing chamber. Measurements of TER and TEP can be used to estimate the permeability of ions through the tight junction and certain properties of ion channels. To this end, the solutions in the two halves of the Ussing chamber can be changed independently and various inhibitors can be introduced. Panel (**a**) was reproduced from Rizzolo (Encyclopedia of the Eye. 4. Oxford: Academic Press; 2010. p. 101–8), with permission

tions. At the other extreme, the paracellular path of systemic capillaries, intestinal mucosa, and the proximal kidney tubule are very leaky. Most epithelia, including RPE of various vertebrate species, fall somewhere along this continuum.

Epithelial barriers depend on a complex of junctions found at the apical end of the lateral membranes, the apical junctional complex (Fig. 2.1). The complex is a ribbon of cell-cell contact between the neighboring cells of an epithelial monolayer. The ribbon completely encircles each cell, like the plastic holder that binds a six-pack of beverage. The apical-most member of the complex is the tight junction (zonula occludens). The basal-most junction is the adherens junction (zonula adherens). Interspersed within the ribbon of tight junctions is a collection of gap junctions. Gap junctions form channels between neighboring cells. They are typically found in clusters all along the lateral membrane of an epithelial cell, but in RPE and endothelial cells they are incorporated into tight junctions [78, 95–97]. The three junctions collaborate as signal transducers to regulate cell size, shape, polarity, and proliferation [98–100]. Tight junctions act as a passive fence to maintain polarity, and the entire complex participates in the intracellular membrane trafficking that establishes polarity [98, 101–105].

Structurally, the proteins of adherens and gap junctions span the paracellular space to interact with their partners in the neighboring cells. Tight junctions differ by fusing neighboring lateral membranes to eliminate the paracellular space. When viewed in cross-section by transmission electron microscopy, the lateral membranes appear as two, parallel electron-dense lines that "kiss" at one or more spots (schematized in Fig. 2.1b). The kisses form pentilaminar structures where the extracellular-facing electron-dense lines of neighboring cells have fused. The lateral membranes can be viewed *en face* by using freeze-fracture electron microscopy. Freeze-fracture splits the phospholipid bilayer along the interface between the two leaflets of the plasma membrane. Transmembrane proteins are represented by "bumps" and "pits" in the image. The transmembrane proteins of tight junctions appear as an anastomosing network of strands. The strands correspond to the kisses observed by transmission electron microscopy. The strands seem to be permanent structures in these static images, but *in vivo* the strands constantly break apart and reseal [101, 106].

Detailed studies of tight junction morphology in chick embryonic RPE illustrate the principles established by studies of tight junctions across species and tissues. Morphology of the junctions loosely correlates with permeability [107], but numerous variables complicate this analysis: the number of parallel strands, the density of anastomotic connections (branch points/unit length), the depth (thickness of the anastomotic network), and especially the protein composition of the junctions. During chick RPE development, strands initially appear as discontinuous clusters of one or two strands that gradually coalesce into a complete network. The number of strands increases from three to five with a corresponding increase in depth [78]. In the later stages of development through adulthood the density of anastomoses increases [108]. A similar morphology was reported in rodent RPE [109]. Because of the role of protein composition, junctions that share morphological features might still differ in their barrier properties [78, 110]. A culture model of RPE development illustrates this latter point (see section "Electrophysiological Assays").

Protein Composition

Aside from specific claudin family members, the composition of RPE tight junctions is similar to that of other epithelia. Tight junctions are composed of transmembrane, adaptor, and effector proteins that form a complicated interacting network [111]. The transmembrane proteins responsible for the strands observed by freeze-fracture electron microscopy are claudin and occludin. Claudins are the principal strand-forming proteins. Of the 27 or more claudin family members, only a subset is expressed by a given epithelium to give that epithelium unique paracellular selectivity and permeability. Occludin can form strands to a small extent, and appears to decrease permeability without affecting selectivity [112]. Occludin is enriched where the membranes of three neighboring cells are in contact. Adaptor proteins link transmembrane proteins to effectors, such as transcription factors, G-proteins, phosphatases and kinases (reviewed in [101, 102, 111]). The zonula occludens family (ZO-1, ZO-2, and ZO-3) were the first adaptors to be identified. Among them they express many protein-binding domains including nine different PDZ domains, which are the most numerous protein-binding domains found in nature [113]. Additional PDZ, and other protein-binding domains are expressed by other adaptor proteins. These adaptors have an enormous capacity to bind diverse effector proteins. A number of these effector proteins are potential regulatory targets, because: their half-lives are short relative to other membrane proteins, they rapidly associate/dissociate from the complex, or they carry signals into the nucleus [114–117]. The many proteins involved together with these dynamic features indicate the tight junction is a major regulatory center that can respond rapidly to pharmacologic agents and physiologic changes [29, 118–120].

The protein composition of tight junctions is conserved among species and different types of epithelia. Examination of published transcriptomes for chick and human RPE show the same proteins are present in RPE [57, 61, 66, 77]. The apical junctional complex contains several protein families including the claudins and those cadherins that are part of the adherens junction. Tissue-specific functions are possible, because a given epithelium expresses only a few members of each family. Birds and mammals express different claudin family members in their RPE, and some family members are restricted to a particular developmental stage [28].

Claudins Are Major Determinants for the Selectivity and Permeability of Tight Junctions

Claudins bind each other within the plane of the membrane and with claudins in the neighboring cells [53, 121–125]. At least 27 claudins have been identified by sequence analysis. The canonical family member has four transmembrane domains, two extracellular loops, and conserved C-terminal amino acids for binding ZO-1 and other adaptor proteins. The first extracellular loop determines the permeability and selectivity of the claudin [126–129]. They can be classified as "pore-forming" or "barrier forming" and each class classified as "anion-selective" or "cation-selective" [125]. Table 2.1 shows the properties of claudins that have been identified in the RPE or epithelium of the choroid plexus. Why does nature require 27 or more unique claudins? The original notion was that with a large family to choose from, an epithelium could fine-tune the barrier function of its tight junctions to match the function of their membrane transporters. Recent data suggests that claudins are also signaling molecules [59, 60, 130]. Therefore, claudins with similar barrier functions might be needed to regulate different signal transduction pathways.

Claudins appear to play a role in the differentiation of the neurosensory retina by changing the barrier properties of the RPE as development proceeds. Comprehensive studies of claudin expression are available for chick and human fetal RPE [28, 66, 77]. The studies of chick embryogenesis revealed that the apical junctional complex is remodeled throughout the maturation of RPE. Focusing on the tight junctions,

Table 2.1 Properties of claudins found in RPE and the epithelium of the choroid plexus

	Claudin		
Selectivity	Choroid plexus	Human RPE	Chick RPE
Pore forming			
Anion			
	–[a]	–	–
Cation			
	2	2[b]	–
	–	10b[b]	–
Barrier forming			
Anion			
	1	1[b]	1
	–	3[c]	–
			5
	11	–	–
Cation			
	–	19[c]	–
Unknown			
	–	–	20[d]

Data compiled from reviews by Günzel and Yu and by Rizzolo et al. [53, 125]

[a]Undetected or detected in trace amounts

[b]Detected in only a subset of cells

[c]Detected in the entire monolayer

[d]Does not appear until the late stage of development

claudin-1 and claudin-5 were expressed early in development, but after the expression of ZO-1, ZO-2 and the formation of adherens junctions. The principal claudin, claudin-20, did not appear until late in development. Claudin-1 and claudin-5 are anion-selective, barrier-forming proteins. Nothing is known regarding the properties of claudin-20. Interestingly, the adaptor protein, ZO-3, appeared at the same time as claudin-20. The functional significance of these changes is unknown, but may reflect changes in the physiology of the developing retina. As noted earlier for non-primate mammals and chicks, the development of the retina, RPE and outer BRB are temporally related, and signals from the retina regulate barrier function and other aspects of RPE development.

We have a more static view of claudin expression in humans, because it would be unethical to perform a detailed study of development and maturation. Claudin-3 and claudin-19 are expressed in all cells of cultured hfRPE [131].

Only removal of claudin-19 resulted in the loss of barrier function and only mutants of claudin-19 cause ocular disease. Apparently, there is insufficient claudin-3 to form tight junctions on its own, and naturally occurring mutations of claudin-3 are unassociated with retinal disease (https://www.genecards.org/). Both claudins are barrier-forming proteins that are slightly cation-selective. Claudin-1, claudin-2, and claudin-10b were detected in subsets of the cultured cells, suggesting that there might be regional variation in claudin expression about the retina. Claudin-2 and claudin-10b are cation-selective, pore-forming proteins. These claudins might modulate barrier function in regions where they are found. Other regional differences in RPE have also been reported for the expression of cadherins and the polarity of the Na^+/K^+-ATPase [132].

Claudins Regulate Additional Pathways of Barrier Function Through Effects on Gene Expression

Besides direct effects on pathway (1), claudin-3 and claudin-19 regulate the expression of genes that enable epithelia to form a tissue barrier [59]. The barrier properties of the human ARPE-19 cell line are rudimentary, especially in cells that have been passaged >20 times, because claudins are detected in very few cells. Claudin-19 is not expressed at all. Exogenous expression of either claudin-3 or claudin-19 increased the TER in a matter of days. Cell behavior was more epithelial-like in wound healing assays. Surprisingly, the gene expression increased for a handful of signature genes and maturation genes that are unrelated to tight junctions. In other words, expression of these claudins partially restored the RPE transcriptome and phenotype. Some of these effects were mediated by an Akt signaling pathway [59]. Insight into this issue comes from studies of the disease familial hypomagnesemia with hypercalciuria and nephrocalcinosis with ocular involvement (FHHNCOI).

FHHNC is a severe renal disease that sometimes affects the eye [133–135]. In the kidney claudin-16 and claudin-19 form an interacting pair, and mutants of either cause the disease. Because claudin-16 is not expressed in RPE [22, 61], only mutants of claudin-19 cause ocular involvement (FHHNCOI) [134–136]. The ocular disease is severe and appears in early childhood, including bilateral macular coloboma, chorioretinal degeneration, nystagmus, strabismus, and visual loss [137–139].

It was unclear why a defect in tight junctions would have such wide-ranging effects. New areas of investigation were opened by the finding that claudin-19 is also a signaling molecule that affects the expression of RPE signature genes [59]. These studies with ARPE-19 were confirmed and expanded using a multipronged approach [60]. Naturally occurring point mutations of CLDN19, the gene for claudin-19, were expressed in hiPSC, mice, ARPE-19 cells, and cultured hfRPE. In hiPSC, mutation of both alleles prevented eyecups from forming to implicate claudin-19 in early steps of ocular differentiation. The expression of many signature genes in the RPE were down-regulated. Expression of the mutations in ARPE-19 accumulated in cytoplasmic vesicles and, when co-expressed with wild-type, blocked wild-type claudin-19 from reaching the cell surface. The same effect was observed in hfRPE, along with a decrease in the expression of neurotrophic growth factors, NGF and PEDF, and visual cycle proteins, including RPE65. In mice, an examination of normal ocular development between birth and 90 days revealed that claudin-19 was transiently expressed in retinal progenitor cells and early retinal ganglion cells. Exogenous expression of the human mutations of CLDN19 beginning at birth resulted in apoptosis of photoreceptors, disorganization of retinal bipolar cells, and loss of function as measured by electroretinography. A common thread to each of these experimental approaches was decreased expression of RPE65, the isomerase that regenerates 11-*cis*-retinal (Fig. 2.2, pathway 5). By circumventing this enzyme and supplying the photoreceptors with the analogue, 9-*cis*-retinal, visual function could be restored. These studies indicate that claudin-19 affects barrier function directly through its effects on tight junctions and indirectly by regulating gene expression of proteins involved in other pathways across the outer BRB.

Analysis of Paracellular Barrier Function

Intravenous injection of the fluorescent tracer, sodium fluorescein, is commonly used to study the integrity of the inner and outer BRB in patients and experimental animals, but is less suitable for detailed analysis of tight junctions. In healthy eyes, the fluorescein should be confined to the inner retinal vasculature and the RPE should attenuate the signal that leaks from the choroidal vasculature. Leaks from micro aneurysms of retinal vessels or compromised RPE are readily detected, however this all-or-none assay reflects a complete disassembly of endothelial or RPE tight junctions. To study how the permeability or semi-selectivity of intact junctions might be modulated, methods are required that can distinguish the contributions of size and electrical charge. Comprehensive assays of tight junctions address these properties by measuring the diffusion of uncharged tracers that vary in size or electrophysiological assays of inorganic ions. The following sections are abbreviated from a detailed description that discusses the assumptions that underlie these measurements and how to mitigate them [53].

A hypothesis that has gained considerable support postulates that solutes use "pore" or "leak" pathways to traverse tight junctions [28, 126, 140]. The hypothesis stemmed from the observation that paracellular flux and TER measure distinct properties that could be regulated independently [141, 142]. The first is a high capacity pathway that can be modeled as pores along the tight junctional strands, or can be regarded as the resin of an ion-exchange column (Fig. 2.1b). In either event, this pathway is available only to solutes that are small. A common measure of size is the Stokes radius, which is the radius of a sphere with the same hydrodynamic properties. The pores can accommodate solutes with a Stokes radius <~4.0 Å [143, 144]. The chemical nature of the pores determines whether they are cation- or anion-selective or neutral. It also determines if they are leaky or tight. Note that tight junctions are orders of magnitude less selective than membrane channels, presumably because of the leak pathway used by larger solutes. The leak pathway is a low capacity path that depends on the dynamics of strand-breaking and resealing [106, 140]. With each strand-break the solutes can diffuse deeper into and eventually across the tight junction. Sodium fluorescein is not the tracer of choice for this analysis, because it is charged and its Stokes radius (4.5 Å) is at the boundary of the leak and pore pathways.

Permeation of Polymeric Solutes

Large polymers and proteins are useful for accessing the leak pathway or a complete disruption of tight junctions. A commonly used polymer is dextran linked to fluorescein. These dextrans are available in various sizes that are all larger than accommodated by the pore pathway. This discussion focuses on another polymer, polyethylene glycol, because they are unaffected by the ionic charge of the pore or leak pathways, and they have a broad range of sizes above and below the 4 Å boundary between the pore and leak pathways. The permeation coefficient is the best way to compare data among laboratories and is measured using the formula:

$$P = (X)_t / (X/ml)_i / A / T \qquad (2.1)$$

where $(X)_t$ = total tracer that crossed the monolayer, $(X/ml)_i$ = the concentration of tracer initially added to one or the other medium chamber, A = surface area of the culture in cm^2, and T = time in hours. The final units are: cm/h [145, 146].

Polyethylene glycols are available as polydisperse mixtures. A seminal experiment that confirmed the size-limitation of the pore pathway added this mixture to one side of an epithelial monolayer and used column chromatography to determine which polymers crossed the monolayer. The permeation coefficient for each length of polyethylene glycol was determined. When graphed against size, a sharp break in the permeation coefficient was observed at a Stokes radius of ~4.0 Å [144].

A simplified application of this method uses methylated polyethylene glycol, which is available as two polydisperse mixtures with an average molecular weight of 550 or 2000. The pore pathway is available to most of the low molecular weight glycol, and unavailable for most of the high molecular weight glycol. The methyl group allows the concentration of the polyethylene glycol to be determined by ELISA assay. The apparent permeation coefficient can be determined for the low and high molecular weight glycols. The ratio of the permeation coefficients reflects the relative size of the pore and leak pathways, and can determine how the leak pathway is affected by experimental conditions. The permeation coefficient measured in the apical-to-basal direction should be the same in the basal-to-apical direction. If not, there may be a transcellular transport mechanism available for that tracer. The disparity observed for VEGF led to the discovery of an apical-to-basal transcytosis pathway for hfRPE [21, 22]. RPE secretion of VEGF is non-polarized, but the transcytosis pathway reduces the concentration of VEGF in the subretinal space to the low levels required by the neurosensory retina [21, 147].

The finding that the size of the pores is ~4.0 Å helps explain studies of tight junction development during the embryogenesis of chick RPE. In a culture model of chick RPE maturation, retinal conditioned medium affected morphology by closing breaks in tight junction strands, and altering the expression of claudins [66, 77, 78]. Sealing the strands greatly reduced the permeation of large tracers, horseradish peroxidase and inulin. The small tracer, mannitol, was minimally affected, because it is small enough to use pore and leak pathways [72]. Changes in claudin expression did not affect the permeation of large tracers, but affected small ions. Subsequent studies using mannitol and charged tracers of equal size 3-*O*-methlyglucose, glucosamine and *N*-acetylneuraminic acid found that the pore pathway selected against negatively-charged *N*-acetylneuraminic acid, but not positively-charged glucosamine [142]. This finding is consistent with electrophysiological assays that indicate that RPE tight junctions are slightly cation selective.

Electrophysiological Assays

There are several ways that ions can cross an epithelial monolayer (Fig. 2.2). Pathway (1) is diffusion through the paracellular space between neighboring cells. Ion selectivity is due to the high-capacity, pore pathway, but as noted above the leak pathway can make a contribution. One way to measure ion permeability is to use a surrogate that is related to permeability, the resistance to an electrical current passed across the monolayer. The electrical resistance offered by pathway (1), the shunt pathway, can be denoted R_S. Pathway (3) illustrates how ions also pass through the cell. The dominant resistance to this pathway is offered by the lipid bilayer of the plasma membrane, but membrane transporters provide a way for ions to cross the bilayer. Because of the polarized distribution of ion pumps, channels, and transporters, the apical plasma membrane offers a different electrical resistance (R_A) than the basolateral membrane (R_B). Although many authors erroneously equate the transepithelial electrical resistance (TER) to resistance of the tight junctions (R_S), TER is actually an amalgam of (R_S), (R_A), and (R_B). TER is related to R_S by Eq. (2.2) [148]:

$$TER = R_S \times \left(\frac{R_A + R_B}{R_A + R_B + R_S} \right) \tag{2.2}$$

In physiological conditions for RPE, TER < R_S, but if membrane transport is inhibited by adding barium and removing CO_2, then $R_A + R_B \gg R_S$ and the TER $\approx R_S$. The equipment used to make these measurements is illustrated in Fig. 2.5.

The transepithelial electrical potential (TEP) is another valuable measure. The asymmetric distribution of pumps, channels and transporters of Fig. 2.2, pathway (3), combine to generate an electrochemical gradient across the epithelial monolayer. As examples, the three epithelia illustrated in Fig. 2.4 generate gradients of different size and polarity based on protein composition and distribution. A clogged filter can generate an artifactual electrical resistance, but only a living cell can convert the energy of ATP into the energy of a TEP by generating an electrochemical gradient across the epithelium. Artificially imposed TEPs can be used to measure the permeation coefficient of an ion (P_{ion}). First, membrane transport is blocked, which increases membrane resistance such that $R_A + R_B \gg R_S$ and TER $\approx R_S$ (see Eq. 2.2). Under these conditions, ions move through the paracellular pathway (Fig. 2.2, pathway 1) down an experimentally imposed electrochemical gradient. A TEP can be generated chemically by placing different concentrations of NaCl on either side of the monolayer (taking care to balance osmolality). This "dilution potential" will reveal whether Na^+ or Cl^- crosses the tight junction more readily and quantify the difference. Alternatively, a TEP can be generated by placing different chloride salts on opposite sides of the monolayer. This "bi-ionic potential" will reveal which cation permeates more readily. Calculation of the permeability coefficient for a given ion can be determined by combining these TEP measurements [149].

In various non-primate species, the TER reported for RPE in physiologic media ranges from 138 to 426 $\Omega \times cm^2$. By contrast, the endothelial portions of the BBB have a TER = 1000–1500 $\Omega \times cm^2$ [25–27, 41]. After inhibiting transport through the plasma membrane, the resistance of RPE tight junctions (R_S) was revealed to be 1.1–7.0× higher than the TER in physiologic medium and ranged from 373 to 1254 $\Omega \times cm^2$. In serum free medium, or serum only in the basolateral chamber, hfRPE has a TER $\approx$ 200 $\Omega \times cm^2$. When incubated in a medium that inhibits transport through the plasma membrane, the TER $\approx$ 330 $\Omega \times cm^2$ [131]. Therefore, effects on TER should be interpreted with caution, before ascribing an effect solely to tight junctions.

Analysis of RPE Tight Junctions by Multiple Assays

In the chick model of RPE maturation, retinal conditioned medium sealed discontinuities in the network of tight junctional strands to decrease diffusion across the leak pathway. Additionally, it modulates the expression of claudins along with a variety of other proteins, including some related to transcellular barrier pathways [72, 77, 142]. The result was an increase in TER. Because the TER in this model was <100 $\Omega \times cm^2$, this effect of retinal conditioned medium was likely due to the observed changes in claudin expression. The active factors in retinal conditioned medium prepared from retinas isolated from E7 were chemically distinct from the active factors prepared from E14 retinas [80]. The retinal secretions responsible for these effects differed from the factors that Mueller cells and pericytes secrete to regulate the inner blood-retinal barrier [27, 80]. E7 retinal conditioned medium tightened the leak and pore pathways of RPE isolated from E7 embryos, but not E14 RPE. E14 retinal conditioned medium tightened these pathways in E7 and E14 embryos. Although E14 conditioned medium furthered the maturation of E7 RPE beyond the effects of E7 conditioned medium, the treated E7 RPE was less mature than untreated E14 RPE. These experiments demonstrate that the retinal secretions that affect the maturation of RPE change as the retina matures. Further, as the RPE matures it expresses new signaling pathways that can respond to the new retinal secretions.

In hfRPE, serum in the apical medium compartment, but not the basal compartment, increased the TER fourfold [22]. In contrast, serum in the basal medium compartment, but not the apical compartment increased the permeation of large polyethylene glycol (R_s > 4.0 Å) by increasing apical-to-basal bulk-phase transcytosis. Apical serum inhibited transcytosis, even if serum was in the basal compartment. The role of transcytosis was revealed by measuring the permeation coefficient in both directions. The permeation coefficient for small polyethylene glycol (R_s < 4.0 Å) was the same in both directions and was unaffected by the presence or absence of serum in either compartment. The permeation coefficient for large polyethylene glycol was greater in the apical-to-basal direction, unless transcytosis was inhibited by NH_4OH. With NH_4OH, serum no longer affected the permeation coefficient despite a large effect on TER. Because TER is an instantaneous measurement, it would be unaffected by the slow process of transcytosis. These data illustrate how the tight and leak pathways of paracellular transport can be regulated independently, and how different mechanisms of barrier function can be affected by apical and basal stimuli.

When these data are combined with electrophysiological measurements, a fuller understanding of the tight junction is achieved. The permeation coefficients of hfRPE for ions indicate that the tight junctions are slightly cation selective: $Na^+/Cl^- \approx 1.4$ [131] versus $Na^+/Cl^- \approx 5.5$ when claudin 2 was over-expressed [131]. (These measurements correct for the different diffusion coefficients of the two ions.) When tumor necrosis factor-alpha (TNFα) was added to the apical, but not basal, side of the monolayer, there was a dramatic decrease in TER and increase in the permeation coefficient for large polyethylene glycol. Both effects were observed regardless of the presence of serum in the culture medium. Despite these large effects, the expression of tight junction proteins and their localization to the apical junctional complex was unaffected.

These studies reveal how the same stimulus can affect barrier properties differently depending on whether they are presented to the apical and basal side of the monolayer. They also demonstrate that despite the ease of TER measurements, effects on barrier properties need to be evaluated by using the full range of available assays.

The Interplay of Tight Junctions and Membrane Transporters

Each epithelium has a distinct tissue- or region-within-a-tissue-specific function (e.g., secrete fluid, absorb fluid, maintain a particular ion gradient). Accordingly, the properties of tight junctions (permeability, selectivity) must be integrated with the particular transcellular transport mechanisms an epithelium expresses to perform an epithelium-wide function [16–18, 148]. The functions of the apical and basolateral membranes are coupled to maintain cell volume, while also transporting ions across the cell to generate electrochemical gradients [148]. For example, if chloride channel in one membrane were blocked, intracellular $[Cl^-]$ would rise and inhibit transport through a $Na^+/K^+/2Cl^-$ symporter located in the opposite membrane, thereby affecting the kinetics of pumping by the Na^+/K^+-ATPase. Membrane coupling also occurs via tight junctions, depending on their permeability and selectivity [148].

RPE uses the high Na^+ concentration in the subretinal space for driving solutes through symporters and antiporters that are polarized to the apical membrane [42, 150, 151]. A symporter transports Na^+, K^+ and Cl^- into the cell (Fig. 2.2, pathway 3). Cl^- passively moves down its concentration gradient to leave the cell via channels polarized to the basolateral membrane. The net effect is Cl^- is actively transported from the apical to the basal side of RPE. The translocation of electrical charge is partially balanced by the passive transepithelial movement of Na^+ [150] or K^+ [151]. There may be a basolateral Na^+ channel, but it should be noted that for RPE tight junctions the permeation coefficient for K^+, Na^+, and Cl^- human is small due to the barrier-forming protein, claudin-19 [131]. Regardless, the osmotic gradient created by the transepithelial transport of chloride salts leads to the absorption of water [150, 151]. A tight junction that retards monovalent cations and Cl^- would help maintain the apical-positive TEP required for this mechanism without expending a lot of ATP.

As a counter example, the choroid plexus redistributes some transporters, lacks some transporters found in RPE and expresses others that are not found in RPE (Fig. 2.4b). Consequently, cerebral spinal fluid is secreted rather than absorbed. In mice, the tight junctions containing claudin-1, -2, and -11 were evident in the epithelium of the choroid plexus [152]. Like claudin-19, claudin-1 and claudin-11 are barrier forming proteins, but unlike the slight cation-selectivity of claudin-19, they are slightly anion selective [125].

Retinal Pathology and RPE

The mechanisms of retinal edema are poorly understood. The many contributors include: RPE, Bruch's membrane, inner and outer limiting membranes, Müller cells, pericytes, and retinal and choroidal vessels. Confounding factors for understanding the disease include the differences between primates and non-primate mammals and the role of barriers such as the outer limiting membrane. In primates, the RPE's ability to pump fluid in the disease state may be adversely affected by the outer limiting membrane.

To understand how the outer limiting membrane might be involved, the thin line in Fig. 2.3a illustrates the continuity of the apical junctional complexes of the neurotube and its derivatives. The apical junctional complex lacks tight junctions in the ependyma and the neurosensory retina (Fig. 2.3b). In the neurosensory retina, the apical junction complex is called the outer limiting membrane. In non-primates, the outer limiting membrane is permeable to proteins as large as albumin, with a Stokes radius <30–36 Å [153], but those proteins can only cross tight junctions by the leak pathway (Fig. 2.2, pathway 2). When albumin was injected into the subretinal space of rabbits, little crossed the RPE, whereas a significant amount entered the vitreous [154]. Primates may differ from non-primate mammals by incorporating tight junction-like properties into the outer limiting membrane [155]. The presence of occludin, but not claudins, was reported. By transmission electron microscopy, tight junction-like structures were observed between Müller cells and photoreceptors, but only traditional adherens junctions were observed between Müller cells. These authors suggested the outer limiting membrane might join the choriocapillaris and RPE as a third component of the outer BRB.

A breakdown in the tight junctions of the outer and inner BRB can lead to retinal edema. In the first case, the pumping capacity of the RPE would be diminished. Disruption of the inner BRB would lead to protein and increased fluid leaking into the interstitium. Protein in the interstitium would increase osmotic pressure to keep fluid in the retina rather than re-enter the capillaries or be removed by the RPE [34, 156, 157]. The strategy of increasing the RPE's ability to remove fluid by stimulating the Na^+/K^+-ATPase is not effective, but has been tried in severe disease [156]. One reason the strategy fails might be that the outer limiting membrane in primates retards diffusion of protein into the subretinal space, and the protein retains fluid in the neurosensory retina. Theoretically, an effective strategy would disrupt the outer limiting membrane and remove protein from the subretinal space by stimulating bulk-phase, apical-to-basal transcytosis in the RPE.

Hyperpermeability of choroidal vessels might also disrupt the pumping ability of the RPE, as observed in central serous chorioretinopathy [158]. Subretinal fluid and even serous retinal detachment associated with this condition often resolves spontaneously. Various hypotheses have been offered, but the mechanism of the disease is unknown. Hyperpermeability of unknown origin increases the hydrostatic pressure in the choroid. The increased pressure might overwhelm apical-to-basal pumping by the RPE with the resultant basal-to-apical flow of fluid. The responses of RPE to the effects of choroidal hydrostatic pressure have not been reported. Treatments for the disease focus on reducing the permeability of the choroidal vasculature. When chronic or recurrent detachments do occur, the RPE degrades and secondary degradation of the retina follows.

Unlike central serous chorioretinopathy, age related macular degeneration (AMD) affects an older population and originates with the RPE and Bruch's membrane. The many mechanisms under investigation are beyond the scope of this chapter, and we will focus on barrier-related studies. In wet AMD, leaky capillaries breach the RPE to invade the subretinal space. Several investigators studied the effects of subretinal serum on tight junctions. Serum added to the apical (subretinal) medium chamber (Fig. 2.5a) increased the permeability of tight junctions in chick and rodent RPE [159, 160]. An increase in permeability might exacerbate retinal edema by dissipating the ion gradients needed to absorb water. The opposite result was obtained with hfRPE. In this case, apical, but not basal serum, decreased the permeability of tight junctions and increased the expression of occludin [22, 61]. The effect might be a defense mechanism to mitigate the effects of subretinal edema.

The inflammation associated with AMD or uveitis might affect RPE tight junctions, as observed in other tight junctions [161–166]. Despite an increase in fluid flux due to interferon-γ [167, 168], proinflammatory cytokines interleukin 1-beta and interferon-γ had no significant effect on hfRPE tight junctions. Tumor necrosis factor-α dramatically decreased the TER, but only if it was applied to the apical side of the monolayer [131]. There was minimal effect on the expression of tight junction proteins or their localization to tight junctions, but there was a large increase in apical stress fibers. These fibers are anchored in the apical junctional complex and cross the cell to link discontinuous regions of the complex. The increased tortuosity of the tight junctions that was observed likely reflects the tension place upon them by the fibers. Tension alone, or the tortuous path of the tight junctions in the plane of the monolayer might account for the decrease in permeability [107, 169]. Nonetheless, tumor necrosis factor-α activated receptors on both sides of the monolayer that induce inhibitors of apoptosis [131, 170]. These two observations suggest there are at least two downstream signal transduction pathways for tumor necrosis factor-α that are localized to one or the other pole of the RPE cell.

Conclusions

Epithelial monolayers form barriers between two tissues. The polarity essential for barrier function is established by signaling from the apical junctional complex and basolateral membranes. Beyond their classical role of determining the selectivity and permeability of tight junctions, claudins have emerged as signaling proteins responsible for tissue-specific properties. Claudin-19 affects the expression level of many mRNAs, including those for several pathways of the RPE barrier. Polarity and barrier function can be modulated by apical interactions, especially if the apical membrane faces a solid tissue. This is the case for a subset of epithelia like the RPE. The effects of the neurosensory retina on RPE polarity are most evident during differentiation, when the molecular definition of an RPE cell is in constant flux. RPE also belongs to a second subset of epithelia that face a fenestrated capillary bed on their basal side. These epithelia secrete VEGF (aka vascular permeability factor) to induce fenestra, but the reverse interaction of the capillaries on the RPE has proven difficult to study and the data are sparse. RPE belongs to a third subset of epithelia, those derived from neuroepithelium. These epithelia presumably begin with a common transcriptome that become specialized by their different basal and apical interactions. Comparisons between RPE with other members of these subsets lead to the view that RPE is part of an integrated unit that includes the neurosensory retina and choriocapillaris.

If the RPE phenotype depends on the neurosensory retina and choriocapillaris for its specialized properties, how does RPE remain differentiated in culture when these tissues are absent? Some clues are provided by the studies of barrier function discussed in this chapter. Notably, RPE isolated from early development is different from RPE isolated later in development. In chick, RPE does not differentiate into late RPE in culture unless provided with secretions of the developing neurosensory retina [77, 142]. For the neurosensory secretions to be effective, RPE must be plated on an extracellular matrix that is appropriate for the age when the RPE was isolated [72]. In mice, barrier function increases when RPE is co-cultured with endothelial cells [73]. Co-culture of stem-cell derived RPE with retinal progenitor cells increases barrier function and promotes the differentiation of each tissue (manuscript in preparation). Therefore, cultured RPE qualitatively resembles native RPE, but co-culture provides a method to create a more accurate model of the RPE barrier and explore the underlying mechanisms.

Given that mono-cultures have yielded many insights into the native RPE barrier, how does RPE retain so many native barrier properties in primary cell culture? Asked other ways, how does RPE isolated from different developmental stages retain stage-specific barrier properties, or why does freshly isolated RPE lose differentiated properties after a few passages in culture? Some insights were gained by comparing gene expression in these various cultures with gene expression of freshly isolated tissue or by manipulating culture conditions. A fresh approach would examine how the epigenetics of RPE changes during differentiation and aging, and in response to pathology. Epigenetics studies how methylation and acetylation of chromosomes opens or closes the transcription of different parts of the genome [171]. These modifications are regulated by environmental interactions and can be passed to daughter cells for a few generations without continued environmental stimuli. Exploring the hypothesis that epigenetic modifications regulate these phenomena would lead to the mechanisms for how an RPE cell "remembers" the developmental stage from which it was isolated, and why RPE loses tissue specific properties in culture with cell passage.

The ultimate goal of these proposed studies is to understand how the various pathways of barrier function are intertwined and regulated. Building this network would identify the central nodes that regulate different barrier functions. These nodes would be the most effective targets for developing new therapeutic agents that treat barrier dysfunction in choroidal and retinal diseases.

References

1. Bok D. Autoradiographic studies on the polarity of plasma membrane receptors in retinal pigment epithelial cells. In: Hollyfield J, editor. The structure of the eye. New York: Elsevier Biomedical; 1982. p. 247–56.
2. Miller SS, Steinberg RH, Oakley B. The electrogenic sodium pump of the frog retinal pigment epithelium. J Membr Biol. 1978;44(3):259–79.
3. Rodriguez-Boulan E, Macara IG. Organization and execution of the epithelial polarity programme. Nat Rev Mol Cell Biol. 2014;15(4):225–42.
4. Nelson WJ, Dickinson DJ, Weis WI. Roles of cadherins and catenins in cell–cell adhesion and epithelial cell polarity. In: van Roy F, editor. Prog Mol Biol Transl Sci, vol. 116: Academic; 2013. p. 3–23.
5. Manninen A. Epithelial polarity—generating and integrating signals from the ECM with integrins. Exp Cell Res. 2015;334(2):337–49.
6. Rizzolo LJ. Polarization of the $Na^{+}K^{+}$-ATPase in epithelia derived from the neuroepithelium. Int Rev Cytol. 1999;185:195–235.
7. Rizzolo LJ, Zhou S, Li Z-Q. The neural retina maintains integrins in the apical membrane of the RPE early in development. Invest Ophthalmol Vis Sci. 1994;35:2567–76.
8. Lehmann GL, Benedicto I, Philp NJ, Rodriguez-Boulan E. Plasma membrane protein polarity and trafficking in RPE cells: past, present and future. Exp Eye Res. 2014;126:5–15.
9. Bok D, O'Day W, Rodriguez-Boulan E. Polarized budding of vesicular stomatitis and influenza virus from cultured human and bovine retinal pigment epithelium. Exp Eye Res. 1992;55:853–60.
10. Gundersen D, Orlowski J, Rodriguez-Boulan E. Apical polarity of Na,K-ATPase in retinal pigment epithelium is linked to a reversal of the ankyrin-fodrin submembrane cytoskeleton. J Cell Biol. 1991;112:863–72.
11. Huotari V, Sormunen R, Lehto VP, Eskelinen S. The polarity of the membrane skeleton in retinal pigment epithelial cells of developing chicken embryos and in primary culture. Differentiation. 1995;58:205–15.
12. Rizzolo LJ, Joshi HC. Apical orientation of the microtubule organizing center and associated γ-tubulin during the polarization of the retinal pigment epithelium in vivo. Dev Biol. 1993;157:147–56.
13. Rizzolo LJ, Zhou S. The distribution of Na^{+},K^{+}-ATPase and 5A11 antigen in apical microvilli of the retinal pigment epithelium is unrelated to α-spectrin. J Cell Sci. 1995;108:3623–33.
14. Goldman EE. Die aussere ind inner sekretion des gesunden und kranken organisimus im lichte der "vitalen farbung". Beitr Klin Chirurg. 1909;64:192–265.
15. Goldman EE. Vitalfarbung am zentralnervensystem. Abh Preuss Akad Wiss Phys Math. 1913;1:1–60.
16. Larre I, Ponce A, Franco M, Cereijido M. The emergence of the concept of tight junctions and physiological regulation by ouabain. Semin Cell Dev Biol. 2014;36(Suppl C):149–56.
17. Frömter E, Diamond JM. Route of passive ion permeation in epithelia. Nat New Biol. 1972;235:9–13.
18. Powell DW. Barrier function of epithelia. Am J Physiol. 1981;241:G275–G88.
19. Anderson JM, Cereijido M. Introduction: evolution of ideas on the tight junction. In: Anderson JM, Cereijido M, editors. Tight junctions. 2nd ed. Boca Raton: CRC Press; 2001. p. 1–18.
20. Rizzolo LJ. Glucose transporters in RPE development. In: Tombran-Tink J, Barnstable C, editors. Ocular transporters in ophthalmic diseases and drug delivery. Totowa: Humana Press; 2008. p. 185–99.
21. Peng S, Adelman RA, Rizzolo LJ. Minimal effects of VEGF and anti-VEGF drugs on the permeability or selectivity of RPE tight junctions. Invest Ophthalmol Vis Sci. 2010;51(6):3216–25.
22. Peng S, Rao VS, Adelman RA, Rizzolo LJ. Claudin-19 and the barrier properties of the human retinal

pigment epithelium. Invest Ophthalmol Vis Sci. 2011;52(3):1392–403.
23. Adijanto J, Banzon T, Jalickee S, Wang NS, Miller SS. CO2-induced ion and fluid transport in human retinal pigment epithelium. J Gen Physiol. 2009;133(6):603–22.
24. Marmor MF, Wolfensberger TJ. The retinal pigment epithelium: function and disease. New York: Oxford University Press; 1998.
25. Butt AM, Jones HC, Abbott NJ. Electrical resistance across the blood-brain barrier in anaesthetized rats: a developmental study. J Physiol. 1990;429:47–62.
26. Kandel ER, Schwartz JH, Jessell TM, editors. Principles of neural science. 4th ed. New York: McGraw-Hill; 2000.
27. Tout S, Chan-Ling T, Hollander H, Stone J. The role of Muller cells in the formation of the blood-retinal barrier. Neuroscience. 1993;55:291–301.
28. Rizzolo LJ. Development and role of tight junctions in the retinal pigment epithelium. Int Rev Cytol. 2007;258:195–234.
29. Wilt SD, Rizzolo LJ. Unique aspects of the blood-brain barrier. In: Anderson JM, Cereijido M, editors. Tight junctions. 2nd ed. Boca Raton: CRC Press; 2001. p. 415–43.
30. Korte GE, Burns MS, Bellhorn RV. Epithelium-capillary interactions in the eye: the retinal pigment epithelium and the choriocapillaris. Int Rev Cytol. 1989;114:221–48.
31. Braekevelt CR. Fine structure of the choriocapillaris, Bruch's membrane and retinal epithelium in the sheep. Anat Embryol (Berl). 1983;166:415–25.
32. Korte GE. Choriocapillaris regeneration in the rabbit. Ultrastructure of new endothelial tube formation. Invest Ophthalmol Vis Sci. 1989;30(9):1938–50.
33. Marmor M. Mechanisms of fluid accumulation in retinal edema. Doc Ophthalmol. 1999;97(3):239–49.
34. Scholl S, Kirchhof J, Augustin AJ. Pathophysiology of macular edema. Ophthalmologica. 2010;224(Suppl 1):8–15.
35. Quinton PM, Wright EM, Tormey JM. Localization of sodium pumps in the choroid plexus epithelium. J Cell Biol. 1973;58(3):724–30.
36. Steinberg RH, Miller S. Aspects of electrolyte transport in frog pigment epithelium. Exp Eye Res. 1973;16(5):365–72.
37. Ernst SA, Palacios JR, Siegel GJ. Immunocytochemical localization of Na^+, K^+-ATPase in mouse choroid plexus. J Histochem Cytochem. 1986;34:189–95.
38. Masuzawa T, Ohta T, Kawakami K, Sato F. Immunocytochemical localization of Na^+, K^+-ATPase in the canine choroid plexus. Brain. 1985;108:625–46.
39. Wright EM. Mechanisms of ion transport across the choroid plexus. J Physiol. 1972;226:545–71.
40. Ostwald TJ, Steinberg RH. Localization of frog retinal pigment epithelium Na+-K+ ATPase. Exp Eye Res. 1980;31(3):351–60.
41. Gallemore RP, Hughes BA, Miller SS. Retinal pigment epithelial transport mechanisms and their contributions to the electroretinogram. Prog Retin Eye Res. 1997;16:509–66.
42. Wimmers S, Karl MO, Strauss O. Ion channels in the RPE. Prog Retin Eye Res. 2007;26(3):263–301.
43. Rajasekaran SA, Hu J, Gopal J, Gallemore R, Ryazantsev S, Bok D, Rajasekaran AK. Na,K-ATPase inhibition alters tight junction structure and permeability in human retinal pigment epithelial cells. Am J Physiol Cell Physiol. 2003;284(6):C1497–507.
44. Marmorstein AD, Finnemann SC, Bonilha VL, Rodriguez-Boulan E. Morphogenesis of the retinal pigment epithelium: toward understanding retinal degenerative diseases. Ann N Y Acad Sci. 1998;857:1–12.
45. Okami T, Yamamoto A, Omori K, Takada T, Uyama M, Tashiro Y. Immunocytochemical localization of Na+,K+-ATPase in rat retinal pigment epithelial cells. J Histochem Cytochem. 1990;38:1267–75.
46. Edelman JL, Sachs G, Adorante JS. Ion transport asymmetry and functional coupling in bovine pigmented and nonpigmented ciliary epithelial cells. Am J Physiol. 1994;266:C1210–C21.
47. Raviola G, Raviola E. Intercellular junctions in the ciliary epithelium. Invest Ophthalmol Vis Sci. 1978;17:958–81.
48. Wiederholt M, Helbig H, Korbmacher C. Ion transport across the ciliary epithelium: lessons from cultured cells and proposed role of the carbonic anhydrase. In: Botre F, Gross G, Storey BT, editors. Carbonic anhydrase. New York: Wiley; 1991. p. 232–44.
49. Coca-Prados M, Fernandez-Cabezudo MJ, Sanchez-Torres J, Crabb JW, Ghosh S. Cell-specific expression of the human Na^+,K^+-ATPase β2 subunit isoform in the nonpigmented ciliary epithelium. Invest Ophthalmol Vis Sci. 1995;36:2717–28.
50. Ghosh S, Freitag AC, Martin-Vasallo P, Coca-Prados M. Cellular distribution and differential gene expression of the three alpha subunit isoforms of the Na,K-ATPase in the ocular ciliary epithelium. J Biol Chem. 1990;265:2935–40.
51. Stroeva OG, Mitashov VI. Retinal pigment epithelium: proliferation and differentiation during development and regeneration. Int Rev Cytol. 1983;83:221–93.
52. Rizzolo LJ. Barrier properties of cultured retinal pigment epithelium. Exp Eye Res. 2014;126:16–26.
53. Rizzolo LJ, Peng S, Luo Y, Xiao W. Integration of tight junctions and claudins with the barrier functions of the retinal pigment epithelium. Prog Retin Eye Res. 2011;30(5):296–323.
54. Maminishkis A, Chen S, Jalickee S, Banzon T, Shi G, Wang FE, Ehalt T, Hammer JA, Miller SS. Confluent monolayers of cultured human fetal retinal pigment epithelium exhibit morphology and physiology of native tissue. Invest Ophthalmol Vis Sci. 2006;47(8):3612–24.
55. Blenkinsop TA, Saini JS, Maminishkis A, Bharti K, Wan Q, Banzon T, Lotfi M, Davis J, Singh D, Rizzolo LJ, Miller S, Temple S, Stern JH. human adult retinal pigment epithelial stem cell-derived RPE monolayers exhibit key physiological characteristics of native tissue. Invest Ophthalmol Vis Sci. 2015;56(12):7085–99.

56. Miyagishima KJ, Wan Q, Corneo B, Sharma R, Lotfi MR, Boles NC, Hua F, Maminishkis A, Zhang C, Blenkinsop T, Khristov V, Jha BS, Memon OS, D'Souza S, Temple S, Miller SS, Bharti K. In pursuit of authenticity: induced pluripotent stem cell-derived retinal pigment epithelium for clinical applications. Stem Cells Transl Med. 2016;5(11):1562–74.
57. Strunnikova NV, Maminishkis A, Barb JJ, Wang F, Zhi C, Sergeev Y, Chen W, Edwards AO, Stambolian D, Abecasis G, Swaroop A, Munson PJ, Miller SS. Transcriptome analysis and molecular signature of human retinal pigment epithelium. Hum Mol Genet. 2010;19:2468–86.
58. Liao J-L, Yu J, Huang K, Hu J, Diemer T, Ma Z, Dvash T, Yang X-J, Travis GH, Williams DS, Bok D, Fan G. Molecular signature of primary retinal pigment epithelium and stem-cell-derived RPE cells. Hum Mol Genet. 2010;19(21):4229–38.
59. Peng S, Wang S-B, Singh D, Zhao PYC, Davis K, Chen B, Adelman RA, Rizzolo LJ. Claudin-3 and claudin-19 partially restore native phenotype to ARPE-19 cells via effects on tight junctions and gene expression. Exp Eye Res. 2016;151:1791–89.
60. Wang S-B, Xu T, Peng S, Singh D, Ghiassi-Nejad M, Adelman RA, Rizzolo LJ. Disease-associated mutations of claudin-19 disrupt retinal neurogenesis and visual function. Commun Biol. 2019;2(1):113.
61. Peng S, Gan G, Qiu C, Zhong M, An H, Adelman RA, Rizzolo LJ. Engineering a blood-retinal barrier with human embryonic stem cell-derived retinal pigment epithelium: transcriptome and functional analysis. Stem Cells Transl Med. 2013;2(7):534–44.
62. Dunn KC, Aotaki-Keen AE, Putkey FR, Hjelmeland LM. ARPE-19, a human retinal pigment epithelial cell line with differentiated properties. Exp Eye Res. 1996;62(2):155–69.
63. Samuel W, Jaworski C, Postnikova OA, Kutty RK, Duncan T, Tan LX, Poliakov E, Lakkaraju A, Redmond TM. Appropriately differentiated ARPE-19 cells regain phenotype and gene expression profiles similar to those of native RPE cells. Mol Vis. 2017;23:60–89.
64. Luo Y, Zhuo Y, Fukuhara M, Rizzolo LJ. Effects of culture conditions on heterogeneity and the apical junctional complex of the ARPE-19 cell line. Invest Ophthalmol Vis Sci. 2006;47(8):3644–55.
65. Rizzolo LJ. Polarity and the development of the outer blood-retinal barrier. Histol Histopathol. 1997;12:1057–67.
66. Rizzolo LJ, Chen X, Weitzman M, Sun R, Zhang H. Analysis of the RPE transcriptome reveals dynamic changes during the development of the outer blood-retinal barrier. Mol Vis. 2007;13:1259–73.
67. Bridges CD. Distribution of retinol isomerase in vertebrate eyes and its emergence during retinal development. Vis Res. 1989;29(12):1711–7.
68. Klein G, Langegger M, Timpl R, Ekblom P. Role of laminin A chain in the development of epithelial cell polarity. Cell. 1988;55:331–41.
69. Sorokin L, Sonnenberg A, Aumailley M, Timpl R, Ekblom P. Recognition of the laminin E8 cell-binding site by an integrin possessing the α6 subunit is essential for epithelial polarization in developing kidney tubules. J Cell Biol. 1990;111:1265–73.
70. Stoker AW, Streuli CH, Martins-Green M, Bissell MJ. Designer microenvironments for the analysis of cell and tissue function. Curr Opin Cell Biol. 1990;2:864–74.
71. Rizzolo LJ. Basement membrane stimulates the polarized distribution of integrins but not the Na,K-ATPase in the retinal pigment epithelium. Cell Regul. 1991;2:939–49.
72. Ban Y, Rizzolo LJ. A culture model of development reveals multiple properties of RPE tight junctions. Mol Vis. 1997;3:18.
73. Benedicto I, Lehmann GL, Ginsberg M, Nolan DJ, Bareja R, Elemento O, Salfati Z, Alam NM, Prusky GT, Llanos P, Rabbany SY, Maminishkis A, Miller SS, Rafii S, Rodriguez-Boulan E. Concerted regulation of retinal pigment epithelium basement membrane and barrier function by angiocrine factors. Nat Commun. 2017;8:15374.
74. Grunwald GB. Cadherin cell adhesion molecules in retinal development and Pathology. Prog Retin Eye Res. 1996;15:363–92.
75. Liu X, Mizoguchi A, Takeichi M, Honda Y, Ide C. Developmental changes in the subcellular localization of R-cadherin in chick retinal pigment epithelium. Histochem Cell Biol. 1997;108:35–43.
76. Sandig M, Kalnins VI. Morphological changes in the zonula adhaerens during embryonic development of chick retinal pigment epithelial cells. Cell Tissue Res. 1990;259:455–61.
77. Sun R, Peng S, Chen X, Zhang H, Rizzolo LJ. Diffusible retinal secretions regulate the expression of tight junctions and other diverse functions of the retinal pigment epithelium. Mol Vis. 2008;14:2237–62.
78. Rahner C, Fukuhara M, Peng S, Kojima S, Rizzolo LJ. The apical and basal environments of the retinal pigment epithelium regulate the maturation of tight junctions during development. J Cell Sci. 2004;117(Pt 15):3307–18.
79. Luo Y, Fukuhara M, Weitzman M, Rizzolo LJ. Expression of JAM-A, AF-6, PAR-3 and PAR-6 during the assembly and remodeling of RPE tight junctions. Brain Res. 2006;1110(1):55–63.
80. Ban Y, Wilt SD, Rizzolo LJ. Two secreted retinal factors regulate different stages of development of the outer blood-retinal barrier. Brain Res Dev Brain Res. 2000;119:259–67.
81. Ozanics V, Jakoviec FA. Prenatal development of the eye and its adenexa. In: Jakoviec FA, editor. Ocular anatomy and teratology. Philadelphia: Harper and Row; 1982.
82. Gamm DM, Melvan JN, Shearer RL, Pinilla I, Sabat G, Svendsen CN, Wright LS. A novel serum-free method for culturing human prenatal retinal pig-

ment epithelial cells. Invest Ophthalmol Vis Sci. 2008;49(2):788–99.
83. Flannery JG, O'Day W, Pfeffer BA, Horwitz J, Bok D. Uptake, processing and release of retinoids by cultured human retinal pigment epithelium. Exp Eye Res. 1990;51:717–28.
84. Buchholz DE, Hikita ST, Rowland TJ, Friedrich AM, Hinman CR, Johnson LV, Clegg DO. Derivation of functional retinal pigmented epithelium from induced pluripotent stem cells. Stem Cells. 2009;27(10):2427–34.
85. Idelson M, Alper R, Obolensky A, Ben-Shushan E, Hemo I, Yachimovich-Cohen N, Khaner H, Smith Y, Wiser O, Gropp M, Cohen MA, Even-Ram S, Berman-Zaken Y, Matzrafi L, Rechavi G, Banin E, Reubinoff B. Directed differentiation of human embryonic stem cells into functional retinal pigment epithelium cells. Cell Stem Cell. 2009;5(4):396–408.
86. Sugino IK, Sun Q, Wang J, Nunes CF, Cheewatrakoolpong N, Rapista A, Johnson AC, Malcuit C, Klimanskaya I, Lanza R, Zarbin MA. Comparison of FRPE and human embryonic stem cell-derived RPE behavior on aged human Bruch's membrane. Invest Ophthalmol Vis Sci. 2011;52(8):4979–97.
87. Gullapalli VK, Sugino IK, Van Patten Y, Shah S, Zarbin MA. Impaired RPE survival on aged submacular human Bruch's membrane. Exp Eye Res. 2005;80(2):235–48.
88. Tezel TH, Del Priore LV. Repopulation of different layers of host human Bruch's membrane by retinal pigment epithelial cell grafts. Invest Ophthalmol Vis Sci. 1999;40(3):767–474.
89. Del Priore LV, Geng L, Tezel TH, Kaplan HJ. Extracellular matrix ligands promote RPE attachment to inner Bruch's membrane. Curr Eye Res. 2002;25(2):79–89.
90. Tezel TH, Del Priore LV, Kaplan HJ. Reengineering of aged Bruch's membrane to enhance retinal pigment epithelium repopulation. Invest Ophthalmol Vis Sci. 2004;45(9):3337–48.
91. Sinha D, Phillips J, Joseph Phillips M, Gamm DM. Mimicking retinal development and disease with human pluripotent stem cellsmimicking retinal development and disease. Invest Ophthalmol Vis Sci. 2016;57(5):ORSFf1–9.
92. Tucker BA, Mullins RF, Streb LM, Anfinson K, Eyestone ME, Kaalberg E, Riker MJ, Drack AV, Braun TA, Stone EM. Patient-specific iPSC-derived photoreceptor precursor cells as a means to investigate retinitis pigmentosa. Elife. 2013;2:e00824.
93. Singh D, Wang S-B, Xia T, Tainsh L, Ghiassi-Nejad M, Xu T, Peng S, Adelman RA, Rizzolo LJ. A biodegradable scaffold enhances differentiation of embryonic stem cells into a thick sheet of retinal cells. Biomaterials. 2018;154:158–68.
94. Dermietzel R, Krause D. Molecular anatomy of the blood-brain barrier as defined by immunocytochemistry. Int Rev Cytol. 1991;127:57–109.
95. Hudspeth AJ, Yee AG. The intercellular junctional complexes of retinal pigment epithelia. Investig Ophthalmol. 1973;12:354–65.
96. Kojima T, Yamamoto T, Murata M, Chiba H, Kokai Y, Sawada N. Regulation of the blood–biliary barrier: interaction between gap and tight junctions in hepatocytes. Med Electron Microsc. 2003;36(3):157–64.
97. Li MWM, Mruk DD, Lee WM, Cheng CY. Connexin 43 is critical to maintain the homeostasis of the blood-testis barrier via its effects on tight junction reassembly. Proc Natl Acad Sci U S A. 2010;107:17998–8003.
98. Mellman I, Nelson WJ. Coordinated protein sorting, targeting and distribution in polarized cells. Nat Rev Mol Cell Biol. 2008;9(11):833–45.
99. Halbleib JM, Nelson WJ. Cadherins in development: cell adhesion, sorting, and tissue morphogenesis. Genes Dev. 2006;20(23):3199–214.
100. Hartsock A, Nelson WJ. Adherens and tight junctions: structure, function and connections to the actin cytoskeleton. Biochim Biophys Acta. 2008;1778(3):660–9.
101. Steed E, Balda MS, Matter K. Dynamics and functions of tight junctions. Trends Cell Biol. 2010;20(3):142–9.
102. Matter K, Aijaz S, Tsapara A, Balda MS. Mammalian tight junctions in the regulation of epithelial differentiation and proliferation. Curr Opin Cell Biol. 2005;17(5):453–8.
103. Caplan MJ, Seo-Mayer P, Zhang L. Epithelial junctions and polarity: complexes and kinases. Curr Opin Nephrol Hypertens. 2008;17(5):506–12.
104. Cereijido M, Contreras RG, Shoshani L, Flores-Benitez D, Larre I. Tight junction and polarity interaction in the transporting epithelial phenotype. Biochim Biophys Acta. 2008;1778(3):770–93.
105. Yeaman C, Grindstaff KK, Nelson WJ. Mechanism of recruiting Sec6/8 (exocyst) complex to the apical junctional complex during polarization of epithelial cells. J Cell Sci. 2004;117(4):559–70.
106. Sasaki H, Matsui C, Furuse K, Mimori-Kiyosue Y, Furuse M, Tsukita S. Dynamic behavior of paired claudin strands within apposing plasma membranes. Proc Natl Acad Sci U S A. 2003;100(7):3971–6.
107. Claude P. Morphological factors influencing transepithelial permeability: a model for the resistance of the zonula occludens. J Membr Biol. 1978;39:219–32.
108. Kniesel U, Wolburg H. Tight junction complexity in the retinal pigment epithelium of the chicken during development. Neurosci Lett. 1993;149:71–4.
109. Caldwell RB, Slapnick SM, McLaughlin BJ. Lanthanum and freeze-fracture studies of retinal pigment epithelial cell junctions in the streptozotocin diabetic rat. Curr Eye Res. 1985;4:215–27.
110. Stevenson BR, Anderson JM, Goodenough DA, Mooseker MS. Tight junction structure and ZO-1 content are identical in two strains of Madin-Darby canine kidney cells which differ in transepithelial resistance. J Cell Biol. 1988;107:2401–8.

111. Paris L, Bazzoni G. The protein interaction network of the epithelial junctional complex: a system-level analysis. Mol Biol Cell. 2008;19(12):5409–21.
112. Cummins PM. Occludin: one protein, many forms. Mol Cell Biol. 2012;32(2):242–50.
113. Venter JC, Adams MD, Myers EW, Li PW, Mural RJ, Sutton GG, Smith HO, Yandell M, Evans CA, Holt RA, Gocayne JD, Amanatides P, Ballew RM, Huson DH, Wortman JR, Zhang Q, Kodira CD, Zheng XH, Chen L, Skupski M, Subramanian G, Thomas PD, Zhang J, Gabor Miklos GL, Nelson C, Broder S, Clark AG, Nadeau J, McKusick VA, Zinder N, Levine AJ, Roberts RJ, Simon M, Slayman C, Hunkapiller M, Bolanos R, Delcher A, Dew I, Fasulo D, Flanigan M, Florea L, Halpern A, Hannenhalli S, Kravitz S, Levy S, Mobarry C, Reinert K, Remington K, Abu-Threideh J, Beasley E, Biddick K, Bonazzi V, Brandon R, Cargill M, Chandramouliswaran I, Charlab R, Chaturvedi K, Deng Z, Di Francesco V, Dunn P, Eilbeck K, Evangelista C, Gabrielian AE, Gan W, Ge W, Gong F, Gu Z, Guan P, Heiman TJ, Higgins ME, Ji RR, Ke Z, Ketchum KA, Lai Z, Lei Y, Li Z, Li J, Liang Y, Lin X, Lu F, Merkulov GV, Milshina N, Moore HM, Naik AK, Narayan VA, Neelam B, Nusskern D, Rusch DB, Salzberg S, Shao W, Shue B, Sun J, Wang Z, Wang A, Wang X, Wang J, Wei M, Wides R, Xiao C, Yan C, Yao A, Ye J, Zhan M, Zhang W, Zhang H, Zhao Q, Zheng L, Zhong F, Zhong W, Zhu S, Zhao S, Gilbert D, Baumhueter S, Spier G, Carter C, Cravchik A, Woodage T, Ali F, An H, Awe A, Baldwin D, Baden H, Barnstead M, Barrow I, Beeson K, Busam D, Carver A, Center A, Cheng ML, Curry L, Danaher S, Davenport L, Desilets R, Dietz S, Dodson K, Doup L, Ferriera S, Garg N, Gluecksmann A, Hart B, Haynes J, Haynes C, Heiner C, Hladun S, Hostin D, Houck J, Howland T, Ibegwam C, Johnson J, Kalush F, Kline L, Koduru S, Love A, Mann F, May D, McCawley S, McIntosh T, McMullen I, Moy M, Moy L, Murphy B, Nelson K, Pfannkoch C, Pratts E, Puri V, Qureshi H, Reardon M, Rodriguez R, Rogers YH, Romblad D, Ruhfel B, Scott R, Sitter C, Smallwood M, Stewart E, Strong R, Suh E, Thomas R, Tint NN, Tse S, Vech C, Wang G, Wetter J, Williams S, Williams M, Windsor S, Winn-Deen E, Wolfe K, Zaveri J, Zaveri K, Abril JF, Guigo R, Campbell MJ, Sjolander KV, Karlak B, Kejariwal A, Mi H, Lazareva B, Hatton T, Narechania A, Diemer K, Muruganujan A, Guo N, Sato S, Bafna V, Istrail S, Lippert R, Schwartz R, Walenz B, Yooseph S, Allen D, Basu A, Baxendale J, Blick L, Caminha M, Carnes-Stine J, Caulk P, Chiang YH, Coyne M, Dahlke C, Mays A, Dombroski M, Donnelly M, Ely D, Esparham S, Fosler C, Gire H, Glanowski S, Glasser K, Glodek A, Gorokhov M, Graham K, Gropman B, Harris M, Heil J, Henderson S, Hoover J, Jennings D, Jordan C, Jordan J, Kasha J, Kagan L, Kraft C, Levitsky A, Lewis M, Liu X, Lopez J, Ma D, Majoros W, McDaniel J, Murphy S, Newman M, Nguyen T, Nguyen N, Nodell M, Pan S, Peck J, Peterson M, Rowe W, Sanders R, Scott J, Simpson M, Smith T, Sprague A, Stockwell T, Turner R, Venter E, Wang M, Wen M, Wu D, Wu M, Xia A, Zandieh A, Zhu X. The sequence of the human genome. Science. 2001;291(5507):1304–51.
114. Van Itallie CM, Colegio OR, Anderson JM. The cytoplasmic tails of claudins can influence tight junction barrier properties through effects on protein stability. J Membr Biol. 2004;199(1):29–38.
115. Shen L, Weber CR, Turner JR. The tight junction protein complex undergoes rapid and continuous molecular remodeling at steady state. J Cell Biol. 2008;181(4):683–95.
116. Sourisseau T, Georgiadis A, Tsapara A, Ali RR, Pestell R, Matter K, Balda MS. Regulation of PCNA and cyclin D1 expression and epithelial morphogenesis by the ZO-1-regulated transcription factor ZONAB/DbpA. Mol Cell Biol. 2006;26(6):2387–98.
117. Gonzalez-Mariscal L, Tapia R, Chamorro D. Crosstalk of tight junction components with signaling pathways. Biochim Biophys Acta. 2008;1778(3):729–56.
118. Bentzel CJ, Palant CE, Fromm M. Physiological and pathological factors affecting the tight junction. Boca Raton: CRC Press; 1992.
119. Rubin LL, Staddon JM. The cell biology of the blood-brain barrier. Annu Rev Neurosci. 1999;22:11–28.
120. Le Moellic C, Boulkroun S, Gonzalez-Nunez D, Dublineau I, Cluzeaud F, Fay M, Blot-Chabaud M, Farman N. Aldosterone and tight junctions: modulation of claudin-4 phosphorylation in renal collecting duct cells. Am J Physiol Cell Physiol. 2005;289(6):C1513–21.
121. Furuse M, Sasaki H, Tsukita S. Manner of interaction of heterogeneous claudin species within and between tight junction strands. J Cell Biol. 1999;147(4):891–903.
122. Tsukita S, Furuse M. Pores in the wall: claudins constitute tight junction strands containing aqueous pores. J Cell Biol. 2000;149:13–6.
123. Elkouby Naor L, Ben Yosef T, Kwang WJ. Functions of claudin tight junction proteins and their complex interactions in various physiological systems. Int Rev Cell Mol Biol. 2010;279:1–32. Academic.
124. Hou J, Renigunta A, Konrad M, Gomes AS, Schneeberger EE, Paul DL, Waldegger S, Goodenough DA. Claudin-16 and claudin-19 interact and form a cation-selective tight junction complex. J Clin Invest. 2008;118(2):619–28.
125. Günzel D, Yu ASL. Claudins and the modulation of tight junction permeability. Physiol Rev. 2013;93(2):525–69.
126. Van Itallie CM, Anderson JM. Claudins and epithelial paracellular transport. Annu Rev Physiol. 2006;68:403–29.
127. Colegio OR, Van Itallie CM, McCrea HJ, Rahner C, Anderson JM. Claudins create charge-selective channels in the paracellular pathway between epithelial cells. Am J Physiol Cell Physiol. 2002;283(1):C142–C7.
128. Hou J, Paul DL, Goodenough DA. Paracellin-1 and the modulation of ion selectivity of tight junctions. J Cell Sci. 2005;118(Pt 21):5109–18.

129. Alexandre MD, Jeansonne BG, Renegar RH, Tatum R, Chen YH. The first extracellular domain of claudin-7 affects paracellular Cl- permeability. Biochem Biophys Res Commun. 2007;357(1):87–91.
130. González-Mariscal L, Domínguez-Calderón A, Raya-Sandino A, Ortega-Olvera JM, Vargas-Sierra O, Martínez-Revollar G. Tight junctions and the regulation of gene expression. Semin Cell Dev Biol. 2014;36:213–23.
131. Peng S, Gan G, Rao VS, Adelman RA, Rizzolo LJ. Effects of proinflammatory cytokines on the claudin-19 rich tight junctions of human retinal pigment epithelium. Invest Ophthalmol Vis Sci. 2012;53(8):5016–28.
132. Burke JM, Hjelmeland LM. Mosaicism of the retinal pigment epithelium: seeing the small picture. Mol Interv. 2005;5(4):241–9.
133. Simon DB, Lu Y, Choate KA, Velazquez H, Al-Sabban E, Praga M, Casari G, Bettinelli A, Colussi G, Rodriguez-Soriano J, McCredie D, Milford D, Sanjad S, Lifton RP. Paracellin-1, a renal tight junction protein required for paracellular Mg2+ resorption. Science. 1999;285(5424):103–6.
134. Muller D, Kausalya PJ, Claverie-Martin F, Meij IC, Eggert P, Garcia-Nieto V, Hunziker W. A novel claudin 16 mutation associated with childhood hypercalciuria abolishes binding to ZO-1 and results in lysosomal mistargeting. Am J Hum Genet. 2003;73(6):1293–301.
135. Konrad M, Schaller A, Seelow D, Pandey AV, Waldegger S, Lesslauer A, Vitzthum H, Suzuki Y, Luk JM, Becker C, Schlingmann KP, Schmid M, Rodriguez-Soriano J, Ariceta G, Cano F, Enriquez R, Juppner H, Bakkaloglu SA, Hediger MA, Gallati S, Neuhauss SC, Nurnberg P, Weber S. Mutations in the tight-junction gene claudin 19 (CLDN19) are associated with renal magnesium wasting, renal failure, and severe ocular involvement. Am J Hum Genet. 2006;79(5):949–57.
136. Naeem M, Hussain S, Akhtar N. Mutation in the tight-junction gene claudin 19 (CLDN19) and familial hypomagnesemia, hypercalciuria, nephrocalcinosis (FHHNC) and severe ocular disease. Am J Nephrol. 2011;34(3):241–8.
137. Claverie-Martín F, García-Nieto V, Loris C, Ariceta G, Nadal I, Espinosa L, Fernández-Maseda Á, Antón-Gamero M, Avila Á, Madrid Á, González-Acosta H, Córdoba-Lanus E, Santos F, Gil-Calvo M, Espino M, García-Martinez E, Sanchez A, Muley R, RenalTube Group. Claudin-19 mutations and clinical phenotype in spanish patients with familial hypomagnesemia with hypercalciuria and nephrocalcinosis. PLoS One. 2013;8(1):e53151.
138. Al-Shibli A, Konrad M, Altay W, Al Masri O, Al-Gazali L, Al Attrach I. Familial hypomagnesemia with hypercalciuria and nephrocalcinosis (FHHNC): report of three cases with a novel mutation in CLDN19 gene. Saudi J Kidney Dis Transpl. 2013;24(2):338–44.
139. Faguer S, Chauveau D, Cintas P, Tack I, Cointault O, Rostaing L, Vargas-Poussou R, Ribes D. Renal, ocular, and neuromuscular involvements in patients with CLDN19 mutations. Clin J Am Soc Nephrol. 2011;6(2):355–60.
140. Liang GH, Weber CR. Molecular aspects of tight junction barrier function. Curr Opin Pharmacol. 2014;19:84–9.
141. Balda MS, Whitney JA, Flores C, González S, Cereijido M, Matter K. Functional dissociation of paracellular permeability and transepithelial electrical resistance and disruption of the apical-basolateral intramembrane diffusion barrier by expression of a mutant tight junction membrane protein. J Cell Biol. 1996;134:1031–49.
142. Ban Y, Rizzolo LJ. Differential regulation of tight junction permeability during development of the retinal pigment epithelium. Am J Physiol. 2000;279:C744–C50.
143. Watson CJ, Rowland M, Warhurst G. Functional modeling of tight junctions in intestinal cell monolayers using polyethylene glycol oligomers. Am J Physiol Cell Physiol. 2001;281(2):C388–97.
144. Van Itallie CM, Holmes J, Bridges A, Gookin JL, Coccaro MR, Proctor W, Colegio OR, Anderson JM. The density of small tight junction pores varies among cell types and is increased by expression of claudin-2. J Cell Sci. 2008;121(Pt 3):298–305.
145. Rochat T, Casale J, Hunninghake GW, Peterson MW. Neutrophil cathepsin G increases permeability of cultured type II pneumocytes. Am J Physiol. 1988;255:C603–11.
146. van Os C, de Jong MD, Slegers JF. Dimensions of polar pathways through rabbit gallbladder epithelium. The effect of phloretin on nonelectrolyte permeability. J Membr Biol. 1974;15:363–82.
147. Saint-Geniez M, Maharaj AS, Walshe TE, Tucker BA, Sekiyama E, Kurihara T, Darland DC, Young MJ, D'Amore PA. Endogenous VEGF is required for visual function: evidence for a survival role on muller cells and photoreceptors. PLoS One. 2008;3(11):e3554.
148. Reuss L. Epithelial transport. In: Hoffman JF, Jamieson JD, editors. Handbook of physiology section 14: cell physiology. New York: Oxford University Press; 1997. p. 309–88.
149. Sugita S, Usui Y, Horie S, Futagami Y, Aburatani H, Okazaki T, Honjo T, Takeuchi M, Mochizuki M. T-cell suppression by programmed cell death 1 ligand 1 on retinal pigment epithelium during inflammatory conditions. Invest Ophthalmol Vis Sci. 2009;50(6):2862–70.
150. Hughes BA, Gallemore RP, Miller SS. Transport mechanisms in the retinal pigment epithelium. In: Marmor MF, Wolfensberger TJ, editors. The retinal pigment epithelium. New York: Oxford University Press; 1998. p. 103–34.
151. Strauss O. The retinal pigment epithelium in visual function. Physiol Rev. 2005;85(3):845–81.

152. Wolburg H, Wolburg-Buchholz K, Liebner S, Engelhardt B. Claudin-1, claudin-2 and claudin-11 are present in tight junctions of choroid plexus epithelium of the mouse. Neurosci Lett. 2001;307(2):77–80.
153. Bunt-Milam AH, Saari JC, Klock IB, Garwin GG. Zonulae adherentes pore size in the external limiting membrane of the rabbit retina. Invest Ophthalmol Vis Sci. 1985;26:1377–80.
154. Takeuchi A, Kricorian G, Marmor MF. Albumin movement out of the subretinal space after experimental retinal detachment. Invest Ophthalmol Vis Sci. 1995;36(7):1298–305.
155. Omri S, Omri B, Savoldelli M, Jonet L, Thillaye-Goldenberg B, Thuret G, Gain P, Jeanny JC, Crisanti P, Behar-Cohen F. The outer limiting membrane (OLM) revisited: clinical implications. Clin Ophthalmol. 2010;4:183–95.
156. de Smet MD, Okada AA. Cystoid macular edema in uveitis. Dev Ophthalmol. 2010;47:136–47.
157. Vinores SA, Derevjanik NL, Ozaki H, Okamoto N, Campochiaro PA. Cellular mechanisms of blood-retinal barrier dysfunction in macular edema. Doc Ophthalmol. 1999;97(3–4):217–28.
158. Iacono P, Battaglia Parodi M, Falcomatà B, Bandello F. Central serous chorioretinopathy treatments: a mini review. Ophthalmic Res. 2015;55(2):76–83.
159. Peng S, Rahner C, Rizzolo LJ. Apical and basal regulation of the permeability of the retinal pigment epithelium. Invest Ophthalmol Vis Sci. 2003;44:808–17.
160. Chang CW, Ye L, Defoe DM, Caldwell RB. Serum inhibits tight junction formation in cultured pigment epithelial cells. Invest Ophthalmol Vis Sci. 1997;38:1082–93.
161. Marchiando AM, Shen L, Graham WV, Weber CR, Schwarz BT, Austin JR, Raleigh DR, Guan Y, Watson AJM, Montrose MH, Turner JR. Caveolin-1–dependent occludin endocytosis is required for TNF induced tight junction regulation in vivo. J Cell Biol. 2010;189(1):111–26.
162. Oshima T, Laroux FS, Coe LL, Morise Z, Kawachi S, Bauer P, Grisham MB, Specian RD, Carter P, Jennings S, Granger DN, Joh T, Alexander JS. Interferon-gamma and interleukin-10 reciprocally regulate endothelial junction integrity and barrier function. Microvasc Res. 2001;61(1):130–43.
163. Bruewer M, Luegering A, Kucharzik T, Parkos CA, Madara JL, Hopkins AM, Nusrat A. Proinflammatory cytokines disrupt epithelial barrier function by apoptosis-independent mechanisms. J Immunol. 2003;171(11):6164–72.
164. Youakim A, Ahdieh M. Interferon-gamma decreases barrier function in T84 cells by reducing ZO-1 levels and disrupting apical actin. Am J Physiol. 1999;276(5 Pt 1):G1279–88.
165. Coyne CB, Vanhook MK, Gambling TM, Carson JL, Boucher RC, Johnson LG. Regulation of airway tight junctions by proinflammatory cytokines. Mol Biol Cell. 2002;13(9):3218–34.
166. Fish SM, Proujansky R, Reenstra WW. Synergistic effects of interferon gamma and tumour necrosis factor alpha on T84 cell function. Gut. 1999;45(2):191–8.
167. Li R, Maminishkis A, Banzon T, Wan Q, Jalickee S, Chen S, Miller SS. IFN{gamma} regulates retinal pigment epithelial fluid transport. Am J Physiol Cell Physiol. 2009;297(6):C1452–65.
168. Miller SS, Maminishkis A, Li R, Adijanto J. Retinal pigment epithelium: cytokine modulation of epithelial physiology. In: Dartt D, editor. Encyclopedia of the eye, vol. 4. Oxford: Academic; 2010. p. 89–100.
169. Madara JL. Regulation of the movement of solutes across tight junctions. Annu Rev Physiol. 1998;60:143–59.
170. Yang P, McKay BS, Allen JB, Jaffe GJ. Effect of NF-kappa B inhibition on TNF-alpha-induced apoptosis in human RPE cells. Invest Ophthalmol Vis Sci. 2004;45(7):2438–46.
171. Seisenberger S, Peat JR, Hore TA, Santos F, Dean W, Reik W. Reprogramming DNA methylation in the mammalian life cycle: building and breaking epigenetic barriers. Philos Trans R Soc Lond Ser B Biol Sci. 2013;368(1609):20110330.

3 RPE Phagocytosis

Claudia Müller and Silvia C. Finnemann

Introduction

The retinal pigment epithelium (RPE) forms a polarized monolayer in the retina. Its basolateral aspect adheres to a specialized basement membrane, Bruch's membrane, and neighbors the choroidal vasculature, while its apical surface extends microvilli into the subretinal space and faces photoreceptor rods and cones of the neural retina. RPE cells perform numerous roles in support of photoreceptors specifically and the neural retina generally that are essential for vision including directed transport of ions, water and metabolites, absorption of light, secretion of growth factors and other signaling proteins, participation in the visual cycle and phagocytosis of spent photoreceptor outer segment fragments (POS) [1]. As both photoreceptors and RPE cells are post-mitotic and non-migratory their interactions persist in the mammalian eye and individual RPE cells must continue to perform their support activities for life.

Clearance phagocytosis of POS by the RPE is a daily task that is critical to maintain photoreceptors. Lack of or abnormal RPE phagocytosis caused by mutations in genes encoding proteins of the RPE phagocytic machinery impairs retinal function and integrity in experimental animal models [2–5] and causes retinitis pigmentosa (RP) in human patients (recently reviewed by Parinot and Nandrot (2016)) [6]. Moreover, failure to efficiently degrade engulfed POS by RPE cells compromised by oxidative stress and likely other age-related changes contributes to accumulation in the RPE of modified proteins and lipids in cytoplasmic lysosome-derived storage organelles known as lipofuscin [5–8]. Excess lipofuscin accumulation is harmful to the aging RPE and retina in human and experimental animals and is thought to contribute to age-related macular degeneration [9, 10].

In the vertebrate retina, the process of photoreceptor outer segment renewal continuously turns over the light sensitive outer segment portions of photoreceptors thought to bear damaged proteins and lipids. Permanent photoreceptor cells rejuvenate but maintain constant length of their outer segments by coordinating shedding of distal, most aged outer segment tips with precisely balanced formation of new membrane disks at the proximal end of outer segments [11]. The RPE participates in this process by removing shed photoreceptor debris by receptor-mediated phagocytosis [12].

Molecular mechanisms that promote synchronized POS tip shedding are only poorly understood. At the time of rod shedding the plasma membrane of POS tips externalizes

C. Müller · S. C. Finnemann (✉)
Department of Biological Sciences, Center for Cancer, Genetic Diseases and Gene Regulation, Fordham University, Bronx, NY, USA
e-mail: Claudia.Mueller@evotec.com; finnemann@fordham.edu

A. K. Klettner, S. Dithmar (eds.), *Retinal Pigment Epithelium in Health and Disease*,
https://doi.org/10.1007/978-3-030-28384-1_3

phosphatidylserine (PS), an "eat me" signal also displayed by cells undergoing apoptosis [13]. RPE cells recognize exposed PS opsonized by extracellular bridge ligands with their phagocytic receptors. Moreover, RPE cells also enhance synchronized PS externalization in a diurnal rhythmic pattern to match the peak of their phagocytic activity. Thus, synchronized outer segment tip shedding is not photoreceptor cell autonomous but requires activities of the RPE.

In mammals, RPE clearance of POS occurs in a diurnal rhythm entrained by light and circadian mechanisms [14]. Both rods and cones shed POS [12, 15–17]. Different mammalian species shed cone POS either at the onset of light or of the dark period [18–25]. In contrast, in all species studied, rods shed POS at light onset. As rods make up the vast majority of photoreceptors in both rodent and human retina, rod POS shedding prompts a burst of phagocytic activity and uptake by the RPE at light onset followed by a period of relative phagocytic inactivity during which RPE cells process engulfed POS in phagolysosomes [5, 14]. RPE cells enzymatically break down POS proteins and POS-derived lipids, some of them for metabolism and others for recycling to photoreceptors [26–30].

Altogether, photoreceptors and RPE collaborate to achieve the necessary coordination of their activities that ensures maintenance of functional outer segments for life. The recurring challenge with spent POS requires RPE cells to engulf and degrade POS daily for life. This unique and enormous phagocytic load renders RPE cells the most highly phagocytic cell type in the body.

Experimental Approaches to Quantify the Phagocytic Function of the RPE

RPE phagocytosis can be investigated either by examining the RPE *in situ* or by feeding experimental phagocytic particles to RPE cells grown in culture. Both approaches have unique advantages that make them complementary. In the following we will discuss advantages of each strategy and the methods used.

Phagocytic challenge of RPE cells in culture has three distinct advantages over examining RPE phagocytosis *in situ*. (1) RPE cells may be manipulated before or during phagocytosis assays using genetic or pharmacological approaches. (2) Feeding wild-type POS to mutant RPE and vice versa will identify if a given genetic change affects activities of RPE or photoreceptors or both during outer segment renewal. (3) Cell culture assays can experimentally separate the distinct phases of the phagocytic process, particle recognition/binding, internalization, and digestion yielding insight into the dependence of each step on particular sets of genes and molecules. RPE cells grown in culture can maintain avid phagocytic activity specifically towards isolated POS [31]. However, phagocytic activity of RPE in culture may vary with cell culture condition. It is thus imperative to maintain strict culture protocols and experimental planning. POS for feeding to RPE in cell culture phagocytic assays can be obtained from fresh retinas e.g. from pig, cow, or rat following established protocols [32, 33]. Larger batches of POS may be prepared and stored as deep-frozen aliquots ensuring that particle quality and quantity show little variation from experiment to experiment. POS may be covalently labeled with a fluorescence dye or radiolabeled before use. Alternatively, POS may be detected labeling fixed samples with antibodies specific to POS, such as transducin or rhodopsin. Most commonly antibodies to rhodopsin are used, as opsin is by far the most abundant protein of POS and reliable monoclonal antibodies against well-defined epitopes of rhodopsin are commercially available [34, 35]. RNA silencing reducing candidate protein levels before or pharmacological modulators before or during phagocytic challenge will help identifying roles for specific molecules in the phagocytic process. Of note, RPE cells require extracellular molecules as stoichiometric bridge ligands between RPE surface receptors and POS (see sections "Recognition and Binding of POS by RPE Cells" and "Cell Surface Receptors and RPE Signaling Pathways Mediating POS Internalization" for more details). While present in the retina at physiological levels, such factors must be supplemented in experimental POS phagocytosis assays to promote POS binding and engulfment, either in the form of purified ligand proteins or by addition of fetal bovine serum, which provides a mix of potent but poorly defined molecules supporting RPE phagocytosis [31, 36].

Examining specifically binding, internalization, and degradation phases of RPE phagocytosis can be accomplished by choosing appropriate duration of POS challenge, POS post-challenge incubation (in a discontinuous, pulse-chase type POS phagocytosis assay) selective addition of binding receptor versus internalization receptor bridge proteins, and taking advantage of the fact that rodent RPE cells in culture bind POS at temperatures above ~17 °C (but now below) while internalization does not proceed at temperatures below ~25 °C [37, 38]. For example, POS incubation in the presence of binding receptor ligand at 20 °C will allow only POS binding allowing studying the binding process in itself or yielding RPE cells with pre-bound POS, which following removal of excess POS may be supplemented with internalization receptor ligand and shifted to 37 °C to monitor specifically the internalization step.

Flow cytometry may be used to quantify the amount of phagocytosed POS by RPE cells in culture. Including manipulations removing or quenching the fluorescence of POS that are bound but not internalized will allow discriminating bound and internalized POS material [39, 40]. Flow cytometry-based analysis may quantify POS uptake by large numbers of cells to yield insight into levels of POS per cell and the fraction of cells in a population that takes up POS.

We prefer to study POS phagocytosis using immunofluorescence microscopy of fixed intact RPE monolayers since it allows us to distinguish bound and internalized POS fragments while monitoring cell morphology in the same sample. Selective immunofluorescence labeling of surface-bound POS after non-permeabilizing fixation can discriminate bound and internalized POS [41]. In RPE cells that are grown to differentiate into polarized monolayers with a cuboidal shape, confocal microscopy can discriminate surface-bound from engulfed fluorescent POS based on their position relative to the tight junction marker ZO-1 or F-actin. To accomplish this analysis, x-y image stacks comprising the entire cell are separated into two non-overlapping apical and central z-stacks. The apical z-stack is chosen such that it shows only POS signal located above tight junction/apical microvilli F-actin marker staining, which are bound POS. The central stack is chosen such that it includes only cell aspects below the tight junction or apical F-actin marker. Maximal projections of these separated stacks allow quantification and counting of bound and engulfed POS in the same sample (Fig. 3.1) [42].

Besides the method outlined above and illustrated in Fig. 3.1, experimental approaches to POS binding and engulfment by RPE cells in culture based on fluorescence microscopy or immunoblotting quantification may provide similar insight or additionally focus on POS phagosome acidification [43, 44].

Unlike POS phagocytosis by RPE cells in culture, the phagocytic activity of the RPE in the retina is directly linked to re-growth and shedding of the photoreceptor outer segments. In the healthy retina, rod POS shedding occurs at light onset prompting immediate POS clearance by the RPE. Any defect in POS shedding will affect POS phagocytosis secondarily. Moreover, animal model studies indicate that, conversely, abnormal RPE phagocytosis secondarily affects POS shedding [13]. Measures of phagocytic uptake by the RPE *in situ* in animal models may thus reflect abnormalities in either or both cell types involved. As intact outer segments and shed POS are located directly adjacent to the apical surface of the RPE a bona fide POS binding process does not take place during RPE phagocytosis *in situ*. However, recognition of extracellular bridge proteins by RPE surface receptors activates the same signaling pathways leading to internalization as in RPE in culture [5]. Studies of RPE phagocytosis *in situ* take advantage of the fact that outer segment renewal is highly synchronized and subjected to a strict diurnal rhythm. In cross sections of the retina, electron microscopy identifies engulfed POS based on morphology and location [7, 45], while

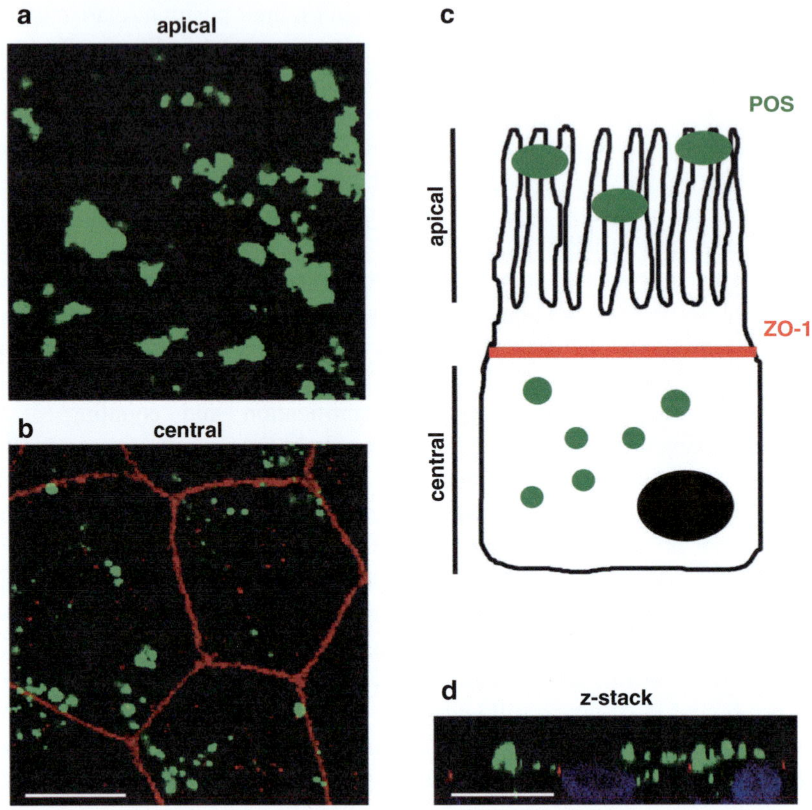

Fig. 3.1 Confocal microscopy analysis of phagocytosed photoreceptor outer segment fragments (POS) distinguishes bound and engulfed particles. (**a**) Apical x-y confocal projection shows POS (green) located above tight junctions indicated by lack of ZO-1 marker labeling in this area. These are quantified as bound POS. (**b**) Central x-y projections show tight junctions (ZO-1 labeling in red) and engulfed POS (green). (**c**) Scheme illustrating separate quantification of bound and engulfed POS based on location relative to tight junction marker labeling by confocal microscopy. The RPE cell nucleus is indicated in black. (**d**) The x-z confocal projection shows relative distribution of nuclei (shown in blue), ZO-1 stained tight junctions (shown in red) and POS (shown in green). POS below the tight junction are engulfed. Reproduced from Davis et al. 2017

light microscopy identifies POS based on POS marker immunoreactivity [46]. Counting POS phagosomes in the RPE of experimental animals at specific time points in relation to light onset allows quantifying the phagocytic load obtained by the RPE at light onset, a measure of phagocytic capacity, and following the decrease in POS phagosomes in the RPE at later time points reflecting progression of POS digestion [47]. Side-by-side comparison of POS phagosome counts with age- and strain-matched control animals provides insight into effects of altering genotypes or experimental treatments. Besides cross sections RPE phagocytosis can be examined in RPE flat mount preparations as well. Following removal of the retina, eyes may be observed live for detection of acidified POS phagosomes [48] or fixed and processed for POS marker immunofluorescence microscopy [47, 49].

Taken together, analysis of RPE phagocytosis in cell culture allows identification of molecular players in this process by separately probing and

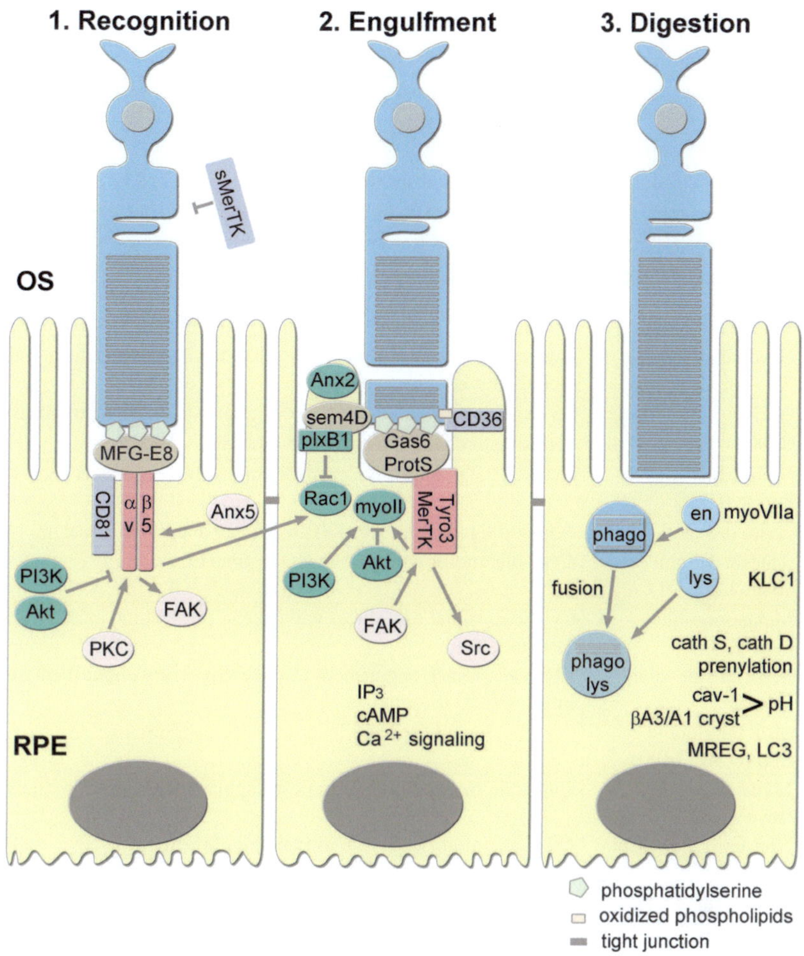

Fig. 3.2 Molecules and mechanisms known to date to contribute to the three different steps of RPE phagocytosis. In each step receptors at the apical RPE surface are highlighted in pink and purple, proteins related with cytoskeletal rearrangement in green, intracellular signaling components in rose, digestion in blue and extracellular ligands in grey. For brief description of protein roles and abbreviations please see Table 3.1. Details of protein roles are provided in the main text. Not all proteins contributing to RPE phagocytosis may be included

interfering with binding/recognition, internalization, and digestion step. In contrast, observation of RPE phagocytosis *in situ* illuminates a molecule's relevance for retinal structure and function under physiological conditions providing important complementary insight.

Molecular Mechanisms of RPE Phagocytosis

RPE phagocytosis belongs to a group of non-inflammatory clearance phagocytosis mechanisms that other phagocytes in the body use to remove apoptotic cells and cell debris and that are conserved from worm to man [38, 50, 51]. Recognition/binding and engulfment steps of phagocytosis require engagement and downstream signaling of specific phagocyte surface receptor proteins. While professional phagocytes of the immune system like macrophages or dendritic cells possess numerous surface receptors that can trigger or participate in clearance phagocytosis, RPE cells possess and use only a limited repertoire of molecules for POS phagocytosis. The scheme in Fig. 3.2 summarizes our current knowledge of the molecular mechanisms of RPE phagocytosis of POS.

Table 3.1 Proteins contributing to RPE phagocytosis as summarized in Fig. 3.2

Protein (abbreviation)	Role	References
AKT kinase (Akt)	Cytosolic signal transducer with functions in F-actin recruitment and POS engulfment	[80]
Annexin A5 (Anx5)	Cytosolic regulator of αvβ5 integrin surface levels	[55]
Annexin A2 (Anx2)	Cytosolic signal transducer with role in POS uptake synchronization	[49]
αvβ5 integrin (αvβ5)	RPE cell surface recognition receptor recognizing PS-bearing POS	[5, 52–54]
βA3/A1 crystallin	Cytosolic signal transducer with role in phagosome maturation (acidification)	[108, 109]
Cathepsin D, cathepsin S	Lysosomal enzymes with roles in POS protein (opsin) degradation	[8, 30, 102, 103]
Caveolin-1 (cav-1)	Cytosolic signal transducer with role in phagosome maturation (acidification)	[47]
CD36	RPE cell surface receptor that recognizes oxidized phospholipids	[73–77]
CD81	Tetraspanin co-receptor of αvβ5 integrin	[57]
Focal adhesion kinase (FAK)	Cytosolic signal transducer mediating activation of MerTK	[5, 36, 78]
Gas6, proteinS	Secreted ligands for MertK/Tyro3 in the subretinal space	[67–70]
Kinesin-1 light chain-1 (KLC1)	Cytosolic motor with role in phagosome transport	[101]
Melanoregulin (MREG)	Cytosolic signal transducer with role in phagosome maturation (LC3 association)	[110, 111]
Mer tyrosine kinase (MerTK)	RPE cell surface engulfment receptor triggering engulfment and limiting POS recognition	[2, 3, 56, 61–64]
Milk fat globule-EGF8 (MFG-E8)	Secreted ligand for αvβ5 integrin in the subretinal space	[36, 58]
Myosin7a (myoVIIA)	Cytosolic motor with role in post-engulfment phagosome transport	[97]
Non-muscle myosin II (myoII)	Cytosolic motor with role in POS engulfment	[79]
Phosphoinositide 3-kinase (PI3K)	Cytosolic signal transducer with role in POS engulfment	[80]
Plexin B1 (plxB1)	RPE cell surface receptor coordinating diurnal termination of RPE phagocytic activity	[96]
Protein kinase C (PKC)	Cytosolic signal transducer regulating αvβ5 integrin anchorage to F-actin	[38]
Rab escort-protein-1 (REP-1)	Cytosolic signal transducer with role in phagosome-lysosome fusion	[104]
Rac1 GTPase	Cytosolic signal transducer regulating F-actin assembly in phagocytic cup	[43]
Semaphorin 4D	Activating ligand of plexin B1 in the subretinal space	[96]
Soluble MerTK extracellular fragment (sMerTK)	Decoy MerTK receptor with inhibitory role in vitro	[70]
Src kinase (Src)	Cytosolic signal transducer with role in POS engulfment	[90]
Tyro3 receptor tyrosine kinase (Tyro3)	MerTK paralog; if expressed by RPE may substitute for MerTK	[65, 66]

Recognition and Binding of POS by RPE Cells

In the recognition/binding step of POS clearance, RPE cells respond to phosphatidylserine (PS) exposed by distal ends of outer segments, which serves as an "eat me" signal [13]. POS recognition requires an active phagocytic machinery at the apical side of RPE cells. The integrin receptor αvβ5 is the only integrin family receptor localized to the apical aspect of RPE cells. *In vivo* and cell culture experiments have provided complementary results indicating that αvβ5 serves as primary POS recognition receptor in human and rodent RPE [5, 52–54]. Ligand binding activity of αvβ5 integrin is highly regulated. RPE cells use a cytosolic protein kinase C (PKC) dependent pathway to promote anchorage of αvβ5 receptors to the F-actin cytoskeleton, which is required for its function in POS recognition [38]. Cell surface levels of αvβ5 integrin are regulated by its interaction with cytosolic annexin A5 (Anx5 in Fig. 3.2) [55]. Moreover, feedback mechanisms between αvβ5 integrin and the internalization machinery impact activity of αvβ5 such that increasing surface levels of αvβ5 integrin does not promote a proportional increase in POS binding [56]. Finally, αvβ5 activity is dependent on its plasma membrane co-receptor, the tetraspanin CD81. CD81 does not function as a binding receptor for POS itself, but inhibition or overexpression of CD81 reduces or increases particle binding by αvβ5 integrin, respectively [57].

Activated αvβ5 receptors do not bind their substrates, PS-bearing POS, directly, but via extracellular bridge proteins that opsonize POS. The subretinal space contains secreted PS-binding glycoproteins, including Protein S, Gas6, and milk fat globule-EGF8 (MFG-E8). Of these, MFG-E8 specifically acts to bridge POS and αvβ5 integrin receptors of the RPE [36]. MFG-E8 may be secreted into the subretinal space by both photoreceptors and RPE [58]. The blockade of αvβ5 integrin as well as lack of αvβ5 or MFG-E8 greatly reduces POS binding by RPE cells. However, a bona fide binding process does not take place in the intact retina, where outer segments, POS and apical surface of the RPE with its αvβ5 receptors are in close contact at all times. However, mice lacking β5 integrin or MFG-E8 do not show the characteristic morning peak of POS phagosomes in the RPE after light onset. Instead, phagocytosis occurs at a reduced but constant level at all times of day [5, 36]. Thus, the binding of MFG-E8-opsonized POS to αvβ5 integrin receptors and their ligation promotes the synchronized peak of POS engulfment. That aged β5 null mice show reduced vision and accumulation of autofluorescent lipofuscin-like material in the RPE illustrates that the rhythmicity of POS clearance is vital to long term health and function of the retina [5].

Cell Surface Receptors and RPE Signaling Pathways Mediating POS Internalization

Antibody blockade of αvβ5 integrin greatly reduces POS binding, but internalization of surface-bound particles is unaffected [53]. Signaling downstream of αvβ5 is necessary but not sufficient for engulfment of αvβ5–bound POS. Thus, the internalization step of POS phagocytosis requires signaling stimulated by POS binding to αvβ5 integrin in addition to a distinct set of surface receptors and their downstream signaling.

Studies on POS phagocytosis and specifically its internalization step have been greatly facilitated by the availability of an animal model that lacks this activity. The Royal College of Surgeons (RCS) rat was first identified in 1938 and has since been widely studied as model of hereditary blindness since [3, 59]. Mullen and LaVail in 1976 showed that RCS retinal degeneration is caused by a defect of clearance phagocytosis by the RPE rather than a photoreceptor defect [3, 41, 60]. In 2000, the causative mutation in the RCS rat was identified to disable the gene for the receptor tyrosine kinase Mer (MerTK). A deletion mutation in the *MERTK* gene in the RCS rat yields a shortened transcript and absence of MerTK protein [61, 62]. Adenoviral delivery of MerTK to RCS RPE rescues the phagocytic defect and improves RCS retinal integrity *in vivo* [63, 64]. Targeted mutation has generated a MerTK knockout mouse model that phenocopies the RCS rat [2]. In both RCS rat and MerTK knockout models photoreceptors continue to grow from the inner segment side, but RPE cells are unable to engulf POS. As a result, outer segments briefly elongate and distort before outer segment debris and possibly shed POS accumulate in the subretinal space further causing distress of photoreceptors, which eventually die. Notably, lack of MerTK does not cause retinal degeneration in mice with increased expression of Tyro3 in the RPE [65], a receptor tyrosine kinase that is very similar in structure and ligand binding activity to MerTK [66]. Altogether these data illustrate the critical importance of MerTK or equivalent RTK activity for POS phagocytosis by RPE cells.

Like αvβ5 integrin, MerTK or Tyro3 do not interact directly with spent or shedding POS but are ligated by soluble bridge proteins. Protein S and Gas6 are members of a protein family with binding domains shared by both RTKs as well as a binding domain for the PS exposed by POS. Gas6 or ProteinS knockout mouse retinas are phenotypically normal but deletion of both ligands leads to photoreceptor cell death as seen in MerTK rats and mice with rapid early onset retinal degeneration [67, 68]. These *in vivo* data suggest overlapping functions for the RTK ligands. Indeed, both proteins may lead to MerTK receptor ligation, activation and POS internalization by RPE in culture [69]. In contrast, other cell culture experiments have suggested that ProteinS and Gas6 may exert distinct MerTK downstream signals [70]. Further unrelated bridge ligands, e.g. tubby and tubby-like protein 1, and galectin-3 have been proposed but their physiological significance remains untested [71, 72]. With ProteinS/Gas6 together evidently necessary and sufficient for POS internalization via MerTK, additional experiments will be needed to clarify role or contributions of additional molecules and mechanisms.

In addition to RTK activity, RPE may employ CD36 receptor ligation to activate POS engulfment. CD36 is expressed at the apical, phagocytic surface [73]. It recognizes oxidized lipids or lipoproteins. In the phagocytic process CD36 acts in a post binding step and independent of the POS binding receptor αvβ5 integrin [74]. Dependence of CD36 on specific oxidized phospholipids that are generated in retina subjected to high intensity light and the possibility of pro-inflammatory signaling downstream of CD36 suggests that CD36 may contribute to RPE phagocytic activity in damaged or distress retina rather than in routine diurnal outer segment renewal in the healthy retina [75–77].

Ligation of phagocytic receptors of the RPE by bridge proteins opsonizing shed POS elicits cytosolic signaling pathways that ultimately reorganize the cell for particle engulfment. Signaling activities downstream of both, αvβ5 integrin and MerTK/Tyro3 are required.

The cytosolic tyrosine kinase focal adhesion kinase (FAK) is a crucial signaling component between αvβ5 integrin and MerTK linking binding and engulfment mechanisms. FAK mediates the activation of MerTK directly or indirectly by increasing phosphorylation and therefore activity of this receptor [78]. FAK resides in a complex with αvβ5 at the apical plasma membrane domain of the RPE, the site of POS phagocytosis. αvβ5 integrin ligation during POS binding first increases FAK recruitment to the apical complex, in which it is phosphorylated at multiple tyrosine residues. Phosphorylated FAK then dissociates from the complex and redistributes from the apical membrane to the RPE cytoplasm. In rodent retina, *in vivo* FAK phosphorylation and activity peak right after light onset. Synchronized tyrosine phosphorylation of MerTK can be detected subsequently, 2 hours after light onset. These activity peaks are absent in β5 integrin and MFG-E8 knockout mice demonstrating the requirement for MFG-E8-αvβ5 signaling for elevating MerTK activity during the diurnal burst of POS clearance [5, 36].

As much as αvβ5 signaling regulates MerTK activity, reverse receptor cross talk also takes place in RPE cells: RPE cells use a MerTK dependent feedback mechanism to limit phagocytic particle binding by αvβ5 integrin [56]. RPE cells that transiently or permanently lack the expression of MerTK bind excessive numbers of POS via surface αvβ5 receptors. A small fraction of MerTK is cleaved and released as soluble extracellular fragment (sMerTK) during POS phagocytosis *in vivo* and *in vitro* and may further contribute to the regulation of the RPE's phagocytic capacity. sMerTK may act as decoy receptor blocking effects of MerTK ligands on RPE cells, but cell culture assays found that sMerTK affects mainly POS binding [70].

Like for all forms of phagocytosis, F-actin cytoskeletal re-arrangement is the cardinal process required for particle engulfment by RPE cells [51]. The RPE's long apical microvilli are based on F-actin and reach into the subretinal space interdigitating with intact photoreceptor outer segments. These structures are likely distinct from the *de novo* F-actin recruitment beneath surface-bound phagocytic particles for formation of structures called "phagocytic cups" that are needed during phagocytic processes. POS internalization requires closure of phagocytic cups, which depends on further F-actin reorganization together with plasma membrane fusion.

Both αvβ5 integrin and MerTK signaling contribute to F-actin dynamics during POS clearance by RPE cells. Activated Rac1, a member of the Rho GTPase family of primary cellular regulators of the F-actin cytoskeleton dynamics, promotes the recruitment of F-actin cytoskeletal elements. MFG-E8-ligated αvβ5 integrin is required for both MerTK activation via FAK and F-actin recruitment via Rac1. Both pathways are required for phagocytic clearance, but Rac1 activation does not require MerTK [43]. Annexin A2 (Anx2 in Fig. 3.2), a cytosolic Ca^{2+}- and phospholipid binding protein and regulator of F-actin dynamics serves in early stages of phagocytosis during phagocytic cup closure [49]. Annexin A2 is recruited to nascent phagocytic cups in RPE cells in culture and dissociates once phagosomes have been internalized. Tyrosine phosphorylation of Annexin A2 is increased at the peak of phagocytic activity in wild-type mice. In annexin A2 knockout mice POS phagocytosis is slightly attenuated and the peak of FAK activation is delayed but not eliminated. These observations suggest that annexin A2 recruitment to the forming phagosome leads to the activation of Src kinase, which is required for the activation of FAK and downstream MerTK activation.

MerTK also directly contributes to F-actin cytoskeletal rearrangement in a way that mobilizes non-muscle myosin II (myoII in Fig. 3.2) from the RPE cell periphery to sites of POS engulfment [79]. Akt signaling contributes to regulation of this process as Akt inhibition increases both the number of phagocytic cups and the recruitment of F-actin and myosin II to individual phagocytic cups in RPE cells in culture [80]. This role of Akt is independent and contrasts with the contribution of PI3 kinase in POS engulfment: PI3 kinase inhibition during POS binding weakens F-actin association with bound POS, has no effect on myosin-II recruitment, and inhibits engulfment. Note that unrelated to their opposing roles in internalization, inhibition of either Akt or PI3 kinase increases POS binding by cultured RPE cells. Taken together, Akt functions downstream of PI3 kinase in POS binding, while its inhibitory role in early events of F-actin assembly and rearrangement beneath bound particles that promotes OS engulfment is distinct from PI3-kinase.

Signaling mediators of the IP_3/Ca^{2+} intracellular signaling system and the cAMP second messenger system have both been reported to regulate RPE phagocytosis *in vitro*. Pharmacological increases in intracellular cAMP levels in cultured RPE reduce phagocytosis of ROS, while similar increases in cGMP had no effect [81–83]. Stimulation of RPE adenosine A2 receptors, which induces generation of intracellular cAMP, also reduce POS internalization by RPE cells in culture [84]. MerTK ligation during POS phagocytosis by RPE cells in culture may increase IP_3, which in turn activates ingestion of bound POS [78, 85, 86]. Elevating IP_3 levels pharmacologically is sufficient to increase phagocytic activity of RCS RPE cells in culture [87]. As expected from RTK/IP_3 signaling, RPE phagocytosis also involves a rise in intracellular free Ca^{2+} [88]. Ca^{2+} oscillations in RPE monolayers in regions with bound POS have been reported [89]. However, the specific and essential targets of IP_3 signaling remain to be uncovered.

Src kinase interacts with MerTK and its phosphorylation and activation is increased after phagocytic challenge of cells and downstream of MerTK [90]. Downstream of Src signaling, MerTK dependent tyrosine phosphorylation of GDP dissociation inhibitor alpha (GDI1) may regulate Rab GTPase dependent membrane dynamics such as vesicle fusion [91].

Another downstream effect of Src kinase signaling during RPE phagocytosis is activation of L-type Ca^{2+} channels [92]. Blocking L-type channels in cultured RPE cells reduces phagocytosis, and ligation of POS binding receptor integrins activates L-type Ca^{2+} channel activity [40]. Further, MaxiK Ca^{2+} dependent K^+ (BK) ion channels, L-type Ca^{2+} channels and bestrophin-1 contribute to intracellular Ca^{2+} homeostasis and affect POS phagocytosis by RPE cells in culture [93]. Lack of BK or $Ca_v1.3$ L-type Ca^{2+} channels in mice leads to a shift in phagocytosis rhythm and shortened outer segments suggesting an imbalance of POS shedding and outer segment growth [94]. Moreover, a recent report showed cAMP dependent circadian rhythms in Ca^{2+} spiking frequencies and bead uptake by human RPE cells in culture [95]. If and how these signaling processes are linked to the known phagocytic machinery for POS remains to be shown.

Altogether, the ligation of αvβ5 integrin and MerTK via the complex signaling mechanisms discussed above result in post-translational protein activity changes through altered protein phosphorylation and changes in GTP load that allow re-arrangement of the cytoskeleton and plasma membrane required for POS intake.

In the eye, these processes occur after light onset in a synchronized and highly coordinated fashion that promote the characteristic phagocytic burst. Importantly, elevated signaling is swiftly terminated by RPE cells at the end of its morning phagocytic activity [5, 43]. The molecular mechanisms used in the retina to inactivate phagocytic signaling after the daily phagocytic burst remain only partly understood. They include the synchronized activation of the RPE surface receptor plexin B1 (plxnB1; plxB1 in Fig. 3.2) by its ligand semaphorin 4D (sema4D; Sem4D in Fig. 3.2), which is found in the rat retina especially in or on cone photoreceptors [96]. In wild-type but not in RCS phagocytosis-defective rat retina, sema4D levels and, likely as a result, plxnB1 phosphorylation are reduced 1 hour after light onset as compared to either 1 hour before or 3 hours after. Mice lacking either plxnB1 or sema4D show increased numbers of POS in the RPE 1 hour after light onset suggesting a physiological function of sema4D/plxnB1 signaling in attenuating the phagocytic burst. Mechanistically, plxnB1 signaling acts on inhibiting F-actin dynamics required for phagocytosis: adding purified Sema4D to RPE cells in culture during POS challenge prevents Rac1 GTPase activation abolishing POS internalization without affecting POS binding.

Processing and Degradation of Phagocytosed POS by RPE Cells

RPE cells need to digest internalized POS material promptly and completely to prevent gradually buildup of undigested debris that is toxic for the RPE and may contribute to age-related retinal dysfunction. Phagosomes (phago in Fig. 3.2) move from apical to basal RPE regions to mature and fuse with lysosomes (lys in Fig. 3.2), forming phagolysosomes (phago lys in Fig. 3.2), and degrade their content. The molecular control of these phagolysosomal digestion processes remains only poorly understood.

Post-engulfment phagosome transport inside RPE cells depends on both F-actin and microtubule dependent processes. In the shaker-1 mouse model, RPE cells lacking functional F-actin motor myosin VIIA (myoVIIa in Fig. 3.2) show delay of phagosomes exit from the F-actin-rich apical region [97, 98]. Human myosin VIIA mutations cause Usher 1B, a deaf-blindness disorder [99, 100].

Having exited the apical F-actin cytoskeleton on their way towards central and basal areas of the RPE cell, POS phagosomes move bidirectionally along microtubules while associated with kinesin-1 light chain 1 (KLC1) [101]. Lack of KLC1 results in defects of phagosome trafficking, possibly decreasing the probability of phagosome fusion with other vesicles. Impaired POS phagosome degradation eventually increases accumulation of RPE and sub-RPE deposits resulting in a pro-oxidative, pro-inflammatory environment.

The degradation of engulfed POS protein and lipid components requires enzymatic hydrolyses. Earlier studies focused on degradation of POS opsin, the by far most abundant protein in POS. Early during maturation und movement towards the cell body phagosomes transiently interact with endosomes (en in Fig. 3.2) such that opsin undergoes limited proteolysis even before bona fide phagosome-lysosome fusion [35]. Activities of cathepsin D and cathepsin S proteases (cath S, cath D in Fig. 3.2) and phagosomal acidification have been shown to be essential for efficient lysosomal opsin degradation [30, 45]. In transgenic mice expressing a mutant form of cathepsin D resulting in impaired processing of internalized POS RPE cells accumulate autofluorescent opsin-positive inclusion [8]. Ultimately, fusion with cathepsin D positive lysosomes promotes step-wise opsin degradation [35]. Synchronized appearance of cathepsin D in phagolysosomes correlates with decreasing levels of detectable opsin and progressive acidification [102]. Cathepsin D activity fluctuates in the RPE with its diurnal maximum at the time of peak phagocytic activity [103].

Recent studies have shed light on the enormous importance of POS lipid digestion. For disposal of POS lipids and recycling of metabolic intermediates back to the outer retina RPE cells use fatty acid β-oxidation and ketogenesis pathways, which support the cells energy demand and prevent buildup of lipid accumulation, which causes oxidative stress and mitochondrial dysfunction. POS phagosome maturation and processing are linked to ketogenesis and release of β-hydroxibutyrate (β-HB) [27]. Cultured RPE cells release increased levels of the ketone body β-HB apically after challenged with POS. Mouse RPE/choroid explants mainly release β-HB levels after light onset at the time of the daily burst of phagocytic activity. Animal models of delayed phagosome processing or abnormal phagosome lipid content show a time shift in the β-HB release illustrating the importance of tight temporal regulation for long term retinal health.

Our understanding of the control of POS phagosomal processing remains limited but there is evidence that it is precisely regulated at the level of organelle fusion. Rab escort-protein-1 (REP-1) supports posttranslational isoprenyl modification of Rab GTPases that control vesicle formation, movement, docking and fusion. RPE cells in culture lacking REP-1 internalize POS like control cells but show delayed POS protein clearance [104]. This suggests that absence of REP-1 inhibits POS specific phagosomal-lysosomal fusion events through aberrant Rab GTPase activities. In general, fusion with lysosomes is a required step in ensuring that the pH of POS phagosomes decreases sufficiently to allow enzymatic hydrolyses. Inhibition of the vacuolar-type ATPase (v-ATPase) proton pump by Bafilomycin A1 prevents POS degradation even if cathepsin D is present in phagosomes [102]. Acidification is affected by signaling through receptors such as adenosine A2 receptors, P2X7 receptors, and CFTR although it remains to be tested if such signaling is dynamic or specifically controlling diurnal POS clearance [105–107]. The scaffolding protein caveolin-1 (cav-1 in Fig. 3.2) contributes to POS phagolysosomal acidification. Caveolin-1 resides on maturing phagolysosomes in RPE cells *in vivo* and in cell culture and is essential for phagolysosomal POS degradation [47]. RPE-specific deletion of caveolin-1 *in vivo* reverses rhythmic profiles of levels and activity of lysosomal enzymes and impairs photoreceptor function. Lowering caveolin-1 protein levels in RPE cells in culture is sufficient to impair lysosomal acidification decreasing lysosomal and phagolysosomal enzyme activities.

Like caveolin-1, βA3/A1 crystallin (βA3/A1 cryst in Fig. 3.2) is localized to lysosomes and required for degradation of POS [108]. In RPE-specific βA3/A1 crystallin knockout mice V-ATPase activity is decreased and lysosomal pH elevated, resulting in undigested POS accumulation. Mechanistically, βA3/A1 crystallin affects lysosomal acidification by interacting with and presumably regulating activity of v-ATPase proton pump components [109].

In addition to completing POS renewal every 24 hours for life, RPE cells must coordinate processes of POS renewal with other cellular maintenance activities. Specifically, regulated routine organelle maintenance and degradation of protein aggregates via autophagic processes also employ and occupy lysosomes. Indeed, molecular mechanisms of POS degradation partly overlap with macroautophagy and the two degradative pathways via shared use of lysosomes influence each other. The shared presence of microtubule-associated protein 1 light chain 3 (LC3) on POS phagosomes and autophagosomes in RPE cells has recently led to a new classification of RPE phagocytosis as belonging to "LC3-associated phagocytosis" (LAP) pathways [110]. A key protein coordinating POS turnover and macroautophagy in RPE cells is melanoregulin (MREG), an intracellular sorting protein that is hypothesized to play a role in organelle biogenesis including lysosome maturation and intracellular trafficking. Lack of MREG results in reduced cathepsin D activity and delayed degradation of engulfed POS by RPE cells *in vivo* and in culture [7]. MREG links and may balance macroautophagic and phagocytic processes by interacting with LC3 and coordinating its association with phagosomes in the RPE [111].

Taken together, RPE cells tightly regulate degradation of engulfed POS to ensure both coordination with autophagy and completion within 24 hours and in time for the next phagocytic burst. How intracellular processing is triggered by phagocytic surface receptors and their signaling pathways remains to be elucidated.

Defects in POS Clearance Phagocytosis by RPE Cells and Human Retinal Disease

Animal models with specific molecular or engineered defects in POS renewal show retinal abnormalities ranging from rapid early onset and complete retinal degeneration of the RCS rat to abnormal but gradual accumulation of undigested POS debris followed by photoreceptor dysfunction [5] or of little impact on visual function within the short life span of a rodent [7]. In human patients, inherited defects in engulfment of POS and subsequent degradation are also associated with inherited retinal degenerative diseases.

Disease causing mutations in the engulfment receptor MerTK were identified in patients with early onset retinitis pigmentosa who suffer from severe retinal degenerations [112]. MerTK mutations have also been linked to rare retinal dystrophies and severe rod cone dystrophy [113, 114]. The very rapid and complete retinal degeneration found in the RCS rat is not seen in human RP due to MerTK mutation found so far, which suggests that POS phagocytosis takes place to some extent in affected patients, either through partly active MerTK or through alternate pathways.

Another progressive degeneration of RPE, photoreceptors and choroid, choroideremia (CHM) is caused by mutations in the CHM gene encoding REP-1 [115]. CHM patients have less or no REP-1 protein [116, 117] and show accumulation of unprocessed POS material in the RPE and excess inflammatory cells in the choroid [104].

RPE cells are post-mitotic with high phagocytic activities and high metabolic demand. Partly degraded and oxidized debris material gradually accumulates in autofluorescent lipofuscin granules in human RPE with age. Lipofuscin is rich in oxidized lipids including retinoid derivatives some of them directly and specifically toxic to RPE and harmful to its phagocytic activity [118, 119]. Lipofuscin arises from gradual and long-term accumulation of incompletely degraded, oxidized remnants of POS phagolysosome and/or autophagosome content. Although still poorly understood, all evidence suggests that excessive lipofuscin accumulation in the aging human eye impairs RPE function and health and secondarily affects vision as support for the neural retina by compromised RPE cells fails.

Outlook

Exciting technical and conceptual progress in understanding POS phagocytosis has provided the foundation for the development of new treatments for RPE pathologic conditions. Specifically, MerTK mutation associated retinal degenerations have been the focus of gene and cell replacement therapeutic approaches as well as drug studies. AAV hMerTK vector treatment introduced photoreceptor rescue in the RCS rat and MerTK null-mouse animal models [120, 121]. Clinical trials for different forms of MerTK-associated retinal dystrophies are on the way [122]. Complete replacement of RPE cells generated from various stem cell sources like pluripotent (hESC), induced pluripotent (iPSC) and adult RPE stem cells (RPESC) is also under development [123]. Further, patient specific iPSC derived RPE models have become available that allow screening approaches to potential new treatments like in a nonsense variant of MerTK-RPE read-through inducing drugs to restore production of a full length protein [124].

On the basic research side, it has become clear that strict coordination of photoreceptor growth and shedding, phagocytosis of spent POS tips and degradation and waste removal must create a precise homeostatic balance that is essential for photoreceptor and RPE health. Many open questions remain on the signaling mechanisms used by both RPE and photoreceptors to communicate and fine tune these processes including how RPE cells contribute to shedding. Much remains to be learned about phagosome processing, degradation, recycling and transport processes towards the retina and the choroid. Recent methodological advances will surely allow addressing these important issues in the near future.

References

1. Strauss O. The retinal pigment epithelium in visual function. Physiol Rev. 2005;85(3):845–81.
2. Duncan JL, LaVail MM, Yasumura D, Matthes MT, Yang H, Trautmann N, et al. An RCS-like retinal dystrophy phenotype in mer knockout mice. Invest Ophthalmol Vis Sci. 2003;44(2):826–38.
3. Dowling JE, Sidman RL. Inherited retinal dystrophy in the rat. J Cell Biol. 1962;14:73–109.
4. Bok D, Hall MO. The role of the pigment epithelium in the etiology of inherited retinal dystrophy in the rat. J Cell Biol. 1971;49(3):664–82.
5. Nandrot EF, Kim Y, Brodie SE, Huang X, Sheppard D, Finnemann SC. Loss of synchronized retinal phagocytosis and age-related blindness in mice lacking αvβ5 integrin. J Exp Med. 2004;200(12):1539–45.
6. Parinot C, Nandrot EF. A comprehensive review of mutations in the MERTK proto-oncogene. Adv Exp Med Biol. 2016;854:259–65.
7. Damek-Poprawa M, Diemer T, Lopes VS, Lillo C, Harper DC, Marks MS, et al. Melanoregulin (MREG) modulates lysosome function in pigment epithelial cells. J Biol Chem. 2009;284(16):10877–89.
8. Rakoczy PE, Zhang D, Robertson T, Barnett NL, Papadimitriou J, Constable IJ, et al. Progressive age-related changes similar to age-related macular degeneration in a transgenic mouse model. Am J Pathol. 2002;161(4):1515–24.
9. Sparrow JR, Boulton M. RPE lipofuscin and its role in retinal pathobiology. Exp Eye Res. 2005;80(5):595–606.
10. Delori FC, Goger DG, Dorey CK. Age-related accumulation and spatial distribution of lipofuscin in RPE of normal subjects. Invest Ophthalmol Vis Sci. 2001;42(8):1855–66.
11. Young RW. The renewal of photoreceptor cell outer segments. J Cell Biol. 1967;33(1):61–72.
12. Young RW, Bok D. Participation of the retinal pigment epithelium in the rod outer segment renewal process. J Cell Biol. 1969;42(2):392–403.
13. Ruggiero L, Connor MP, Chen J, Langen R, Finnemann SC. Diurnal, localized exposure of phosphatidylserine by rod outer segment tips in wild-type but not Itgb5$^{-/-}$ or Mfge8$^{-/-}$ mouse retina. Proc Natl Acad Sci U S A. 2012;109(21):8145–8.
14. LaVail MM. Rod outer segment disk shedding in rat retina: relationship to cyclic lighting. Science. 1976;194(4269):1071–4.
15. Steinberg RH, Wood I, Hogan MJ. Pigment epithelial ensheathment and phagocytosis of extrafoveal cones in human retina. Philos Trans R Soc Lond Ser B Biol Sci. 1977;277(958):459–74.
16. Anderson DH, Fisher SK. Disc shedding in rodlike and conelike photoreceptors of tree squirrels. Science. 1975;187(4180):953–5.
17. Anderson DH, Fisher SK, Erickson PA, Tabor GA. Rod and cone disc shedding in the rhesus monkey retina: a quantitative study. Exp Eye Res. 1980;30(5):559–74.
18. Bobu C, Craft CM, Masson-Pevet M, Hicks D. Photoreceptor organization and rhythmic phagocytosis in the nile rat Arvicanthis ansorgei: a novel diurnal rodent model for the study of cone pathophysiology. Invest Ophthalmol Vis Sci. 2006;47(7):3109–18.
19. Bobu C, Hicks D. Regulation of retinal photoreceptor phagocytosis in a diurnal mammal by circadian clocks and ambient lighting. Invest Ophthalmol Vis Sci. 2009;50(7):3495–502.
20. Immel JH, Fisher SK. Cone photoreceptor shedding in the tree shrew (Tupaia belangerii). Cell Tissue Res. 1985;239(3):667–75.

21. Fisher SK, Pfeffer BA, Anderson DH. Both rod and cone disc shedding are related to light onset in the cat. Invest Ophthalmol Vis Sci. 1983;24(7):844–56.
22. Young RW. The daily rhythm of shedding and degradation of cone outer segment membranes in the lizard retina. J Ultrastruct Res. 1977;61(2):172–85.
23. Young RW. The daily rhythm of shedding and degradation of rod and cone outer segment membranes in the chick retina. Invest Ophthalmol Vis Sci. 1978;17(2):105–16.
24. O'Day WT, Young RW. Rhythmic daily shedding of outer-segment membranes by visual cells in the goldfish. J Cell Biol. 1978;76(3):593–604.
25. Tabor GA, Fisher SK, Anderson DH. Rod and cone disc shedding in light-entrained tree squirrels. Exp Eye Res. 1980;30(5):545–57.
26. Bibb C, Young RW. Renewal of fatty acids in the membranes of visual cell outer segments. J Cell Biol. 1974;61(2):327–43.
27. Reyes-Reveles J, Dhingra A, Alexander D, Bragin A, Philp NJ, Boesze-Battaglia K. Phagocytosis-dependent ketogenesis in retinal pigment epithelium. J Biol Chem. 2017;292(19):8038–47.
28. Bazan NG, Gordon WC, Rodriguez de Turco EB. Docosahexaenoic acid uptake and metabolism in photoreceptors: retinal conservation by an efficient retinal pigment epithelial cell-mediated recycling process. Adv Exp Med Biol. 1992;318:295–306.
29. Rodriguez de Turco EB, Parkins N, Ershov AV, Bazan NG. Selective retinal pigment epithelial cell lipid metabolism and remodeling conserves photoreceptor docosahexaenoic acid following phagocytosis. J Neurosci Res. 1999;57(4):479–86.
30. Rakoczy PE, Mann K, Cavaney DM, Robertson T, Papadimitreou J, Constable IJ. Detection and possible functions of a cysteine protease involved in digestion of rod outer segments by retinal pigment epithelial cells. Invest Ophthalmol Vis Sci. 1994;35(12):4100–8.
31. Mayerson PL, Hall MO. Rat retinal pigment epithelial cells show specificity of phagocytosis in vitro. J Cell Biol. 1986;103(1):299–308.
32. Parinot C, Rieu Q, Chatagnon J, Finnemann SC, Nandrot EF. Large-scale purification of porcine or bovine photoreceptor outer segments for phagocytosis assays on retinal pigment epithelial cells. J Vis Exp. 2014;94:52100.
33. Molday RS, Molday LL. Identification and characterization of multiple forms of rhodopsin and minor proteins in frog and bovine rod outer segment disc membranes. Electrophoresis, lectin labeling, and proteolysis studies. J Biol Chem. 1979;254(11):4653–60.
34. Esteve-Rudd J, Lopes VS, Jiang M, Williams DS. In vivo and in vitro monitoring of phagosome maturation in retinal pigment epithelium cells. Adv Exp Med Biol. 2014;801:85–90.
35. Wavre-Shapton ST, Meschede IP, Seabra MC, Futter CE. Phagosome maturation during endosome interaction revealed by partial rhodopsin processing in retinal pigment epithelium. J Cell Sci. 2014;127(Pt 17):3852–61.
36. Nandrot EF, Anand M, Almeida D, Atabai K, Sheppard D, Finnemann SC. Essential role for MFG-E8 as ligand for αvβ5 integrin in diurnal retinal phagocytosis. Proc Natl Acad Sci U S A. 2007;104(29):12005–10.
37. Mazzoni F, Safa H, Finnemann SC. Understanding photoreceptor outer segment phagocytosis: use and utility of RPE cells in culture. Exp Eye Res. 2014;126:51–60.
38. Finnemann SC, Rodriguez-Boulan E. Macrophage and retinal pigment epithelium phagocytosis: apoptotic cells and photoreceptors compete for αvβ3 and αvβ5 integrins, and protein kinase C regulates αvβ5 binding and cytoskeletal linkage. J Exp Med. 1999;190(6):861–74.
39. Westenskow PD, Moreno SK, Krohne TU, Kurihara T, Zhu S, Zhang ZN, et al. Using flow cytometry to compare the dynamics of photoreceptor outer segment phagocytosis in iPS-derived RPE cells. Invest Ophthalmol Vis Sci. 2012;53(10):6282–90.
40. Karl MO, Kroeger W, Wimmers S, Milenkovic VM, Valtink M, Engelmann K, et al. Endogenous Gas6 and Ca^{2+}-channel activation modulate phagocytosis by retinal pigment epithelium. Cell Signal. 2008;20(6):1159–68.
41. Chaitin MH, Hall MO. Defective ingestion of rod outer segments by cultured dystrophic rat pigment epithelial cells. Invest Ophthalmol Vis Sci. 1983;24(7):812–20.
42. Davis RJ, Alam NM, Zhao C, Muller C, Saini JS, Blenkinsop TA, et al. The developmental stage of adult human stem cell-derived retinal pigment epithelium cells influences transplant efficacy for vision rescue. Stem Cell Reports. 2017;9(1):42–9.
43. Mao Y, Finnemann SC. Essential diurnal Rac1 activation during retinal phagocytosis requires αvβ5 integrin but not tyrosine kinases focal adhesion kinase or Mer tyrosine kinase. Mol Biol Cell. 2012;23(6):1104–14.
44. Guha S, Coffey EE, Lu W, Lim JC, Beckel JM, Laties AM, et al. Approaches for detecting lysosomal alkalinization and impaired degradation in fresh and cultured RPE cells: evidence for a role in retinal degenerations. Exp Eye Res. 2014;126:68–76.
45. Bosch E, Horwitz J, Bok D. Phagocytosis of outer segments by retinal pigment epithelium: phagosome-lysosome interaction. J Histochem Cytochem. 1993;41(2):253–63.
46. Sethna S, Finnemann SC. Analysis of photoreceptor rod outer segment phagocytosis by RPE cells in situ. Methods Mol Biol. 2013;935:245–54.
47. Sethna S, Chamakkala T, Gu X, Thompson TC, Cao G, Elliott MH, et al. Regulation of phagolysosomal digestion by caveolin-1 of the retinal pigment epithelium is essential for vision. J Biol Chem. 2016;291(12):6494–506.
48. Mao Y, Finnemann SC. Live imaging of lysotracker-labelled phagolysosomes tracks diurnal phagocy-

tosis of photoreceptor outer segment fragments in rat RPE tissue ex vivo. Adv Exp Med Biol. 2016;854:717–23.
49. Law AL, Ling Q, Hajjar KA, Futter CE, Greenwood J, Adamson P, et al. Annexin A2 regulates phagocytosis of photoreceptor outer segments in the mouse retina. Mol Biol Cell. 2009;20(17):3896–904.
50. Penberthy KK, Ravichandran KS. Apoptotic cell recognition receptors and scavenger receptors. Immunol Rev. 2016;269(1):44–59.
51. Mao Y, Finnemann SC. Regulation of phagocytosis by Rho GTPases. Small GTPases. 2015;6(2):89–99.
52. Miceli MV, Newsome DA, Tate DJ Jr. Vitronectin is responsible for serum-stimulated uptake of rod outer segments by cultured retinal pigment epithelial cells. Invest Ophthalmol Vis Sci. 1997;38(8):1588–97.
53. Finnemann SC, Bonilha VL, Marmorstein AD, Rodriguez-Boulan E. Phagocytosis of rod outer segments by retinal pigment epithelial cells requires αvβ5 integrin for binding but not for internalization. Proc Natl Acad Sci U S A. 1997;94(24):12932–7.
54. Lin H, Clegg DO. Integrin αvβ5 participates in the binding of photoreceptor rod outer segments during phagocytosis by cultured human retinal pigment epithelium. Invest Ophthalmol Vis Sci. 1998;39(9):1703–12.
55. Yu C, Munoz LE, Boeltz S, Finnemann SC. Contribution of annexin A5 to diurnal phagocytosis by the retinal pigment epithelium. ARVO Annual Meeting Abstract. Invest Ophthalmol Vis Sci. 2016;57(12):237.
56. Nandrot EF, Silva KE, Scelfo C, Finnemann SC. Retinal pigment epithelial cells use a MerTK-dependent mechanism to limit the phagocytic particle binding activity of αvβ5 integrin. Biol Cell. 2012;104(6):326–41.
57. Chang Y, Finnemann SC. Tetraspanin CD81 is required for the αvβ5-integrin-dependent particle-binding step of RPE phagocytosis. J Cell Sci. 2007;120(Pt 17):3053–63.
58. Burgess BL, Abrams TA, Nagata S, Hall MO. MFG-E8 in the retina and retinal pigment epithelium of rat and mouse. Mol Vis. 2006;12:1437–47.
59. Bourne MC, Campbell DA, Tansley K. Hereditary degeneration of the rat retina. Br J Ophthalmol. 1938;22(10):613–23.
60. Mullen RJ, LaVail MM. Inherited retinal dystrophy: primary defect in pigment epithelium determined with experimental rat chimeras. Science. 1976;192(4241):799–801.
61. D'Cruz PM, Yasumura D, Weir J, Matthes MT, Abderrahim H, LaVail MM, et al. Mutation of the receptor tyrosine kinase gene Mertk in the retinal dystrophic RCS rat. Hum Mol Genet. 2000;9(4):645–51.
62. Nandrot E, Dufour EM, Provost AC, Pequignot MO, Bonnel S, Gogat K, et al. Homozygous deletion in the coding sequence of the c-mer gene in RCS rats unravels general mechanisms of physiological cell adhesion and apoptosis. Neurobiol Dis. 2000;7(6 Pt B):586–99.
63. Feng W, Yasumura D, Matthes MT, LaVail MM, Vollrath D. Mertk triggers uptake of photoreceptor outer segments during phagocytosis by cultured retinal pigment epithelial cells. J Biol Chem. 2002;277(19):17016–22.
64. Vollrath D, Feng W, Duncan JL, Yasumura D, D'Cruz PM, Chappelow A, et al. Correction of the retinal dystrophy phenotype of the RCS rat by viral gene transfer of Mertk. Proc Natl Acad Sci U S A. 2001;98(22):12584–9.
65. Vollrath D, Yasumura D, Benchorin G, Matthes MT, Feng W, Nguyen NM, et al. Tyro3 modulates Mertk-associated retinal degeneration. PLoS Genet. 2015;11(12):e1005723.
66. Lew ED, Oh J, Burrola PG, Lax I, Zagorska A, Traves PG, et al. Differential TAM receptor-ligand-phospholipid interactions delimit differential TAM bioactivities. Elife. 2014;3:e03385.
67. Prasad D, Rothlin CV, Burrola P, Burstyn-Cohen T, Lu Q, Garcia de Frutos P, et al. TAM receptor function in the retinal pigment epithelium. Mol Cell Neurosci. 2006;33(1):96–108.
68. Burstyn-Cohen T, Lew ED, Traves PG, Burrola PG, Hash JC, Lemke G. Genetic dissection of TAM receptor-ligand interaction in retinal pigment epithelial cell phagocytosis. Neuron. 2012;76(6):1123–32.
69. Hall MO, Obin MS, Heeb MJ, Burgess BL, Abrams TA. Both protein S and Gas6 stimulate outer segment phagocytosis by cultured rat retinal pigment epithelial cells. Exp Eye Res. 2005;81(5):581–91.
70. Law AL, Parinot C, Chatagnon J, Gravez B, Sahel JA, Bhattacharya SS, et al. Cleavage of Mer tyrosine kinase (MerTK) from the cell surface contributes to the regulation of retinal phagocytosis. J Biol Chem. 2015;290(8):4941–52.
71. Caberoy NB, Zhou Y, Li W. Tubby and tubby-like protein 1 are new MerTK ligands for phagocytosis. EMBO J. 2010;29(23):3898–910.
72. Caberoy NB, Alvarado G, Bigcas JL, Li W. Galectin-3 is a new MerTK-specific eat-me signal. J Cell Physiol. 2012;227(2):401–7.
73. Ryeom SW, Sparrow JR, Silverstein RL. CD36 participates in the phagocytosis of rod outer segments by retinal pigment epithelium. J Cell Sci. 1996;109(Pt 2):387–95.
74. Finnemann SC, Silverstein RL. Differential roles of CD36 and αvβ5 integrin in photoreceptor phagocytosis by the retinal pigment epithelium. J Exp Med. 2001;194(9):1289–98.74.
75. Sun M, Finnemann SC, Febbraio M, Shan L, Annangudi SP, Podrez EA, et al. Light-induced oxidation of photoreceptor outer segment phospholipids generates ligands for CD36-mediated phagocytosis by retinal pigment epithelium: a potential mechanism for modulating outer segment phagocytosis under oxidant stress conditions. J Biol Chem. 2006;281(7):4222–30.

76. Picard E, Houssier M, Bujold K, Sapieha P, Lubell W, Dorfman A, et al. CD36 plays an important role in the clearance of oxLDL and associated age-dependent sub-retinal deposits. Aging (Albany NY). 2010;2(12):981–9.
77. Gnanaguru G, Choi AR, Amarnani D, D'Amore PA. Oxidized lipoprotein uptake through the CD36 receptor activates the NLRP3 inflammasome in human retinal pigment epithelial cells. Invest Ophthalmol Vis Sci. 2016;57(11):4704–12.
78. Finnemann SC. Focal adhesion kinase signaling promotes phagocytosis of integrin-bound photoreceptors. EMBO J. 2003;22(16):4143–54.
79. Strick DJ, Feng W, Vollrath D. Mertk drives myosin II redistribution during retinal pigment epithelial phagocytosis. Invest Ophthalmol Vis Sci. 2009;50(5):2427–35.
80. Bulloj A, Duan W, Finnemann SC. PI 3-kinase independent role for AKT in F-actin regulation during outer segment phagocytosis by RPE cells. Exp Eye Res. 2013;113:9–18.
81. Edwards RB, Bakshian S. Phagocytosis of outer segments by cultured rat pigment epithelium. Reduction by cyclic AMP and phosphodiesterase inhibitors. Invest Ophthalmol Vis Sci. 1980;19(10):1184–8.
82. Hall MO, Abrams TA, Mittag TW. The phagocytosis of rod outer segments is inhibited by drugs linked to cyclic adenosine monophosphate production. Invest Ophthalmol Vis Sci. 1993;34(8):2392–401.
83. Edwards RB, Flaherty PM. Association of changes in intracellular cyclic AMP with changes in phagocytosis in cultured rat pigment epithelium. Curr Eye Res. 1986;5(1):19–26.
84. Gregory CY, Abrams TA, Hall MO. Stimulation of A2 adenosine receptors inhibits the ingestion of photoreceptor outer segments by retinal pigment epithelium. Invest Ophthalmol Vis Sci. 1994;35(3):819–25.
85. Heth CA, Schmidt SY. Protein phosphorylation in retinal pigment epithelium of Long-Evans and Royal College of Surgeons rats. Invest Ophthalmol Vis Sci. 1992;33(10):2839–47.
86. Heth CA, Marescalchi PA. Inositol triphosphate generation in cultured rat retinal pigment epithelium. Invest Ophthalmol Vis Sci. 1994;35(2):409–16.
87. Heth CA, Marescalchi PA, Ye L. IP3 generation increases rod outer segment phagocytosis by cultured Royal College of Surgeons retinal pigment epithelium. Invest Ophthalmol Vis Sci. 1995;36(6):984–9.
88. Wimmers S, Karl MO, Strauss O. Ion channels in the RPE. Prog Retin Eye Res. 2007;26(3):263–301.
89. Kindzelskii AL, Elner VM, Elner SG, Yang D, Hughes BA, Petty HR. Toll-like receptor 4 (TLR4) of retinal pigment epithelial cells participates in transmembrane signaling in response to photoreceptor outer segments. J Gen Physiol. 2004;124(2):139–49.
90. Shelby SJ, Colwill K, Dhe-Paganon S, Pawson T, Thompson DA. MERTK interactions with SH2-domain proteins in the retinal pigment epithelium. PLoS One. 2013;8(2):e53964.
91. Shelby SJ, Feathers KL, Ganios AM, Jia L, Miller JM, Thompson DA. MERTK signaling in the retinal pigment epithelium regulates the tyrosine phosphorylation of GDP dissociation inhibitor alpha from the GDI/CHM family of RAB GTPase effectors. Exp Eye Res. 2015;140:28–40.
92. Strauss O, Buss F, Rosenthal R, Fischer D, Mergler S, Stumpff F, et al. Activation of neuroendocrine L-type channels (alpha1D subunits) in retinal pigment epithelial cells and brain neurons by pp60(c-src). Biochem Biophys Res Commun. 2000;270(3):806–10.
93. Strauss O, Reichhart N, Gomez NM, Muller C. Contribution of ion channels in calcium signaling regulating phagocytosis: maxiK, cav1.3 and bestrophin-1. Adv Exp Med Biol. 2016;854:739–44.
94. Müller C, Mas Gomez N, Ruth P, Strauss O. CaV1.3 L-type channels, maxiK Ca(2+)-dependent K(+) channels and bestrophin-1 regulate rhythmic photoreceptor outer segment phagocytosis by retinal pigment epithelial cells. Cell Signal. 2014;26(5):968–78.
95. Ikarashi R, Akechi H, Kanda Y, Ahmad A, Takeuchi K, Morioka E, et al. Regulation of molecular clock oscillations and phagocytic activity via muscarinic Ca^{2+} signaling in human retinal pigment epithelial cells. Sci Rep. 2017;7:44175.
96. Bulloj A, Maminishkis A, Mizui M, Finnemann SC. Semaphorin4D-PlexinB1 signaling attenuates photoreceptor outer segment phagocytosis by reducing Rac1 activity of RPE cells. Mol Neurobiol. 2017;55(5):4320–32.
97. Gibbs D, Kitamoto J, Williams DS. Abnormal phagocytosis by retinal pigmented epithelium that lacks myosin VIIa, the Usher syndrome 1B protein. Proc Natl Acad Sci U S A. 2003;100(11):6481–6.
98. Udovichenko IP, Gibbs D, Williams DS. Actin-based motor properties of native myosin VIIa. J Cell Sci. 2002;115(Pt 2):445–50.
99. Weil D, Blanchard S, Kaplan J, Guilford P, Gibson F, Walsh J, et al. Defective myosin VIIA gene responsible for Usher syndrome type 1B. Nature. 1995;374(6517):60–1.
100. Petit C. Usher syndrome: from genetics to pathogenesis. Annu Rev Genomics Hum Genet. 2001;2:271–97.
101. Jiang M, Esteve-Rudd J, Lopes VS, Diemer T, Lillo C, Rump A, et al. Microtubule motors transport phagosomes in the RPE, and lack of KLC1 leads to AMD-like pathogenesis. J Cell Biol. 2015;210(4):595–611.
102. Deguchi J, Yamamoto A, Yoshimori T, Sugasawa K, Moriyama Y, Futai M, et al. Acidification of phagosomes and degradation of rod outer segments in rat retinal pigment epithelium. Invest Ophthalmol Vis Sci. 1994;35(2):568–79.
103. Kim IT, Kwak JS. Degradation of phagosomes and diurnal changes of lysosomes in rabbit retinal pigment epithelium. Korean J Ophthalmol. 1996;10(2):82–91.

104. Gordiyenko NV, Fariss RN, Zhi C, MacDonald IM. Silencing of the CHM gene alters phagocytic and secretory pathways in the retinal pigment epithelium. Invest Ophthalmol Vis Sci. 2010;51(2):1143–50.
105. Guha S, Baltazar GC, Coffey EE, Tu LA, Lim JC, Beckel JM, et al. Lysosomal alkalinization, lipid oxidation, and reduced phagosome clearance triggered by activation of the P2X7 receptor. FASEB J. 2013;27(11):4500–9.
106. Liu J, Lu W, Guha S, Baltazar GC, Coffey EE, Laties AM, et al. Cystic fibrosis transmembrane conductance regulator contributes to reacidification of alkalinized lysosomes in RPE cells. Am J Physiol Cell Physiol. 2012;303(2):C160–9.
107. Liu J, Lu W, Reigada D, Nguyen J, Laties AM, Mitchell CH. Restoration of lysosomal pH in RPE cells from cultured human and ABCA4$^{(-/-)}$ mice: pharmacologic approaches and functional recovery. Invest Ophthalmol Vis Sci. 2008;49(2):772–80.
108. Zigler JS Jr, Zhang C, Grebe R, Sehrawat G, Hackler L Jr, Adhya S, et al. Mutation in the betaA3/A1-crystallin gene impairs phagosome degradation in the retinal pigmented epithelium of the rat. J Cell Sci. 2011;124(Pt 4):523–31.
109. Valapala M, Wilson C, Hose S, Bhutto IA, Grebe R, Dong A, et al. Lysosomal-mediated waste clearance in retinal pigment epithelial cells is regulated by CRYBA1/betaA3/A1-crystallin via v-ATPase-mTORC1 signaling. Autophagy. 2014;10(3):480–96.
110. Kim JY, Zhao H, Martinez J, Doggett TA, Kolesnikov AV, Tang PH, et al. Noncanonical autophagy promotes the visual cycle. Cell. 2013;154(2):365–76.
111. Frost LS, Lopes VS, Bragin A, Reyes-Reveles J, Brancato J, Cohen A, et al. The Contribution of melanoregulin to microtubule-associated protein 1 Light Chain 3 (LC3) associated phagocytosis in retinal pigment epithelium. Mol Neurobiol. 2015;52(3):1135–51.
112. Gal A, Li Y, Thompson DA, Weir J, Orth U, Jacobson SG, et al. Mutations in MERTK, the human orthologue of the RCS rat retinal dystrophy gene, cause retinitis pigmentosa. Nat Genet. 2000;26(3):270–1.
113. Thompson DA, McHenry CL, Li Y, Richards JE, Othman MI, Schwinger E, et al. Retinal dystrophy due to paternal isodisomy for chromosome 1 or chromosome 2, with homoallelism for mutations in RPE65 or MERTK, respectively. Am J Hum Genet. 2002;70(1):224–9.
114. McHenry CL, Liu Y, Feng W, Nair AR, Feathers KL, Ding X, et al. MERTK arginine-844-cysteine in a patient with severe rod-cone dystrophy: loss of mutant protein function in transfected cells. Invest Ophthalmol Vis Sci. 2004;45(5):1456–63.
115. Seabra MC, Brown MS, Goldstein JL. Retinal degeneration in choroideremia: deficiency of rab geranylgeranyl transferase. Science. 1993;259(5093):377–81.
116. MacDonald IM, Mah DY, Ho YK, Lewis RA, Seabra MC. A practical diagnostic test for choroideremia. Ophthalmology. 1998;105(9):1637–40.
117. Sergeev YV, Smaoui N, Sui R, Stiles D, Gordiyenko N, Strunnikova N, et al. The functional effect of pathogenic mutations in Rab escort protein 1. Mutat Res. 2009;665(1–2):44–50.
118. Vives-Bauza C, Anand M, Shiraz AK, Magrane J, Gao J, Vollmer-Snarr HR, et al. The age lipid A2E and mitochondrial dysfunction synergistically impair phagocytosis by retinal pigment epithelial cells. J Biol Chem. 2008;283(36):24770–80.
119. Lakkaraju A, Finnemann SC, Rodriguez-Boulan E. The lipofuscin fluorophore A2E perturbs cholesterol metabolism in retinal pigment epithelial cells. Proc Natl Acad Sci U S A. 2007;104(26):11026–31.
120. LaVail MM, Yasumura D, Matthes MT, Yang H, Hauswirth WW, Deng WT, et al. Gene therapy for MERTK-associated retinal degenerations. Adv Exp Med Biol. 2016;854:487–93.
121. Conlon TJ, Deng WT, Erger K, Cossette T, Pang JJ, Ryals R, et al. Preclinical potency and safety studies of an AAV2-mediated gene therapy vector for the treatment of MERTK associated retinitis pigmentosa. Hum Gene Ther Clin Dev. 2013;24(1):23–8.
122. Ghazi NG, Abboud EB, Nowilaty SR, Alkuraya H, Alhommadi A, Cai H, et al. Treatment of retinitis pigmentosa due to MERTK mutations by ocular subretinal injection of adeno-associated virus gene vector: results of a phase I trial. Hum Genet. 2016;135(3):327–43.
123. Yvon C, Ramsden CM, Lane A, Powner MB, da Cruz L, Coffey PJ, et al. Using stem cells to model diseases of the outer retina. Comput Struct Biotechnol J. 2015;13:382–9.
124. Ramsden CM, Nommiste B, Lane AR, Carr AF, Powner MB, Smart MJK, et al. Rescue of the MERTK phagocytic defect in a human iPSC disease model using translational read-through inducing drugs. Sci Rep. 2017;7(1):51.

4 Ion Channels of the Retinal Pigment Epithelium

Nadine Reichhart and Olaf Strauß

Introduction

From the beginning, the evolution of light-sensory organs included the functional association of a pigmented and a light-sensitive cell. This association has developed a complex cooperation between the photoreceptors and the RPE in the vertebrate retina [1–4]. The partnership requires special functions of the RPE that include transepithelial transport of ions and water across the RPE, K^+ buffering in the subretinal space, phagocytosis of daily shed photoreceptor outer segments, and secretion of a variety of factors including neurotrophic, growth or immune modulatory factors. At the same time these RPE functions are strongly depending on ionic mechanisms and therefore on the orchestrated activity of a large variety of ion channels [5, 6]. Since the failure of one of the RPE functions listed above leads to degeneration of photoreceptors and therefore to loss of vision, the investigation of ion channel activity in health and disease is of outmost importance to understand RPE physiology and pathology. This book chapter describes ion channels of the RPE and their roles in RPE function to develop a molecular model of ionic mechanisms in the RPE.

In general, ion channels were identified as targets in a large number of diseases. The research area that investigates the role of ion channels in disease has developed the term "channelopathies" for this group of disease conditions [7–10]. Ion channels contribute to disease by two major causalities. One is that the ion channel cause the disease either by loss or gain of function. Mostly these channelopathies are hereditary diseases where the gene mutant causes either directly the loss/gain of function or indirectly because the mutation affects proteins that regulate ion channel function. Prominent examples for directly caused channelopathies are mutations in ion channels expressed in the myocard to cause longQT syndrome (voltage-gated Ca^{2+}, K^+ and Na^+ channels) [9, 10], myotonia (Cl channels) [7] or cystic fibrosis (ATP-gated Cl channel) [11]. Another way by which ion channels cause diseases is that cells or tissues develop over-activities of ion channels that in turn lead to the pathology. Examples for this condition are cancer cells that promote their own growth by Ca^{2+} channel driven growth factor secretion [12] or upregulation of the $P2X_7$ ATP-receptor channel in immune associated diseases [13, 14]. Thus, given the robust knowledge about the role of ion channels in disease, we have to expect that also in RPE-related diseases ion channels might play a prominent role.

N. Reichhart · O. Strauß (✉)
Experimental Ophthalmology, Department of Ophthalmology, Charité – Universitätsmedizin Berlin, a corporate member of Freie Universität, Humboldt-University, The Berlin Institute of Health, Berlin, Germany
e-mail: Nadine.reichhart@charite.de; olaf.strauss@charite.de

A. K. Klettner, S. Dithmar (eds.), *Retinal Pigment Epithelium in Health and Disease*,
https://doi.org/10.1007/978-3-030-28384-1_4

Ionic Mechanisms of RPE Function

Epithelial Transport

Extracellular fluid is accumulated in the retina by water that moves from the anterior parts of the eye towards the retina driven by intraocular pressure and by local production through the metabolic activity of the retinal neurons. Concomitant to the neuronal activity, the extracellular volume varies with changes of illumination. In the outer retina the RPE keeps the extracellular volume small by a constant transport of water across the epithelium which can be as high as 10.1 μL/cm²/h in the human retina [3, 15]. Mechanisms of ion transport adaptation enable the compensation of changes in extracellular volume in response to illumination changes. Illumination of the retina leads to a transient increase in extracellular volume that shortly recovers [16]. The transport of water is driven by a transepithelial transport of Cl^- across the RPE that generates an osmotic gradient [17–24] (Fig. 4.1). This gradient in turn pulls the water through aquaporin water channels across the RPE [25]. The transepithelial Cl^- transport is an active transport requiring the degradation of ATP, the energy source for the transport activity of Na^+/K^+-ATPases. The apically localized Na^+/K^+-

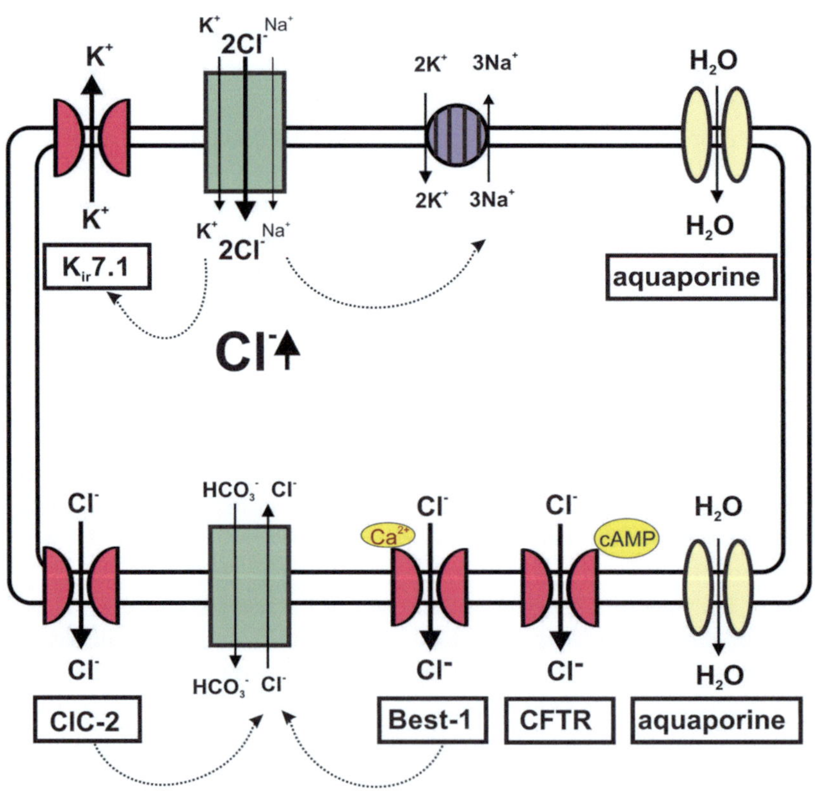

Fig. 4.1 Apical and basolateral mechanisms in epithelial transport of Cl^- and water by the RPE. The apical Na^+/K^+-ATPase generates a Na^+ gradient from extra- to intracellular space that is used by the apical $Na^+/2Cl^-/K^+$-co-transporter to accumulate Cl^- in the intracellular space. K^+ is recycled back to the extracellular space across the apical membrane through inward rectifier channels (Kir.7.1) and keeps the K^+ gradient across the apical membrane small to facilitate the transport processes. Cl^- leaves the cell across the basolateral membrane through divers Cl channels in the basolateral membrane. CCl-2 (member 2 of the CCl chloride channel family) seems to provide the basal conductance; bestrophin-1 (BEST1) and CFTR (cystic fibrosis transmembrane regulator) that are regulated by intracellular messengers can adopt the Cl^- transport. The Cl transport osmotically drives water via the transcellular route through water channels across the RPE

ATPase eliminates Na^+ from intracellular space of the RPE and in turn transports K^+ into RPE cells across its apical membrane. Apically localized K^+ channels led K^+ recycle back to extracellular space that faces the photoreceptors, the subretinal space. As a result, a gradient for Na^+ between the intracellular and the extracellular space of the RPE is generated. The apically localized $Na^+/2Cl^-/K^+$-co-transporter to take up Na^+, K^+ and Cl^- from subretinal space and to transport these ions into the RPE across the apical membrane use that gradient. Since Na^+ and K^+ leave the RPE cell across the apical membrane by the activity of the Na^+/K^+-ATPase and apical K^+ channels, the transport activity of $Na^+/2Cl^-/K^+$-co-transporter results in an accumulation of Cl^- inside the RPE cells leading to intracellular Cl^- concentrations of about 40–60 mM [15, 26, 27]. Finally, the high intracellular Cl^- concentration drives Cl^- out of the RPE across the basolateral membrane to the blood side of the RPE resulting in transepithelial transport of Cl^-.

Ion Channels That Contribute to Transepithelial Ion Transport by the RPE

Apical mechanisms: The key transport activity in the apical membrane is mediated by the $Na^+/2Cl^-/K^+$-co-transporter. The apical Na^+/K^+-ATPase counteracts the uptake of Na^+ into the RPE and at the same time provides the energy for transepithelial ion transport [28]. For Cl^- accumulation inside the cell, K^+ must leave the RPE. This is enabled by a high K^+ conductance of the apical membrane that supports both the activity of the Na^+/K^+-ATPase and the $Na^+/2Cl^-/K^+$-cotransporter. The Na^+/K^+-ATPase removes Na^+ from the intracellular space of the RPE and would accumulate K^+ in the intracellular compartment. However, since K^+ can flow back across the apical membrane through K^+ channels into subretinal space and since the transport capacity of K^+ channels is much higher than that of the Na^+/K^+-ATPase, the K^+ gradient across the apical membrane is kept small. This small K^+ gradient subsequently facilitates the transport activity of the Na^+/K^+-ATPase. Indeed, a non-specific inhibition of apical K^+ channels with blockers such as Ba^{2+} reduces the transepithelial transport by the RPE [20, 29, 30]. In the same way, the apical K^+ channels support the activity of the $Na^+/2Cl^-/K^+$-cotransporter with the difference that its activity is additionally energized by the Na^+/K^+-ATPase. The K^+ channels that provide this function display a large conductance over the resting membrane potential of the RPE and permit outward currents of K^+. These are properties of inwardly rectifying K^+ channels. The most compelling evidence demonstrates the expression of Kir7.1 channels in the RPE.

Basolateral mechanisms: As described above, the transepithelial transport of Cl^- largely depends on the Cl^- efflux pathway across the basolateral membrane of the RPE [31–33]. The activity of a large variety of Cl channels in the basolateral membrane provides this efflux pathway. So far the expression of the Cl channels ClC2 [34, 35], Ano2 (anoctamin-2 or TMEM16B), bestrophin-1 and CFTR (cystic fibrosis transmembrane regulator) was found. This variety of different Cl channels provides a basic conductance on one-hand and Cl^- efflux pathways that adopt the transport activity to the various metabolic needs on the other hand. It is likely that ClC2 is responsible for the basic transport activity. The RPE in ClC2 knockout mice shows no transepithelial potential [34]. Since transepithelial transport of Cl^- and water is linked to pH regulation [36] and transport of lactic acid [37], the pH-dependent ClC2 might is capable to fulfill this task [34]. The other above listed Cl channels are activated by different intracellular second messengers and are therefore Cl channels that adopt the Cl^- transport to different metabolic needs of the retina. The literature identified two major second-messengers: cAMP and Ca^{2+}. Increasing the intracellular cAMP concentration by application of IBMX/forskolin leads to enhanced transepithelial Cl^- transport [38–43]. It is likely that activation of the cAMP-dependent Cl channel CFTR in the RPE is responsible for that mechanism [44]. Several lines of evidence also identified increases in intracellular free Ca^{2+} to stimulate the transepithelial transport of Cl^- across the RPE. For example, application of extracellular ATP increases intracellular free Ca^{2+}

via activation of purinergic receptors and stimulates the Cl^- transport across the RPE. Ca^{2+}-dependent Cl channels represent the key molecules for this effect [45, 46]. Two Ca^{2+}-dependent Cl channels are known to be expressed in the RPE. These are bestrophin-1 [47, 48] and anoctamin-2 [49, 50]. Bestrophin-1 was the first candidate discussed to represent the Ca^{2+}-dependent Cl channel in the RPE [51]. The bestrophin-1 gene, first known as the VMD2 gene (now BEST1), was discovered as the gene that causes the Best vitelliforme macular degeneration [47, 48]. The hallmark of Best's disease is a reduced light-peak of the electro-oculogram. Since the light-peak originates from the depolarization of RPE basolateral membrane that is caused by an increase in the basolateral Cl^- conductance, bestrophin-1 was a very likely candidate [32, 33, 52]. Bestrophin-1 was found to function as a Ca^{2+}-dependent Cl channel in heterologous expression systems [47, 48, 51]. However, RPE cells from either a bestrophin-1 knockout or a mutant bestrophin-1 knock-in mouse model that carries a mutation leading to a loss of function, did not show alterations in the membrane conductance for Cl^- [53, 54]. Thus, endogenously expressed bestrophin-1 does not seem to contribute directly to the Ca^{2+}-dependent Cl conductance. Another candidate to provide the Ca^{2+}-dependent basolateral Cl conductance is anoctamin-2 (Ano2 or TMEM16B) [49, 50]. Ano2 localizes to the basolateral membrane of the RPE and its activity is demonstrated in isolated RPE cells from the mouse or in human cells. It is likely that the list is not complete. Older publications have shown that a considerable number of channels of the ClC family are expressed in the RPE [35, 55]. However, the clarification of their functional relevance needs further clarification.

Several lines of evidence have indicated that the transepithelial Cl^- transport is accompanied by an additional transepithelial transport of K^+ from the apical to the basolateral side of the RPE [15, 17, 20, 24, 29, 56–59]. K^+ enters the RPE at the apical site via the activity of the Na^+/K^+-ATPase. A K^+ channel that provides the efflux pathway across the basolateral membrane might be the so-called M-type currents (muscarinic activated currents) [60]. These ion channels are weakly outwardly rectifying and are active close to the resting membrane voltage of the RPE. The group of Hughes and colleagues could find the expression and activity of KCNQ4 and KCNQ5 channels [61–63]. Most importantly, KCNQ4 and KCNQ5 localize to the basolateral membrane of the RPE and are therefore most likely the K^+ channels that are involved in transepithelial transport of K^+. Another role of these channels might be in the maintenance of the subretinal K^+ homeostasis as will be described below.

Volume-dependent mechanisms: The transport of water across the RPE requires also an efficient volume regulation. That is achieved in the apical membrane by the volume sensitivity of the $Na^+/2Cl^-/K^+$-co-transporter [17, 64]. In the basolateral membrane, volume-sensitive Cl channel help to maintain a stable cell volume. Data from independent groups demonstrated that bestrophin-1 regulates directly or permits the volume regulation via influx of Cl^- into the cell [65, 66].

K^+ Buffering in the Subretinal Space

Light is transduced into changes of the membrane potential of the photoreceptors by the light transduction cascade [67]. In the presence of light, the membrane potential of the photoreceptors is depending on the extracellular and intracellular K^+ concentration difference of the photoreceptors. Thus, precise transduction of light perception depends on stable extracellular K^+ concentrations. Changes in the illumination of photoreceptors, however, principally lead to changes in the extracellular K^+ concentration [3, 29, 56, 68–70]. In the dark, cation channels are open in the photoreceptor outer segments. The inflow of cations into the photoreceptor outer segments is counter-balanced by an outflow of K^+ from the inner segment. When light hits the photoreceptor outer segment, the cation channels there are closed and the outflow of K^+ out of the inner segments becomes smaller. Consequently, the extracellular K^+ concentration in the subretinal space decreases from 5 to 2 mM. When switching from light to darkness the reversed process occurs leading to an increase in subretinal K^+ concentration. These changes are compensated for by the transport activities of the RPE across the apical membrane that occur in response to light-dependent changes in extracellular K^+ concentration [58, 71] (Fig. 4.2). This compensation is enabled by a voltage-dependent modulation of the K^+-conductance of the apical membrane. The compensating activity by the RPE can be measured as a signal in the electroretinogram, the c-wave [3].

These apical compensation mechanisms are only one part of the process of maintenance of the subretinal K^+ homeostasis. According to the model of Dornonville de LaCour, the compensation of subretinal K^+ changes is coupled to the transepithelial transport of K^+ across the RPE

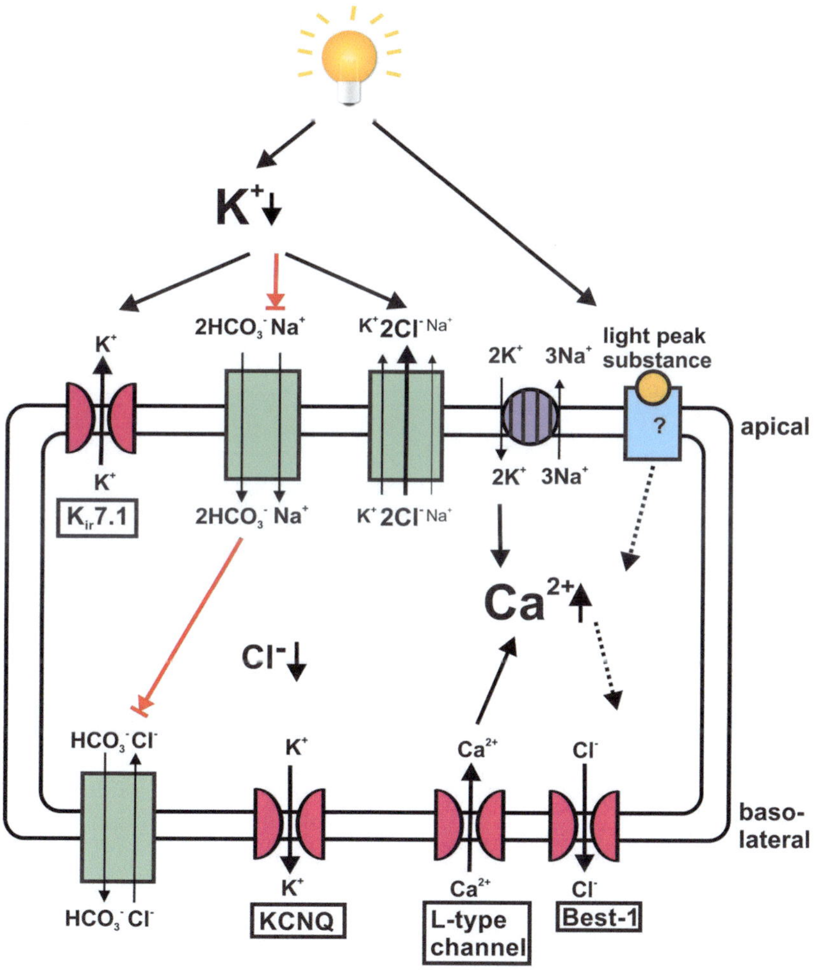

Fig. 4.2 Light-dependent mechanisms of ion transport. Stimulation of photoreceptors by light leads to a decrease of the subretinal K^+ concentration. This change is compensated for by cycling back a proportion of transepithelial transported K^+ across the apical membrane through Kir7.1 channels. The uptake of K^+ via the apical $Na^+/2Cl^-/K^+$-co-transporter and K^+ efflux through basolateral KCNQ voltage-dependent K^+ channels establish the transportation route of K^+ across the RPE. Illumination of the retina releases a so unknown light-peak substance that bind to a receptor at the RPE's apical membrane. This leads to an increase in intracellular free Ca^{2+} under the contribution of L-type Ca^{2+} channels. Ca^{2+} in turn activates Ca^{2+}-dependent Cl channel BEST-1 or Ano2 leading to an increase in transepithelial Cl^- transport and higher transepithelial basolateral negative potential that contributes the electro-oculogram

[58, 71]. This is a sustained transport activity of K^+ from the apical to the basolateral side of the RPE. In the case of illumination of the retina and a subsequent decrease of the subretinal K^+ concentration, the apical membrane hyperpolarizes and the apical K^+ conductance increases [72]. In consequence, an efflux of K^+ across the apical membrane compensates for the decrease in the subretinal K^+ concentration. At the same time, a short-delayed hyperpolarization of the basolateral membrane and a decrease of basolateral K^+ conductance occurs. Thus, the decrease in the subretinal K^+ concentration is compensated by a decrease in transepithelial K^+ transport. In the case of a transition from light to dark, subretinal K^+ increases. The apical membrane conductance decreases, leading to depolarization of apical membrane; this leads to a decrease of the apical K^+ conductance and a reduction of the K^+ efflux across the apical membrane. The basolateral membrane conductance in general and specifically the K^+ efflux via the basolateral membrane increases and thus, stimulates the transepithelial K^+ transport across the RPE. Since the outwardly rectifying K^+ channels KCNQ4 and KCNQ5 that localize to the basolateral membrane increase their conductance with depolarization, they are the ideal candidates for that function. As the Cl^- efflux across the basolateral membrane, that occurs during the transepithelial transport of Cl^- across the RPE, leads to depolarization of the basolateral membrane, the transepithelial transport of K^+ is functionally connected to Cl^- [17, 73].

Ion Channels Contributing to the Control of Subretinal K^+ Homeostasis

The ion channels that contribute to the maintenance of the subretinal K^+ concentration must display inward and outward conductance for K^+ over a large voltage range. These are properties of inward rectifier K^+ channels (family of Kir channels). Furthermore, the inward rectifier should show only a mild rectification and the unique property of increasing conductance with decreasing extracellular K^+ concentrations. Indeed the expression of such an inward rectifier was described from the beginning of the patch-clamp analysis of the RPE of many species [74–79]. The group of Hughes and colleagues were the one who identified the molecular identity of the inward rectifier being Kir7.1 [80–82]. Furthermore, Kir1.7 localizes to the apical processes in the RPE which confirms it functional role [83]. The detection of a mutation in the Ki7.1 channel gene that causes the snowflake vitreoretinal degeneration demonstrates the importance of this channel for the RPE function and retinal stability [84].

Ca^{2+}-Signaling to Regulate RPE Functions

Ca^{2+} ions show a very high affinity to proteins. For that reason, the intracellular free Ca^{2+} concentration in cells is 10,000 times smaller than that of the extracellular space. The high binding affinity of Ca^{2+} to proteins leads to conformational changes of proteins and can be used therefore to regulate protein function [85]. Changes in the concentration of intracellular free Ca^{2+} therefore serve as second-messenger of membrane bound receptors to transfer extracellular signals into changes of cell function. Ca^{2+} as second-messenger stimulates cell proliferation, apoptosis, secretion, neurotransmitter release, phagocytosis, contraction or motility of cells. Indeed, many RPE cell functions are regulated by increases in intracellular changes: regulation of transepithelial transport of ions and water, phagocytosis and secretion [4, 6, 86]. Basically, the RPE contains in melanosomes high intracellular concentrations of Ca^{2+} [87]. It further expresses the NQX1 Na^+/Ca^{2+} exchanger to remove Ca^{2+} from the cytosol [88, 89]. That transporter is the same one that also controls the Ca^{2+} homeostasis in the heart highlighting the ability of the RPE to generate Ca^{2+} signals. Furthermore, a Ca^{2+}-ATPase keeps the cytosolic Ca^{2+} concentration small [90]. Since the RPE shows a rather high basal Ca^{2+} conductance by the activity of TRPC (transient receptor potential channels; canonical subtype) channels [91], the RPE's metabolic investment to the cytosolic Ca^{2+} concentration is comparatively high. The physiological role of this is not known.

With the above-described role of Ca^{2+}, the question arises, how only one single ion, Ca^{2+}, can regulate so many different functions. Specific reactions are coded by the spatial and temporal pattern of the Ca^{2+} signal [85]. The recruitment of different Ca^{2+} transporting mechanisms and Ca^{2+} sources generate specific patterns for control of different cellular functions [92] (Fig. 4.3). Intracellular Ca^{2+} stores can provide very fast Ca^{2+} rises but only for a limited duration. These Ca^{2+} stores are on one hand endoplasmatic Ca^{2+} stores that release Ca^{2+} by stimulation of different mediators such as inositol-1,4,5,-trisphosphate (IP3) or cyclic-ADP-ribose, both reaction products of phospholipases that are activated by G-protein coupled membrane bound receptors. On the other hand, also specialized mitochondria can serve as Ca^{2+} stores and contribute to the spatial and temporal pattern of Ca^{2+} signals. Ca^{2+} signals of longer duration are generated by an influx of extracellular Ca^{2+} into the cell via Ca^{2+}-conducting ion channels in the plasma membrane. The release of Ca^{2+} from Ca^{2+} stores can be coupled to an influx of Ca^{2+} into the cell (store-operated Ca^{2+} entry or SOCE) by a Ca^{2+} sensing protein of Ca^{2+} stores, stim-1 (stromal interacting molecule-1) that directly binds to Ca^{2+} channels in the plasma membrane [93, 94]. Stim-1

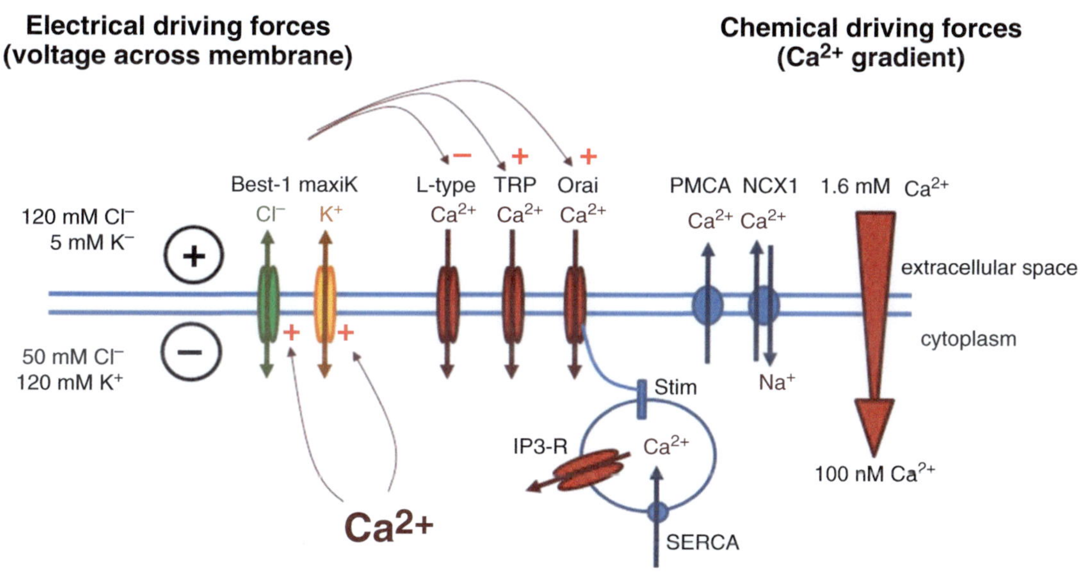

Fig. 4.3 Driving-forces, Ca^{2+} sources and Ca^{2+} channels that define intracellular Ca^{2+} signals. The driving forces that generate Ca^{2+} signals are the transmembranal potential (left) resulting from the activity of Cl and K^+ channels and the extra- and intracellular Cl^- and K^+ concentrations plus the steep Ca^{2+} gradient extra- and intra-cellular space (right). For that gradient various Ca^{2+} transport mechanisms keep the intracellular Ca^{2+} concentration small: Ca^{2+}-ATPases and the Na^+/Ca^{2+}-exchanger in the plasma membrane remove Ca^{2+} from the cytosol by transport into the extracellular space and Ca^{2+}-ATPases that take up Ca^{2+} into cytosolic Ca^{2+}-stores further support by the activity of plasma membrane transporters. Increases in cytosolic free Ca^{2+} result from activation of ion channels in the Ca^{2+}-stores or/and in the plasma membrane. Plasma membrane channels can be voltage-dependent or voltage- independent. Activation of voltage-dependent Ca^{2+} channels (L-type) increase intracellular free Ca^{2+} which in turns activate Ca^{2+}-dependent K^+ channels (maxiK) and terminates the activity of the voltage-dependent Ca^{2+} channel. On the other hand, the activation of non-voltage-dependent Ca^{2+} channels (TRP) activates Ca^{2+}-dependent K^+ channel in the same way but this time it leads to an increase of the driving forces of Ca^{2+} into the cell and larger Ca^{2+} signals. Release of Ca^{2+} from cytosolic Ca^{2+} stores activates the Ca^{2+}-conducting Orai channels via Stim-1 interaction. *Best-1* bestrophin-1, *L-type* L-type channels, *IP3-R* inositol-1,4,5-trisphosphate receptor, *maxiK* Ca^{2+}-dependent K^+ channel of large conductance, *NCX1* Na^+/Ca^{2+}-exchanger-1, *Orai* Icrac channel, *PMCA* plasma membrane Ca^{2+}-ATPase, *SERCA* sarcoplasmic Ca^{2+}-ATPase, *Stim-1* stromal interacting molecule-1, *TRP* transient receptor potential Ca^{2+}-conducting channel. From Strauss [92]

becomes active by a decrease of the Ca^{2+} concentration inside the Ca^{2+} store. Ca^{2+} channels can also be activated by changes in the membrane potential of the cell, mediated by G-proteins, serine/threonine or tyrosine protein kinases. Once a Ca^{2+} conducting ion channel is activated, the amount of Ca^{2+} that enters the cell depends on the electrochemical driving force.

Mechanisms of SOCE have been also described in the RPE. Increasing intracellular IP3 concentration leads to activation of Ca^{2+}-dependent Cl channels via depletion of Ca^{2+} stores and generation of SOCE [95, 96]. This mechanism might be important for the regulation of transepithelial transport of Cl^- across the RPE. For SOCE involved ion channels, the RPE functionally expresses Orai-1 channels and stim-2 [97]. The Ca^{2+}-dependent Cl channel bestrophin-1 seems to play an additional role in this mechanism. A proportion of bestrophin-1 is expressed in the intracellular membranes, those of cytosolic Ca^{2+} stores that are IP3 sensitive [97]. In bestrophin-1 knockout cells ATP-generated Ca^{2+} rises become either smaller or are completely diminished [98]. Bestrophin-1 knockdown by siRNA further reduced the amount of Ca^{2+} that can be released from cytosolic Ca^{2+} stores [97]. Thus bestrophin-1 acts in cytosolic Ca^{2+} stores as Cl channel that transports the counter ion to facilitate movements of Ca^{2+} either in or out of the store.

An important regulator of the Ca^{2+} signals that result from Ca^{2+} influx into the cell is the membrane potential. The more negative the membrane potential gets, the larger is the amplitude of the resulting Ca^{2+} signal [85]. On the other hand, many Ca^{2+} channels are voltage-dependent and activated by depolarization; Ca^{2+} signals become larger with more positive membrane potentials. Also, non-Ca^{2+} conducting ion channels that interact with Ca^{2+} conducting ion channels can determine the amplitude or duration of Ca^{2+} signals via the membrane potential. Ca^{2+}-activated K^+ channels hyperpolarize the membrane potential in response to an increase in intracellular Ca^{2+}. In case the underlying Ca^{2+} signals result from voltage-dependent Ca^{2+} channels, activation of Ca^{2+}-dependent K^+ channels leads to termination of the Ca^{2+} signal. On the other hand, if the K^+ channel activating Ca^{2+} signals results from voltage-independent Ca^{2+} channels, the hyperpolarization leads to a further increase in the Ca^{2+} signal. As will be explained in more detail below, the RPE expresses voltage-dependent L-type Ca^{2+} channels and the Ca^{2+}-dependent K^+ channel maxiK [86, 99–106]. Their activity is closely linked to each other in the RPE. Inhibition of maxiK channels by specific blockers leads to an increase in L-type channel activity [106]. Also for Ca^{2+} signaling mediated by L-type channels, bestrophin-1 acts as a regulator [53, 107–110]. Bestrophin-1 can directly bind to β-subunits of L-type channels and modulate their biophysical properties such as voltage-dependence or surface expression [107, 108, 110]. With bestrophin-1, the overall activity of L-type channels becomes smaller. Ca^{2+}-dependent Cl channels can also interact with Ca^{2+} channels by modulation of the membrane voltage. Their effects, however, depend on the intracellular Cl^- concentration that may vary from cell to cell or may even be heterogeneously distributed over the cell body. Considering the RPE, the intracellular Cl^- concentration is with quite high (40–60 mM). Thus, in the RPE, activation of Cl channels leads to depolarization of the cell membrane and subsequent increase of Ca^{2+} conductance through voltage-dependent Ca^{2+} channels. Since both L-type channels and Ca^{2+}-dependent Cl channels localize to the basolateral membrane [49, 107] their interaction is likely but so far not investigated.

Summary: The RPE expresses a large variety of Ca^{2+} transporters and channels. Furthermore, the electrochemical gradients of K^+ and Cl^- permit indirect regulation of Ca^{2+} transport mechanisms via K^+ and Cl channels. Their complex interplay results in the generation of very specific Ca^{2+} signals that in turn permit a precise regulation of the different functions of the RPE by Ca^{2+} as second-messenger. In the following, Ca^{2+} conducting ion channels and their contribution to regulation of RPE functions will be explained in detail.

Secretion

The RPE is able to secrete a large variety of different growth-factors or cytokines [4, 111]. These factors enable the RPE to interact with its neighboring tissues: the photoreceptors at the apical side and the endothelium of the choriocapillaris and systemic immune cells at the basolateral side. Among these factors, VEGF-A (vascular-endothelial growth factor-A) [111–113] and PEDF (pigment-epithelium-derived factor) [114, 115] are the most prominent ones. VEGF-A is secreted to the basolateral side of the RPE towards the endothelial cells of the choriocapillaris. This constant secretion is required to maintain the stability but also to maintain the fenestrated structure of choroidal endothelium [112]. On the other hand, PEDF is secreted to apical side of the RPE where it acts as a neurotrophic factor to maintain the structural and functional integrity of photoreceptors and retinal neurons [114, 115]. As in many secreting tissues or in the presynaptic terminals, Ca^{2+} signaling regulates the exocytosis process and the secretion underlying changes in the gene expression. So far, two Ca^{2+} conducting ion channels were found to increase intracellular free Ca^{2+} to increase the release of VEGF-A (Fig. 4.4).

L-type Ca^{2+} channels: Originally, L-type channels were defined by their long-lasting currents and the fact that they are activated by a low-voltage; two properties that had given the "L" in

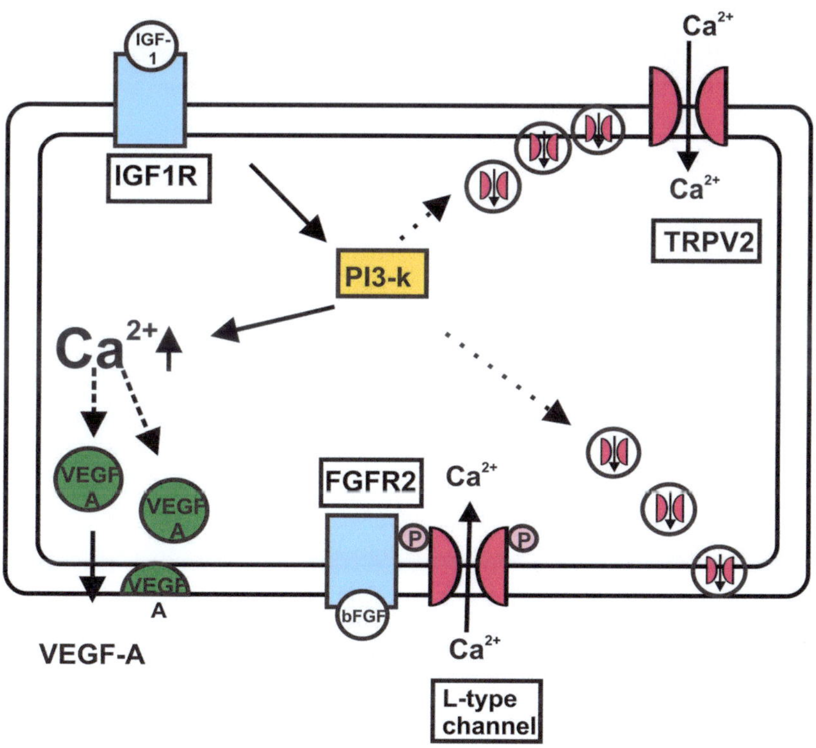

Fig. 4.4 Regulation of secretion by the Ca^{2+} channels L-type and TRPV2. Increase in intracellular free Ca^{2+} represents the trigger for the release of VEGF-A from the RPE cell in to the extracellular space. The underlying Ca^{2+} signals are either generated by activation of L-type Ca^{2+} channels or TRPV2 channels. L-type channels are generally activated by tyrosine kinases. bFGF stimulates VEGF-A secretion by direct interaction of the bFGF receptor FGFR2 and the L-type channel protein that leads to phosphorylation of the L-type channel protein. IGF-1 leads to increased VEGF-A secretion by activation of TRPV2 channels through activation of the PI3-kinase that in turn increases the TRPV2 channel activity and the surface expression of the TRPV2 channel protein in the plasma membrane. *bFGF* basic fibroblast growth-factor or fibroblast growth-factor-2, *FGFR2* receptor for fibroblast growth-factor 2, *IGF1R* receptor for insulin-like growth factor, *L-type channel* L-type voltage-dependent Ca^{2+} channel, *PI3-k* phosphoinosit-3-kinase, *TRPV2* transient receptor potential channel—vanilloid subtype 2, *VEGF-A* vascular endothelial growth-factor-A

L-type [116]. These channels belong to a family of four genes coding for the pore-forming α-subunit that define their biophysical/pharmacological properties: $Ca_V1.1$ (formerly α1S subunit) expressed mainly in the skeletal muscle, $Ca_V1.2$ (formerly α1C subunit) expressed mainly in smooth-muscle cells and neurons, $Ca_V1.3$ (formerly the α1D subunit) expressed in neuroendocrine cells and the $Ca_V1.4$ subunit (formerly α1D) uniquely expressed in photoreceptor terminals [116]. Earliest investigations of ion channels in the RPE indicated the expression of L-type channels that was confirmed by many groups and for RPE cells of many species [86, 100, 102–104, 117]. L-type channels of the RPE were identified as the $Ca_V1.3$ subunit [86, 100, 104] that is also expressed for example in neuroendocrine cells such as the β-cells of the pancreas. Thus, the L-type channels are good candidates for the regulation of secretion by the RPE. The influence of L-type channels on cell function can be rather easily investigated by the use of substances that represent specific blockers, the dihydropyridine derivatives [116]. Indeed the basal secretion of VEGF-A depends on the activity of these channels as it can be shown by measuring the concentration of VEGF-A in the supernatant of RPE cells in the presence of dihydropyridines [86, 118, 119]. Also stimuli that increase the secretion of VEGF-A act partly via the activation of L-type channels in the RPE. For example, bFGF (basic fibroblast growth factor or fibroblast growth factor-2) can increase intracellular free Ca^{2+} and VEGF-A secretion via the activation of L-type channels [120]. This occurs by a mechanism that involves the direct interaction of the L-type channel protein with bFGF-receptor FGFR2. The stimulation of FGFR2 in RPE cells leads to direct binding of FGFR2 to the $Ca_V1.3$ subunit which in turns lead to tyrosine-phosphorylation of the $Ca_V1.3$ subunit. This in turn shifts the voltage-dependence of these channels and the activation threshold closer towards the resting potential of RPE cells that increase its activity and intracellular free Ca^{2+} [120]. Both tyrosine-kinase and L-type channel inhibition lead to a reduction of the bFGF stimulated VEGF-A secretion. The shift in the voltage-dependence by tyrosine-phosphorylation represents an important mechanism for the regulation of L-type channel activity in the RPE. Tyrosine-kinase activity by the src-kinase is required to maintain the basic activity [100]. Without the constant phosphorylation, the channel shows a quick run-down of its activity. This regulation of the activity of L-type channels and subsequently the VEGF-A secretion might also play a role in the development of choroidal neovascularization (CNV), the most severe complication of wet AMD. Investigation of ion channels in RPE cells that were freshly isolated from CNV membranes indicated different kinetic properties and higher activity [121]. Indeed these cells showed a higher VEGF-A secretion that was dependent on the activity of L-type channels. Thus, it was concluded that an environment of growth-factors and extracellular matrix proteins might lead to higher tyrosine-phosphorylation activity and therefore L-type channel activity leading to higher secretion rates. Not only might the control of the angiogenic activity in the outer retina by the RPE be under influence of L-type channel-dependent secretion. The control of local immune responses by the RPE to maintain the immune privilege of the eye depends also on the secretion of immune suppressive factors by the RPE. Since L-type channels of $Ca_V1.3$ subtype that are prominent regulators of secretion are expressed in the RPE these Ca^{2+} channels might be also involved in that function. Indeed complement signaling at the RPE is supporting this hypothesis [122, 123]. Exposure of RPE cells to active complement components increases intracellular free Ca^{2+} as second messenger by activation of endogenously expressed ion channels. Although this has not been investigated in detail, it appears that activation of L-type channels via ryanodine-receptors plays an important role. Exposure of RPE cells to human serum as source of complement leads to an increase in intracellular free Ca^{2+} that can be blocked by dihydropyridines. Analysis of complement-driven secretion of VEGF-A shows that complement-dependent activation of L-type channels represents a major pathway and stimulates secretion [124–126].

TRPV2 channels: The human body expresses a large variety of Ca^{2+}- conducting ion channels of the TRP (transient receptor potential) channel family [127]. These TRP channels are multimodal channels by their activation mechanisms and are involved in signal transduction in sensory cells or regulate a plethora of different cells functions. In addition, the RPE expresses a variety of TRP channels, among them the TRPV2 channel (TRP-vanilloid subtype-2) [128–130]. In the RPE it serves to increase intracellular free Ca^{2+} in response to a variety of extracellular stimuli. For example the activation of angiotensin-2-receptors of the subtype 1 (AT1) generate Ca^{2+} signals via activation of TRPV2 channels via a signaling cascade that requires the activation of phospholipase-C, the generation of inositol-1,4,5-trisphosphate and activation of PI3-kinase (phosphoinosit-3-kinase) [128]. The same pathway activates TRPV2 channels in response to stimulation of RPE cells by IGF-1 (insulin-growth-factor-1) [129, 130]. IGF-1 leads not only to an increase of the channel activity per se but also to an increase in the number TRPV2 channel proteins in the RPE plasma membrane [130]. Interestingly, IGF-1 is a strong activator of the VEGF-A secretion by the RPE. In fact, the potency of IGF-1 to stimulate the VEGF-A secretion is larger than that by bFGF. Using blockers or siRNA approaches against TRPV2 it could be demonstrated that indeed the IGF-1-dependent activation of TRPV2 leads to an increased release of VEGF-A by RPE cells [129]. TRPV2 seems also to have an impact in retinal degenerations by its activation mechanisms. First, IGF-1 signaling might be an important player in the pathomechanisms leading to age-related macular degeneration [131–134]. IGF-1 expression in photoreceptors is upregulated in eyes from patients with age-related macular degeneration but not in age-matched controls [132]. Since the RPE expresses IGF-1 receptors, it is implied that IGF-1 secretion by photoreceptors gives a signal to the RPE. Since IGF-1 can activate VEGF-A secretion via TRPV2 activation this signal from the photoreceptors might be one of the triggers for the development of CNV. Second, TRPV2 channels are heat-sensitive [129]. This property might not be the physiological role of TRPV2 channels in the RPE because they are mainly involved in AngII or IGF-1 signaling. However, the heat-sensitivity implies an explanation for the therapeutic effects of laser treatments in the outer retina. RPE cells that are not directly exposed to the laser beam but are in the close neighborhood are heated up enough to activate TRPV2 channels. This in turn might provoke the secretion of growth-factors such as VEGF-A or cytokines. This might be even more effective in the pro-angiogenic environment in age-related macular degeneration. Here the presence of IGF-1 would increase the number of TRPV2 channels in the RPE plasma membrane and the heat pulse will affect the RPE function much stronger.

Summary: The RPE's expression of Ca^{2+}-conducting ion channels is that of a secreting cell. So far, two Ca^{2+}-conducting ion channels have been reported to regulate the secretion of VEGF-A, L-type channel $Ca_V1.3$ and TRPV2. These channels are activated by different signaling pathways and link therefore the VEGF-A secretion to different specialized extracellular stimuli.

Epithelial Transport

The basic mechanism of epithelial transport and the involvement of ion channels is described above. A key-role in the transepithelial transport of Cl^- across the RPE plays the Cl^- conductance of the basolateral membrane. An increase in the basolateral Cl^- conductance increases the transepithelial transport. Thus, the regulation of basolateral Cl channels provides the most important control of the transepithelial transport. This task might be dependent on the activity of the Ca^{2+}-dependent Cl channel anoctamin-2 (see above). The Ca^{2+}-signaling that controls Ca^{2+}-dependent Cl channels of the RPE involves release of Ca^{2+} from cytosolic Ca^{2+} stores and Ca^{2+} channels. Indeed direct intracellular application of IP3 in a patch-clamp experiment via the recording pipette leads to activation of Ca^{2+}-dependent Cl channels in RPE cells by both Ca^{2+} from intracellular stores and SOCE [95, 96]. This might be the underlying mechanism how extracellular ATP increases transepithelial transport of Cl^- across the RPE [45, 46]. ATP binds to P2Y receptors that in turn lead to releases of Ca^{2+} from cytosolic Ca^{2+} stores. The ion channel that provides the Ca^{2+} influx into cell to generate longer lasting signals is not known. It might by the L-type Ca^{2+} channel because its voltage-dependence can be changed by intracellular IP3 application towards higher ion channel activity [135]. This in turn leads to an increase in cytosolic free Ca^{2+}. Measurements of the DC-ERG in mice that correspond with the electro-oculogram in humans [136] support this hypothesis *in vivo* [3, 53]. These recordings measure the amplitude of the so-called light rise that results from a more negative potential between the cornea and the posterior pole of the eye [136]. This potential is determined from the Cl^- efflux across the basolateral membrane of the RPE [32, 33, 52, 137] (Fig. 4.2). The DC-ERG in L-type channel $Ca_V1.3$ knockout mice shows a smaller amplitude than that of the wild-type littermates [138]. Thus, the activity of L-type channels is required to increase the basolateral Cl^- conductance. Another regulator of the basolateral Cl^- conductance is bestrophin-1 [53, 54, 109, 139]. It can directly interact with the L-type channel protein and reduce the L-type channel activity [107, 108, 110]. Furthermore, bestrophin-1 interferes with the Ca^{2+} homeostasis of intracellular Ca^{2+} stores that in turn mediates the regulation of transepithelial Cl^- transport [97, 98, 140]. Again, measurements of the DC-ERG in mice might support this hypothesis. The light-rise becomes larger in bestrophin-1 knockout mice compared to the wild-type littermates [53]. Considering bestrophin-1 being an inhibitor of the L-type channels, then the loss of bestrophin-1 leads to higher activity and stronger activation of transepithelial transport of Cl^-. Since a decreased light-rise in the electro-oculogram represents the hallmark for the diagnosis of Best's vitelliforme macular dystrophy that is caused by mutations in the gene of bestrophin-1, these mechanisms might play a role in degenerative diseases of the macula [47, 48]. However, the precise patho-mechanisms are not yet understood.

Summary: Together with CFTR the Ca^{2+}-dependent Cl channel anoctamin-2 is a regulator of transepithelial Cl^- transport. The underlying regulation Ca^{2+} signaling involves the activation of purinergic receptors, release of Ca^{2+} from cytosolic stores and SOCE. Ion channels that are involved in the regulation of transepithelial transport are likely bestrophin-1 and L-type channels.

Phagocytosis

One of the most important function of the RPE is its involvement in the daily regeneration of the photoreceptor outer segments [1, 2, 4, 141]. New outer segments are formed from the base of the photoreceptor cilium and the destroyed tips are phagocytosed by the RPE. This process is regulated in a circadian manner and takes place in the morning after opening of the eyes [142, 143]. Ion channels are directly involved in this process by contributing to the required volume regulation (Fig. 4.5). Here bestrophin-1 might be the most important ion channel [65, 66]. The ability of the RPE to increase the Cl^- conductance in response to volume increase depends on the presence of bestrophin-1. The role of bestrophin-1 might be either the formation of the volume-dependent Cl channel or the contribution to regulate volume-dependent Cl channels. The exact mechanism is not clear but the hypothesis that bestrophin-1 forms the volume-activated Cl channel seems to be in favor.

Ionic mechanisms probably regulate the interaction between the photoreceptors and the RPE in this process. An important role might play ATP-dependent signaling via purinergic receptors and the release of ATP from the RPE serving for autocrine and paracrine stimulation [144–146]. Here, the activation of P2Y receptors in particular plays the most important role. The intracellular effects in the RPE are the regulation and preparation of the lysosomal system to establish the requirements for digestion of phagocytosed material. As described above ion channels contribute directly in P2Y signaling such as Ano2. In this process, the Cl^- channel CFTR has the double role to participate the process of ATP release by the RPE [147] and in the establishment of an acidic pH in lysosomes [148].

Another role of ion channels in the regulation of phagocytosis might be the control of the circadian rhythm of the phagocytosis [99] (Fig. 4.5). Analysis of the phagocytosis of maxiK knockout

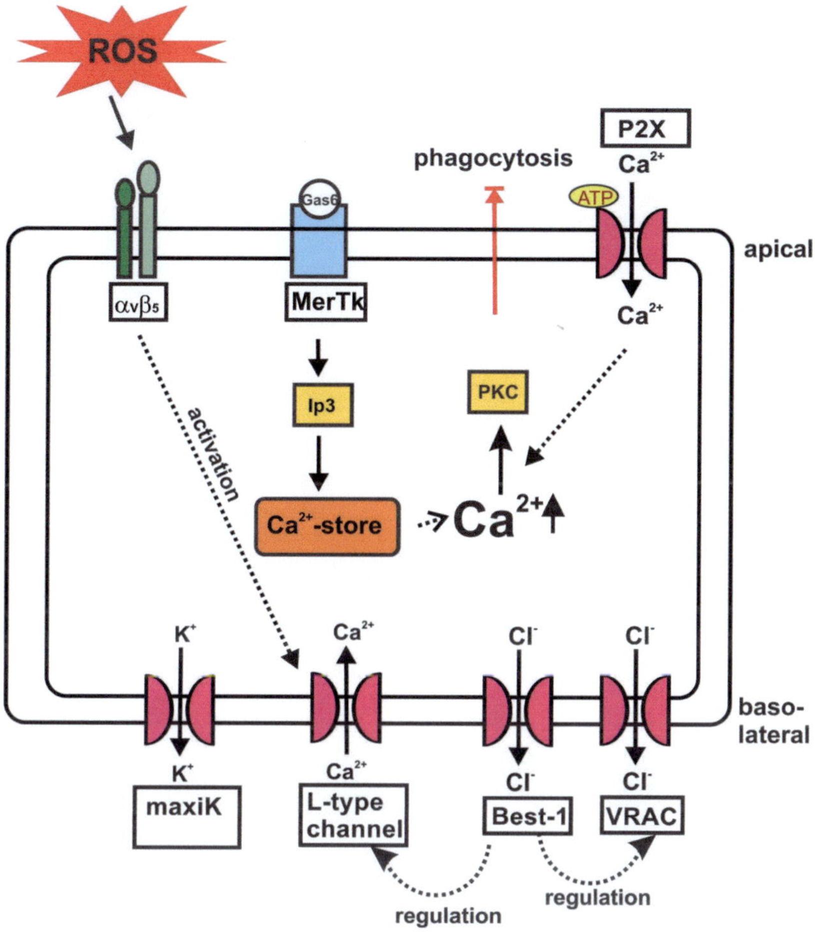

Fig. 4.5 Potential role of ion channels in the regulation of phagocytosis. Role of direct activation: Activation of MerTK probably by Gas6 represents one of the most important trigger for the uptake of photoreceptor outer segments. Since MerTK activation leads to generation of IP3 it is likely that activation of IP3-receptor ion channels in cytosolic Ca^{2+} stores is involved in the process. Volume regulation: uptake of large amounts of phagocytosed material requires an efficient volume regulation. The underlying volume-regulatory increase in the membrane conductance provides bestrophin-1 either directly as ion channel or as regulator of volume-activated ion channels. Circadian rhythm: Knockout mice indicate that L-type channels and Ca^{2+}-dependent maxiK channels contribute to the circadian regulation of phagocytosis. L-type channels might activated by $\alpha_V\beta_5$ integrins and regulated by bestrophin-1. A possible but unproven involvement comes from the ATP receptor P2X which is a ligand gated Ca^{2+} channel. *Gas6* Growth-arrest-specific gene-6, *IP3* inositol-1,4,5-trisphosphate, *L-type channel* L-type voltage-dependent Ca^{2+} channel, *MerTK* tyrosine kinase Mer, *PKC* protein kinase-C, *P2X* purinergic receptor 2X

mice shows an earlier rise of the phagocytic activity in the morning [99]. On the other hand, $Ca_V1.3$ knockout mice display a smaller peak of phagocytic activity in the morning but a higher resting activity in the afternoon [99]. Interestingly, the $Ca_V1.3$ mRNA expression varies over time. It is higher in the afternoon compared to the morning meaning that a lower $Ca_V{\cdot}1.3$ activity is required for the increase in phagocytic activity in the morning. Studies about the role of integrins in the regulation of phagocytosis might provide a mechanistic link for this hypothesis. $\alpha_V\beta5$ integrin knockout mice show a loss of circadian rhythm of phagocytosis that is characterized by the absence of the morning peak and increased activity during the day [149]. In vitro studies showed that soluble vitronectin is a ligand of α_V-integrin inhibits the activity of L-type channels in the RPE via src-kinase-dependent phosphorylation [150]. However, the exact mechanism needs further clarification. The role of ATP signaling at the RPE might imply the participation of another ion channel, the P2X receptor. The P2X receptor is an ATP-gated ion channel that conducts Ca^{2+} and is expressed by the RPE [151]. If ATP signaling is required for phagocytosis then Ca^{2+} signals evoked by stimulation of P2X receptors might play a role in the ionic mechanisms that control phagocytosis.

The interaction of bestrophin-1 and $Ca_V1.3$ Ca^{2+} channels and the observation that these two proteins are likely involved in phagocytosis possibly identify a function of the RPE that might be disturbed in the development of Best's vitelliforme macular degeneration [99]. It might be that a disturbed regulation of phagocytosis leads to the accumulation of lipofuscin in the RPE and to retinal degeneration.

Summary: The role of ion channels in phagocytosis is less understood. There might be a direct contribution by volume regulation and an indirect contribution by regulation of the circadian rhythm of phagocytosis.

Summary

Activation or deactivation of ion channels permit or regulate almost every function of cells. Analysis of the RPE *in vivo* and *in vitro* revealed a large variety of ion channels expressed in the RPE. The profile of this ion channel expression is tailor-made to participate in the RPE functions K^+ homeostasis in the RPE surrounding environment, transepithelial transport of water driven by transport of Cl^- ions, secretion and phagocytosis. The analysis how these ion channels contribute to RPE function does not only permit a better understanding of these functions including new insights but helps also to decipher new pathomechanisms that lead to retinal degeneration. The analysis of ion channels of the RPE in relation to their functional role will help to understand RPE function and probably lead to new targets to treat disease.

References

1. Bok D. The retinal pigment epithelium: a versatile partner in vision. J Cell Sci Suppl. 1993;17:189–95.
2. Sparrow JR, Hicks D, Hamel CP. The retinal pigment epithelium in health and disease. Curr Mol Med. 2010;10(9):802–23.
3. Steinberg RH. Interactions between the retinal pigment epithelium and the neural retina. Doc Ophthalmol. 1985;60(4):327–46.
4. Strauss O. The retinal pigment epithelium in visual function. Physiol Rev. 2005;85(3):845–81.
5. Reichhart N, Strauss O. Ion channels and transporters of the retinal pigment epithelium. Exp Eye Res. 2014;126:27–37. https://doi.org/10.1016/j.exer.2014.05.005.
6. Wimmers S, Karl MO, Strauss O. Ion channels in the RPE. Prog Retin Eye Res. 2007;26(3):263–301. https://doi.org/10.1016/j.preteyeres.2006.12.002.
7. Jentsch TJ, Pusch M. CLC chloride channels and transporters: structure, function, physiology, and disease. Physiol Rev. 2018;98(3):1493–590. https://doi.org/10.1152/physrev.00047.2017.
8. Jurkat-Rott K, Lerche H, Weber Y, Lehmann-Horn F. Hereditary channelopathies in neurology. Adv Exp Med Biol. 2010;686:305–34. https://doi.org/10.1007/978-90-481-9485-8_18.
9. Lehmann-Horn F, Jurkat-Rott K. Voltage-gated ion channels and hereditary disease. Physiol Rev. 1999;79(4):1317–72. https://doi.org/10.1152/physrev.1999.79.4.1317.
10. Skinner JR, Winbo A, Abrams D, Vohra J, Wilde AA. Channelopathies that lead to sudden cardiac death: clinical and genetic aspects. Heart Lung Circ. 2019;28(1):22–30. https://doi.org/10.1016/j.hlc.2018.09.007.
11. Mehta A. CFTR: more than just a chloride channel. Pediatr Pulmonol. 2005;39(4):292–8. https://doi.org/10.1002/ppul.20147.
12. Mergler S, Drost A, Bechstein WO, Neuhaus P, Wiedenmann B. Ca(2+) channel properties in neuroendocrine tumor cell cultures investigated by whole-cell patch-clamp technique. Ann N Y Acad Sci. 2004;1014:137–9.
13. De Marchi E, Orioli E, Dal Ben D, Adinolfi E. P2X7 receptor as a therapeutic target. Adv Protein Chem Struct Biol. 2016;104:39–79. https://doi.org/10.1016/bs.apcsb.2015.11.004.
14. Savio LEB, de Andrade Mello P, da Silva CG, Coutinho-Silva R. The P2X7 receptor in inflammatory diseases: Angel or Demon? Front Pharmacol. 2018;9:52. https://doi.org/10.3389/fphar.2018.00052.
15. Hughes BA, Gallemore RP, Miller SS. Transport mechanisms in the retinal pigment epithelium. In: Marmor MF, Wolfensberger TJ, editors. The retinal pigment epithelium. New York, Oxford: Oxford University Press; 1998. p. 103–34.

16. Li JD, Gallemore RP, Dmitriev A, Steinberg RH. Light-dependent hydration of the space surrounding photoreceptors in chick retina. Invest Ophthalmol Vis Sci. 1994;35(6):2700–11.
17. Bialek S, Miller SS. K+ and Cl- transport mechanisms in bovine pigment epithelium that could modulate subretinal space volume and composition. J Physiol. 1994;475(3):401–17.
18. DiMattio J, Degnan KJ, Zadunaisky JA. A model for transepithelial ion transport across the isolated retinal pigment epithelium of the frog. Exp Eye Res. 1983;37(5):409–20.
19. Edelman JL, Lin H, Miller SS. Potassium-induced chloride secretion across the frog retinal pigment epithelium. Am J Physiol. 1994;266(4 Pt 1):C957–66.
20. Gallemore RP, Hernandez E, Tayyanipour R, Fujii S, Steinberg RH. Basolateral membrane Cl- and K+ conductances of the dark-adapted chick retinal pigment epithelium. J Neurophysiol. 1993;70(4):1656–68.
21. Hu JG, Gallemore RP, Bok D, Frambach DA. Chloride transport in cultured fetal human retinal pigment epithelium. Exp Eye Res. 1996;62(4):443–8.
22. Joseph DP, Miller SS. Apical and basal membrane ion transport mechanisms in bovine retinal pigment epithelium. J Physiol. 1991;435:439–63.
23. La Cour M. Cl- transport in frog retinal pigment epithelium. Exp Eye Res. 1992;54(6):921–31.
24. Miller SS, Edelman JL. Active ion transport pathways in the bovine retinal pigment epithelium. J Physiol. 1990;424:283–300.
25. Hamann S. Molecular mechanisms of water transport in the eye. Int Rev Cytol. 2002;215:395–431.
26. Wiederholt M, Zadunaisky JA. Decrease of intracellular chloride activity by furosemide in frog retinal pigment epithelium. Curr Eye Res. 1984;3(4):673–5.
27. Yamashita H, Yamamoto T. Changes in distribution of chloride ions in embryonic chicken retinal pigment epithelium. Jpn J Ophthalmol. 1990;34(1):22–9.
28. Frambach DA, Roy CE, Valentine JL, Weiter JJ. Precocious retinal adhesion is affected by furosemide and ouabain. Curr Eye Res. 1989;8(6):553–6.
29. Griff ER, Shirao Y, Steinberg RH. Ba2+ unmasks K+ modulation of the Na+-K+ pump in the frog retinal pigment epithelium. J Gen Physiol. 1985;86(6):853–76.
30. Hughes BA, Shaikh A, Ahmad A. Effects of Ba2+ and Cs+ on apical membrane K+ conductance in toad retinal pigment epithelium. Am J Physiol. 1995;268(5 Pt 1):C1164–72.
31. Gallemore RP, Griff ER, Steinberg RH. Evidence in support of a photoreceptoral origin for the "light-peak substance". Invest Ophthalmol Vis Sci. 1988;29(4):566–71.
32. Gallemore RP, Steinberg RH. Effects of DIDS on the chick retinal pigment epithelium. I. Membrane potentials, apparent resistances, and mechanisms. J Neurosci. 1989;9(6):1968–76.
33. Gallemore RP, Steinberg RH. Effects of DIDS on the chick retinal pigment epithelium. II. Mechanism of the light peak and other responses originating at the basal membrane. J Neurosci. 1989;9(6):1977–84.
34. Bosl MR, Stein V, Hubner C, Zdebik AA, Jordt SE, Mukhopadhyay AK, Davidoff MS, Holstein AF, Jentsch TJ. Male germ cells and photoreceptors, both dependent on close cell-cell interactions, degenerate upon ClC-2 Cl(-) channel disruption. EMBO J. 2001;20(6):1289–99.
35. Wills NK, Weng T, Mo L, Hellmich HL, Yu A, Wang T, Buchheit S, Godley BF. Chloride channel expression in cultured human fetal RPE cells: response to oxidative stress. Invest Ophthalmol Vis Sci. 2000;41(13):4247–55.
36. Keller SK, Jentsch TJ, Janicke I, Wiederholt M. Regulation of intracellular pH in cultured bovine retinal pigment epithelial cells. Pflugers Arch. 1988;411(1):47–52.
37. Hamann S, la Cour M, Lui GM, Bundgaard M, Zeuthen T. Transport of protons and lactate in cultured human fetal retinal pigment epithelial cells. Pflugers Arch. 2000;440(1):84–92.
38. Hughes BA, Miller SS, Farber DB. Adenylate cyclase stimulation alters transport in frog retinal pigment epithelium. Am J Physiol. 1987;252(4 Pt 1):C385–95.
39. Hughes BA, Miller SS, Joseph DP, Edelman JL. cAMP stimulates the Na+-K+ pump in frog retinal pigment epithelium. Am J Physiol. 1988;254(1 Pt 1):C84–98.
40. Hughes BA, Miller SS, Machen TE. Effects of cyclic AMP on fluid absorption and ion transport across frog retinal pigment epithelium. Measurements in the open-circuit state. J Gen Physiol. 1984;83(6):875–99.
41. Hughes BA, Segawa Y. cAMP-activated chloride currents in amphibian retinal pigment epithelial cells. J Physiol. 1993;466:749–66.
42. Miller S, Farber D. Cyclic AMP modulation of ion transport across frog retinal pigment epithelium. Measurements in the short-circuit state. J Gen Physiol. 1984;83(6):853–74.
43. Nao-i N, Gallemore RP, Steinberg RH. Effects of cAMP and IBMX on the chick retinal pigment epithelium. Membrane potentials and light-evoked responses. Invest Ophthalmol Vis Sci. 1990;31(1):54–66.
44. Blaug S, Quinn R, Quong J, Jalickee S, Miller SS. Retinal pigment epithelial function: a role for CFTR? Doc Ophthalmol. 2003;106(1):43–50.
45. Maminishkis A, Jalickee S, Blaug SA, Rymer J, Yerxa BR, Peterson WM, Miller SS. The P2Y(2) receptor agonist INS37217 stimulates RPE fluid transport in vitro and retinal reattachment in rat. Invest Ophthalmol Vis Sci. 2002;43(11):3555–66.
46. Peterson WM, Meggyesy C, Yu K, Miller SS. Extracellular ATP activates calcium signaling, ion, and fluid transport in retinal pigment epithelium. J Neurosci. 1997;17(7):2324–37.

47. Hartzell HC, Qu Z, Yu K, Xiao Q, Chien LT. Molecular physiology of bestrophins: multifunctional membrane proteins linked to best disease and other retinopathies. Physiol Rev. 2008;88(2):639–72. https://doi.org/10.1152/physrev.00022.2007.
48. Johnson AA, Guziewicz KE, Lee CJ, Kalathur RC, Pulido JS, Marmorstein LY, Marmorstein AD. Bestrophin 1 and retinal disease. Prog Retin Eye Res. 2017;58:45–69. https://doi.org/10.1016/j.preteyeres.2017.01.006.
49. Keckeis S, Reichhart N, Roubeix C, Strauss O. Anoctamin2 (TMEM16B) forms the Ca2+-activated Cl- channel in the retinal pigment epithelium. Exp Eye Res. 2017;154:139–50. https://doi.org/10.1016/j.exer.2016.12.003.
50. Schreiber R, Kunzelmann K. Expression of anoctamins in retinal pigment epithelium (RPE). Pflugers Arch. 2016;468(11–12):1921–9. https://doi.org/10.1007/s00424-016-1898-2.
51. Sun H, Tsunenari T, Yau KW, Nathans J. The vitelliform macular dystrophy protein defines a new family of chloride channels. Proc Natl Acad Sci U S A. 2002;99(6):4008–13.
52. Gallemore RP, Steinberg RH. Light-evoked modulation of basolateral membrane Cl- conductance in chick retinal pigment epithelium: the light peak and fast oscillation. J Neurophysiol. 1993;70(4):1669–80.
53. Marmorstein LY, Wu J, McLaughlin P, Yocom J, Karl MO, Neussert R, Wimmers S, Stanton JB, Gregg RG, Strauss O, Peachey NS, Marmorstein AD. The light peak of the electroretinogram is dependent on voltage-gated calcium channels and antagonized by bestrophin (best-1). J Gen Physiol. 2006;127(5):577–89. https://doi.org/10.1085/jgp.200509473.
54. Zhang Y, Stanton JB, Wu J, Yu K, Hartzell HC, Peachey NS, Marmorstein LY, Marmorstein AD. Suppression of Ca2+ signaling in a mouse model of Best disease. Hum Mol Genet. 2010;19(6):1108–18. https://doi.org/10.1093/hmg/ddp583.
55. Weng TX, Godley BF, Jin GF, Mangini NJ, Kennedy BG, Yu AS, Wills NK. Oxidant and antioxidant modulation of chloride channels expressed in human retinal pigment epithelium. Am J Physiol Cell Physiol. 2002;283(3):C839–49.
56. Bialek S, Joseph DP, Miller SS. The delayed basolateral membrane hyperpolarization of the bovine retinal pigment epithelium: mechanism of generation. J Physiol. 1995;484(Pt 1):53–67.
57. Dornonville de la Cour M. Ion transport in the retinal pigment epithelium. A study with double barrelled ion-selective microelectrodes. Acta Ophthalmol Suppl. 1993;(209):1–32.
58. la Cour M. The retinal pigment epithelium controls the potassium activity in the subretinal space. Acta Ophthalmol Suppl. 1985;173:9–10.
59. Quinn RH, Miller SS. Ion transport mechanisms in native human retinal pigment epithelium. Invest Ophthalmol Vis Sci. 1992;33(13):3513–27.
60. Takahira M, Hughes BA. Isolated bovine retinal pigment epithelial cells express delayed rectifier type and M-type K+ currents. Am J Physiol. 1997;273(3 Pt 1):C790–803.
61. Pattnaik BR, Hughes BA. Effects of KCNQ channel modulators on the M-type potassium current in primate retinal pigment epithelium. Am J Physiol Cell Physiol. 2012;302(5):C821–33. https://doi.org/10.1152/ajpcell.00269.2011.
62. Zhang X, Hughes BA. KCNQ and KCNE potassium channel subunit expression in bovine retinal pigment epithelium. Exp Eye Res. 2013;116:424–32.
63. Zhang X, Yang D, Hughes BA. KCNQ5/K(v)7.5 potassium channel expression and subcellular localization in primate retinal pigment epithelium and neural retina. Am J Physiol Cell Physiol. 2011;301(5):C1017–26. https://doi.org/10.1152/ajpcell.00185.2011.
64. Adorante JS, Miller SS. Potassium-dependent volume regulation in retinal pigment epithelium is mediated by Na,K,Cl cotransport. J Gen Physiol. 1990;96(6):1153–76.
65. Fischmeister R, Hartzell C. Volume-sensitivity of the bestrophin family of chloride channels. J Physiol. 2005;562(Pt 2):477–91.
66. Milenkovic A, Brandl C, Milenkovic VM, Jendryke T, Sirianant L, Wanitchakool P, Zimmermann S, Reiff CM, Horling F, Schrewe H, Schreiber R, Kunzelmann K, Wetzel CH, Weber BH. Bestrophin 1 is indispensable for volume regulation in human retinal pigment epithelium cells. Proc Natl Acad Sci U S A. 2015;112(20):E2630–9. https://doi.org/10.1073/pnas.1418840112.
67. Baylor D. How photons start vision. Proc Natl Acad Sci U S A. 1996;93(2):560–5.
68. Griff ER. Potassium-evoked responses from the retinal pigment epithelium of the toad Bufo marinus. Exp Eye Res. 1991;53(2):219–28.
69. Schneck ME, Fortune B, Adams AJ. The fast oscillation of the electrooculogram reveals sensitivity of the human outer retina/retinal pigment epithelium to glucose level. Vis Res. 2000;40(24):3447–53.
70. Steinberg RH, Linsenmeier RA, Griff ER. Three light-evoked responses of the retinal pigment epithelium. Vis Res. 1983;23(11):1315–23.
71. la Cour M, Lund-Andersen H, Zeuthen T. Potassium transport of the frog retinal pigment epithelium: autoregulation of potassium activity in the subretinal space. J Physiol. 1986;375:461–79.
72. Oakley B 2nd. Potassium and the photoreceptor-dependent pigment epithelial hyperpolarization. J Gen Physiol. 1977;70(4):405–25.
73. Linsenmeier RA, Steinberg RH. A light-evoked interaction of apical and basal membranes of retinal pigment epithelium: c-wave and light peak. J Neurophysiol. 1983;50(1):136–47.
74. Hughes BA, Steinberg RH. Voltage-dependent currents in isolated cells of the frog retinal pigment epithelium. J Physiol. 1990;428:273–97.

75. Strauss O, Richard G, Wienrich M. Voltage-dependent potassium currents in cultured human retinal pigment epithelial cells. Biochem Biophys Res Commun. 1993;191(3):775–81.
76. Strauss O, Weiser T, Wienrich M. Potassium currents in cultured cells of the rat retinal pigment epithelium. Comp Biochem Physiol A Physiol. 1994;109(4):975–83.
77. Strauss O, Wienrich M. Cultured retinal pigment epithelial cells from RCS rats express an increased calcium conductance compared with cells from non-dystrophic rats. Pflugers Arch. 1993;425(1–2):68–76.
78. Tao Q, Rafuse PE, Kelly ME. Potassium currents in cultured rabbit retinal pigment epithelial cells. J Membr Biol. 1994;141(2):123–38.
79. Wen R, Lui GM, Steinberg RH. Whole-cell K+ currents in fresh and cultured cells of the human and monkey retinal pigment epithelium. J Physiol. 1993;465:121–47.
80. Shimura M, Yuan Y, Chang JT, Zhang S, Campochiaro PA, Zack DJ, Hughes BA. Expression and permeation properties of the K(+) channel Kir7.1 in the retinal pigment epithelium. J Physiol. 2001;531(Pt 2):329–46.
81. Yang D, Pan A, Swaminathan A, Kumar G, Hughes BA. Expression and localization of the inwardly rectifying potassium channel Kir7.1 in native bovine retinal pigment epithelium. Invest Ophthalmol Vis Sci. 2003;44(7):3178–85.
82. Yuan Y, Shimura M, Hughes BA. Regulation of inwardly rectifying K+ channels in retinal pigment epithelial cells by intracellular pH. J Physiol. 2003;549(Pt 2):429–38.
83. Kusaka S, Inanobe A, Fujita A, Makino Y, Tanemoto M, Matsushita K, Tano Y, Kurachi Y. Functional Kir7.1 channels localized at the root of apical processes in rat retinal pigment epithelium. J Physiol. 2001;531(Pt 1):27–36.
84. Pattnaik BR, Tokarz S, Asuma MP, Schroeder T, Sharma A, Mitchell JC, Edwards AO, Pillers DA. Snowflake vitreoretinal degeneration (SVD) mutation R162W provides new insights into Kir7.1 ion channel structure and function. PLoS One. 2013;8(8):e71744. https://doi.org/10.1371/journal.pone.0071744.
85. Berridge MJ, Bootman MD, Roderick HL. Calcium signalling: dynamics, homeostasis and remodelling. Nat Rev Mol Cell Biol. 2003;4(7):517–29.
86. Rosenthal R, Strauss O. Ca2+-channels in the RPE. Adv Exp Med Biol. 2002;514:225–35.
87. Drager UC. Calcium binding in pigmented and albino eyes. Proc Natl Acad Sci U S A. 1985;82(19):6716–20.
88. Fijisawa K, Ye J, Zadunaisky JA. A Na+/Ca2+ exchange mechanism in apical membrane vesicles of the retinal pigment epithelium. Curr Eye Res. 1993;12(3):261–70.
89. Mangini NJ, Haugh-Scheidt L, Valle JE, Cragoe EJ Jr, Ripps H, Kennedy BG. Sodium-calcium exchanger in cultured human retinal pigment epithelium. Exp Eye Res. 1997;65(6):821–34.
90. Kennedy BG, Mangini NJ. Plasma membrane calcium-ATPase in cultured human retinal pigment epithelium. Exp Eye Res. 1996;63(5):547–56.
91. Wimmers S, Strauss O. Basal calcium entry in retinal pigment epithelial cells is mediated by TRPC channels. Invest Ophthalmol Vis Sci. 2007;48(12):5767–72. https://doi.org/10.1167/iovs.07-0412.
92. Strauss O. Transport mechanisms of the retinal pigment epithelium to maintain of visual function. Heat Mass Transf. 2014;50:303–13.
93. Berna-Erro A, Jardin I, Salido GM, Rosado JA. Role of STIM2 in cell function and physiopathology. J Physiol. 2017;595(10):3111–28. https://doi.org/10.1113/JP273889.
94. Rosado JA, Diez R, Smani T, Jardin I. STIM and Orai1 variants in store-operated calcium entry. Front Pharmacol. 2015;6:325. https://doi.org/10.3389/fphar.2015.00325.
95. Strauss O, Steinhausen K, Mergler S, Stumpff F, Wiederholt M. Involvement of protein tyrosine kinase in the InsP3-induced activation of Ca2+-dependent Cl- currents in cultured cells of the rat retinal pigment epithelium. J Membr Biol. 1999;169(3):141–53.
96. Strauss O, Wiederholt M, Wienrich M. Activation of Cl- currents in cultured rat retinal pigment epithelial cells by intracellular applications of inositol-1,4,5-triphosphate: differences between rats with retinal dystrophy (RCS) and normal rats. J Membr Biol. 1996;151(2):189–200.
97. Gomez NM, Tamm ER, Straubeta O. Role of bestrophin-1 in store-operated calcium entry in retinal pigment epithelium. Pflugers Arch. 2013;465(4):481–95. https://doi.org/10.1007/s00424-012-1181-0.
98. Neussert R, Muller C, Milenkovic VM, Strauss O. The presence of bestrophin 1 modulates the Ca2+ recruitment from Ca2+ stores in the ER. Pflugers Arch. 2010;460(1):163–75. https://doi.org/10.1007/s00424-010-0840-2.
99. Muller C, Mas Gomez N, Ruth P, Strauss O. CaV1.3 L-type channels, maxiK Ca(2+)-dependent K(+) channels and bestrophin-1 regulate rhythmic photoreceptor outer segment phagocytosis by retinal pigment epithelial cells. Cell Signal. 2014;26(5):968–78. https://doi.org/10.1016/j.cellsig.2013.12.021.
100. Strauss O, Buss F, Rosenthal R, Fischer D, Mergler S, Stumpff F, Thieme H. Activation of neuroendocrine L-type channels (alpha1D subunits) in retinal pigment epithelial cells and brain neurons by pp60(c-src). Biochem Biophys Res Commun. 2000;270(3):806–10.
101. Strauss O, Wienrich M. Ca(2+)-conductances in cultured rat retinal pigment epithelial cells. J Cell Physiol. 1994;160(1):89–96.
102. Ueda Y, Steinberg RH. Voltage-operated calcium channels in fresh and cultured rat retinal pig-

ment epithelial cells. Invest Ophthalmol Vis Sci. 1993;34(12):3408–18.

103. Ueda Y, Steinberg RH. Dihydropyridine-sensitive calcium currents in freshly isolated human and monkey retinal pigment epithelial cells. Invest Ophthalmol Vis Sci. 1995;36(2):373–80.
104. Wimmers S, Coeppicus L, Rosenthal R, Strauss O. Expression profile of voltage-dependent Ca2+ channel subunits in the human retinal pigment epithelium. Graefes Arch Clin Exp Ophthalmol. 2008;246(5):685–92. https://doi.org/10.1007/s00417-008-0778-7.
105. Wimmers S, Coeppicus L, Strauss O. Cloning and molecular characterization of L type Ca2+ channels in the retinal pigment epithelium. Invest Ophthalmol Vis Sci. 2004;45:e-abstract 3688.
106. Wimmers S, Halsband C, Seyler S, Milenkovic V, Strauss O. Voltage-dependent Ca2+ channels, not ryanodine receptors, activate Ca2+-dependent BK potassium channels in human retinal pigment epithelial cells. Mol Vis. 2008;14:2340–8.
107. Milenkovic VM, Krejcova S, Reichhart N, Wagner A, Strauss O. Interaction of bestrophin-1 and Ca2+ channel beta-subunits: identification of new binding domains on the bestrophin-1 C-terminus. PLoS One. 2011;6(4):e19364. https://doi.org/10.1371/journal.pone.0019364.
108. Reichhart N, Milenkovic VM, Halsband CA, Cordeiro S, Strauss O. Effect of bestrophin-1 on L-type Ca2+ channel activity depends on the Ca2+ channel beta-subunit. Exp Eye Res. 2010;91(5):630–9. https://doi.org/10.1016/j.exer.2010.08.001.
109. Rosenthal R, Bakall B, Kinnick T, Peachey N, Wimmers S, Wadelius C, Marmorstein A, Strauss O. Expression of bestrophin-1, the product of the VMD2 gene, modulates voltage-dependent Ca2+ channels in retinal pigment epithelial cells. FASEB J. 2006;20(1):178–80. https://doi.org/10.1096/fj.05-4495fje.
110. Yu K, Xiao Q, Cui G, Lee A, Hartzell HC. The best disease-linked Cl- channel hBest1 regulates Ca V 1 (L-type) Ca2+ channels via src-homology-binding domains. J Neurosci. 2008;28(22):5660–70. https://doi.org/10.1523/JNEUROSCI.0065-08.2008.
111. Strauss O. Pharmacology of the retinal pigment epithelium, the interface between retina and body system. Eur J Pharmacol. 2016;787:84–93. https://doi.org/10.1016/j.ejphar.2016.03.066.
112. Blaauwgeers HG, Holtkamp GM, Rutten H, Witmer AN, Koolwijk P, Partanen TA, Alitalo K, Kroon ME, Kijlstra A, van Hinsbergh VW, Schlingemann RO. Polarized vascular endothelial growth factor secretion by human retinal pigment epithelium and localization of vascular endothelial growth factor receptors on the inner choriocapillaris. Evidence for a trophic paracrine relation. Am J Pathol. 1999;155(2):421–8.
113. Witmer AN, Vrensen GF, Van Noorden CJ, Schlingemann RO. Vascular endothelial growth factors and angiogenesis in eye disease. Prog Retin Eye Res. 2003;22(1):1–29.
114. Cao W, Tombran-Tink J, Elias R, Sezate S, Mrazek D, McGinnis JF. In vivo protection of photoreceptors from light damage by pigment epithelium-derived factor. Invest Ophthalmol Vis Sci. 2001;42(7):1646–52.
115. Dawson DW, Volpert OV, Gillis P, Crawford SE, Xu H, Benedict W, Bouck NP. Pigment epithelium-derived factor: a potent inhibitor of angiogenesis. Science. 1999;285(5425):245–8.
116. Striessnig J. Pharmacology, structure and function of cardiac L-type Ca(2+) channels. Cell Physiol Biochem. 1999;9(4–5):242–69.
117. Sakai H, Saito T. Na+ and Ca2+ channel expression in cultured newt retinal pigment epithelial cells: comparison with neuronal types of ion channels. J Neurobiol. 1997;32(4):377–90.
118. Rosenthal R, Strauss O. Investigations of RPE cells of choriodal neovascular membranes from patients with age-related macula degeneration. Adv Exp Med Biol. 2003;533:107–13.
119. Strauss O, Heimann H, Foerster MH, Agostini H, Hansen LL, Rosenthal R. Activation of L-type Ca2+ channels is necessary for growth factor-dependent stimulation of VEGF secretion by RPE cells. Invest Ophthalmol Vis Sci. 2003;(44):e-abstract 3926.
120. Rosenthal R, Thieme H, Strauss O. Fibroblast growth factor receptor 2 (FGFR2) in brain neurons and retinal pigment epithelial cells act via stimulation of neuroendocrine L-type channels (Ca(v)1.3). FASEB J. 2001;15(6):970–7.
121. Rosenthal R, Heimann H, Agostini H, Martin G, Hansen LL, Strauss O. Ca2+ channels in retinal pigment epithelial cells regulate vascular endothelial growth factor secretion rates in health and disease. Mol Vis. 2007;13:443–56.
122. Busch C, Annamalai B, Abdusalamova K, Reichhart N, Huber C, Lin Y, Jo EAH, Zipfel PF, Skerka C, Wildner G, Diedrichs-Mohring M, Rohrer B, Strauss O. Anaphylatoxins activate Ca2+, Akt/PI3-kinase, and FOXO1/FoxP3 in the retinal pigment epithelium. Front Immunol. 2017;8:703. https://doi.org/10.3389/fimmu.2017.00703.
123. Genewsky A, Jost I, Busch C, Huber C, Stindl J, Skerka C, Zipfel PF, Rohrer B, Strauss O. Activation of endogenously expressed ion channels by active complement in the retinal pigment epithelium. Pflugers Arch. 2015;467(10):2179–91. https://doi.org/10.1007/s00424-014-1656-2.
124. Kunchithapautham K, Bandyopadhyay M, Dahrouj M, Thurman JM, Rohrer B. Sublytic membrane-attack-complex activation and VEGF secretion in retinal pigment epithelial cells. Adv Exp Med Biol. 2012;723:23–30. https://doi.org/10.1007/978-1-4614-0631-0_4.
125. Kunchithapautham K, Rohrer B. Sublytic membrane-attack-complex (MAC) activation alters regulated rather than constitutive vascular endothelial growth factor (VEGF) secretion in retinal

pigment epithelium monolayers. J Biol Chem. 2011;286(27):23717–24. https://doi.org/10.1074/jbc.M110.214593.
126. Rohrer B, Kunchithapautham K, Genewsky A, Strauss O. Prolonged SRC kinase activation, a mechanism to turn transient, sublytic complement activation into a sustained pathological condition in retinal pigment epithelium cells. Adv Exp Med Biol. 2014;801:221–7. https://doi.org/10.1007/978-1-4614-3209-8_29.
127. Nilius B, Szallasi A. Transient receptor potential channels as drug targets: from the science of basic research to the art of medicine. Pharmacol Rev. 2014;66(3):676–814. https://doi.org/10.1124/pr.113.008268.
128. Barro-Soria R, Stindl J, Muller C, Foeckler R, Todorov V, Castrop H, Strauss O. Angiotensin-2-mediated Ca2+ signaling in the retinal pigment epithelium: role of angiotensin-receptor-associated-protein and TRPV2 channel. PLoS One. 2012;7(11):e49624. https://doi.org/10.1371/journal.pone.0049624.
129. Cordeiro S, Seyler S, Stindl J, Milenkovic VM, Strauss O. Heat-sensitive TRPV channels in retinal pigment epithelial cells: regulation of VEGF-A secretion. Invest Ophthalmol Vis Sci. 2010;51(11):6001–8. https://doi.org/10.1167/iovs.09-4720.
130. Reichhart N, Keckeis S, Fried F, Fels G, Strauss O. Regulation of surface expression of TRPV2 channels in the retinal pigment epithelium. Graefes Arch Clin Exp Ophthalmol. 2015;253(6):865–74. https://doi.org/10.1007/s00417-014-2917-7.
131. Kondo T, Vicent D, Suzuma K, Yanagisawa M, King GL, Holzenberger M, Kahn CR. Knockout of insulin and IGF-1 receptors on vascular endothelial cells protects against retinal neovascularization. J Clin Invest. 2003;111(12):1835–42.
132. Rosenthal R, Wohlleben H, Malek G, Schlichting L, Thieme H, Bowes Rickman C, Strauss O. Insulin like growth factor-1 contributes to neovascularization in age-related macular degeneration. Biochem Biophys Res Commun. 2004;323:1203–8.
133. Slomiany MG, Rosenzweig SA. Autocrine effects of IGF-1 induced VEGF and IGFBP-3 secretion in retinal pigment epithelial cell line ARPE-19. Am J Physiol Cell Physiol. 2004;287(3):C746–53.
134. Slomiany MG, Rosenzweig SA. IGF-1-induced VEGF and IGFBP-3 secretion correlates with increased HIF-1 alpha expression and activity in retinal pigment epithelial cell line D407. Invest Ophthalmol Vis Sci. 2004;45(8):2838–47.
135. Mergler S, Strauss O. Stimulation of L-type Ca(2+) channels by increase of intracellular InsP3 in rat retinal pigment epithelial cells. Exp Eye Res. 2002;74(1):29–40.
136. Arden GB, Constable PA. The electro-oculogram. Prog Retin Eye Res. 2006;25(2):207–48. https://doi.org/10.1016/j.preteyeres.2005.11.001.
137. Fujii S, Gallemore RP, Hughes BA, Steinberg RH. Direct evidence for a basolateral membrane Cl- conductance in toad retinal pigment epithelium. Am J Physiol. 1992;262(2 Pt 1):C374–83.
138. Wu J, Marmorstein AD, Striessnig J, Peachey NS. Voltage-dependent calcium channel CaV1.3 subunits regulate the light peak of the electroretinogram. J Neurophysiol. 2007;97(5):3731–5. https://doi.org/10.1152/jn.00146.2007.
139. Marmorstein AD, Marmorstein LY, Rayborn M, Wang X, Hollyfield JG, Petrukhin K. Bestrophin, the product of the Best vitelliform macular dystrophy gene (VMD2), localizes to the basolateral plasma membrane of the retinal pigment epithelium. Proc Natl Acad Sci U S A. 2000;97(23):12758–63.
140. Strauss O, Neussert R, Muller C, Milenkovic VM. A potential cytosolic function of bestrophin-1. Adv Exp Med Biol. 2012;723:603–10. https://doi.org/10.1007/978-1-4614-0631-0_77.
141. Mazzoni F, Safa H, Finnemann SC. Understanding photoreceptor outer segment phagocytosis: use and utility of RPE cells in culture. Exp Eye Res. 2014;126:51–60. https://doi.org/10.1016/j.exer.2014.01.010.
142. Besharse JC, Hollyfield JG, Rayborn ME. Photoreceptor outer segments: accelerated membrane renewal in rods after exposure to light. Science. 1977;196(4289):536–8.
143. Young RW, Bok D. Participation of the retinal pigment epithelium in the rod outer segment renewal process. J Cell Biol. 1969;42(2):392–403.
144. Mitchell CH. Release of ATP by a human retinal pigment epithelial cell line: potential for autocrine stimulation through subretinal space. J Physiol. 2001;534(Pt 1):193–202.
145. Mitchell CH, Reigada D. Purinergic signalling in the subretinal space: a role in the communication between the retina and the RPE. Purinergic Signal. 2008;4(2):101–7. https://doi.org/10.1007/s11302-007-9054-2.
146. Sanderson J, Dartt DA, Trinkaus-Randall V, Pintor J, Civan MM, Delamere NA, Fletcher EL, Salt TE, Grosche A, Mitchell CH. Purines in the eye: recent evidence for the physiological and pathological role of purines in the RPE, retinal neurons, astrocytes, Muller cells, lens, trabecular meshwork, cornea and lacrimal gland. Exp Eye Res. 2014;127:270–9. https://doi.org/10.1016/j.exer.2014.08.009.
147. Reigada D, Mitchell CH. Release of ATP from retinal pigment epithelial cells involves both CFTR and vesicular transport. Am J Physiol Cell Physiol. 2005;288(1):C132–40. https://doi.org/10.1152/ajpcell.00201.2004.
148. Liu J, Lu W, Guha S, Baltazar GC, Coffey EE, Laties AM, Rubenstein RC, Reenstra WW, Mitchell CH. Cystic fibrosis transmembrane conductance regulator contributes to reacidification of alkalinized lysosomes in RPE cells. Am J Physiol Cell Physiol. 2012;303(2):C160–9. https://doi.org/10.1152/ajpcell.00278.2011.
149. Finnemann SC, Bonilha VL, Marmorstein AD, Rodriguez-Boulan E. Phagocytosis of rod outer

segments by retinal pigment epithelial cells requires alpha(v)beta5 integrin for binding but not for internalization. Proc Natl Acad Sci U S A. 1997;94(24):12932–7.
150. Karl MO, Kroeger W, Wimmers S, Milenkovic VM, Valtink M, Engelmann K, Strauss O. Endogenous Gas6 and Ca2+-channel activation modulate phagocytosis by retinal pigment epithelium. Cell Signal. 2008;20(6):1159–68. https://doi.org/10.1016/j.cellsig.2008.02.005.
151. Ryan JS, Baldridge WH, Kelly ME. Purinergic regulation of cation conductances and intracellular Ca2+ in cultured rat retinal pigment epithelial cells. J Physiol. 1999;520(Pt 3):745–59.

RPE and the Vascular Endothelial Growth Factor

5

Alexa Karina Klettner

Vascular Endothelial Growth Factor

The Vascular endothelial growth factor (VEGF) family consists of several members, such as VEGF-A–F and placental growth factor [1], but only VEGF-A will be covered in this chapter and hitherto referred to as VEGF. VEGF, originally identified in 1983 (then termed Vascular Permeability Factor) [2] and cloned in 1989 [3, 4], is considered the most important angiogenic growth factor in angiogenesis [5]. Early studies concerning VEGF showed its importance for the vascularization of the developing embryo, as even the loss of a single allele of VEGF is lethal [6, 7]. The VEGF gene consists of eight exons and seven introns and several isoforms exit due to alternative splicing (and enzymatic cleavage). The isoforms are designated by the number of amino acids they contain, the most abundant being $VEGF_{121}$, $VEGF_{165}$, $VEGF_{186}$ and $VEGF_{206}$ [8]. Of note, several other isoforms have been described [9]. The isoforms differ in their solubility and their ability to bind to heparan sulfate proteoglycans (HS) and the VEGF co-receptor neuropilin. While $VEGF_{165}$ has an intermediate solubility, the longer isoforms are sequestered to the extracellular matrix and can be cleaved by plasmin or matrix metalloproteases, resulting in short isoforms like $VEGF_{111}$ or $VEGF_{113}$ [10]. In addition, inhibitory isoforms of VEGF have been described, $VEGF_{xxxb}$, which are additionally alternatively spliced in exon 8 [9].

VEGF expression is tightly regulated on several levels (Fig. 5.1). Depending on cell type, VEGF can for example be induced by hypoxia, which is the major inducing factor [11], oxidative stress or cytokines [12–14]. In addition, autocrine regulation has been suggested [15–17]. The different regulation pathways are dependent on the stimulus, and differences can be found between constitutive and induced expression (see below). On a transcriptional level, the VEGF promotor region is special, as it does not contain a TATA box as an initiation recognition sequence, but a GC-rich region. In addition, the 5′UTR region is very long with various promotor binding sites, including but not limited to SP-1, AP-1, AP-2, Stat3, NFkB or Hypoxia inducible factor (HIF) 1α [8, 18, 19]. In addition to the canonical pathway, mediated by eukaryotic initiation factor, VEGF translation can be mediated by internal ribosome binding sites (IRES), which enables ribosomes to translate independently of the 7-methyguanosine cap and eukaryotic initiation factor, allowing e.g. translation under hypoxic conditions [20, 21]. Post-transcriptionally, VEGF is regulated via its mRNA half-life. Due to instability elements, VEGF is predisposed to mRNA degradation by endonucleases. Under hypoxic

A. K. Klettner (✉)
Department of Ophthalmology, University of Kiel, University Medical Center, Kiel, Schleswig-Holstein, Germany
e-mail: AlexaKarina.Klettner@uksh.de

A. K. Klettner, S. Dithmar (eds.), *Retinal Pigment Epithelium in Health and Disease*,
https://doi.org/10.1007/978-3-030-28384-1_5

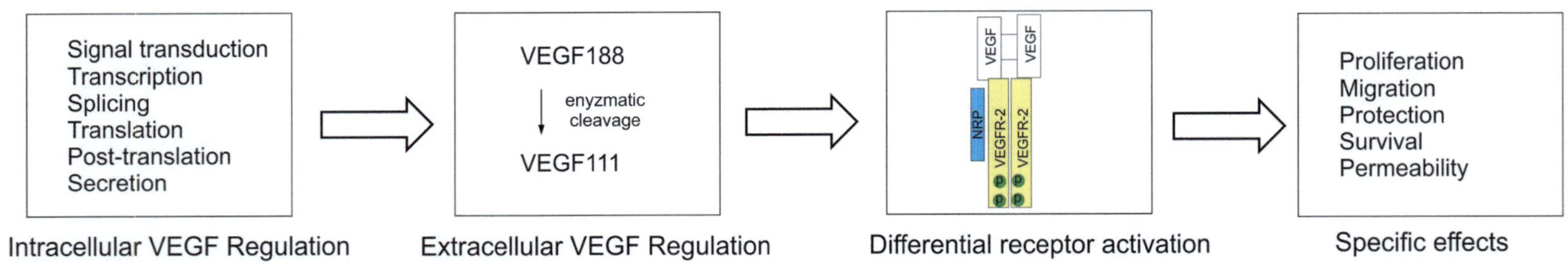

Fig. 5.1 VEGF and its effects are regulated on many levels, including intracellular mechanisms inducing VEGF expression of differentially spliced isoforms, extracellular cleavage creating further isoforms, and consequent differential receptor activation, inducing the specific cellular VEGF responses

conditions, however, the mRNA is stabilized by the RNA-binding protein HuR, protecting the mRNA from degradation [22–24]. Finally, VEGF secretion is regulated in the endoplasmic reticulum and the Golgi apparatus, with chaperones like ORP1 50 and αB-cystallin involved [25–27]. Important factors in the signal transduction of VEGF regulation are the Mitogen activated protein kinases (MAPK) p38, extracellular signal-regulated kinase (ERK) 1/2 and c-Jun N-terminal kinases (JNK) [17, 28].

In order to exert its function, VEGF binds to its receptors, VEGFR-1 and VEGFR-2. In addition, neuropilins act as co-receptors. VEGFR-1 has a higher affinity for VEGF than VEGFR-2, but its signal transduction activity is considered to be weaker [29]. The role of VEGFR-1 is not conclusive, but generally considered to be a negative regulator of angiogenesis, though not exclusively [30]. The main receptor for the angiogenic properties of VEGF is VEGFR-2. Binding of VEGF leads to a dimerization of the receptor, which, in turn, results in the phosphorylation of specific tyrosine residues. The specific phosphorylation patterns depend on the VEGF isoform, leading differential cellular responses [31]. Both receptor are expressed in the outer retina, with VEGFR-1 shown to be expressed on the inner segments of photoreceptors and the inner choriocapillaries, while VEGFR-2 is expressed on the retinal pigment epithelium (RPE) and the endothelium of the choriocapillaris on the side facing the RPE [32–35]. Neuropilins, on the other hand, are transmembrane glycoproteins lacking intracellular activity, considered to be co-receptors to modulate VEGF receptor response. These may be connected to internalization of the receptor [36–38].

RPE Derived VEGF Function in the Healthy Retina

VEGF can be produced by many different cells of the eye, such as Müller cells, astrocytes, and even neuronal cells, but the RPE is considered the major source of VEGF of the outer retina [39]. RPE cells secrete high amounts of VEGF, with $VEGF_{165}$ being the most abundant, followed by $VEGF_{121}$ and, to a much lesser extent, $VEGF_{189}$ [40–43].

Development

While VEGF is a major factor in the development of the retinal vasculature and also in the development of the neuroretina, the source of the VEGF is not considered to be the RPE, but rather astrocytes and Müller cells [44–47]. Nevertheless, the RPE has been shown to be important for the development of the neuroretina [48]. For the development of choroid, on the other hand, the RPE as a source of VEGF is indispensable [49, 50]. Indeed, ablation of VEGF expression in the RPE results in a complete absence of the choriocapillaris and a consequent loss of visual function [49]. The expression of VEGF in the RPE correlates with the proliferation activity in the choroid, while VEGF mRNA is only found in the RPE, but not in the choroid, while the VEGF protein is found in the RPE as well as in choroidal vascular endothelial cells, suggesting a paracrine effect of the VEGF [51, 52]. In concordance, VEGFR-2 is expressed in the vascular endothelium but not in RPE cells at this developmental stage, where it develops postnatally [42, 47, 53, 54]. Indeed, loss of RPE derived VEGF at embryonic day 10–12 but not 16–18 displayed defects on the choroidal vasculature in mice, stressing the time-dependent requirement of RPE-derived VEGF in choroidal development [55]. Furthermore, during this time window, a loss of photoreceptor function can be observed. Of note, the developmental expression of VEGF by the RPE in the course of choroidal development is not dependent on the transcription factor HIF1α [49].

Adult Retina

A major role for RPE derived VEGF is the maintenance of the choriocapillaris. The photoreceptors have a high demand for oxygen and nutrients, which is applied to them by the choriocapillaris.

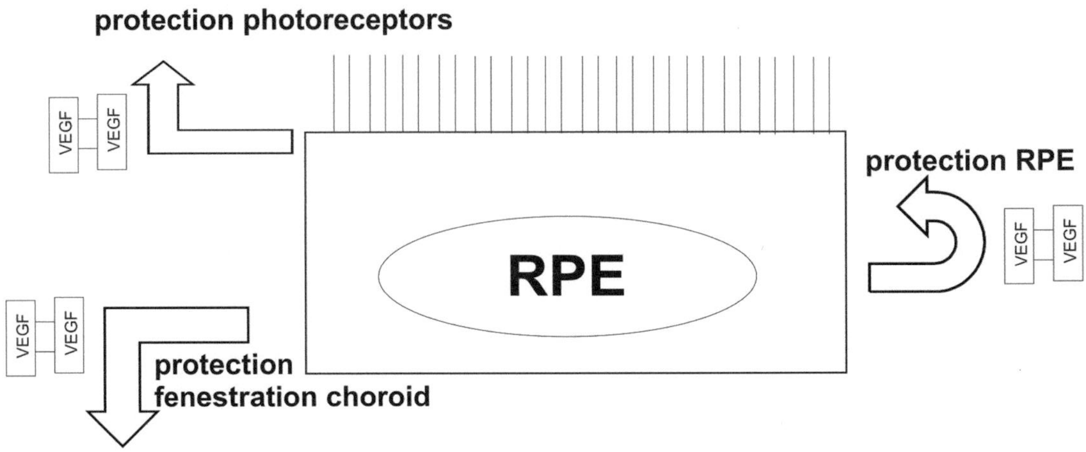

Fig. 5.2 The RPE constitutively secretes VEGF in apical and basal direction. Apical RPE-derived VEGF protects the photoreceptors and the RPE, while basally secreted VEGF upholds the fenestration and protects the endothelial cells of the choriocapillaris

The endothelium of the choriocapillaris is fenestrated and highly permeable for nutrients and other low molecular weight proteins [56]. RPE cells protect choroidal vascular endothelial cells and preserve the capillary fenestration, with VEGF being the major factor for this function [57]. RPE cells secrete VEGF predominantly on the basal side (while there also apical secretion) [12, 32, 58], and the adjacent endothelial express VEGFR-2 on the side facing the RPE [32, 42]. If VEGF from the RPE is inhibited, either by anti-VEGF compounds or conditional knock-down of RPE-specific VEGF, the fenestration disappears and an atrophy of the choriocapillaris may follow [59–61]. Of note, soluble VEGF is needed, as mice expressing only $VEGF_{188}$ develop an atrophy of the choriocapillaris over time, followed by photoreceptor cell death [57]. Indeed, VEGF has been shown to protect endothelial cells from a variety of insults, such as starvation or oxidative stress [62, 63]. VEGF may even be indispensable for adult vision, as a RPE-specific knock-out of VEGF in the adult mice results in a rapid vision loss, dysfunction of cone photoreceptors and ablation of the choriocapillaris [59]. Indeed, VEGF has been shown to be directly protective on neuronal cells of the retina, such as ganglion cells or photoreceptors [35, 64–66]. RPE derived VEGF also exerts autocrine function. Adult RPE cells express VEGFR-2 [42] and VEGF may be involved in RPE proliferation and migration [67–69]. In addition, VEGF can act as a survival factor for RPE cells, protecting them from oxidative stress (Fig. 5.2). The protection is mediated via VEGFR-2 signaling and involves phosphatidylinositol 3 kinase (PI3K) and Akt activation [33]. Indeed, long term treatment with anti-VEGF can change the ultrastructure of the RPE *in vivo*, such as reduced microvilli, reduction of melanin granules, or reduced basal infoldings [49, 53]. The question whether long-term inhibition of VEGF induce direct damage and cell death in RPE cells is under debate, with increased apoptosis being found but no general decreased cell viability seen for long-term treatment in vitro [53, 70]. VEGF inhibition seems to induce transient damage in RPE [53]. Also, in our hands, long term treatment with anti-VEGF did not change the ultrastructure of mitochondria or induced premature aging in the cells [70]. Also, care has to be taken when interpreting results obtained with anti-VEGF compounds, as their effects may be unrelated to their anti-VEGF properties. For example, anti-VEGF compounds bevacizumab and aflibercept have been shown to reduce phagocytic ability of RPE cells, but this may be related more to their Fc-fragment than to their anti-VEGF binding abilities [68, 69, 71].

An important function of the RPE is its barrier properties [72]. The exact influence of VEGF on the permeability of RPE cells in under debate, as the literature is conflicting. VEGF has been described to tighten the barrier of the RPE cells [73], e.g. via regulation of tight junction protein expression [74], to have no effect [75] as well as to break the RPE cell barrier [76, 77]. Recently, a role of VEGF in complement regulation in the RPE has been proposed, as VEGF has been shown to increase complement factor H (CFH) and CD46 expression in the RPE, while, conversely, VEGF inhibition reduced their expression, and, moreover, resulted in an increased C3d deposits [78].

While the effects of long-term deletion of VEGF on the retina is under debate [53, 59, 79], the loss of the physiological functions VEGF may be one of the causes of the atrophy development found after long-term use of anti-VEGF therapy in many AMD patients [80].

RPE Derived VEGF in the Diseased Retina

VEGF is a major pathological factor in a series of retinal diseases, such as diabetic retinopathy and age-related macular degeneration [81], but also retinopathy of prematurity, retinal vein occlusion, and others [82, 83]. RPE cells in close connections to choroidal neovascularization express high levels of VEGF [84, 85] and proliferative RPE cells displaying elevated VEGF expression are seen in subretinal vascular membrane of AMD patients [86]. Overproduction of VEGF by RPE cells in transgenic mice can lead to new blood vessel formation in the choroid, strongly indicating the importance for RPE derived VEGF for the development of choroidal neovascularizations [87, 88]. However, it should be noted that increased VEGF alone may not be enough to induce pathology, and further factors and disruption of the RPE or the Bruch's membrane may be needed [87, 89]. Concerning diabetic retinopathy, Müller cells are considered the main source of pathologic VEGF [90]. However, some studies indicate that VEGF derived from the RPE may also contribute to the barrier dysfunction in diabetic macular edema [91, 92] and directly reduce the fluid resorption capacity in RPE cells [93].

While VEGF is generally considered a survival factor for the RPE and the retina and important if not vital for its function (see above) [33, 59], there are some studies that claim a deleterious effect of increased VEGF on cells of the retina, indicating a pathological role of VEGF not only in exudative, but also atrophic age-related macular degeneration. In mice, overexpression of VEGF can result in an RPE barrier breakdown and accumulation of macrophages [76]. These barrier breakdowns may also serve as entry points for neovascularizations. RPE degenerations can be seen in these VEGF overexpressing mice, with increased retinal atrophy, correlating with visual cycle defects and reduced rhodopsin contents [76]. Similarly, in light induced retinal injury, VEGF is has been indicated to be involved in barrier breakdown and secondary photoreceptor degeneration [77]. Furthermore, VEGF overexpression activated inflammasomes, which mediated photoreceptor degeneration in these mice [94].

Regulation of VEGF in the RPE

The RPE is a major source of VEGF and VEGF is constitutively secreted by the RPE [32]. On a developmental level, the major factor for RPE differentiation is Microphthalmia-associated transcription factor (MITF) [95]. MITF also participates in the expression of VEGF in the RPE [96], and VEGF expression and secretion is considered a differentiation marker of RPE cells [96, 97]. In addition, the secretion of VEGF by the RPE is polarized, with a higher amount of VEGF secreted to basal, as compared to the apical side [32, 58]. As described above, the regulation of VEGF is regulated on many levels and this regulation is dependent on the stimulus. As RPE cells constitutively express VEGF, different pathways are involved in physiological and induced VEGF secretion (Fig. 5.3).

Constitutive VEGF

The constitutive expression of VEGF in the RPE is mainly mediated by the transcription factor NFkB and, to a lesser extent, the transcription

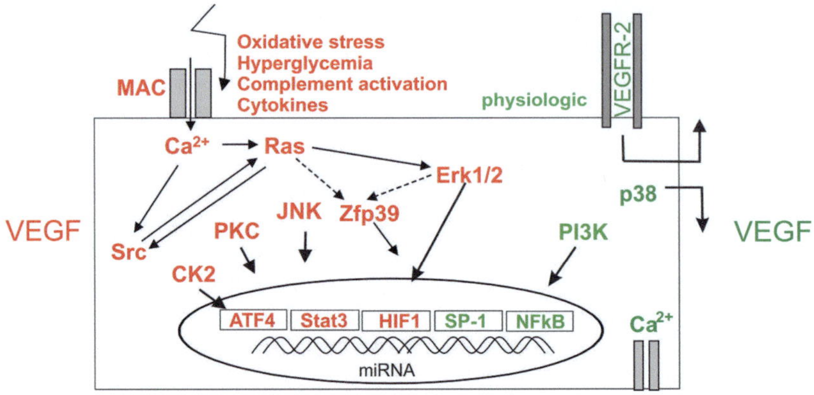

Fig. 5.3 Selected pathways of VEGF regulation in the RPE. While constitutive VEGF regulation in the RPE may be mediated by the transcription factors SP-1 and NFkB, Calcium channels, PI3K, the MAPK p38 (basal) and autocrine VEGFR-2 activation (apical) (all green), different stimuli can induce VEGF via several transcription factors, such as ATF4, Stat3 or HIF1α, via different kinases such as CK2, JNK, ERK1/2, Src or PKC, Calcium influx and downregulation of mRNA destabilizers such as Zfp39 (all red). Please note that these pathways are exemplary and that pathways involved in physiologic regulation may also contribute to pathologic elevation. For more specific information please refer to the text

factor SP-1, while neither HIF1α nor Stat3 are involved [17]. Considering signal transduction pathways, we could show that p38 partly mediated the constitutive expression of VEGF. Interestingly, p38 pathways seem to be independent from the transcription factor NFkB, as an inhibition of both abolished VEGF secretion in our model system [17]. Furthermore, p38 was involved primarily in the secretion on the basal, not the apical side, while the transcription factors NFkB and SP-1 influenced basal as well as apical secretion [58]. In addition, there seems to be a positive autoregulatory mechanism to constitutive VEGF secretion in the RPE as the inhibition of the VEGFR-2 reduces VEGF secretion [17], mainly at the apical side [58]. This mechanisms may explain why several VEGF inhibitors, which act by impeding VEGF binding to their receptor, actually reduce VEGF expression in the RPE, as shown for bevacizumab, ranibizumab and fucoidan [16, 98]. The signal transduction pathway in VEGFR-2 regulated VEGF secretion is mediated via PI3K, and not via phosphokinase C (PKC) [17]. Interestingly, the protective effect of VEGF has been described to be mediated by VEGFR-2 and PI3K [66]. Constitutive VEGF expression has also been shown to be regulated by of L-type, high-voltage activated Ca^{2+} channels in the RPE [99]. These channels may also be involved in hyperthermia and IGF-1 mediated VEGF upregulation (see below) [100].

Hypoxia

The primary stimulus for VEGF upregulation is hypoxia [43, 101]. Experimentally, hypoxia can be generated via low oxygen pressure or chemically via cobalt chloride. Cobalt chloride increases VEGF expression in the RPE [102]. Hypoxia-induced elevation of VEGF is mediated via activation and translocation of the transcription factors HIF1α (via PI3K/Akt) and NFkB, and the p38 MAPK pathway [103–105]. HIF1α is the major transcription factor for hypoxia-related genes and also involved in hyperglycemic VEGF regulation. Of interest, VEGF and HIF1α are regulated by a common set of MicroRNAs (miRNAs) which bind to the 3′UTR of both genes, resulting in a cross-talk between VEGF and HIF1α, with one gene positively regulating the other [106]. miRNAs are noncoding RNA molecules that affect the stability and translation of mRNA by binding to a specific miRNA response element [107]. In addition, hypoxia upregulates VEGF via the Wnt/β-catenin pathway, most likely via the T cell factor (TCF)-4 binding element, and via hypoxia-induced tissue factor [14]. Also, dsRNA-activated protein kinase (PKR) has been implicated in hypoxia mediated VEGF expression, via the PI3K/Akt signaling pathway [108]. Furthermore, CXC-chemokine receptor 4 (CXCR4) has been implicated, most likely downstream of NFkB [109]. Additionally, PKC has been shown to take part in hypoxia mediated VEGF upregulation [110]. In a recent study, C9 mRNA was shown to induce VEGF in hypoxia, while the C9 protein inhibited it, suggesting a direct regulatory effect of the C9 mRNA [111].

Oxidative Stress and Hyperglycemia

Oxidative stress is an important stimulus for VEGF secretion in the RPE [12, 112]. Interestingly, in polarized RPE cells the secretion of VEGF seems to be more strongly induced on the apical side, indicating a protective effect directed towards the photoreceptors [12]. Both oxidative stress and hyperglycemia can induce a secretion of VEGF in exosomes [113] which is in concordance with the release of the anti-VEGF therapeutic in exosomes [114]. In oxidative stress induced VEGF upregulation, the MAPK ERK1/2 is involved in short term VEGF upregulation [115, 116]. In addition, NFkB has been implicated in oxidative stress induced VEGF upregulation [113, 117]. Oxidized phospholipids, which accumulate in the RPE in the aged eye, also stimulate VEGF expression in RPE cells. This is mediated by the transcription factor ATF4 via the protein kinase CK2 [118]. ATF4 is a contributor of the unfolded protein response, a form of endoplasmic reticulum (ER) stress response, which aims to restore ER homeostasis when the protein load is too high and the protein folding in the ER is disturbed [119]. ER stress has been shown to induce VEGF in the RPE via the transcription factor OASIS [120]. Furthermore, VEGF-induction by amyloid β [121] has been described to be mediated by ER stress [122]. Amyloid β induced upregulation of VEGF may be connected to mitochondrial reactive oxygen species, and to the activation of TLR-4 (see below) [123, 124]. Receptor for advanced glycation end products (RAGE) can act as a receptor for amyloid β, and RAGE-mediated VEGF upregulation is NFkB dependent [125].

VEGF is an important pathological factor in the diabetic retina. Indeed, high glucose has been described to increase the release of VEGF from retinal pigment epithelial cells [113, 126, 127]. Interestingly, also a sharp drop of glucose concentration may induce VEGF secretion [127]. The transcription factors HIF1α, NFkB and Stat3 have been indicated to be involved in VEGF increase after high glucose insult [110, 128, 129]. Also, PKC seems to take part in VEGF regulation after in high glucose [110]. The increase may be related to an oxidative stress challenge of these cells as high glucose content of the cell medium may lead to an elevated production of ROS [113]. The insulin-like growth factor (IGF)-1 is an inducer of VEGF in the RPE [130]. This can be inhibited by somatostatin [131]. The upregulation is mediated via Ca^{2+}channels [100], HIF1α [132] and the MAPK ERK1/2 [133]. Insulin itself also elevates VEGF transcription [134].

Inflammation

VEGF is also involved in inflammation. In order to detect pathogen associated molecular patterns (PAMPs) or danger associated molecular patters (DAMPs), RPE cells express Toll-like receptors (TLR) [135]. TLR are central for pathogen detection in innate immunity. Activation of TLR induces the expression and secretion of pro-inflammatory cytokines to induce inflammatory reaction and to augment the activation of the adaptive immune system. Among the TLR, TLR-2 detects peptidoglycan of gram positive bacteria, TLR-3 is able to detected double stranded RNA, which is a hallmark of certain viruses, and TLR-4 senses lipopolysaccharide which is found on gram-negative bacteria [136, 137]. RPE cells express moderate levels of TLR-2, and its activation by Chlamydia pneumoniae induces a VEGF response in RPE cells [138]. RPE cells abundantly express TLR-3, and the activation of the receptor induces a pro-inflammatory cytokine release in these cells [139], including VEGF [140]. MAPK did not participate in the regulation of VEGF in this setting. Also, the activation of TLR-4 has been shown to induce the secretion of VEGF, via NFkB [123]. Also, cytokines can induce VEGF secretion in RPE cells, as shown for Tumor necrosis factor (TNF) α [14]. This pathway may be correlated to oxidative stress-induced VEGF increase and may be mediated via Wnt/β-catenin [14]. Of interest, NFkB was not involved in this particular upregulation [14]. The influence of TNFα, however, may be related to the differentiation of the cells, as another study showed that the increase was only seen in non-polarized cells, while in polarized cells, VEGF secretion was, conversely, reduced by TNFα [141].

The cytokine transforming growth factor (TGF) β, on the other hand, is considered to be immunoregulatory in the retina [142] and pro-angiogenic, and is constitutively secreted by RPE cells in high amounts [70, 143]. TGFβ in different isoforms induces VEGF in the RPE. TGFβ induces VEGF expression in RPE cells via de-novo protein synthesis [28, 144]. Of interest, VEGF expression increases synergistically if cells are stimulated with TGFβ2 and TNFα, which is most likely to be regulated at a transcriptional level [28]. While all major MAPK (p38, ERK1/2 and, shown for TGFβ2, JNK) seem to be involved in TGFβ induced VEGF upregulation, the major MAPK appears to be p38, especially when TNFα is also involved. A difference between TGFβ1 and TGFβ2 can be seen regarding NFkB and PKC, as both are involved in VEGF upregulation caused by TGFβ2, but not TGFβ1 [28, 144]. Also, TGFβ2 and thrombin show a synergistic VEGF induction [145]. Thrombin is formed at hemorrhagic sites, and is elevated e.g. in retinal ischemia and proliferative diabetic retinopathy [146, 147]. While similar pathways are involved in thrombin mediated upregulation of VEGF, such as ERK1/2, p38, JNK, NFkB, PI3K, PTK and PKC, JNK seems to be a major factor here [145]. Thrombin also acts synergistically with TNFα. In contrast to TNFα, however, thrombin induces VEGF in polarized and non-polarized cells alike [148].

Interestingly, a marker for age-associated inflammation, miR-146a, which is upregulated in the aged RPE/choroid, reduces the expression of VEGF in RPE cells [149]. Also inflammasomes, which are key mediators of the innate immune system and which induce the secretion of several pro-inflammatory cytokines in the RPE, reduce VEGF secretion both via and independent of IL-18 [150, 151].

Complement factors have also been shown to induce VEGF secretion, shown for complement factor 5a [152], complement factor 3a [153] or sublytic C5b-9 membrane attack complex [116, 154, 155]. For the sublytic, C5b—9 mediated VEGF increase, Ras, ERK1/2 and Src, but not p38 were shown to be involved. In addition, the stabilization of VEGF mRNA by a reduction of the destabilizing protein zfp36 was shown [116].

Hyperthermia

Several studies have shown that the secretion of VEGF is temperature dependent. Hyperthermia induces expression and secretion of VEGF, which was mediated by p38 and the c-Jun Kinase (JNK) [156] and PI3K [100]. In addition, hyperthermia induces VEGF secretion via Ca^{2+} channels [100]. In concordance, hypothermia reduces VEGF secretion by the RPE, while it shows no effect on Pigment epithelium-derived factor (PEDF) expression, which is an anti-angiogenic cytokine [157, 158]. Interestingly, hyperthermia induces VEGF expression in laser exhibited some protection against subsequent oxidative-stress induced VEGF expression [159].

More factors have been described to induce VEGF expression in the RPE, such as retinoid acid [160, 161], lysosomal stress [41], loss of cell-cell contact [162], or senescence [163]. More research is needed to elucidate the pathways which regulate these elevations.

Conclusion

RPE derived VEGF exerts many functions in the physiological and diseased retina. While VEGF-inhibitors are an established therapy and widely used for several diseases [164–166], the consequences of long-term inhibition of VEGF are not sufficiently known and just being assessed. Further research is warranted to disclose the consequences of anti-VEGF therapy, not only in the elderly, but also in the working-age and infant population [167–169].

The regulation of VEGF is complex and highly dependent on the stimulus. This might hold new avenues for a more targeted therapy, concentrating on the pathological stimulus rather than on broad VEGF secretion, possibly sparing the physiologic functions. More research is needed in elucidating the different regulatory pathways.

References

1. Witmer AN, Vrensen GF, Van Noorden CJ, Schlingemann RO. Vascular endothelial growth factors and angiogenesis in eye disease. Prog Retin Eye Res. 2003;22:1–2.
2. Senger DR, Galli SJ, Dvorak AM, Perruzzi CA, Harvey VS, Dvorak HF. Tumor cells secrete a vascular permeability factor that promotes accumulation of ascites fluid. Science. 1983;219:983–5.
3. Keck PJ, Hauser SD, Krivi G, Sanzo K, Warren T, Feder J, Connolly DT. Vascular permeability factor, an endothelial cell mitogen related to PDGF. Science. 1989;246:1309–12.
4. Leung DW, Cachianes G, Kuang WJ, Goeddel DV, Ferrara N. Vascular endothelial growth factor is a secreted angiogenic mitogen. Science. 1989;246:1306–9.
5. Ferrara N. VEGF-A: a critical regulator of blood vessel growth. Eur Cytokine Netw. 2009;20:158–63.
6. Carmeliet P, Ferreira V, Breier G, Pollefeyt S, Kieckens L, Gertsenstein M, Fahrig M, Vandenhoeck A, Harpal K, Eberhardt C, Declercq C, Pawling J, Moons L, Collen D, Risau W, Nagy A. Abnormal blood vessel development and lethality in embryos lacking a single VEGF allele. Nature. 1996;380:435–9.
7. Ferrara N, Carver-Moore K, Chen H, Dowd M, Lu L, O'Shea KS, Powell-Braxton L, Hillan KJ, Moore MW. Heterozygous embryonic lethality induced by targeted inactivation of the VEGF gene. Nature. 1996;380:439–42.
8. Tischer E, Mitchell R, Hartman T, Silva M, Gospodarowicz D, Fiddes JC, Abraham JA. The human gene for vascular endothelial growth factor. Multiple protein forms are encoded through alternative exon splicing. J Biol Chem. 1991;266:11947–54.
9. Dehghanian F, Hojati Z, Kay M. New insights into VEGF-A alternative splicing: key regulatory switching in the pathological process. Avicenna J Med Biotechnol. 2014;6:192–9.
10. Lee S, Jilani SM, Nikolova GV, Carpizo D, Iruela-Arispe ML. Processing of VEGF-A by matrix metalloproteinases regulates bioavailability and vascular patterning in tumors. J Cell Biol. 2005;169:681–91.
11. Aiello LP, Northrup JM, Keyt BA, Takagi H, Iwamoto MA. Hypoxic regulation of vascular endothelial growth factor in retinal cells. Arch Ophthalmol. 1995;113:1538–44.
12. Kannan R, Zhang N, Sreekumar PG, Spee CK, Rodriguez A, Barron E, Hinton DR. Stimulation of apical and basolateral VEGF-A and VEGF-C secretion by oxidative stress in polarized retinal pigment epithelial cells. Mol Vis. 2006;12:1649–59.
13. Klettner A, Roider J. Mechanisms of pathological VEGF production in the retina and modification with VEGF-antagonists. In: Stratton RD, Hauswirth WW, Gardner TW, editors. Oxidative stress in applied basic research and clincial practice, studies on retinal and choroidal disorders. Springer; 2012. p. 277–306.
14. Wang H, Han X, Wittchen ES, Hartnett ME. TNF-α mediates choroidal neovascularization by upregulating VEGF expression in RPE through ROS-dependent β-catenin activation. Mol Vis. 2016;22:116–28.
15. Deudero JJ, Caramelo C, Castellanos MC, Neria F, Fernández-Sánchez R, Calabia O, Peñate S, González-Pacheco FR. Induction of hypoxia-inducible factor 1alpha gene expression by vascular endothelial growth factor. J Biol Chem. 2008;283:11435–44.
16. Klettner A, Roider J. Comparison of bevacizumab, ranibizumab, and pegaptanib in vitro: efficiency and possible additional pathways. Invest Ophthalmol Vis Sci. 2008;49:4523–7.
17. Klettner A, Westhues D, Lassen J, Bartsch S, Roider J. Regulation of constitutive vascular endothelial growth factor secretion in retinal pigment epithelium/choroid organ cultures: p38, nuclear factor κB, and the vascular endothelial growth factor receptor-2/phosphatidylinositol 3 kinase pathway. Mol Vis. 2013;19:281–91.
18. Forsythe JA, Jiang BH, Iyer NV, Agani F, Leung SW, Koos RD, Semenza GL. Activation of vascular endothelial growth factor gene transcription by hypoxia-inducible factor 1. Mol Cell Biol. 1996;16:4604–13.
19. Pagès G, Pouysségur J. Transcriptional regulation of the Vascular Endothelial Growth Factor gene—a concert of activating factors. Cardiovasc Res. 2005;65:564–73.

20. Akiri G, Nahari D, Finkelstein Y, Le SY, Elroy-Stein O, Levi BZ. Regulation of vascular endothelial growth factor (VEGF) expression is mediated by internal initiation of translation and alternative initiation of transcription. Oncogene. 1998;17:227–36.
21. Huez I, Créancier L, Audigier S, Gensac MC, Prats AC, Prats H. Two independent internal ribosome entry sites are involved in translation initiation of vascular endothelial growth factor mRNA. Mol Cell Biol. 1998;18:6178–90.
22. Levy AP, Levy NS, Goldberg MA. Post-transcriptional regulation of vascular endothelial growth factor by hypoxia. J Biol Chem. 1996;271:2746–53.
23. Levy NS, Chung S, Furneaux H, Levy AP. Hypoxic stabilization of vascular endothelial growth factor mRNA by the RNA-binding protein HuR. J Biol Chem. 1998;273:6417–23.
24. Yoo PS, Mulkeen AL, Cha CH. Post-transcriptional regulation of vascular endothelial growth factor: implications for tumor angiogenesis. World J Gastroenterol. 2006;12:4937–42.
25. Abcouwer SF, Marjon PL, Loper RK, Vander Jagt DL. Response of VEGF expression to amino acid deprivation and inducers of endoplasmic reticulum stress. Invest Ophthalmol Vis Sci. 2002;43:2791–8.
26. Kase S, He S, Sonoda S, Kitamura M, Spee C, Wawrousek E, Ryan SJ, Kannan R, Hinton DR. alphaB-crystallin regulation of angiogenesis by modulation of VEGF. Blood. 2010;115:3398–406.
27. Ozawa K, Kondo T, Hori O, Kitao Y, Stern DM, Eisenmenger W, Ogawa S, Ohshima T. Expression of the oxygen-regulated protein ORP150 accelerates wound healing by modulating intracellular VEGF transport. J Clin Invest. 2001;108:41–50.
28. Bian ZM, Elner SG, Elner VM. Regulation of VEGF mRNA expression and protein secretion by TGF-beta2 in human retinal pigment epithelial cells. Exp Eye Res. 2007;84:812–22.
29. Waltenberger J, Claesson-Welsh L, Siegbahn A, Shibuya M, Heldin CH. Different signal transduction properties of KDR and Flt1, two receptors for vascular endothelial growth factor. J Biol Chem. 1994;269:26988–95.
30. Rahimi N. VEGFR-1 and VEGFR-2: two non-identical twins with a unique physiognomy. Front Biosci. 2006;11:818–29.
31. Chen TT, Luque A, Lee S, Anderson SM, Segura T, Iruela-Arispe ML. Anchorage of VEGF to the extracellular matrix conveys differential signaling responses to endothelial cells. J Cell Biol. 2010;188:595–609.
32. Blaauwgeers HG, Holtkamp GM, Rutten H, Witmer AN, Koolwijk P, Partanen TA, Alitalo K, Kroon ME, Kijlstra A, van Hinsbergh VW, Schlingemann RO. Polarized vascular endothelial growth factor secretion by human retinal pigment epithelium and localization of vascular endothelial growth factor receptors on the inner choriocapillaris. Evidence for a trophic paracrine relation. Am J Pathol. 1999;155:421–8.
33. Byeon SH, Lee SC, Choi SH, Lee HK, Lee JH, Chu YK, Kwon OW. Vascular endothelial growth factor as an autocrine survival factor for retinal pigment epithelial cells under oxidative stress via the VEGF-R2/PI3K/Akt. Invest Ophthalmol Vis Sci. 2010;51:1190–7.
34. Kim I, Ryan AM, Rohan R, Amano S, Agular S, Miller JW, Adamis AP. Constitutive expression of VEGF, VEGFR-1, and VEGFR-2 in normal eyes. Invest Ophthalmol Vis Sci. 1999;40:2115–21.
35. Saint-Geniez M, Maharaj AS, Walshe TE, Tucker BA, Sekiyama E, Kurihara T, Darland DC, Young MJ, D'Amore PA. Endogenous VEGF is required for visual function: evidence for a survival role on Müller cells and photoreceptors. PLoS One. 2008;3:e3554.
36. Bachelder RE, Crago A, Chung J, Wendt MA, Shaw LM, Robinson G, Mercurio AM. Vascular endothelial growth factor is an autocrine survival factor for neuropilin-expressing breast carcinoma cells. Cancer Res. 2001;61:5736–40.
37. Grünewald FS, Prota AE, Giese A, Ballmer-Hofer K. Structure-function analysis of VEGF receptor activation and the role of coreceptors in angiogenic signaling. Biochim Biophys Acta. 2010;1804:567–80.
38. Wang L, Zeng H, Wang P, Soker S, Mukhopadhyay D. Neuropilin-1-mediated vascular permeability factor/vascular endothelial growth factor-dependent endothelial cell migration. J Biol Chem. 2003;278:48848–60.
39. Klettner A. Physiological functions of VEGF in the retina and its possible implications of prolonged anti-VEGF therapy. In: Parker ML, editor. Vascular endothelial growth factor: biology, regulation and clinical significance. Nova Publishing; 2013. p. 117–36.
40. Adamis AP, Shima DT, Yeo KT, Yeo TK, Brown LF, Berse B, D'Amore PA, Folkman J. Synthesis and secretion of vascular permeability factor/vascular endothelial growth factor by human retinal pigment epithelial cells. Biochem Biophys Res Commun. 1993;193:631–8.
41. Bergmann M, Holz F, Kopitz J. Lysosomal stress and lipid peroxidation products induce VEGF-121 and VEGF-165 expression in ARPE-19 cells. Graefes Arch Clin Exp Ophthalmol. 2011;249:1477–83.
42. Saint-Geniez M, Maldonado AE, D'Amore PA. VEGF expression and receptor activation in the choroid during development and in the adult. Invest Ophthalmol Vis Sci. 2006;47:3135–42.
43. Watkins WM, McCollum GW, Savage SR, Capozzi ME, Penn JS, Morrison DG. Hypoxia-induced expression of VEGF splice variants and protein in four retinal cell types. Exp Eye Res. 2013;116:240–6.
44. Gerhardt H, Golding M, Fruttiger M, Ruhrberg C, Lundkvist A, Abramsson A, Jeltsch M, Mitchell C, Alitalo K, Shima D, Betsholtz C. VEGF guides

angiogenic sprouting utilizing endothelial tip cell filopodia. J Cell Biol. 2003;161:1163–77.
45. Scott A, Powner MB, Gandhi P, Clarkin C, Gutmann DH, Johnson RS, Ferrara N, Fruttiger M. Astrocyte-derived vascular endothelial growth factor stabilizes vessels in the developing retinal vasculature. PLoS One. 2010;5:e11863.
46. Stone J, Itin A, Alon T, Pe'er J, Gnessin H, Chan-Ling T, Keshet E. Development of retinal vasculature is mediated by hypoxia-induced vascular endothelial growth factor (VEGF) expression by neuroglia. J Neurosci. 1995;15:4738–47.
47. Yi X, Mai LC, Uyama M, Yew DT. Time-course expression of vascular endothelial growth factor as related to the development of the retinochoroidal vasculature in rats. Exp Brain Res. 1998;118:155–60.
48. Raymond SM, Jackson IJ. The retinal pigmented epithelium is required for development and maintenance of the mouse neural retina. Curr Biol. 1995;5:1286–95.
49. Marneros AG, Fan J, Yokoyama Y, Gerber HP, Ferrara N, Crouch RK, Olsen BR. Vascular endothelial growth factor expression in the retinal pigment epithelium is essential for choriocapillaris development and visual function. Am J Pathol. 2005;167:1451–9.
50. Zhao S, Overbeek PA. Regulation of choroid development by the retinal pigment epithelium. Mol Vis. 2001;7:277–82.
51. Lutty GA, Hasegawa T, Baba T, Grebe R, Bhutto I, McLeod DS. Development of the human choriocapillaris. Eye (Lond). 2010;24:408–15.
52. Zhao J, Song Y, Wang Y, Zhang X. Regulation effect of vascular endothelial growth factor on human fetal choroid vascularization. Yan Ke Xue Bao. 2000;16:11–4.
53. Ford KM, Saint-Geniez M, Walshe T, Zahr A, D'Amore PA. Expression and role of VEGF in the adult retinal pigment epithelium. Invest Ophthalmol Vis Sci. 2011;52:9478–87.
54. Gogat K, Le Gat L, Van Den Berghe L, Marchant D, Kobetz A, Gadin S, Gasser B, Quéré I, Abitbol M, Menasche M. VEGF and KDR gene expression during human embryonic and fetal eye development. Invest Ophthalmol Vis Sci. 2004;45:7–14.
55. Le YZ, Bai Y, Zhu M, Zheng L. Temporal requirement of RPE-derived VEGF in the development of choroidal vasculature. J Neurochem. 2010;112:1584–92.
56. Nickla DL, Wallman J. The multifunctional choroid. Prog Retin Eye Res. 2010;29:144–68.
57. Saint-Geniez M, Kurihara T, Sekiyama E, Maldonado AE, D'Amore PA. An essential role for RPE-derived soluble VEGF in the maintenance of the choriocapillaris. Proc Natl Acad Sci U S A. 2009;106:18751–6.
58. Klettner A, Kaya L, Flach J, Lassen J, Treumer F, Roider J. Basal and apical regulation of VEGF-A and placenta growth factor in the RPE/choroid and primary RPE. Mol Vis. 2015;21:736–48.
59. Kurihara T, Westenskow PD, Bravo S, Aguilar E, Friedlander M. Targeted deletion of Vegfa in adult mice induces vision loss. J Clin Invest. 2012;122:4213–7.
60. Peters S, Heiduschka P, Julien S, Ziemssen F, Fietz H, Bartz-Schmidt KU, Tübingen Bevacizumab Study Group, Schraermeyer U. Ultrastructural findings in the primate eye after intravitreal injection of bevacizumab. Am J Ophthalmol. 2007;143:995–1002.
61. Shimomura Y, Hirata A, Ishikawa S, Okinami S. Changes in choriocapillaris fenestration of rat eyes after intravitreal bevacizumab injection. Graefes Arch Clin Exp Ophthalmol. 2009;247:1089–94.
62. el-Remessy AB, Bartoli M, Platt DH, Fulton D, Caldwell RB. Oxidative stress inactivates VEGF survival signaling in retinal endothelial cells via PI 3-kinase tyrosine nitration. J Cell Sci. 2005;118:243–52.
63. Gerber HP, McMurtrey A, Kowalski J, Yan M, Keyt BA, Dixit V, Ferrara N. Vascular endothelial growth factor regulates endothelial cell survival through the phosphatidylinositol 3′-kinase/Akt signal transduction pathway. Requirement for Flk-1/KDR activation. J Biol Chem. 1998;273:30336–43.
64. Brar VS, Sharma RK, Murthy RK, Chalam KV. Bevacizumab neutralizes the protective effect of vascular endothelial growth factor on retinal ganglion cells. Mol Vis. 2010;16:1848–53.
65. Kilic U, Kilic E, Järve A, Guo Z, Spudich A, Bieber K, Barzena U, Bassetti CL, Marti HH, Hermann DM. Human vascular endothelial growth factor protects axotomized retinal ganglion cells in vivo by activating ERK-1/2 and Akt pathways. J Neurosci. 2006;26:12439–46.
66. Suzuki M, Ozawa Y, Kubota S, Hirasawa M, Miyake S, Noda K, Tsubota K, Kadonosono K, Ishida S. Neuroprotective response after photodynamic therapy: role of vascular endothelial growth factor. J Neuroinflammation. 2011;8:176.
67. Kehler AK, Andersen C, Andreasen JR, Vohra R, Junker N, Poulsen KA, Kolko M. Interaction between VEGF and calcium-independent phospholipase A2 in proliferation and migration of retinal pigment epithelium. Curr Eye Res. 2012;37:500–7.
68. Klettner A, Möhle F, Roider J. Intracellular bevacizumab reduces phagocytotic uptake in RPE cells. Graefes Arch Clin Exp Ophthalmol. 2010;248:819–24.
69. Klettner A, Tahmaz N, Dithmer M, Richert E, Roider J. Effects of aflibercept on primary RPE cells: toxicity, wound healing, uptake and phagocytosis. Br J Ophthalmol. 2014;98:1448–52.
70. Schottler J, Randoll N, Lucius R, Caliebe A, Roider J, Klettner A. Long-term treatment with anti-VEGF does not induce cell aging in primary retinal pigment epithelium. Exp Eye Res. 2018;171:1–11.
71. Dithmer M, Hattermann K, Pomarius P, Aboul Naga SH, Meyer T, Mentlein R, Roider J, Klettner A. The role of Fc-receptors in the uptake and transport of therapeutic antibodies in the retinal pigment epithelium. Exp Eye Res. 2016;145:187–205.

72. Rizzolo LJ. Barrier properties of cultured retinal pigment epithelium. Exp Eye Res. 2014;126:16–26.
73. Miura Y, Klettner A, Roider J. VEGF antagonists decrease barrier function of retinal pigment epithelium in vitro: possible participation of intracellular glutathione. Invest Ophthalmol Vis Sci. 2010;51:4848–55.
74. Ghassemifar R, Lai CM, Rakoczy PE. VEGF differentially regulates transcription and translation of ZO-1alpha+ and ZO-1alpha- and mediates trans-epithelial resistance in cultured endothelial and epithelial cells. Cell Tissue Res. 2006;323:117–25.
75. Peng S, Adelman RA, Rizzolo LJ. Minimal effects of VEGF and anti-VEGF drugs on the permeability or selectivity of RPE tight junctions. Invest Ophthalmol Vis Sci. 2010;51:3216–25.
76. Ablonczy Z, Dahrouj M, Marneros AG. Progressive dysfunction of the retinal pigment epithelium and retina due to increased VEGF-A levels. FASEB J. 2014;28:2369–79.
77. Cachafeiro M, Bemelmans AP, Samardzija M, Afanasieva T, Pournaras JA, Grimm C, Kostic C, Philippe S, Wenzel A, Arsenijevic Y. Hyperactivation of retina by light in mice leads to photoreceptor cell death mediated by VEGF and retinal pigment epithelium permeability. Cell Death Dis. 2013;4:e781.
78. Keir LS, Firth R, Aponik L, Feitelberg D, Sakimoto S, Aguilar E, Welsh GI, Richards A, Usui Y, Satchell SC, Kuzmuk V, Coward RJ, Goult J, Bull KR, Sharma R, Bharti K, Westenskow PD, Michael IP, Saleem MA, Friedlander M. VEGF regulates local inhibitory complement proteins in the eye and kidney. J Clin Invest. 2017;127:199–214.
79. Ueno S, Pease ME, Wersinger DM, Masuda T, Vinores SA, Licht T, Zack DJ, Quigley H, Keshet E, Campochiaro PA. Prolonged blockade of VEGF family members does not cause identifiable damage to retinal neurons or vessels. J Cell Physiol. 2008;217:13–22.
80. Gemenetzi M, Lotery AJ, Patel PJ. Risk of geographic atrophy in age-related macular degeneration patients treated with intravitreal anti-VEGF agents. Eye. 2016;31:1–9.
81. Miller JW, Le Couter J, Strauss EC, Ferrara N. Vascular endothelial growth factor a in intraocular vascular disease. Ophthalmology. 2013;120:106–14.
82. Cornel S, Adriana ID, Mihaela TC, Speranta S, Algerino S, Mehdi B, Jalaladin HR. Anti-vascular endothelial growth factor indications in ocular disease. Rom J Ophthalmol. 2015;59:235–42.
83. Wu AL, Wu WC. Anti-VEGF for ROP and pediatric retinal diseases. Asia Pac J Ophthalmol (Phila). 2018;7:145–51.
84. Amin R, Puklin JE, Frank RN. Growth factor localization in choroidal neovascular membranes of age-related macular degeneration. Invest Ophthalmol Vis Sci. 1994;35:3178–88.
85. Kvanta A, Algvere PV, Berglin L, Seregard S. Subfoveal fibrovascular membranes in age-related macular degeneration express vascular endothelial growth factor. Invest Ophthalmol Vis Sci. 1996;37:1929–34.
86. Ikeda Y, Yonemitsu Y, Onimaru M, Nakano T, Miyazaki M, Kohno R, Nakagawa K, Ueno A, Sueishi K, Ishibashi T. The regulation of vascular endothelial growth factors (VEGF-A, -C, and -D) expression in the retinal pigment epithelium. Exp Eye Res. 2006;83:1031–40.
87. Schwesinger C, Yee C, Rohan RM, Joussen AM, Fernandez A, Meyer TN, Poulaki V, Ma JJ, Redmond TM, Liu S, Adamis AP, D'Amato RJ. Intrachoroidal neovascularization in transgenic mice overexpressing vascular endothelial growth factor in the retinal pigment epithelium. Am J Pathol. 2001;158:1161–72.
88. Spilsbury K, Garrett KL, Shen WY, Constable IJ, Rakoczy PE. Overexpression of vascular endothelial growth factor (VEGF) in the retinal pigment epithelium leads to the development of choroidal neovascularization. Am J Pathol. 2000;157:135–44.
89. Oshima Y, Oshima S, Nambu H, Kachi S, Hackett SF, Melia M, Kaleko M, Connelly S, Esumi N, Zack DJ, Campochiaro PA. Increased expression of VEGF in retinal pigmented epithelial cells is not sufficient to cause choroidal neovascularization. J Cell Physiol. 2004;201:393–400.
90. Le YZ. VEGF production and signaling in Müller glia are critical to modulating vascular function and neuronal integrity in diabetic retinopathy and hypoxic retinal vascular diseases. Vis Res. 2017;139:108–14.
91. Ponnalagu M, Subramani M, Jayadev C, Shetty R, Das D. Retinal pigment epithelium-secretome: a diabetic retinopathy perspective. Cytokine. 2017;95:126–35.
92. Xu HZ, Song Z, Fu S, Zhu M, Le YZ. RPE barrier breakdown in diabetic retinopathy: seeing is believing. J Ocul Biol Dis Infor. 2011;4:83–92.
93. Dahrouj M, Alsarraf O, McMillin JC, Liu Y, Crosson CE, Ablonczy Z. Vascular endothelial growth factor modulates the function of the retinal pigment epithelium in vivo. Invest Ophthalmol Vis Sci. 2014;55:2269–75.
94. Marneros AG. Increased VEGF-A promotes multiple distinct aging diseases of the eye through shared pathomechanisms. EMBO Mol Med. 2016;8:208–31.
95. Nguyen M, Arnheiter H. Signaling and transcriptional regulation in early mammalian eye development: a link between FGF and MITF. Development. 2000;127:3581–91.
96. Ford KM, D'Amore PA. Molecular regulation of vascular endothelial growth factor expression in the retinal pigment epithelium. Mol Vis. 2012;18:519–27.
97. Miura Y, Klettner A, Noelle B, Hasselbach H, Roider J. Change of morphological and functional characteristics of retinal pigment epithelium cells during cultivation of retinal pigment epithelium-choroid perfusion tissue culture. Ophthalmic Res. 2010;43:122–33.

98. Dithmer M, Fuchs S, Shi Y, Schmidt H, Richert E, Roider J, Klettner A. Fucoidan reduces secretion and expression of vascular endothelial growth factor in the retinal pigment epithelium and reduces angiogenesis in vitro. PLoS One. 2014;9:e89150.
99. Rosenthal R, Heimann H, Agostini H, Martin G, Hansen LL, Strauss O. Ca2+ channels in retinal pigment epithelial cells regulate vascular endothelial growth factor secretion rates in health and disease. Mol Vis. 2007;13:443–56.
100. Cordeiro S, Seyler S, Stindl J, Milenkovic VM, Strauss O. Heat-sensitive TRPV channels in retinal pigment epithelial cells: regulation of VEGF-A secretion. Invest Ophthalmol Vis Sci. 2010;51:6001–8.
101. Levy AP, Levy NS, Goldberg MA. Hypoxia-inducible protein binding to vascular endothelial growth factor mRNA and its modulation by the von Hippel-Lindau protein. J Biol Chem. 1996;271:25492–7.
102. Wang B, Zou Y, Yuan ZL, Xiao JG. Genistein suppressed upregulation of vascular endothelial growth factor expression by cobalt chloride and hypoxia in rabbit retinal pigment epithelium cells. J Ocul Pharmacol Ther. 2003;19:457–64.
103. Park H, Lee DS, Yim MJ, Choi YH, Park S, Seo SK, Choi JS, Jang WH, Yea SS, Park WS, Lee CM, Jung WK, Choi IW. 3,3′-Diindolylmethane inhibits VEGF expression through the HIF-1α and NF-κB pathways in human retinal pigment epithelial cells under chemical hypoxic conditions. Int J Mol Med. 2015;36:301–8.
104. Xiao Q, Zeng S, Ling S, Lv M. Up-regulation of HIF-1alpha and VEGF expression by elevated glucose concentration and hypoxia in cultured human retinal pigment epithelial cells. J Huazhong Univ Sci Technolog Med Sci. 2006;26:463–5.
105. Yang XM, Wang YS, Zhang J, Li Y, Xu JF, Zhu J, Zhao W, Chu DK, Wiedemann P. Role of PI3K/Akt and MEK/ERK in mediating hypoxia-induced expression of HIF-1alpha and VEGF in laser-induced rat choroidal neovascularization. Invest Ophthalmol Vis Sci. 2009;50:1873–9.
106. Ling S, Birnbaum Y, Nanhwan MK, Thomas B, Bajaj M, Ye Y. MicroRNA-dependent cross-talk between VEGF and HIF1α in the diabetic retina. Cell Signal. 2013;25:2840–7.
107. Bartel DP. MicroRNAs: target recognition and regulatory functions. Cell. 2009;136:215–33.
108. Zhu M, Liu X, Wang S, Miao J, Wu L, Yang X, Wang Y, Kang L, Li W, Cui C, Chen H, Sang A. PKR promotes choroidal neovascularization via upregulating the PI3K/Akt signaling pathway in VEGF expression. Mol Vis. 2016;22:1361–74.
109. Seong H, Ryu J, Jeong JY, Chung IY, Han YS, Hwang SH, Park JM, Kang SS, Seo SW. Resveratrol suppresses vascular endothelial growth factor secretion via inhibition of CXC-chemokine receptor 4 expression in ARPE-19 cells. Mol Med Rep. 2015;12:1479–84.
110. Young TA, Wang H, Munk S, Hammoudi DS, Young DS, Mandelcorn MS, Whiteside CI. Vascular endothelial growth factor expression and secretion by retinal pigment epithelial cells in high glucose and hypoxia is protein kinase C-dependent. Exp Eye Res. 2005;80:651–62.
111. Hollborn M, Ackmann C, Kuhrt H, Doktor F, Kohen L, Wiedemann P, Bringmann A. Osmotic and hypoxic induction of the complement factor C9 in cultured human retinal pigment epithelial cells: regulation of VEGF and NLRP3 expression. Mol Vis. 2018;24:518–35.
112. Sreekumar PG, Kannan R, de Silva AT, Burton R, Ryan SJ, Hinton DR. Thiol regulation of vascular endothelial growth factor-A and its receptors in human retinal pigment epithelial cells. Biochem Biophys Res Commun. 2006;346:1200–6.
113. Maisto R, Oltra M, Vidal-Gil L, Martínez-Gil N, Sancho-Pelluz J, Filippo CD, Rossi S, D Amico M, Barcia JM, Romero FJ. ARPE-19-derived VEGF-containing exosomes promote neovascularization in HUVEC: the role of the melanocortin receptor 5. Cell Cycle. 2019;18:413–24.
114. Aboul Naga SH, Dithmer M, Chitadze G, Kabelitz D, Lucius R, Roider J, Klettner A. Intracellular pathways following uptake of bevacizumab in RPE cells. Exp Eye Res. 2015;131:29–41.
115. Klettner A, Roider J. Constitutive and oxidative-stress-induced expression of VEGF in the RPE are differently regulated by different mitogen-activated protein kinases. Graefes Arch Clin Exp Ophthalmol. 2009;247:1487–92.
116. Kunchithapautham K, Rohrer B. Sublytic membrane-attack-complex (MAC) activation alters regulated rather than constitutive vascular endothelial growth factor (VEGF) secretion in retinal pigment epithelium monolayers. J Biol Chem. 2011;286:23717–24.
117. Luo X, Gu S, Zhang Y, Zhang J. Kinsenoside ameliorates oxidative stress-induced RPE cell apoptosis and inhibits angiogenesis via Erk/p38/NF-κB/VEGF signaling. Front Pharmacol. 2018;9:240.
118. Pollreisz A, Afonyushkin T, Oskolkova OV, Gruber F, Bochkov VN, Schmidt-Erfurth U. Retinal pigment epithelium cells produce VEGF in response to oxidized phospholipids through mechanisms involving ATF4 and protein kinase CK2. Exp Eye Res. 2013;116:177–84.
119. Sano R, Reed JC. ER stress-induced cell death mechanisms. Biochim Biophys Acta. 2013;1833:3460–70.
120. Miyagi H, Kanemoto S, Saito A, Asada R, Iwamoto H, Izumi S, Kido M, Gomi F, Nishida K, Kiuchi Y, Imaizumi K. Transcriptional regulation of VEGFA by the endoplasmic reticulum stress transducer OASIS in ARPE-19 cells. PLoS One. 2013;8:e55155.
121. Yoshida T, Ohno-Matsui K, Ichinose S, Sato T, Iwata N, Saido TC, Hisatomi T, Mochizuki M, Morita I. The potential role of amyloid beta in the pathogenesis of age-related macular degeneration. J Clin Invest. 2005;115:2793–800.

122. Matsui A, Kaneko H, Kachi S, Ye F, Hwang SJ, Takayama K, Nagasaka Y, Sugita T, Terasaki H. Expression of vascular endothelial growth factor by retinal pigment epithelial cells induced by amyloid-β is depressed by an endoplasmic reticulum stress inhibitor. Ophthalmic Res. 2015;55:37–44.
123. Chen L, Bai Y, Zhao M, Jiang Y. TLR4 inhibitor attenuates amyloid-β-induced angiogenic and inflammatory factors in ARPE-19 cells: implications for age-related macular degeneration. Mol Med Rep. 2016;13:3249–56.
124. Wu L, Tan X, Liang L, Yu H, Wang C, Zhang D, Kijlstra A, Yang P. The role of mitochondria-associated reactive oxygen species in the amyloid β induced production of angiogenic factors by ARPE-19 cells. Curr Mol Med. 2017;17:140–8.
125. Ma W, Lee SE, Guo J, Qu W, Hudson BI, Schmidt AM, Barile GR. RAGE ligand upregulation of VEGF secretion in ARPE-19 cells. Invest Ophthalmol Vis Sci. 2007;48:1355–61.
126. Cai Y, Li X, Wang YS, Shi YY, Ye Z, Yang GD, Dou GR, Hou HY, Yang N, Cao XR, Lu ZF. Hyperglycemia promotes vasculogenesis in choroidal neovascularization in diabetic mice by stimulating VEGF and SDF-1 expression in retinal pigment epithelial cells. Exp Eye Res. 2014;123:87–96.
127. Sone H, Kawakami Y, Okuda Y, Kondo S, Hanatani M, Suzuki H, Yamashita K. Vascular endothelial growth factor is induced by long-term high glucose concentration and up-regulated by acute glucose deprivation in cultured bovine retinal pigmented epithelial cells. Biochem Biophys Res Commun. 1996;221:193–8.
128. Chang ML, Chiu CJ, Shang F, Taylor A. High glucose activates ChREBP-mediated HIF-1α and VEGF expression in human RPE cells under normoxia. Adv Exp Med Biol. 2014;801:609–21.
129. Li X, Cai Y, Wang YS, Shi YY, Hou W, Xu CS, Wang HY, Ye Z, Yao LB, Zhang J. Hyperglycaemia exacerbates choroidal neovascularisation in mice via the oxidative stress-induced activation of STAT3 signalling in RPE cells. PLoS One. 2012;7:e47600.
130. Punglia RS, Lu M, Hsu J, Kuroki M, Tolentino MJ, Keough K, Levy AP, Levy NS, Goldberg MA, D'Amato RJ, Adamis AP. Regulation of vascular endothelial growth factor expression by insulin-like growth factor I. Diabetes. 1997;46:1619–26.
131. Sall JW, Klisovic DD, O'Dorisio MS, Katz SE. Somatostatin inhibits IGF-1 mediated induction of VEGF in human retinal pigment epithelial cells. Exp Eye Res. 2004;79:465–76.
132. Slomiany MG, Rosenzweig SA. Autocrine effects of IGF-I-induced VEGF and IGFBP-3 secretion in retinal pigment epithelial cell line ARPE-19. Am J Physiol Cell Physiol. 2004;287:C746–53.
133. Smith LE, Shen W, Perruzzi C, Soker S, Kinose F, Xu X, Robinson G, Driver S, Bischoff J, Zhang B, Schaeffer JM, Senger DR. Regulation of vascular endothelial growth factor-dependent retinal neovascularization by insulin-like growth factor-1 receptor. Nat Med. 1999;5:1390–5.
134. Lu M, Amano S, Miyamoto K, Garland R, Keough K, Qin W, Adamis AP. Insulin-induced vascular endothelial growth factor expression in retina. Invest Ophthalmol Vis Sci. 1999;40:3281–6.
135. Kumar MV, Nagineni CN, Chin MS, Hooks JJ, Detrick B. Innate immunity in the retina: toll-like receptor (TLR) signaling in human retinal pigment epithelial cells. J Neuroimmunol. 2004;153:7–15.
136. Akira S, Takeda K, Kaisho T. Toll-like receptors: critical proteins linking innate and acquired immunity. Nat Immunol. 2001;2:675–80.
137. Takeda K, Kaisho T, Akira S. Toll-like receptors. Annu Rev Immunol. 2003;21:335–76.
138. Fujimoto T, Sonoda KH, Hijioka K, Sato K, Takeda A, Hasegawa E, Oshima Y, Ishibashi T. Choroidal neovascularization enhanced by Chlamydia pneumoniae via Toll-like receptor 2 in the retinal pigment epithelium. Invest Ophthalmol Vis Sci. 2010;51:4694–702.
139. Ebihara N, Chen L, Tokura T, Ushio H, Iwatsu M, Murakami A. Distinct functions between toll-like receptors 3 and 9 in retinal pigment epithelial cells. Ophthalmic Res. 2007;39:155–63.
140. Klettner A, Koinzer S, Meyer T, Roider J. Toll-like receptor 3 activation in retinal pigment epithelium cells—mitogen-activated protein kinase pathways of cell death and vascular endothelial growth factor secretion. Acta Ophthalmol. 2013;91:e211–8.
141. Terasaki H, Kase S, Shirasawa M, Otsuka H, Hisatomi T, Sonoda S, Ishida S, Ishibashi T, Sakamoto T. TNF-α decreases VEGF secretion in highly polarized RPE cells but increases it in non-polarized RPE cells related to crosstalk between JNK and NF-κB pathways. PLoS One. 2013;8:e69994.
142. Sugita S, Futagami Y, Smith SB, Naggar H, Mochizuki M. Retinal and ciliary body pigment epithelium suppress activation of T lymphocytes via transforming growth factor beta. Exp Eye Res. 2006;83:1459–71.
143. Kvanta A. Expression and secretion of transforming growth factor-beta in transformed and nontransformed retinal pigment epithelial cells. Ophthalmic Res. 1994;26:361–7.
144. Nagineni CN, Samuel W, Nagineni S, Pardhasaradhi K, Wiggert B, Detrick B, Hooks JJ. Transforming growth factor-beta induces expression of vascular endothelial growth factor in human retinal pigment epithelial cells: involvement of mitogen-activated protein kinases. J Cell Physiol. 2003;197:453–62.
145. Bian ZM, Elner SG, Elner VM. Thrombin-induced VEGF expression in human retinal pigment epithelial cells. Invest Ophthalmol Vis Sci. 2007;48:2738–46.
146. Bastiaans J, van Meurs JC, Mulder VC, Nagtzaam NM, Smits-te Nijenhuis M, Dufour-van den Goorbergh DC, van Hagen PM, Hooijkaas H, Dik WA. The role of thrombin in proliferative vitreoretinopathy. Invest Ophthalmol Vis Sci. 2014;55:4659–66.

147. Sagripanti A, Romani A, Ferretti A, Ragone MC, Baicchi U, Carpi A, Nardi M. Blood coagulation parameters in retinal arterial occlusion. Graefes Arch Clin Exp Ophthalmol. 1999;237:480–3.
148. Terasaki H, Shirasawa M, Otsuka H, Yamashita T, Uchino E, Hisatomi T, Sonoda S, Sakamoto T. Different effects of thrombin on VEGF secretion, proliferation, and permeability in polarized and non-polarized retinal pigment epithelial cells. Curr Eye Res. 2015;40:936–45.
149. Hao Y, Zhou Q, Ma J, Zhao Y, Wang S. miR-146a is upregulated during retinal pigment epithelium (RPE)/choroid aging in mice and represses IL-6 and VEGF-A expression in RPE cells. J Clin Exp Ophthalmol. 2016;7:562.
150. Doyle SL, Campbell M, Ozaki E, Salomon RG, Mori A, Kenna PF, Farrar GJ, Kiang AS, Humphries MM, Lavelle EC, O'Neill LA, Hollyfield JG, Humphries P. NLRP3 has a protective role in age-related macular degeneration through the induction of IL-18 by drusen components. Nat Med. 2012;18:791–8.
151. Mohr LK, Hoffmann AV, Brandstetter C, Holz FG, Krohne TU. Effects of inflammasome activation on secretion of inflammatory cytokines and vascular endothelial growth factor by retinal pigment epithelial cells. Invest Ophthalmol Vis Sci. 2015;56:6404–13.
152. Cortright DN, Meade R, Waters SM, Chenard BL, Krause JE. C5a, but not C3a, increases VEGF secretion in ARPE-19 human retinal pigment epithelial cells. Curr Eye Res. 2009;34:57–61.
153. Long Q, Cao X, Bian A, Li Y. C3a increases VEGF and decreases PEDF mRNA levels in human retinal pigment epithelial cells. Biomed Res Int. 2016;2016:6958752.
154. Li W, Chen S, Ma M, Qian J, Ma X. Complement 5b-9 complex-induced alterations in human RPE cell physiology. Med Sci Monit. 2010;16:BR17–23.
155. Lueck K, Wasmuth S, Williams J, Hughes TR, Morgan BP, Lommatzsch A, Greenwood J, Moss SE, Pauleikhoff D. Sub-lytic C5b-9 induces functional changes in retinal pigment epithelial cells consistent with age-related macular degeneration. Eye. 2011;25:1074–82.
156. Faby H, Hillenkamp J, Roider J, Klettner A. Hyperthermia-induced upregulation of vascular endothelial growth factor in retinal pigment epithelial cells is regulated by mitogen-activated protein kinases. Graefes Arch Clin Exp Ophthalmol. 2014;252:1737–45.
157. Coassin M, Duncan KG, Bailey KR, Singh A, Schwartz DM. Hypothermia reduces secretion of vascular endothelial growth factor by cultured retinal pigment epithelial cells. Br J Ophthalmol. 2010;94:1678–83.
158. Takeyama M, Yoneda M, Gosho M, Iwaki M, Zako M. Decreased VEGF-A and sustained PEDF expression in a human retinal pigment epithelium cell line cultured under hypothermia. Biol Res. 2015;48:42.
159. Iwami H, Pruessner J, Shiraki K, Brinkmann R, Miura Y. Protective effect of a laser-induced sublethal temperature rise on RPE cells from oxidative stress. Exp Eye Res. 2014;124:37–47.
160. Chen JT, Liang JB, Chou CL, Shyu RC, Lu DW. Retinoic acid induces VEGF gene expression in human retinal pigment epithelial cells (ARPE-19). J Ocul Pharmacol Ther. 2005;21:413–9.
161. Tokarz P, Piastowska-Ciesielska AW, Kaarniranta K, Blasiak J. All-trans retinoic acid modulates DNA damage response and the expression of the VEGF-A and MKI67 genes in ARPE-19 cells subjected to oxidative stress. Int J Mol Sci. 2016;17:E898.
162. Farjood F, Vargis E. Physical disruption of cell-cell contact induces VEGF expression in RPE cells. Mol Vis. 2017;23:431–46.
163. Marazita MC, Dugour A, Marquioni-Ramella MD, Figueroa JM, Suburo AM. Oxidative stress-induced premature senescence dysregulates VEGF and CFH expression in retinal pigment epithelial cells: implications for age-related macular degeneration. Redox Biol. 2016;7:78–87.
164. Eldweik L, Mantagos IS. Role of VEGF inhibition in the treatment of retinopathy of prematurity. Semin Ophthalmol. 2016;31:163–8.
165. Schmidt-Erfurth U, Chong V, Loewenstein A, Larsen M, Souied E, Schlingemann R, Eldem B, Monés J, Richard G, Bandello F, European Society of Retina Specialists. Guidelines for the management of neovascular age-related macular degeneration by the European Society of Retina Specialists (EURETINA). Br J Ophthalmol. 2014;98:1144–67.
166. Schmidt-Erfurth U, Garcia-Arumi J, Bandello F, Berg K, Chakravarthy U, Gerendas BS, Jonas J, Larsen M, Tadayoni R, Loewenstein A. Guidelines for the management of diabetic macular edema by the European Society of Retina Specialists (EURETINA). Ophthalmologica. 2017;237:185–222.
167. Kniggendorf VF, Novais EA, Kniggendorf SL, Xavier C, Cole ED, Regatieri CV. Effect of intravitreal anti-VEGF on choroidal thickness in patients with diabetic macular edema using spectral domain OCT. Arq Bras Oftalmol. 2016;79:155–8.
168. Quinn GE, Darlow BA. Concerns for development after bevacizumab treatment of ROP. Pediatrics. 2016;137:e20160057.
169. Rofagha S, Bhisitkul RB, Boyer DS, Sadda SR, Zhang K, SEVEN-UP Study Group. Seven-year outcomes in ranibizumab-treated patients in ANCHOR, MARINA, and HORIZON: a multicenter cohort study (SEVEN-UP). Ophthalmology. 2013;120:2292–9.

The RPE Cell and the Immune System

6

Barbara Detrick and John J. Hooks

Introduction

In addition to its indispensable role in the visual system, immunologically the RPE cell is a pivotal retinal cell that participates in the ocular immunity. Recent discoveries have highlighted the importance of this cell in regulating health and disease and our understanding about immunity in the ocular microenvironment has grown exponentially in the last several years. The RPE cell orchestrates both innate and adaptive immunity and contains a plethora of factors to regulate the immune response [1]. Compelling evidence now suggests that immune activation of the RPE cell may have far reaching effects in retinal infections, autoimmunity and retinal degenerations, i.e. age related macular degeneration (AMD) and diabetic retinopathy. As we review the varied ways in which the RPE cell influences ocular immunity, we will highlight possible mechanisms to explain how these responses impact vision.

B. Detrick (✉)
Department of Pathology and Medicine, School of Medicine, The Johns Hopkins University, Baltimore, MD, USA
e-mail: bdetrick@jhmi.edu

J. J. Hooks
Laboratory of Immunology, National Eye Institute, National Institutes of Health, Bethesda, MD, USA

RPE Cell: Role in Ocular Innate Immunity

The immune system is composed of two major recognition systems: innate immunity and adaptive immunity. Innate immunity is considered the immediate immune response to an insult or pathogen, is nonspecific and does not confer long-lasting protective immunity. Nevertheless, it often determines the fate of the adaptive immune response. Once engaged, innate immunity can activate a series of immune components: such as, microbial sensors (Toll-like receptors (TLRs), NOD-like receptors, NLR, RIG-1 like helicases), certain critical cell types, cytokines, chemokines as well as a group of complement components; all directed to assist the host with eliminating the current insult (Table 6.1).

Over the last several decades, tremendous progress has taken place in the field of immunology. Many of these advances have enhanced our understanding of how the immune response impacts human health and disease and have uncovered novel therapeutic approaches to treat many human disorders [2]. In this chapter, we will not attempt to identify all of the new immunologic developments that have been reported. Rather, we have chosen to highlight a few discoveries that have relevance within the retina that better inform about mechanisms of ocular diseases and potential treatment strategies. Current reviews will be included in areas not covered in detail.

A. K. Klettner, S. Dithmar (eds.), *Retinal Pigment Epithelium in Health and Disease*,
https://doi.org/10.1007/978-3-030-28384-1_6

Table 6.1 RPE cell participation in innate immunity

RPE cell component	Immune responses generated
Immune sensors (TLRs, NOD-like receptors)	– Cytokine/chemokine production
	– Pro-inflammatory responses
	– TLR3 leads to photoreceptor and RPE modulation
	– VEGF production
	– Cell death or protection
Cytokines	– IL-6, IL-1β—inflammatory activity
	– IFN-β, IL-11, TGF-β—immunosuppressive activity
	– IL-6, MCP-1—influence angiogenesis
Chemokines	– CXCL9, CXCL10—Attract T and NK cells
	– CXCL8—Attracts neutrophils
	– MCP-1—Attracts monocytes, dendritic cells and memory T cells
Growth factor production	– VEGF—Induces neovascularization
	– PDGF
Complement components	– CD46, CD55, CD59—Downregulates complement activation
	– C3a and C5a receptors—Induces inflammation
	– Associated with alterations in AMD and other dystrophies

Components of Innate Immunity

Toll-Like Receptors

TLRs are a family of evolutionary conserved innate immune recognition molecules that sense molecular patterns associated with microbial pathogens. TLR recognition of these microbial patterns leads to a signal transduction cascade that generates a rapid and robust inflammatory response marked by cellular activation and the production of a variety of cytokines, including pro-inflammatory cytokines, cytokines that promote T cell differentiation, type 1 interferons and chemokines. Since their discovery in 1980, the TLR molecules have been described in numerous cell types throughout the body [3]. Currently, the human TLR family comprises ten TLRs and each is distinguished by their ligand specificity [3]. Also, each TLR has a unique location and expression pattern within the cell. For example, TLR3, 7 and 9 are located manly within the cellular endosome while the remaining TLRs (TLR2, 4, 5, 6) are found on the cell membrane. Overall, TLRs located on the cell membrane recognize bacterial products (i.e. TLR4 recognizes bacterial lipid A from Gram negative bacteria) while the intracellular TLRs detect viral or bacterial nucleic acids (i.e. TLR3 interacts with dsRNA formed during virus replication).

These sentinel molecules were originally described on the RPE cell well over 10 years ago [4]. It is not surprising that the RPE cell is endowed with many of the TLRs, since it is strategically situated and can provide a rapid defense system for the retina [4]. Analysis of TLR gene expression identified the presence of TLR1 through 7, 9 and 10 on human RPE cells. Interestingly, TLR3, a vital TLR for defense against virus infection, is the most highly expressed TLR on the RPE cell. TLR3 recognizes a dsRNA motif, an intermediate product of virus replication or an analog of dsRNA, polyinosinic:polycytidylic acid (Poly I:C). Analysis of signaling through TLR3 revealed that the RPE cell secreted several pro-inflammatory mediators, including, IL-6, IL-8 (CXCL8), MCP-1, ICAM-1, CXCL9, CXCL10 and VEGF [5]. These molecules provide signals for immune and retinal resident cells to activate and initiate inflammatory pathways. An important immunosuppressive cytokine, that is selectively upregulated by TLR3, is IFN-β. This cytokine and its unique interaction with the RPE cell will be discussed later.

Interest in the retinal TLRs has continued at a rapid pace and recent work has demonstrated a potential involvement of TLRs in a variety of retinal diseases. For example, TLR polymorphisms have been associated with AMD [6, 7]. Investigations exploring the utility of siRNA treatment for AMD, identified that siRNA signaled through TLR3 [8, 9]. This signaling process results in the inhibition of vascular endothelial growth factor (VEGF) expression. These studies suggest a mechanism by which siRNA molecules can inhibit neovascularization in AMD. Also, the critical importance of the

TLRs is underscored by recent investigations evaluating deficiencies in TLR. In a mouse model of diabetic retinopathy it was reported that a deficiency in TLR7 inhibits inflammation and this lack of TLR7 results in an attenuation of diabetic retinopathy [10].

Several investigators have identified that activation of TLR3 within RPE cells is associated with RPE cell damage that may contribute to retinal degenerations in AMD and other retinal disorders [11, 12]. Klettner and associates found that TLR3 activation in RPE cells results in cell death partly mediated by JNK [13, 14]. Alternatively, studies have also demonstrated a protective role for TLR3 signaling. Patel and associates have shown that TLR3 signaling through a STAT3 dependent mechanism protects RPE cells from oxidative stress [15, 16]. Taken together, these studies illustrate the major position of the RPE in innate immunity and stress the plethora of responses TLR signaling affects. Future experiments are needed to better define the role of TLRs in human ocular diseases and to pinpoint additional strategies that limit or boost their function [12].

Cytokines

Cytokines are potent, low molecular-weight protein cell regulators often produced transiently and locally by many cell types. Following their initial discovery nearly 60 years ago, the cytokine definition has grown to include their multiple effects as pleiotropic proteins whose biological properties support key roles in hematopoiesis, immunity, infectious disease, tumorigenesis, homeostasis, cellular development and growth. Thus, because of their varied participatory roles, we recognize these molecules as powerful agents that control many aspects of health and disease and as potential therapeutic tools for variety of immune based disorders. Immunologically, cytokines have emerged as mediators that bridge innate and adaptive immunity, as molecules that participate in both inflammatory and anti-inflammatory activities and as regulators that influence numerous diseases.

The body is filled with cells that produce cytokines and each cell is strategically designed and ready to generate a cytokine signature when needed. Within the retina, the RPE cell serves as a rich source of cytokines. Many of the cytokines produced, such as, IL-6, IL-8, MCP-1, CXCL9 and CXCL10 are pro-inflammatory and will be highlighted here. The immunosuppressive cytokines produced by the RPE cell will be discussed in the immunoregulation section.

In the early and mid 1980s, IL-6 was first described as a lymphocyte stimulating factor that activated T cells and differentiated B cells. Now some 40 years later, we appreciate that IL-6 exerts its effects on a broad variety of responses ranging from acute and chronic inflammation to vascular disease and because of these multiple activities, this cytokine is now considered a primary target for clinical intervention [17].

In the eye, numerous cells generate IL-6. The RPE cell produces high levels of IL-6 in response to several stimuli, such as, infectious agents, other cytokines (IL-1 β, TNF-α and IFNs) and TLR ligation [18, 19]. As we have witnessed elsewhere in the body, the release of IL-6 by the RPE cell may be an important component of a chronic as well as acute inflammatory response in the retina. Based on the analysis of systemic diseases several studies have implicated the persistent production of IL-6 as a cytokine involved with the onset and development of autoimmunity [20, 21]. In order to better understand pathogenic mechanisms in autoimmune retinopathy (AIR), we evaluated the presence of cytokine markers in AIR patients. Recently, our laboratory identified the increased presence of IL-6 and CXCL9 in AIR patient sera and show that these elevated levels correlate with augmented disease severity. These studies provide evidence that IL-6 and CXCL9 may participate in AIR pathology [22]. A previous study using flow cytometric immunophenotyping to analyze this same cohort of patients noted that B-lymphocyte anomalies were described in AIR patient plasma compared to normal and uveitic patient samples [23]. Both of these observations hint that the immune response may play a role AIR. Nevertheless, additional investigations are needed to unravel the involvement of the immune response in this rare disease with the hope that more definitive guidelines for diagnosis and treatment strategy will be developed.

Chemokines are a superfamily of small diffusible protein molecules (8–14 kDa) secreted by various cell types in response to inflammatory, infectious and autoimmune disease signals [24]. Chemokines participate in inflammation by regulating neutrophil, macrophage and lymphocyte trafficking to the pathologic site. The presence of chemokine expression in the retina has been associated with a number of retinal disorders. Numerous studies have revealed that within the retina, the RPE cell provides high levels of IL-8, MCP-1 and CXCL9 and CXCL10. IL-8, often identified as one of the early inflammatory mediators following injury, is a potent chemoattractant and activator of neutrophils. In addition, IL-8 promotes the migration and proliferation of endothelial cells and possesses strong angiogenic properties within the eye. Another chemokine that directs monocytes, memory T cells and dendritic cells to an inflammatory site and is associated with neovascularization, is CCL2 (MCP-1). Like IL-8, this chemokine has also been implicated in number of disorders within the retina. Not long ago, Chan and colleagues demonstrated in an animal model that CCL2 was associated with AMD. The authors show that mice deficient in CCL2 develop a retinal disease that mimics human AMD [25].

As a result of extensive work examining the immunoregulatory role of the IFN molecules in the immune response, a group of chemokines was discovered. CXCL9 and CXCL10 are interferon inducible chemokines that interact with their receptor, CXCR3, on the surface of T cells and NK cells resulting in the migration and activation of these cells into inflamed sites. Following the first description of these two chemokines by Detrick et al., in a degenerative disease, experimental coronavirus retinopathy (ECOR), Nawaz and collaborators also detected both CXCL9 and CXCL10 on retinal endothelial cells in human diabetic retinopathy [26, 27]. Additional chemokine signaling studies were reported in a rodent model of degeneration by Rutar and associates. These investigators found that CXCL10 was present in this model system and was responsible for the chemokine mediated inflammation observed [28, 29].

Chronic inflammation and exaggerated VEGF production are important hallmarks of choroidal neovascularization in AMD and other vitreoretinal disorders. Moreover, the RPE is a key pathologic site in this disease. Reports from several investigators have shown in vitro that stimulation of RPE cells with cytokines, such as, IL-1β, TNF-α and IFN-γ results in the production of high levels of VEGF [30, 31]. This example emphasizes the potent influence of immune activated RPE cells and the detrimental consequence of this upregulation of inflammatory cytokines. Based on such findings, strategies to block VEGF production have been developed and anti-VEGF is now considered standard care for AMD. For a more detailed description of VEGF treatment and AMD, we refer the reader to [32].

This is an exciting time in cytokine biology. As a result of these new discoveries, it is anticipated that continued research will further our understanding and offer new options for therapeutic interventions.

Complement

The complement system, a complex and sophisticated network of various proteins, regulators and receptors, is an integral component of innate and adaptive immunity. Over the years there has been a rebirth of interest related to the complement system. The complement system in the immune privileged-eye plays a critical role in retinal hemostasis by providing the retina neuroprotection. This dynamic proteolytic cascade is tightly regulated and constantly monitors inflammation via its complement regulatory proteins while continuing to eliminate invading pathogens [32].

The RPE cell manufactures and possess on its cell surface many of the complement components. For example, both C3a and C5a receptors are expressed on the RPE membrane. When C5a interacts with the RPE C5a receptor, TLR4 is activated to produce pro-inflammatory cytokines, such as IL-1β, IL-6, IL-8, MCP-1 and GM-CSF [33, 34]. In this way the complement system drives inflammation in the retina.

Alternatively, as mentioned above, the complement system also has designed ways to downregulate its activity through three major membrane complement regulatory proteins, CD46, CD55 and CD59. CD46 and CD55 act early in the complement cascade to inhibit C3 and C5 convertase. CD59 acts later in complement pathway to block C9 and the membrane attack complex, MAC. All three of these regulatory proteins are found on the RPE cell [35]. Pro-inflammatory cytokines, for example, IL1β and TNF-α, amplify the expression of CD46 and CD59 and thus may provide protection to the RPE cell from complement-mediated cytolysis. Thus, the RPE cell is responsible for maintaining a delicate balance between initiating inflammation and suppressing complement-medicated inflammation.

Based on a number of eloquent studies, there is significant evidence that altered regulation of the complement system may be associated with AMD and Stargardt's disease [36, 37]. These exciting reports identified a strong genetic component that links complement regulatory protein polymorphisms and MAC formation. During the course of AMD, both MAC and C5a have been described to accumulate in drusen and in RPE [34, 35]. These studies add to our current understanding that chronic inflammation and dysregulation of complement regulatory proteins promote inflammation and thus contribute to a retinal degenerative process. Another RPE associated factor, Apolipoprotein E (APoE) has been shown to participate in lipid metabolism and neurodegeneration. Complement activation induces ApoE accumulation in RPE cell and ApoE is commonly detected in the RPE and drusen component in AMD [38].

RRPE Cell: A Sentinel Cell and Innate Immunity

Since the RPE cell is endowed with many of the components of the innate immune response, it can serve as a first responder to infectious insults. When one reviews the literature on examples of retinal infections, it becomes apparent that the varied infectious agents used the RPE cell as a refuge. This is true for systemic cytomegalovirus infection, cytomegalovirus retinopathy, coronavirus in experimental coronavirus retinopathy (ECOR), HIV in AIDS, and ocular infections associated with mycobacterium tuberculi and Toxoplasma gondii [39–43]. As discussed above, the RPE cell provides the first line of defense and is posed to eliminate the pathogen with its multiple TLR molecules, interactions with immune cells and production of soluble mediators [5]. However, for many infectious agents, activation of the adaptive immune response is required.

RPE Cell and Microglia Interactions

Microglia are resident macrophage cells in the brain and retina. These cells participate in a number of immunologic activities, such as, the production of both pro- and anti-inflammatory cytokines and molecules. Microglia cells are therefore important immunoregulatory cells that are capable of rapidly responding to a variety of warning signals. Numerous studies have identified that microglia activation in the brain is associated with a variety of neurodegenerative and neuroinflammatory diseases. Not surprisingly, these cells in the retina, are also activated in retinal degenerative and inflammatory conditions.

Thus, both the RPE cell and the retinal microglia cells are capable of participating in inflammatory and degenerative processes. Within the retina, studies have shown that the RPE cells and the microglia may interact, and cross talk with one another, especially through the production of cytokines [15]. As we have seen, the RPE cells are activated by TLR3 stimulation and produce a variety of potent cytokines [5]. Klettner and associates showed that supernatant fluids from TLR3 activated RPE cells can up-regulate microglia cells to produce IL-1β, IL-6 and Cox-2. These studies provide evidence that RPE cells may act as an inflammatory signal for microglia cells.

These initial studies have been expanded to investigate the cross-talk between RPE and microglia. Jo and associated demonstrated that interaction between these cells determines the integrity of the outer blood-retinal barrier in murine diabetic retinopathy [44]. This interaction was mediated by the presence of IL-6 and the production of TNF-α by the microglia cells. In a rat model of photo oxidative damage, which has similarities with AMD, IL-1β produced by microglia was associated with increased expression of the chemokines, CCL2, CXCL1 and CXCL10 in the RPE cell. The authors stress the potential importance of these chemokines in AMD. Using the human ARPE-19 in vitro, it was demonstrated that activation of microglia cells triggered inflammasome activation in RPE cells with resultant lysosomal destabilization [45]. In summary, these exciting studies substantiate significant immunologic collaboration between the RPE cell and the microglia cell within the retina. Moreover, these studies highlight the need for continued studies exploring the relationship between these cells and their potential role in a variety of retinal disorders.

RPE Cell Participation in Immunoregulation

Inflammation in the retina is a critical response of the host to retinal insults and is outlined in Fig. 6.1. Regulation of the immune system is clearly an important area of research. In fact, studies identifying how tumor cells escape immune destruction by the PD-L1 pathway has led to exciting novel cancer treatment strategies. The concept of regulatory mechanisms in the ocular microenvironment that restrain immune-mediated inflammation is not new. Over 70 years ago, Sir Peter Medawar identified the concept of immune privilege in the brain, eye and the pregnant uterus [46]. Today, we know that immune privilege extends to the anterior chamber as well as the retina where an array of regulatory mechanisms act in concert to prevent immunologic inflammation and maintain tissue integrity [47, 48]. Some of these mechanisms include the presence of a blood-retinal barrier, a lack of lymphatic drainage, the presence of immunosuppressive cytokines and regulatory T cells. Controlling unnecessary inflammation is not an immunologically inert activity but rather a very active process that allows the eye to escape the damage associated with a full blown inflammatory response. Today, we recognize that the RPE cell is a major player in this dynamic regulatory pathway.

The eye has evolved suppressive mechanisms to down-regulate the immuneresponse and one way in which this RPE cell participates to control unwanted activation is by producing cytokines. An outline of the immune-protective role of the RPE cell is seen in Figs. 6.2, 6.3, and 6.4. The RPE cell releases three suppressive factors including TGF-β, IL-11 and IFN-β. One of these molecules highly expressed in the RPE cell is IFN-β [5, 6]. It is well known that the IFNs are involved in numerous immune reactions and induction of type 1 IFN gene expression is an essential part of innate immunity [4]. Since the RPE cell continuously expresses high levels of IFN-β through IRF-7 up-regulation, our laboratory explored ways in which this molecule may function in the retinal microenvironment (Fig. 6.2). In vitro experiments and in vivo studies show that IFN-β acts as an immunosuppressive cytokine to block immune reactivity and thus protect the retinal tissue from excessive damage and visual loss [6]. IFN-β provides this protection in two ways. IFN-β can down-regulate CXCL9 and the adhesion molecule, ICAM-1. The net effect of this activity would be a "tightening" of the blood retinal barrier and decreased ocular inflammation [49].

IL-11 is another interesting member of the IL-6 family of cytokines and is produced in elevated levels by the RPE cell [50]. This pleiotropic cytokine has anti-inflammatory and cytoprotective actions [51]. Under normal conditions the RPE cell does not produce IL-11, however, following treatment with TGF-β, IL-1β or TNF-α, an up-regulation of gene expression and protein production of IL-11 is observed (Fig. 6.3). Therefore, during inflammation, IL-11 is produced by the RPE cell and then participates by limiting inflammation and providing cytoprotection to the RPE and other retinal cells [52].

TGF-β is a potent multifunctional cytokine that has been shown to provide immunosuppressive actions in the eye [53]. These studies have shown that TGF-β down-regulates APC function and inhibits several T cell functions contributing to ocular immune privilege. Several investigators have also shown that the presence of TGF-β is associated with retinal disorders, such as retinal detachments, proliferative vitreoretinopathy and choroidal neovascularization. As noted above,

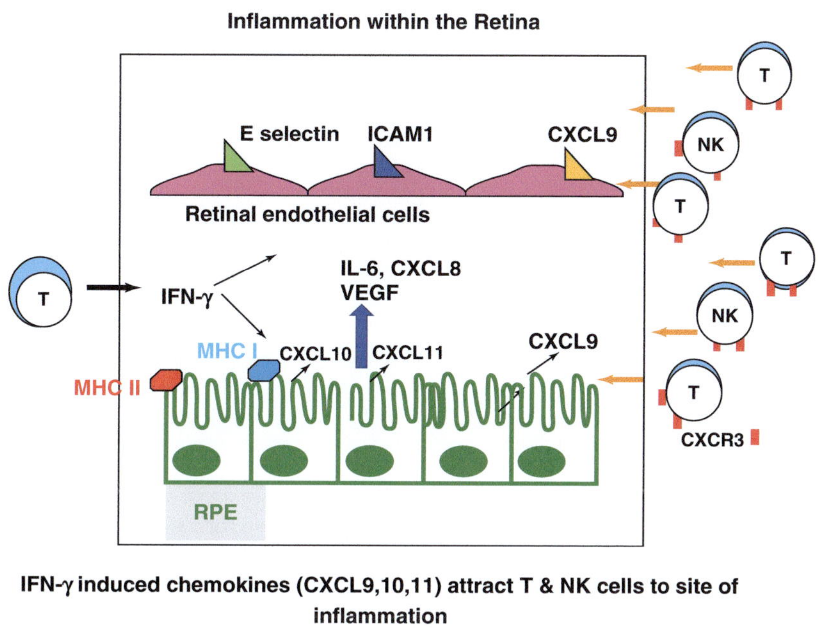

Fig. 6.1 Inflammation within the retina. IFN-γ generated by activated T cells induces RPE cells to express MHC class I and II molecules and to produce proinflammatory cytokines such as IL-6, CXCL8 (attract neutrophils), CXCL9, CXCL10, CXCL11 (attract T cells). CXCL9 is also produced by retinal vessel endothelial cells

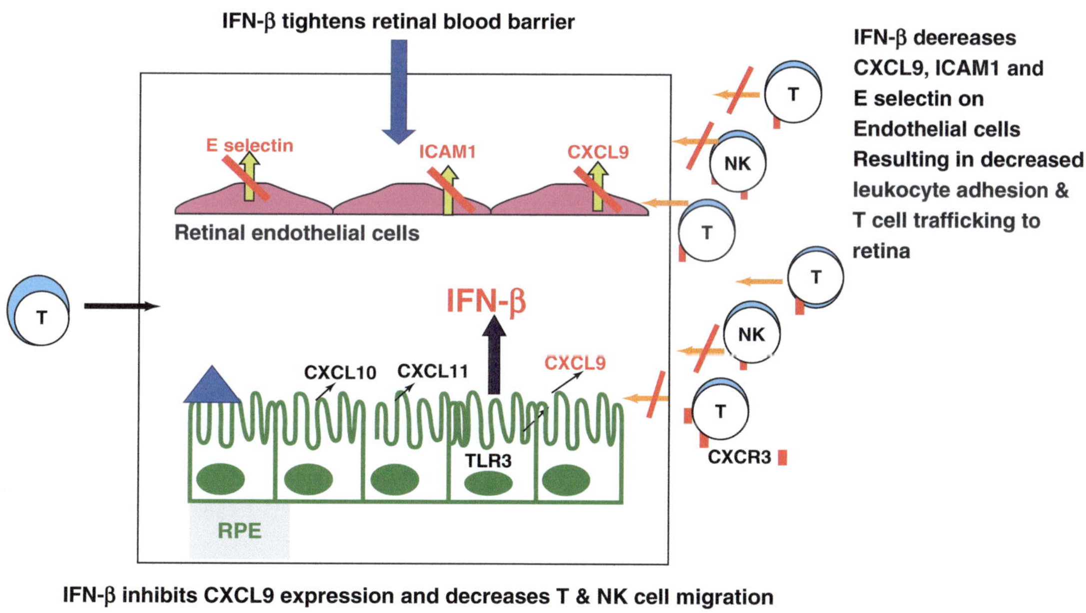

Fig. 6.2 IFN-β inhibits CXCL9 expression and decreases T and Natural Killer (NK) cell migration. High levels of IFN-β are produced by the RPE cells through the activation of TLR3 within the RPE cell. IFN–β decreases CXCL9, ICAM-1 and E selectin on endothelial cells. This results in a dramatic tightening of the retinal-blood barrier. This also results in decreased leukocyte adhesion and T cell trafficking into the retina

the RPE cell is a major source of TGF-β. Moreover, TGF-β can act upon RPE cell causing the release of VEGF, PDGF and hemooxygenase [20, 54, 55].

The manner by which RPE cellular receptor for complement and PD-L1 regulate the immune response have been described and are outlined in Fig. 6.4.

Fig. 6.3 TGF-β and IL-11 support Treg formation and decreases activated T cell migration. When activated, the RPE cell produces two additional anti-inflammatory cytokines, TGF-β and IL-11. TGF-β stimulate CD4+ T cells to differentiate into Tregs. These cells suppress effector T cell activation and proliferation. IL-11 provides protection of Tregs

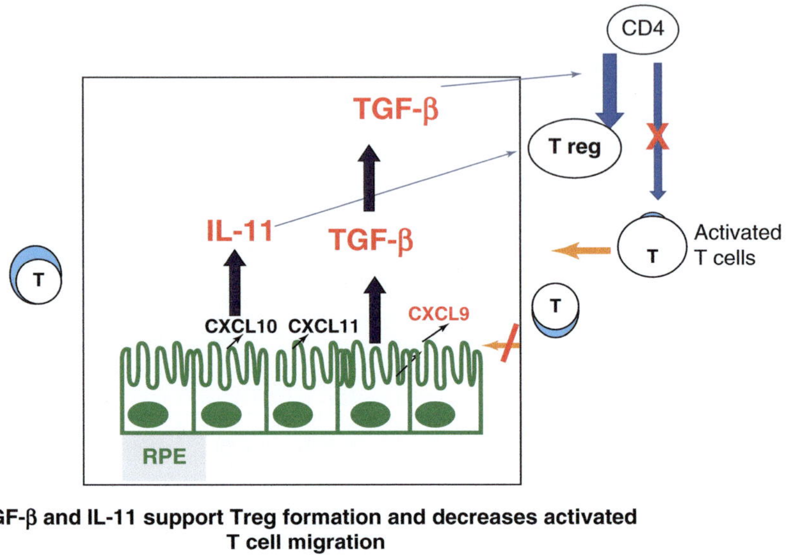

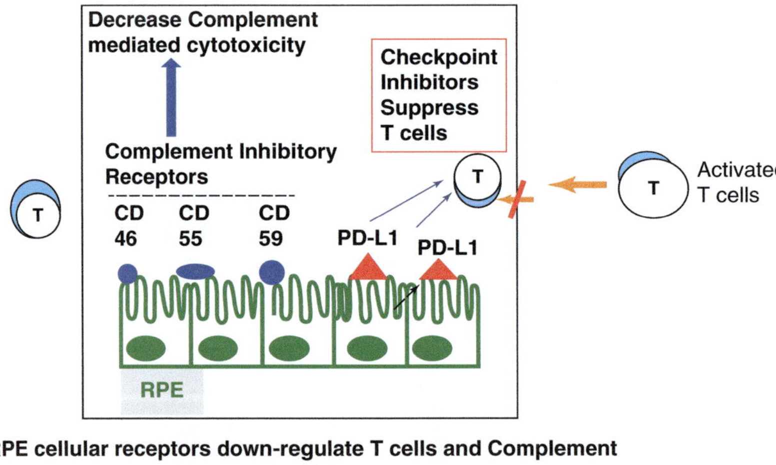

Fig. 6.4 RPE cellular receptors down-regulate T cells and Complement. Activated RPE cells express three complement inhibitory receptors. CD46 is a complement regulatory protein that inactivates C3b and C4b. CD55 is a complement decay accelerating factor that indirectly blocks MAC formation. CD59 directly blocks MAC formation. Activated RPE cells also express the immune checkpoint inhibitor, PD-L1. Interaction of T cells with this receptor on the RPE cell results in suppression of T cell activity

RPE Cell: Role in Ocular Adaptive Immunity

Unlike the innate immune response, the adaptive response is highly specific, has immunologic memory, and can respond rapidly and vigorously to a second antigen exposure. The adaptive immune response involves antibody-mediated and cell–mediated immune responses (Table 6.2). Antigen processing and presentation represent the hallmark of the adaptive immune response. An overview of all the components and their interactions during the adaptive immune response is not possible here however, early experiments establishing the RPE as an APC will be briefly mentioned. We direct the reader to the following review, [56].

Major Histocompatibility Complex, MHC, class I and II molecules, which serve as the recognition system capable of distinguishing self

Table 6.2 RPE cell participation in adaptive immunity

RPE cell component	Immune responses generated
MHC class I	– Role in antigen presentation
	– Modulated by IFNs
	– Participation in NK and T cell killing
MHC class II and costimulatory molecules (CD80, CD86)	– Role in antigen presentation
	– Modulated by IFN-γ
Cytokines	– See Table 6.1
RPE cytokine receptors	– Stimulate RPE pro-inflammatory and immunoregulatory cytokines as well as VEGF
Complement	– See Table 6.1
PD-L1 (programed death ligand)	– Tolerance
	– Regulation of T cells

from non-self, bind peptide antigens, present them to appropriate T cells and initiate the first step in antigen recognition. Cells armed with these molecules are capable of becoming antigen presenting cells, APC. Resident APCs can be found in various areas throughout the body, including the retina. Depending on the cell type, these molecules may require activation by IFN-γ. Both T cells and NK cells can serve as the source of INF-γ.

Since antigen presentation is the central component of adaptive immunity, our laboratories explored the expression and function of MHC molecules within the retina. When one evaluates the normal retina, MHC class I and II molecules are not expressed. We noted that when retinal tissue obtained from patients with uveitis, retinitis pigmentosa or Sympathic Ophthalmia were evaluated, the RPE cell expressed MHC class I and II molecules and the infiltrating T cells contained IL-2 and IFN-γ [57–59]. Next, our in vitro studies demonstrated that IFN-γ treatment up-regulated both class I and class II molecules on normal RPE cells and hence equipped the cell to participate as a resident APC in the retina [60, 61]. In a series of in vitro studies we demonstrated that both retinal and non-retinal (BCG) antigens can be processed and presented by the activated RPE cell [60]. These finding were an essential first step underscoring the important role of the RPE cell in inflammatory, infectious and degenerative disorders. In order to further evaluate the RPE cells in vivo, we explored two animal models systems that are described below.

Animal models have been invaluable to assist in uncovering fundamental mechanisms of disease pathogenesis. One of the first animal models to explore retinal inflammation was experimental autoimmune uveitis, EAU, which is a T cell-mediated disease that mimics human uveitis [62]. Using this model system, our laboratory tracked the expression of the MHC class II molecules on RPE cells and recorded the entry of inflammatory cells into the retina [63]. Moreover, following the administration of anti-MHC class II antibody prior to EAU induction, we observed that this treatment limited the expression of MHC class II molecules on RPE cells, reduced the severity of disease and significantly delayed the onset of EAU. Collectively, these studies helped to establish the critical role of the RPE cells in ocular autoimmunity and inflammation.

Another animal model system used to clarify basic mechanisms involved in retinal degenerations was experimental coronavirus retinopathy (ECOR) [1]. This is the first retinal model to demonstrate a virus-induced degeneration, viral persistence, a genetic predisposition to virus-induced tissue damage and a virus triggered autoimmune response. ECOR is a retinal degenerative disease that is composed of three basic components; a virus component, a genetic component and an immunologic component [64–66]. Our early studies showed that inoculation of the neurotrophic JHM strain of mouse hepatitis virus (MHV) into the vitreous or anterior chamber of BALB/c mice resulted in two distinct patterns of retinal pathology. The early phase of the disease, day 1–8, was characterized by retinal vasculitis and perivasculitis. The late phase of the disease, after day 10, was characterized by retinal degenerative changes. The retinal layers revealed disorganization with large areas of outer and inner segment loss. In addition, the RPE cells were morphologically abnormal with foci of RPE cell swelling, proliferation and cell atrophy [67, 68]. During this infection, we also noted that the RPE cell was the first cell infected by the virus [64, 65, 69, 70]. This was not unexpected since the RPE cell serves as an excellent reservoir for numerous pathogens. Analysis of retinal gene expression and protein expression identified the early upregulation of cytokines and chemokines, including, IL-6, TNF-α, IFNs, CXCL9, CXCL10 and ICAM-1 [26, 71]. The presence of IFN-γ was also detected in the serum and served as the rational for the enhanced expression of MHC class I and II molecules on the RPE cell.

The genetic constitution of the host can be a critical factor in determining the outcome of a viral infection and this was also observed in ECOR [72]. The susceptible strain of mice, BALB/c, were not the only rodent strain examined. CD-1 mice were extensively studied after coronavirus infection. During the early phase of the disease (day 1–8) both strains of mice showed that the virus infected and replicated within the retina and this was associated with a typical retinal vasculitis. However, on day 10–140, only the BALB/c mice experienced the late phase of the disease marked by retinal degeneration. In contrast, in the resistant strain, CD-1 mice, the retina reverted to a normal architecture. We have identified two key differences between the mouse strains that contributed to this retinal degeneration. First, a distinct difference in the intensity of the innate immune response was observed in these mice that developed a retinopathy compared to the mice without late retinal disease. At day 2 and 3 the BALB/c mice had extremely high levels of IFN-γ, CXCL9 and CXCL10 which was measured by retinal gene expression. These same elevated levels of cytokines were found in the serum [26]. When CXCL9 and CXCL10 interact with its receptor, CXCR3 on T cells and NK cells, immune cells migrate to specific targets, in this case to the retina. The second distinct difference was the observation that the retinal degenerative process in BALB/c mice was associated with the presence of antiretinal autoantibodies. These antibodies were directed against the neural retina and the RPE cell. In contrast, these autoantibodies were not detected in the sera from normal or mock injected BALB/c mice. Likewise, none of the CD-1 mice developed antiretinal antibodies [66]. These mice also produced significantly lower levels of CXCL9 and CXCL10. Therefore, the mice that failed to develop antiretinal antibodies also failed to develop a retinal degeneration. These findings suggest a role for autoimmunity in the pathogenesis of ECOR and illustrate how a robust innate immune response may contribute to a heightened adaptive immune response that leads to a retinal degeneration. This model recapitulates key elements of human retinal degenerative diseases and serves as a template for exploring basic mechanisms of this degenerative process.

Immunologic Tools That Translate into RPE Discoveries

Development of new powerful technologies to support translational studies in human immunology have led to significant findings in basic and clinical immunology as well as in visual science. We initially investigated the RPE cell by developing monoclonal antibodies to identify epitopes that were unique to the RPE cell [73]. One evolutionally conserved epitope that we identified that was specific only to RPE cells was termed, RPE65 [73, 74]. This molecule has subsequently been the subject of active genetic research. Mutations in the RPE65 gene have been identified in Leber's Congenital Amaurosis. Recently, RPE65 adenoviral vector expressing RPE65 cDNA was used successfully in 12 pediatric patients with this disease [75, 76].

Future Directions and Clinical Applications

In summary, the RPE cell plays a pivotal role in retina immunity. The RPE cell orchestrates both innate and adaptive immunity and possesses molecules that can limit these responses. The regulation of immunity and hemostasis within the retina through cytokine production, TLR activation, complement regulators and APC properties are all key elements in the RPE cell's inventory. Continuing investigations of these immune related components, their complex regulatory networks and their various antagonists will allow even more discoveries and provide additional clues to inform about mechanisms that can lead to future treatments for many human retinal diseases.

References

1. Detrick B, Hooks JJ. Immune regulation in the retina. Immunol Res [Internet]. 2010;47(1–3):153–61. https://doi.org/10.1007/s12026-009-8146-1. https://www.ncbi.nlm.nih.gov/pubmed/20082152.
2. Detrick B, Schmitz JL, Hamilton RG. Manual of molecular and clinical laboratory immunology. 8th ed. Washington, DC: ASM Press; 2016.
3. Hunter CA, Jones SA. IL-6 as a keystone cytokine in health and disease. Nat Immunol [Internet]. 2015;16(5):448–57. https://doi.org/10.1038/ni.3153. http://www.nature.com/ni/journal/v16/n5/abs/ni.3153.html?foxtrotcallback=true.
4. Sabroe I, Parker LC, Dower SK, Whyte MK. The role of TLR activation in inflammation. J Pathol [Internet]. 2008;214(2):126–35. https://www.ncbi.nlm.nih.gov/pubmed/18161748.
5. Kumar MV, Nagineni CN, Chin MS, Hooks JJ, Detrick B. Innate immunity in the retina: toll-like receptor (TLR) signaling in human retinal pigment epithelial cells. J Neuroimmunol [Internet]. 2004;153(1–2):7–15. https://www.ncbi.nlm.nih.gov/pubmed/15265658.
6. Hooks JJ, Nagineni CN, Hooper LC, Hayashi K, Detrick B. IFN-beta provides immuno-protection in the retina by inhibiting ICAM-1 and CXCL9 in retinal pigment epithelial cells. J Immunol [Internet]. 2008;180(6):3789–96. https://www.ncbi.nlm.nih.gov/pubmed/18322185.
7. Edwards AO, Chen D, Fridley BL, James KM, Wu Y, Abercasis G, et al. Toll-like receptor polymorphisms and age-related macular degeneration. Invest Ophthalmol Vis Sci [Internet]. 2008;49(4):1652–9. https://doi.org/10.1167/iovs.07-1378. https://www.ncbi.nlm.nih.gov/pubmed/18385087.
8. Cho Y, Wang JJ, Chew EY, Ferris FL, Mitchell P, Chan CC, Tuo J. Toll-like receptor polymorphisms and age-related macular degeneration: replication in three case-control samples. Invest Ophthalmol Vis Sci [Internet]. 2009;50(12):5614–8. https://doi.org/10.1167/iovs.09-3688. https://www.ncbi.nlm.nih.gov/pubmed/19628747.
9. Kleinman ME, Yamaada K, Takeda A, Chandrasekaran V, Nozaki M, Baffi JZ, et al. Sequence- and target-independent angiogenesis suppression by siRNA via TLR3. Nature [Internet]. 2008;452(7187):591–7. https://doi.org/10.1038/nature06765. https://www.ncbi.nlm.nih.gov/pubmed/18368052.
10. Kleinman ME, Ambati J. A window to innate neuroimmunity: toll-like receptor-mediated cell responses in the retina. Adv Exp Med Biol. 2012;723:3–9. https://doi.org/10.1007/978-1-4614-0631-0_1.
11. Liao YR, Li ZJ, Zeng P, Lan YQ. TLR7 deficiency contributes to attenuated diabetic retinopathy via inhibition of inflammatory response. Biochem Biophys Res Commun [Internet]. 2017;493:1136–42. https://doi.org/10.1016/j.bbrc.2017.08.085. pii: S0006-291X(17): 1644–3. https://www.ncbi.nlm.nih.gov/pubmed/28843858.
12. Yang Z, Stratton C, Francis PJ, Kleinman ME, Tan PL, Gibbs D, et al. Toll-like receptor 3 and geographic atrophy in age-related macular degeneration. New Engl J Med [Internet]. 2008;359(14):1456–63. https://doi.org/10.1056/NEJMoa0802437. https://www.ncbi.nlm.nih.gov/pubmed/18753640.
13. Wörnle M, Merkle M, Wolf A, Ribeiro A, Himmelein S, Kemt M, et al. Inhibition of TLR3-mediated proinflammatory effects by Alkylphosphocholines in human retinal pigment epithelial cells. Invest Ophthalmol Vis Sci [Internet]. 2011;52(9):6536–44. https://doi.org/10.1167/iovs.10-6993. https://www.ncbi.nlm.nih.gov/pubmed?holding=jhumlib_fft_ndi&otool=jhumlib&term=IOVS+2011+52%3A6536-6544.
14. Klettner A, Koinzer S, Meyer T, Roider J. Toll-like receptor 3 activation in retinal pigment epithelium cells—mitogen-activated protein kinase pathways of cell death and vascular endothelial growth factor secretion. Acta Ophthalmol [Internet]. 2013;91(3):e211–8. https://doi.org/10.1111/aos.12031. https://www.ncbi.nlm.nih.gov/pubmed/23387336.
15. Klettner A, Hamann T, Schlüter K, Lucius R, Roider J. Retinal pigment epithelium cells alter the pro-inflammatory response of retinal microglia to TLR-3 stimulation. Acta Ophthalmol [Internet]. 2014;92(8):e621–9. https://doi.org/10.1111/aos.12472. https://www.ncbi.nlm.nih.gov/pubmed/24930695.
16. Patel AK, Hackam AS. Toll-like receptor 3 (TLR3) protects retinal pigmented epithelium (RPE) cells from oxidative stress through a STAT3-dependent mechanism. Mol Immunol [Internet]. 2013;54(2):122–31. https://doi.org/10.1016/j.molimm.2012.11.005. https://www.ncbi.nlm.nih.gov/pubmed/23267850.
17. Patel AK, Hackam AS. A novel protective role for the innate immunity Toll-Like Receptor 3 (TLR3) in the retina via Stat3. Mol Cell Neurosci [Internet]. 2014;63:38–48. https://doi.org/10.1016/j.mcn.2014.09.004. https://www.ncbi.nlm.nih.gov/pubmed/25264029.
18. Lai S, Fishman EK, Lai H, Pannu H, Detrick B. Serum IL-6 levels are associated with significant coronary stenosis in cardiovascularly asymptomatic inner-city black adults in the US. Inflamm Res [Internet]. 2009;58(1):15–21. https://doi.org/10.1007/s00011-008-8150-2. https://www.ncbi.nlm.nih.gov/pubmed?holding=jhumlib_fft_ndi&otool=jhumlib&term=Lai+S+Inflamm+Res+2009+58%3A15-21.

19. Nagineni CN, Detrick B, Hooks JJ. Toxoplasma gondii infection induces gene expression and secretion of interleukin 1 (IL-1), IL-6, granulocyte-macrophage colony-stimulating factor, and intercellular adhesion molecule 1 by human retinal pigment epithelial cells. Infect Immun [Internet]. 2000;68(1):407–10. https://doi.org/10.1128/IAI.68.1.407-410.2000. http://iai.asm.org/content/68/1/407.short.
20. Nagineni CN, Cherukuri KS, Kutty V, Detrick B, Hooks JJ. Interferon-gamma differentially regulates TGF-beta1 and TGF-beta2 expression in human retinal pigment epithelial cells through JAK-STAT pathway. J Cell Physiol [Internet]. 2007;210(1):192–200. https://www.ncbi.nlm.nih.gov/pubmed/17013806.
21. Hirano T. Interleukin 6 in autoimmune and inflammatory diseases: a personal memoir. Proc Jpn Acad Ser B Phys Biol Sci [Internet]. 2010;86(7):717–30. https://www.ncbi.nlm.nih.gov/pubmed/20689230.
22. Detrick B, Gangapuutra S, Palsgrove DN, Heaney CD, Hooks JJ, Sen HN. Elevated serum levels of IL-6 and CXCL9 in autoimmune retinopathy (AIR) patients. J Neuroimmunol. 2018;316:74–9. https://doi.org/10.1016/j.jneuroim.2017.12.014.
23. Stansky E, Biancotto A, Dagur PK, Gangaputra S, Chaigne-Delalande B, Nussenblatt R, et al. B cell anomalies in autoimmune retinopathy (AIR). Invest Ophthalmol Vis Sci [Internet]. 2017;58(9):3600–7. https://doi.org/10.1167/iovs.17-21704. https://www.ncbi.nlm.nih.gov/labs/articles/28715846.
24. Griffith JW, Sokol CL, Luster AD. Chemokines and chemokine receptors: positioning cells for host defense and immunity. Annu Rev Immunol [Internet]. 2014;32:659–702. https://doi.org/10.1146/annurev-immunol-032713-120145. https://www.ncbi.nlm.nih.gov/pubmed/24655300.
25. Chan CC, Ross RJ, Shen D, Ding X, Majumdar Z, Bojanowski CM, et al. Ccl2/Cx3cr1-Deficient mice: an animal model for age-related macular degeneration. Ophthalmic Res [Internet]. 2008;40(3–4):124–8. https://www.karger.com/Article/Abstract/119862.
26. Detrick B, Lee MT, Chin MS, Hooper LC, Chan CC, Hooks JJ. Experimental coronavirus retinopathy (ECOR): retinal degeneration susceptible mice have an augmented interferon and chemokine (CXCL9, CXCL10) response early after virus infection. J Neuroimmunol [Internet]. 2008;193(1–2):28–37. https://doi.org/10.1016/j.jneuroim.2007.09.032. https://www.ncbi.nlm.nih.gov/pmc/articles/PMC2562577.
27. Nawaz MI, Van Raemdonck K, Mohammad G, Kangave D, Van Damme J, Abu El-Asrar AM, et al. Autocrine CCL2, CXCL4, CXCL9 and CXCL 10 signal in retinal endothelial cells and are enhanced in diabetic retinopathy. Exp Eye Res [Internet]. 2013;109:67–76. https://doi.org/10.1016/j.exer.2013.01.008. https://www.ncbi.nlm.nih.gov/pubmed/23352833.
28. Rutar M, Natoli R, Chia RX, Valter K, Provis JM. Chemokine-mediated inflammation in the degenerating retina is coordinated by Müller cells, activated microglia, and retinal pigment epithelium. J Neuroinflamm [Internet]. 2015;12:8. https://doi.org/10.1186/s12974-014-0224-1. https://jneuroinflammation.biomedcentral.com/articles/10.1186/s12974-014-0224-1.
29. Natoli R, Fernando N, Madigan M, Chu-Tan JA, Valter K, Provis J, et al. Microglia-derived IL1β promotes chemokine expression by Müller cells and RPE in focal retinal degeneration. Mol Neurodegener [Internet]. 2017;12:31. https://doi.org/10.1186/s13024-017-0175-y. https://molecularneurodegeneration.biomedcentral.com/articles/10.1186/s13024-017-0175-y.
30. Nagineni CN, Kommineni VK, William A, Detrick B, Hooks JJ. Regulation of VEGF expression in human retinal cells by cytokines: implications for the role of inflammation in age-related macular degeneration. J Cell Physiol [Internet]. 2012;227(1):116–26. https://doi.org/10.1002/jcp.27708. http://onlinelibrary.wiley.com/doi/10.1002/jcp.22708.
31. Nagineni CN, Raju R, Nagineni KK, Kommineni VK, Cherukuri A, Kutty RK, et al. Resveratrol suppresses expression of VEGF by human retinal pigment epithelial cells: potential nutraceutical for age-related macular degeneration. Aging Dis [Internet]. 2014;5(2):88–100. https://doi.org/10.14366/AD.2014.050088. https://www.ncbi.nlm.nih.gov/pubmed/24729934.
32. Miller JW. Beyond VEGF—the Weisenfeld lecture. Invest Ophthalmol Vis Sci. 2016;57:6911–8.
33. Fukuoka Y, Strainic M, Medof ME. Differential cytokine expression of human retinal pigment epithelial cells in response to stimulation by C5a. Clin Exp Immunol [Internet]. 2003;131(2):248–53. https://doi.org/10.1046/j.1365-2249.2003.02087.x. https://www.ncbi.nlm.nih.gov/pmc/articles/PMC1808636.
34. Zhu Y, Dai B, Li Y, Peng H. C5a and toll-like receptor 4 crosstalk in retinal pigment epithelial cells. Mol Vis [Internet]. 2015;21:1122–9. https://www.ncbi.nlm.nih.gov/pubmed/26487798. PMC 4588711.
35. Yang P, Tyrrell J, Han I, Jaffe GJ. Expression and modulation of RPE cell membrane complement regulatory proteins. Invest Ophthalmol Vis Sci [Internet]. 2009;50(7):3473–81. https://doi.org/10.1167/iovs.08-3111. http://iovs.arvojournals.org/article.aspx?articleid=2165307.
36. Hageman GS, Anderson DH, Johnson LV, Hancox LS, et al. A common haplotype in the complement regulatory gene factor H (HF1/CFH) predisposes individuals to age-related macular degeneration. Proc Natl Acad Sci U S A. 2005;102:7227–32.
37. Lenis TL, Sarfare S, Jiang Z, Lloyd MB, Bok D, Radu RA. Complement modulation in the retinal pigment epithelium rescues photoreceptor degeneration in a mouse model of Stargardt disease. Proc Natl Acad Sci U S A [Internet]. 2017;114(15):3987–92. https://doi.org/10.1073/pnas.1620299114. http://www.pnas.org/content/114/15/3987.
38. Yang P, Skiba NP, Tewkesbury GM, Treboschi M, Basciu P, Jaffe GJ. Complement-mediated regulation

of apolipoprotein E in cultured human RPE cells. Invest Ophthalmol Vis Sci [Internet]. 2017;58(7):3073–85. https://doi.org/10.1167/iovs.16-20083. https://www.ncbi.nlm.nih.gov/pubmed/28632844.
39. Detrick B, Rhame J, Wang Y, Nagineni CN, Hooks JJ. Cytomegalovirus replication in human retinal pigment epithelial cells. Altered expression of viral early proteins. Invest Ophthalmol Vis Sci [Internet]. 1996;37(5):814–25. https://www.ncbi.nlm.nih.gov/pubmed/8603866.
40. Hooks JJ, Chin MS, Srinivasan K, Momma Y, Hooper LC, Nagineni CN, et al. Human cytomegalovirus induced cyclooxygenase-2 in human retinal pigment epithelial cells augments viral replication through a prostaglandin pathway. Microbes Infect [Internet]. 2006;8(8):2236–44. https://www.ncbi.nlm.nih.gov/pubmed/16782382.
41. Detrick B, Nagineni CN, Grillone LR, Anderson KP, Henry SP, Hooks JJ. Inhibition of human cytomegalovirus replication in a human retinal epithelial cell model by antisense oligonucleotides. Invest Ophthalmol Vis Sci [Internet]. 2001;42(1):163–9. https://www.ncbi.nlm.nih.gov/pubmed/11133862.
42. Rao NA, Saraswathy S, Smith RE. Tuberculous Uveitis: distribution of mycobacterium tuberculosis in retinal pigment epithelium. Arch Ophthalmol [Internet]. 2006;124(12):1777–9. https://doi.org/10.1001/archopth.124.12.1777. https://www.ncbi.nlm.nih.gov/pubmed/17159041.
43. Smith JR, Todd S, Ashander LM, Charitou T, Ma Y, Yeh S, et al. Retinal pigment epithelial cells are a potential reservoir for ebola virus in the human eye. Transl Vis Sci Technol [Internet]. 2017;6(4):12. https://doi.org/10.1167/tvst.4.12. https://www.ncbi.nlm.nih.gov/pmc/articles/PMC5512973.
44. Jo DH, Yun JH, Cho CS, Kim JH, Kim JH, Cho CH. Interaction between microglia and retinal pigment epithelial cells determines the integrity of outer blood retinal barrier in diabetic retinopathy. Glia. 2019;67(2):321–31. https://doi.org/10.1002/glia.23542.
45. Nebel C, Aslanidis A, Rashid K, Langmann T. Activated microglia trigger inflammasome activation and lysosomal destabilization in human RPE cells. Biochem Biophys Res Commun. 2017;484:681–6.
46. Medawar PB. Immunity to homologous grafted skin; the fate of skin homografts transplanted to the brain, to subcutaneous tissue, and other anterior chamber of the eye. Br J Exp Pathol [Internet]. 1948;29(1):58–69. https://www.ncbi.nlm.nih.gov/pubmed/18865105.
47. Forrester JV, Xu H, Lambe T, Cornall R. Immune privilege or privileged immunity? Mucosal Immunol [Internet]. 2008;1:372–81. https://search.proquest.com/docview/1782984727?pq-origsite=gscholar.
48. Dick AD. Doyne lecture 2016: intraocular health and the many faces of inflammation. Eye (Lond) [Internet]. 2017;31:87–96. https://doi.org/10.1038/eye.2016.17. https://www.ncbi.nlm.nih.gov/pubmed/27636226.
49. Morrell CN, Srivastava K, Swaim AM, Lee MT, Chen J, Nagineni CN, et al. Beta interferon suppresses the development of experimental cerebral malaria. Infect Immun [Internet]. 2011;79(4):1750–8. https://doi.org/10.1128/IAI.00810-10. http://iai.asm.org/content/79/4/1750.short.
50. Nagineni CN, Kommineni VK, William A, Hooks JJ, Detrick B. IL-11 expression in retinal and corneal cells is regulated by interferon-gamma. Biochem Biophys Res Commun [Internet]. 2010;391(1):287–92. https://doi.org/10.1016/jbbrc.2009.11.051. https://www.ncbi.nlm.nih.gov/pubmed/19913506.
51. Gurfein BT, Zhang Y, Lopez CB, Argaw AT, Zameer A, Moran TM, et al. IL-11 regulates autoimmune demyelination. J Immunol [Internet]. 2009;183(7):4229–40. https://doi.org/10.4049/jimmunol.0900622. https://www.ncbi.nlm.nih.gov/pubmed/19734214.
52. Xu DH, Zhu Z, Wakefield MR, Xiao H, Bai Q, Fang Y. The role of IL-11 in immunity and cancer. Cancer Lett [Internet]. 2016;373(2):156–73. https://doi.org/10.1016/j.canlet.2016.01.004. https://www.ncbi.nlm.nih.gov/pubmed/26826523.
53. Sugita S. Role of ocular pigment epithelial cells in immune privilege. Arch Immunol Ther Exp (Warsz) [Internet]. 2009;57(4):263–8. https://doi.org/10.1007/s00005-009-0030-0. https://www.ncbi.nlm.nih.gov/pubmed/19568919.
54. Nagineni CN, Samuel W, Nagineni S, Pardhasaradhi K, Wiggert B, Detrick B, et al. Transforming growth factor-beta indices expression of vascular endothelial growth factor in human retinal pigment epithelial cells: involvement in mitogen-activated protein kinases. J Cell Physiol [Internet]. 2003;197:453–62. https://doi.org/10.1002/jcp.10378. http://onlinelibrary.wiley.com/doi/10.1002/jcp.10378/full.
55. Nagineni CN, Kutty V, Detrick B, Hooks JJ. Expression of PDGF and their receptors in human retinal pigment epithelial cells and fibroblasts: regulation by TGF-beta. J Cell Physiol [Internet]. 2005;203(1):35–43. https://www.ncbi.nlm.nih.gov/pubmed/15368539.
56. Roche PA, Furuta K. The ins and outs of MHC Class II—mediated antigen processing and presentation. Nat Rev Immunol. 2015;15:203–16.
57. Detrick B, Rodrigues M, Chan CC, Tso MO, Hooks JJ. Expression of HLA-DR antigen on retinal pigment epithelial cells in retinitis pigmentosa. Am J Ophthalmol [Internet]. 1986;101(5):584–90. https://www.ncbi.nlm.nih.gov/pubmed/3518466.
58. Chan CC, Detrick B, Nussenblatt RB, Palestine AG, Fujikawa LS, Hooks JJ. HLA-DR antigens on retinal pigment epithelial cells from patients with uveitis. Arch Ophthalmol [Internet]. 1986;104(5):725–9. https://www.ncbi.nlm.nih.gov/pubmed/3518683.
59. Hooks JJ, Chan CC, Detrick B. Identification of the lymphokines, interferon-gamma and interleukin-2 in inflammatory eye diseases. Invest Ophthalmol Vis Sci [Internet]. 1988;29(9):1444–51. https://www.ncbi.nlm.nih.gov/pubmed/3138201.
60. Percopo CM, Hooks JJ, Shinohara T, Caspi R, Detrick B. Cytokine-mediated activation of a neuronal retinal resident cell provokes antigen presentation. J Immunol [Internet]. 1990;145(12):4101–7. https://www.ncbi.nlm.nih.gov/pubmed/2147935.

61. Hamel CP, Detrick B, Hooks JJ. Evaluation of Ia expression in rat ocular tissues following inoculation with interferon-gamma. Exp Eye Res [Internet]. 1990;50(2):173–82. https://www.ncbi.nlm.nih.gov/pubmed/2107092.
62. Caspi RR. Understanding autoimmunity in the eye: from animal models to novel therapies. Discov Med [Internet]. 2014;17(93):155–62. https://www.ncbi.nlm.nih.gov/pmc/articles/PMC4573559.
63. Wetzig R, Hooks JJ, Percopo CM, Nussenblatt R, Chan CC, Detrick B. Anti-Ia antibody diminishes ocular inflammation in experimental autoimmune uveitis. Curr Eye Res [Internet]. 1988;7(8):809–18. https://www.ncbi.nlm.nih.gov/pubmed/3263258.
64. Robbins SG, Hamel CP, Detrick B, Hooks JJ. Murine coronavirus induces an acute and long-lasting disease of the retina. Lab Invest [Internet]. 1990;62(4):417–26. https://www.ncbi.nlm.nih.gov/pubmed/2159082.
65. Robbins SC, Detrick B, Hooks JJ. Ocular tropisms of murine coronavirus (strain JHM) after inoculation by various routes. Invest Ophthalmol Vis Sci [Internet]. 1991;32(6):1883–93. https://www.ncbi.nlm.nih.gov/pubmed/1851734.
66. Hooks JH, Percopo C, Wang Y, Detrick B. Retina and retinal pigment epithelial cell autoantibodies are produced during murine coronavirus retinopathy. J Immunol [Internet]. 1993;151(6):3381–9. https://www.ncbi.nlm.nih.gov/pubmed/8397257.
67. Robbins SC, Wiggert B, Kutty G, Chader GJ, Detrick B, Hooks JJ. Redistribution and reduction of interphotoreceptor retinoid-binding protein during ocular coronavirus infection. Invest Ophthalmol Vis Sci [Internet]. 1992;33(1):60–7. https://www.ncbi.nlm.nih.gov/pubmed/1309730.
68. Vinores SA, Wang Y, Vinores MA, Derevjanik NL, Shi A, Klein DA, et al. Blood-retinal barrier breakdown in experimental coronavirus retinopathy: association with viral antigen, inflammation, and VEGF in sensitive and resistant strains. J Neuroimmunol [Internet]. 2001;119(2):175–82. https://www.ncbi.nlm.nih.gov/pubmed/11585619.
69. Komurasaki Y, Nagineni CN, Wang Y, Hooks JJ. Virus RNA persists within the retina in coronavirus-induced retinopathy. Virology [Internet]. 1996;222(2):446–50. https://doi.org/10.1006/viro.1996.0442. http://www.sciencedirect.com/science/article/pii/S0042682296904420.
70. Wang Y, Detrick B, Hooks JJ. Coronavirus (JHM) replication within the retina: analysis of cell tropism in mouse retinal cell cultures. Virology [Internet]. 1993;193(1):124–37. https://www.ncbi.nlm.nih.gov/pubmed/8382393.
71. Hooks JJ, Wang Y, Detrick B. The critical role of IFN-gamma in experimental coronavirus retinopathy. Invest Ophthalmol Vis Sci [Internet]. 2003;44(8):3402–8. https://www.ncbi.nlm.nih.gov/pubmed/12882788.
72. Wang Y, Burnier M, Detrick B, Hooks JJ. Genetic predisposition to coronavirus-induced retinal disease. Invest Ophthalmol Vis Sci [Internet]. 1996;37(1):250–4. https://www.ncbi.nlm.nih.gov/pubmed/8550331.
73. Hooks JJ, Detrick B, Percopo C, Hamel C, Siraganian RP. Development and characterization of monoclonal antibodies directed against the retinal pigment epithelial cell. Invest Ophthalmol Vis Sci [Internet]. 1989;30(10):2106–13. https://www.ncbi.nlm.nih.gov/pubmed/2477341.
74. Hamel CP, Tsilou E, Pfeffer BA, Hooks JJ, Detrick B, Redmond TM. Molecular cloning and expression of RPE65, a novel retinal pigment epithelium-specific microsomal protein that is post-transcriptionally regulated in vitro. J Biol Chem [Internet]. 1993;268(21):15751–7. https://www.ncbi.nlm.nih.gov/pubmed/8340400.
75. Morimura H, Fishman GA, Grover SA, Fulton AB, Berson EL, Dryja TP. Mutations in the RPE65 gene in patients with autosomal recessive retinitis pigmentosa or Leber congenital amaurosis. Proc Natl Acad Sci U S A [Internet]. 1998;95(6):3088–93. https://www.ncbi.nlm.nih.gov/pubmed/9501220.
76. Bainbridge JW, Smith AJ, Barker SS, Robbie S, Henderson R, Balaggan K, et al. Effect of gene therapy on visual function in Leber's congenital amaurosis. N Engl J Med [Internet]. 2008;358:2231–9. https://doi.org/10.1056/NEJMoa0802268. http://www.nejm.org/doiI/full/10.1056/NEJMoa0802268#t=article.

Part II

The RPE in Disease

The RPE in Myopia Development

7

Yan Zhang and Christine F. Wildsoet

Introduction

Myopia, or near-sightedness, is one of the most common types of refractive error, which are major causes of visual impairment and blindness worldwide [1–3]. Refractive errors occur when there is a mismatch between the refractive state or focusing power of the eye and its axial length. They reflect the product of complex developmental interactions between various ocular tissues and compartments, including the cornea and crystalline lens, which together provide refracting power, and the anterior and vitreous chambers, which are the major determinants of overall eye length [4, 5]. Myopia describes the case when the eye is relatively too long and the image plane for distant objects falls in front of the retina. Most myopia is axial rather than refractive in nature and the product of excessive elongation of the vitreous chamber [5, 6]. While the problem of blurred distance vision resulting from such focusing errors can be corrected, for example, with optical appliances, the excessive eye growth carries an increased risk of a number of ocular pathologies, including cataract, retinal detachment, myopic maculopathy, glaucoma and choroidal neovascularization, many of which can lead to irreversible vision loss, with no evidence of a safe threshold level of myopia [7, 8].

In recent years, both the prevalence and severity of myopia have increased rapidly worldwide, albeit with variations between regions and ethnic groups [9–12]. While the estimated global prevalence of myopia was only 28% in 2010, it is now projected to increase to 50% by 2050 [10]. In some subpopulations of East Asia, the reported prevalence of myopia has already reached 80–95% [9, 13, 14]. While there has also been a tendency to view such prevalence figures as an Asian problem, Western countries are not exempt from this myopia epidemic [12, 15]. For example, one United States-based study reported an increase in the prevalence of myopia from 25 to 42% over a 30-year period [12]. The global prevalence of high myopia is also increasing, with a projected figure of 10% by 2050, up from 4% in 2010 [10]. As the risk of secondary ocular complications increases with the level of myopia, the latter figures represent a major public health concern. Indeed, myopia is now recognized as a significant public health problem, both socially and economically [2, 13, 16, 17].

What is the origin of the myopia epidemic? It is generally accepted that myopia is likely a product of gene-environment interactions, rather than being determined by either genetic or environmental factors alone [18–22]. Genetic contributions to myopia have been investigated for both familial non-syndromic (simple) and syndromic

Y. Zhang · C. F. Wildsoet (✉)
School of Optometry, University of California, Berkeley, CA, USA
e-mail: wildsoet@berkeley.edu

A. K. Klettner, S. Dithmar (eds.), *Retinal Pigment Epithelium in Health and Disease*,
https://doi.org/10.1007/978-3-030-28384-1_7

forms. Linkage studies have mapped two dozen loci and identified mutations in a few genes. More recently, genome-wide association studies (GWAS) have been used to screen for myopia candidate genes. Many of the identified candidate genes have been linked to biological processes, with plausible connections to retina-sclera signaling cascades and thus local eye growth modulation. Examples include retinal neurotransmission, ion transport, extracellular matrix (ECM) and connective tissue remodeling [23–25]. Nonetheless, variants identified in GWAS studies explain only ~3% of the variation in myopia prevalence [26]. On the other hand, human epidemiological studies have provided convincing evidence for influences of environmental factors, such as excessive near work and outdoor activities in myopia development and prevention, respectively [27–30]. However, contributing factors are poorly understood and it is likely that interactions between genes and environmental factors at least partly explain the apparent complexities associated with predicting human myopia.

Despite the now general acceptance of the seriousness of the climbing myopia prevalence statistics from a public health perspective, treatments for preventing myopia and/or slowing its progression and thus controlling this epidemic remain limited in both options and overall efficacy [31]. Currently, therapeutic interventions are confined to methods of slowing myopia progression and thus limiting the level of myopia and risk of pathology [32]. While standard optical appliances (spectacles and contact lenses) and refractive surgeries are able to restore sharp distance vision, they have no positive benefits on myopia progression. Nonetheless, some specialized spectacles and contact lenses with multifocal optics have been shown to slow myopia progression [33, 34], and another contact lens modality, orthokeratology, which induces multifocal ocular changes after overnight wear, has also been shown to slow myopia progression [35–37]. In terms of drug therapies for controlling myopia progression, trials of topical ophthalmic medications have been limited to two muscarinic receptor antagonists, atropine and pirenzepine, both of which have been shown to slow myopia progression [38–42]. However, the underlying mechanisms for their therapeutic actions, including their site of action, remain the subject of debate. The same is true for a third drug, 7-methylxanthine, which has been approved for use as an oral medication in Denmark [43]. Among reported limitations and side-effects of the above treatments are ocular infections, due to poor handling of contact lenses and corneal changes with orthokeratology, as well as loss of efficacy and rebound effects with more traditional, higher concentrations of topical atropine [31]. Apart from the more conventional optical and pharmacological interventions, the results of epidemiological studies showing an apparent protective effect of outdoor activities against myopia onset and to a less extent, against progression, await a better understanding of contributing factors for their translation into behavioral recommendations [27, 29, 30].

RPE Changes in Human High Myopia and Related Pathology

Although few pathological changes have been reported in patients with mild to moderate myopia, these changes increase significantly with high myopia (generally defined as <−5 or −6 diopters [D]) [44–46]. Since the major ocular change in myopia is an enlargement of the posterior vitreous chamber, it is not surprising that pathological changes in high myopia are also largely limited to posterior ocular tissues, including retina, retinal pigment epithelium (RPE), Bruch's membrane, choroid and sclera. In myopic maculopathy, RPE changes, including RPE atrophy or loss, are among the frequently described features contributing to the characteristic fundus appearance [45]. Lacquer cracks, another commonly encountered fundus feature of high myopia, are believed to be caused by mechanical linear breaks in Bruch's membrane, and in patchy chorioretinal atrophy, holes in Bruch's membrane have been detected with new imaging technologies, such as swept-source optical coherence tomography

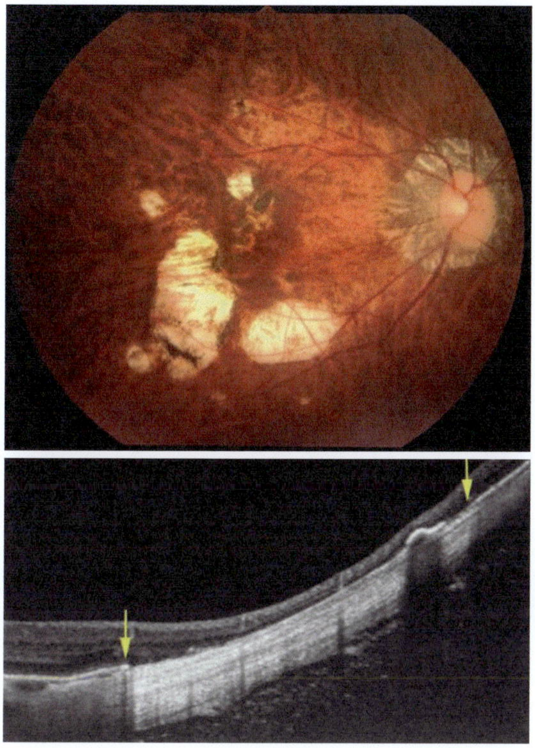

Fig. 7.1 Fundus photograph from a myopia patient with chorioretinal atrophy showing multiple patchy lesions. An OCT image from the same patient shows a RPE defect in the area of atrophy (between arrows). (Images courtesy of Professor Kyoko Ohno-Matsui (Tokyo Medical and Dental University, Tokyo, Japan))

(SS-OCT) (Fig. 7.1) [45, 47]. Such findings are also consistent with observations from more classical, histological studies of highly myopic eyes, of RPE losses and Bruch's membrane defects [48].

Role of RPE in Eye Growth Regulation and Myopia: Experimental Studies

Local Regulation of Eye Growth and RPE as a Relay Station

Although changes in the RPE are commonly observed in high myopia, such changes are usually considered to be secondary to the stretching of posterior ocular tissues as the vitreous chamber enlarges. The active contributions of RPE to later complications, as well as myopia onset and early progression are not very well understood.

Research studies on key ocular tissues such as retina, RPE, choroid, and sclera from myopic patients have been limited by the availability of tissue [49–51]. As substitutes, researchers have relied on a number of different animal models for myopia, including chicks, guinea pigs, tree shrews, marmosets and monkeys, with mice and zebrafish having been also featured in some more recent studies [19, 52–59]. Compared to the more widely studied earlier models, the latter models offer advantages of well-characterized genomes, as well as the availability of genetically modified animals.

Studies using animal models have provided convincing evidence for the role of visual environmental factors in eye growth regulation and myopia development. Most animals exhibit refractive errors at birth and, under normal conditions, these neonatal refractive errors are eliminated through a process of active, vision-dependent emmetropization, which involves the coordinated growth of key ocular components. Evidence for the latter comes from studies involving manipulations of the visual experience of young animals experimentally, using either optical defocusing lenses or form depriving diffusers. All of these disrupt this emmetropization process, with refractive errors being the net result. Specifically, hyperopic optical defocus (imposed with negative lenses) and form-deprivation (wearing diffusers) represent robust methods for stimulating excessive eye elongation, inducing myopia, while myopic defocus (imposed with positive lenses) slows eye elongation in most models. These experimental paradigms have been capitalized on in animal model studies aimed at understanding underlying mechanisms. Two lines of evidence point to these altered eye growth patterns being largely controlled locally, within the eye itself (Fig. 7.2) [19, 60–67]. Neural lesioning studies involving optic nerve section offer the strongest evidence for local ocular control; specifically, while the retina-brain link is thus disrupted, the usual response to negative lenses and diffusers, of increased eye elongation and myopia, is not [63, 65, 67]. Additional evidence comes from studies involv-

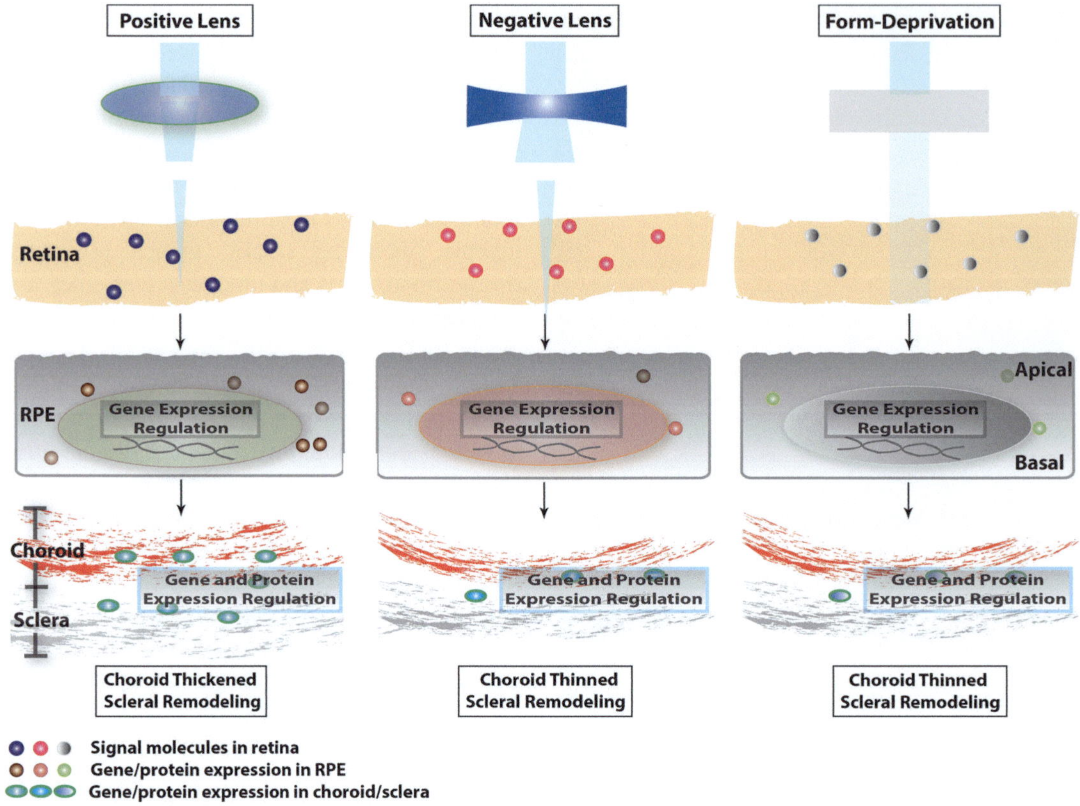

Fig. 7.2 Schematic diagram illustrating the presumed retina-sclera growth modulatory signaling cascades mediating positive lens-induced hyperopia, negative lens-induced myopia, and form-deprivation-induced myopia

ing localized manipulation of retinal images; in these cases, ocular growth changes are confined to the affected segment of the vitreous chamber [60, 64, 68]. The most parsimonious explanation for these observations relies on the assumption that the neural retina is linked via one or more local molecular signal cascades, directed at and mediating the morphological changes in the two outer layers of the eye wall—the choroid and sclera, which ultimately determine the physical dimensions of the vitreous chamber and thus eye length. By manipulating the retinal image and thus neural activity within the retina, the growth modulating signals are altered, with refractive errors being the net result (Fig. 7.2) [19, 69–73].

The RPE is a monolayer of hexagonal-shape pigmented epithelial cells positioned between the neural retina and the choroid (Fig. 7.3). Interconnected by tight junctions, the RPE cells form a key component of the blood-retina barrier, which tightly regulates the exchange between the retina and choroid of ions and water, as well as many molecules, including nutrients, and waste products (Fig. 7.4). The polarized nature of the RPE necessitates orientation labeling; the so-called apical membrane refers to the microvillus surface into which photoreceptor outer segments project, while the basal membrane refers to the surface facing the choroid and abutting Bruch's membrane. Many of the functions of RPE exhibit directionality, including the secretion of growth factors and cytokines, and there are also asymmetries in the distributions of neurotransmitter receptors, ion channels and transporters across the apical versus basal membranes [74–78]. Due to its unique location, juxtaposed between the retina and choroid, and barrier function, the RPE not only plays essential roles in maintaining retinal homeostasis and functions, but also plays important roles in maintaining choroidal

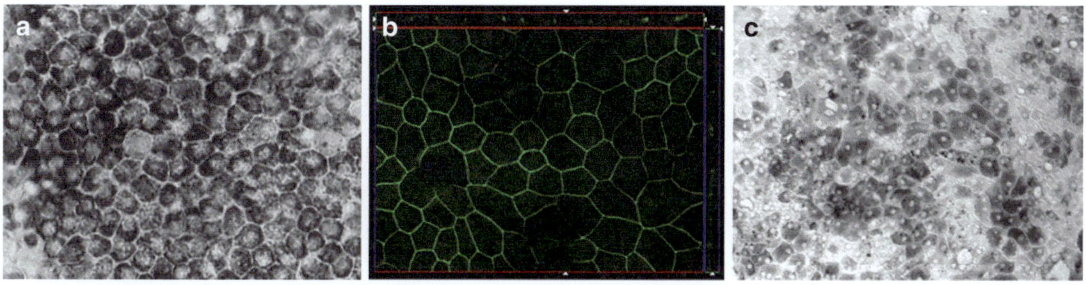

Fig. 7.3 Primary culture of human fetal RPE cells (**a**, **b**) and chick RPE cells (**c**). Confluent primary human fetal RPE cells in culture form tight junctions, as revealed with immunohistochemistry (ZO-1 labelling, **b**)

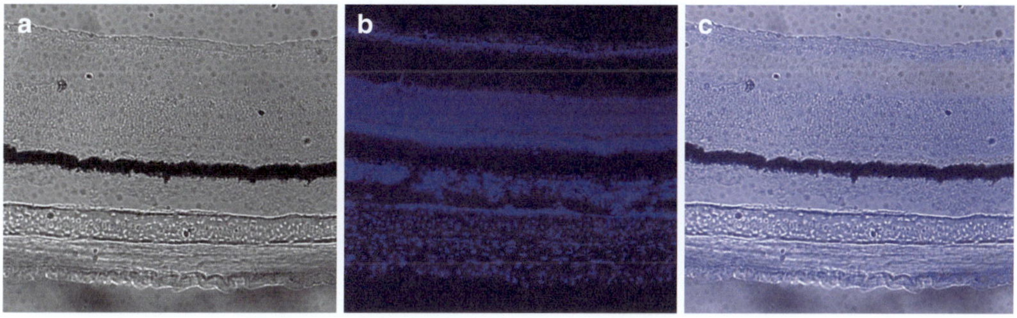

Fig. 7.4 Histology sections of the posterior wall of the chick eye, showing retina, RPE, choroid (CHO), and bilayered sclera (cartilage layer, SC-C; fibrous layer, SC-F) viewed under light microscopy (**a**), after nuclear staining with DAPI (**b**), and merged (**c**)

morphology and physiology [77, 79–81]. In the context of eye growth regulation and myopia, there seems little doubt that the RPE also serves as a relay or conduit for retina-derived growth modulatory signals directed at the choroid and sclera. It is thus also highly likely to play a critical role in the eye growth regulation and refractive error development, although the possibility has been the focus of attention only recently and thus this field of knowledge is still evolving [72].

Growth Factors and Eye Growth Regulation

The RPE is the source of a wide variety of growth factors essential to the maintenance of the structural integrity and functions of retina and choroid [81]. Pigment epithelium-derived factor (PEDF) and transforming growth factor-β (TGF-β) are among the growth and neurotrophic factors secreted predominantly from the apical (retinal) side, while vascular endothelial growth factor (VEGF) appears to be predominantly secreted from the basolateral (choroidal) side, with a presumed role in maintaining the survival and fenestrated morphology of the choriocapillaris [77, 79, 82–84]. The fact that the RPE also expresses receptors for a number of growth factors implies also direct autocrine regulation of some of its functions [85–87]. Some growth factors are also likely to contribute to pathological changes, as the RPE is known to respond to changes and injuries by differentially modulating the synthesis and secretion of certain ones [88, 89]. In the context of eye growth regulation and myopia, there has been only limited study of the roles of RPE-derived growth factors. Nonetheless, a number of multifunctional growth factors, including TGF-βs, bone morphogenetic proteins (BMPs), basic fibroblast growth factor (bFGF), and insulin-like growth factors (IGFs) have been investigated to this end.

TGF-βs

TGF-βs are probably the most studied growth factors in myopia research. They belong to a superfamily of structurally-related, multifunctional growth factors; apart from isoforms of TGF-β, it also includes BMPs, growth differentiation factors (GDFs), activins, inhibins, nodal and anti-Müllerian hormone (AMH) [90, 91]. Outside the eye, TGF-βs are known to be secreted by many cell types and involved in a wide variety of physiological and pathological processes, including embryonic development, organogenesis, immune modulation, cancer progression, wound healing and extracellular matrix remodeling [90, 91]. TGF-β has three isoforms, TGF-β1, TGF-β2, and TGF-β3; all are secreted as dimeric precursor proteins, from which active TGF-β is subsequently released in target tissues [92]. The known molecules involved in TGF-β activation include matrix metalloproteinase 2 (MMP2), MMP9, thrombospondin 1 (THBS1), and integrin [92–95]. Upon ligand binding to TGF-β receptors, intermediate steps involving the formation of heterotetrameric receptor complexes and then phosphorylation of receptors lead to activation of down-stream canonical or non-canonical signaling pathways to induce expression of target genes [90, 96].

Investigations into the roles of TGF-βs in eye growth regulation and myopia encompass both chick and mammalian models and different visual manipulations, with focuses on changes in either or both gene and protein expression of TGF-βs and/or their receptors in a variety of ocular tissues [97–109]. Scleral fibroblasts have been the focus of a number of such *in vivo* studies, as well as *in vitro* studies, which have linked TGF-β to cell proliferation, synthesis and secretion of proteoglycans, collagen production, cell contraction and cell phenotype alteration [100, 101, 110–112]. In terms of investigations into the ocular growth effects of exogenous TGF-β in animal models, one involving the chick form-deprivation model found subconjunctival injection of TGF-β1 to inhibit the myopia rescue effect of bFGF [113].

Chick, tree shrew and marmoset models have all been used in investigations into the role of RPE-derived TGF-β on eye growth regulation. Key results from relevant studies involving TGF-β isoforms and RPE are summarized in Table 7.1. In chicks, mRNA for all three TGF-β isoforms and all three TGF-β receptors (TGFBR1, TGFBR2, TGFBR3), was found to be expressed in the RPE, which also showed isoform-specific, defocus-sensitive changes in TGF-β gene expression [109]. Specifically, short-term exposure to myopic defo-

Table 7.1 Summary of key findings in animal models of eye growth regulation in relation to TGF-β expression changes in RPE alone, or combined with adjacent tissues

Animal	Visual treatments	Ocular tissues	TGF-β isoforms	Methods	Main results	References
Chick	FD for 12 days	Retina-RPE-choroid	TGF-β2	Protein (ELISA)	↑	Seko et al. [107]
Chick	FD for 10 days	Retina-RPE-choroid Retina-RPE-choroid	TGF-β1 TGF-β1, 2, 3, 5	tRNA (PCR) Protein, active form (WB)	↓ ↓	Honda et al. [100]
Chick	+7 or −7 D lens for 15, 30, 120 min	Retina-RPE	TGF-β2	mRNA (qPCR)	NS	Simon et al. [108]
Chick	−10 or +10 D for 2 or 48 h	RPE	TGF-β1, 2, 3	mRNA (qPCR)	NS with −10 D ↑TGF-β2 with +10 D	Zhang et al. [109]
Tree shrew	−5 D lens for 6 or 24 h	RPE Retina-RPE	TGF-β1, 2 TGF-β1, 2	mRNA (qPCR) mRNA (qPCR)	↓TGF-β2 24 h NS	He et al. [114]

FD Form-deprivation, *WB* Western blot, *NS* no significant change in treated versus control, ↑ increase in treated versus control, ↓ decreased treated versus control cus (e.g., with +10 D lenses) resulted in selective up-regulation of TGF-β2, up to 3.5- and 7.5-fold after 2 and 48 hours exposures, respectively. The 2 hours short-term treatment was used to identify genes important for the initiation of altered eye growth, before detectable changes in eye growth can occur, while genes showing differential expression with the 48 hours treatment are likely involved in maintaining the altered growth pattern, as by this time altered growth is detectable with biometry. As imposed myopic defocus inhibits ocular growth, these results suggest that RPE-derived TGF-β2 serves as an inhibitor of ocular elongation. In the broader context of myopia control, they identify TGF-β2 as a gene of interest. In the tree shrew, 24 hours of −5 D lens resulted in a 1.4-fold down-regulation of TGF-β1 gene expression in RPE, but had no effect on TGF-β2 [114]. Interestingly, no differential gene expression of TGF-β1 was observed in combined retina-RPE tissues in the same study, perhaps reflecting opposing retinal expression changes. Nonetheless, differential gene expression of TGFβ-induced (TGFBI) in retina-RPE combined samples was detected in a microarray study involving marmosets [115].

Direct supporting evidence for ocular growth inhibition by RPE-derived TGF-β is still lacking, in part due to design features of relevant earlier studies that render their results inconclusive. Specifically, TGF-βs are secreted proteins that exist in both latent and active forms, yet these properties were not generally taken into account in previous studies in the choice of protein expression assays, which were also mostly undertaken on combinations of ocular tissues, as were gene expression measurements [100, 102, 107, 108].

BMPs

The roles of BMPs in eye growth regulation and myopia development have been the subject of a number of recent investigations. As already noted, BMPs belong to the TGF-β superfamily. As the largest subfamily of this superfamily, it contains more than 20 members, which are typically further grouped into four subfamilies, based on their sequence similarity and known functions [116, 117]. Their name—bone morphogenetic protein—reflects their initial recognition as proteins involved in ectopic bone formation, although BMPs are now known to play important roles in many biological events, including embryogenesis, postnatal homeostasis, stem cell regulation and regeneration, as well as in various pathological events, including neovascularization and some cancers [88, 118–123]. BMPs are synthesized as precursor proteins, which are then secreted in dimeric form with or without their prodomain, or packaged into vesicles for release from cells [124]. Secreted BMPs may interact directly with neighboring cells, be released into the bloodstream, or bind with extracellular antagonist proteins, such as noggin, which regulate their activity. BMPs signal through two different types of serine/threonine kinase receptors, type I and type II receptors, with Smad proteins playing an important intracellular role in the transduction to the nucleus of signals from activated receptor complexes [118, 124].

During embryonic development, BMPs and their receptors are widely expressed in ocular tissues, with diverse roles, including lens induction, ciliary body morphogenesis, RPE specification, retinal patterning, retinotectal projection and retinal stem cell differentiation [125–137]. In the postnatal eye, BMPs play important roles in maintaining physiology hemostasis and they have also been implicated in a number of ocular diseases [25, 88, 121, 122, 138–140]. To date, expression patterns for BMPs and BMP receptors have been described for three commonly used myopia animal models—chicks, tree shrews and guinea pigs [99, 141–146]. Consistent with roles in ocular growth regulation, BMP gene and/or protein expression changes have been detected in one or more posterior ocular tissues in response to commonly used visual manipulations in all three models [99, 141, 142, 145–149]. Of potentially greater relevance to eye growth regulation, BMP2 has been found to induce the gene expression of four inhibitor of DNA binding proteins (IDs) in cultured chick scleral fibroblast; it also influences cell proliferation and extracellular matrix (ECM) synthesis and degradation, with reported effects in a cultured human scleral fibroblast model on collagen, glycosaminoglycan (GAG), and aggrecan synthesis, as well as MMP2, TIMP2 and chondrogenesis-associated gene expression [142, 150–152]. Interestingly, increased BMP2 gene expression in human sclera fibroblasts was also found in response to mechanical loading, to which intraocular pressure contributes *in vivo* [153]. Collectively, these observations suggest a key role for BMP2 in scleral remodeling and thus in eye growth regulation.

The most direct evidence implicating BMPs in the eye growth modulating signal pathways linking the retina with the choroid and sclera comes from studies involving chick and tree shrew models [114, 143, 145, 146]. Key results for relevant BMP gene expression studies involving the RPE are summarized in Table 7.2. In relation to the RPE, defocus, sign-dependent differential regulation of BMP gene expression has been described in response to short-term negative or positive lens treatments in chicks [145, 146]. Changes in BMP2 gene expression are most robust although two other members of the BMP family, BMP4 and BMP7, also show similar bidirectional changes in gene expression, in accord with the direction of experimentally-induced eye growth changes. Specifically, expression is down-regulated in eyes showing accelerated growth, as in myopia progression, and up-regulated in eyes showing slowed (anti-myopia) growth. Other related gene expression studies did not find any defocus-induced changes in the retina and reported only small-scale changes in BMP gene expression in choroid relative to changes in RPE [144]. These observations together strongly suggest critical roles of RPE-derived BMPs in defocus-driven eye growth regulation, with BMPs serving as growth inhibitors. They also offer additional insight into the results of two other chick studies that examined gene expression in combinations of ocular tissues that included RPE. In one of these studies involving retina-RPE, BMP2 gene expression was reported to be down-regulated after 6 hours and 3 days of form-deprivation, in the same direction as that induced by negative lenses, with both treatments leading to accelerated eye growth [143]. The other study involving retina-RPE-choroid reported early, bidirectional BMP2 gene expression under conditions inducing myopia and hyperopia, and as described above for isolated RPE [154]. While similar roles for RPE-derived BMPs in eye growth regulation in mammals await confirmation, a recent study involving tree shrews reported down-regulation of BMP2 gene expression in retina-RPE after 24 hours of −5 D lens treatment [114]. Recent confirmation of BMP2 expression in normal guinea pig RPE (unpublished observation), also represents a promising first step in a line of research that has

Table 7.2 Summary of key findings in animal models of eye growth regulation in relation to BMP expression changes in RPE alone, or combined with adjacent tissues

Animal	Visual treatments	Ocular tissues	BMPs	Methods	Main results	References
Chick	FD for 6 h or 3 days	Retina-RPE	BMP2	mRNA (microarray, qPCR)	↓	McGlinn et al. [143]
Chick	−15 or +15 D for 6 h or 3 days	Retina-RPE	BMP2	mRNA (microarray, qPCR)	↓ with −15 D	Stone et al. [155]
Chick	−10 or +10 D for 2 or 48 h	RPE	BMP2	mRNA (qPCR)	↑ with +10 D ↓ with −10 D	Zhang et al. [146]
Chick	−10 or +10 D for 2 or 48 h	RPE	BMP4, 7	mRNA (qPCR)	↑ with +10 D ↓ with −10 D	Zhang et al. [145]
Chick	−10 or +10 D for 1, 2, or 3 days	Retina-RPE-choroid	BMP2	mRNA (RNA sequencing)	↑ with +10 D ↓ with −10 D	Riddell et al. [154]
Tree shrew	−5 D lens for 6 or 24 h	RPE Retina-RPE	BMP2, 4 BMP2, 4	mRNA (qPCR) mRNA (qPCR)	NS ↓	He et al. [114]

FD Form-deprivation, *WB* Western blot, *NS* no significant change in treated versus control, ↑ increase in treated versus control, ↓ decreased treated versus control potential to open up new therapeutic avenues for myopia control.

Other Growth Factors

In addition to TGF-βs and BMPs, two other growth factors that have also attracted the interest of myopia researchers are IGFs and bFGF. Currently, relatively little is known about their signaling pathways, including whether or not the RPE is an important player, either as a site of synthesis or as a target. Nonetheless, studies that offer some evidence implicating the RPE are summarized below.

Insulin-like growth factors (IGFs) are polypeptide growth factors of the insulin family that consists of two members, IGF1 and IGF2, which play important roles in development and diseases [156–158]. Both IGFs and IGF receptors (IGF1R and IGF2R) are also widely expressed in ocular tissues [159–162]. For example, in chicks, IGF receptors have been detected in all posterior ocular tissues, i.e., retina, RPE, choroid, and sclera [161, 162]. IGFs and their receptors have also been implicated in altered eye growth in animal models. For example, in chicks, IGF1R is reported to be differentially regulated in RPE after 4 hours of positive lens wear and intravitreal injection of IGF1, to induce myopic eye growth [161–163]. Differential regulation of IGF2 was also observed in retina-RPE in tree shrews, after 24 hours of negative lens wear, although no change in IGF1 gene expression was detected [114]. Results from *in vitro* studies involving cultured human RPE cells also support a role for the RPE in IGF-mediated eye growth regulation; they were found to express both IGFs and their receptors and also secrete IGFs into the culture medium [164–166].

RPE is one of a number of ocular tissues that synthesize bFGF and its receptors and also secrete bFGF [167]. The retina and choroid were among other ocular tissues found to express bFGF and its receptors in one study in chicks, although due to the technique used and the dense pigmentation of the RPE, it was not possible to characterize bFGF receptor expression profile in this study [168]. Since both intravitreal and subconjunctival injections of bFGF are effective in inhibiting the excessive eye elongation induced by form-deprivation, the retina, RPE, choroid and sclera all represent potential sites of action [113, 169]. Other indirect evidence supporting a role for bFGF as an important regulator of eye growth includes an observed decrease in bFGF in the chick sclera after 2 weeks of form-deprivation. However, that no change in bFGF was found in combined retina-RPE-choroid in the same study tends to argue against the RPE as the source of bFGF [107]. Results of other studies involving guinea pigs also tend to point away from the RPE. For example, inhibition of lens-induced myopia with a peribulbar injection of bFGF has been linked to altered scleral expression of both collagen and integrin and expression of bFGF was reported to be reduced in scleral desmocytes isolated and cultured from experimentally (lens)-induced myopic eyes [110, 170]. Thus, while these results in chicks and guinea pigs are consistent with a role for bFGF as a "stop" signal in growing eyes, the exact details of the growth modulating signal pathway, including the identity of the cells mediating the action of bFGF, await further study.

Neurotransmitters and Eye Growth Regulation

A number of neurotransmitters have been implicated in eye growth regulation and the RPE is known to both express receptors for some of these neurotransmitters and also synthesize and secrete some of them [72, 171]. Therefore it is possible that the RPE is involved in neurotransmitter-related eye growth regulation and myopia development. Retinal neurotransmitters, including dopamine (DA), acetylcholine (Ach), glucagon and vasoactive intestinal peptide (VIP) are the most studied of these molecules in myopia research. Related studies targeting DA and Ach are reviewed below.

Dopamine

Dopamine is one of the most studied neurotransmitters in the context of eye growth regulation and myopia development [172–174]. Dopamine is widely expressed in both the central nervous system and retina where it plays important roles in development. In the postnatal retina, dopamine has been linked to retinomotor movements and the uncoupling of gap junctions on horizontal cells, both of which affect visual sensitivity [175–177]. Dopaminergic receptors represent a large family of G protein-coupled receptors (D1–D5), with members grouped into two subfamilies, D1-like (D1, D5) and D2-like (D2–D4) receptors, based on their biochemical and pharmacological properties [178]. Evidence supporting the role of dopamine in eye growth regulation comes mainly from two lines of research showing that: (1) retinal levels of dopamine and its metabolites are decreased in animals with visual manipulations that accelerate eye growth, and (2) locally administered exogenous dopamine receptor agonists inhibit the excessive eye elongation that underlies myopia, with more recent studies involving wild type, and genetically modified mice models offering further confirmatory evidence [52, 173, 179–197]. The evidence linking reduced dopamine levels and turnover with myopia comes from studies involving young chicks, guinea pigs, tree shrews and monkeys, which report consistent reductions with form-deprivation or lens induced models [181, 183, 187, 188, 196]. Further indirect evidence tying these changes to eye growth comes from studies of eyes allowed to recover from form-deprivation myopia, when both retinal dopamine and DOPAC levels return to levels comparable to those of contralateral control eyes [198]. Interestingly, low vitreal concentrations of dihydroxyphenylacetic acid (DOPAC), a dopamine metabolite, have also been linked to the use of low light intensity in rearing and associated myopia development in chicks [199]. Studies involving chicks, guinea pigs, tree shrews and monkeys are also the source of supporting evidence that the development of myopia can be inhibited by dopamine agonists, delivered by either intravitreal or subconjunctival injection, or by topical application [180, 184–186, 189–192, 194, 195, 197]. While retinal dopamine receptors are potential sites of action for the latter effects, the RPE is also known to express both D1- and D2-like receptors [176, 200, 201]. Furthermore, the RPE appears to be a readily accessible target for applied drugs. For example, both intravitreal and subconjunctival injections of radioactively-labeled spiperone, a D2 receptor antagonist, were found to reach the RPE [192]. That the RPE is a plausible site of action for dopaminergic effects on eye growth is further supported by other *in vitro* studies. One such study reported physiological responses, including hyperpolarization, in response to dopamine applied to either apical or basolateral membranes of cultured RPE [202]. In another *in vitro* co-culture study, apomorphine, a dopamine receptor agonist, dramatically inhibited the growth-stimulatory effect of RPE cells on scleral chondrocytes [203]. Nonetheless, there remain many unanswered questions in relation to the signal pathway mediating the anti-myopia action of dopamine, given that in yet two other studies, RPE was found to both synthesize and secrete dopamine [204, 205].

Acetylcholine (Ach)

Acetylcholine is a ubiquitous yet important neurotransmitter with critical roles in retina development and functions [206, 207]. Retinal cholinergic cells comprise several subsets of amacrine cells, which are known to synapse with other neurotransmitter networks in the retina, including dopaminergic cells [208–210]. Acetylcholine (Ach) receptors fall into two broad categories, muscarinic acetylcholine receptors (mAChRs) and nicotinic acetylcholine receptors (nAchRs) [211, 212]. Muscarinic receptors (mAChRs), which are widely distributed throughout the eye, represent a family of G protein-coupled receptors, with five receptor subtypes (M1–M5) described in mammals [211, 212]. Consistent with the reports of mAchR on RPE as well as in retina, *in vitro* studies have shown that intracellular signal pathways in RPE can be activated by mAchR agonists [206, 209, 213–216]. Different from the finding with dopamine of reduced retinal turnover in form-deprived myopic eyes, levels of retinal Ach and its metabolite, choline, appear unaffected by the development of myopia in both chicks and tree shrews [188]. On the other hand, intervention studies have shown antimuscarinic drugs to be effective inhibitors of myopia development in both humans and animal models. In animal studies, drugs were administrated via either intravitreal or subconjunctival injection, while topical drops have been the norm for human studies, which have also been limited to atropine, a nonselective antagonist, and pirenzepine, a M1-receptor antagonist [195, 217–225]. Reports in more recent human studies of inhibitory effects with much lower concentrations of topical atropine than used in earlier studies (e.g., 0.01 and 0.1% compared to 1%) [42], argue against inner ocular tissues, including the retina and RPE, as sites of action, based on pharmacokinetic principles. The relatively high intravitreal doses needed to achieve treatment efficacy in another comparative study of eighteen antimuscarinic drugs tested in form-deprived chicks, also challenges the notion of a muscarinic receptor-mediated mechanism involving retina or RPE [226], leading to more recent speculation on possible nonmuscarinic mechanisms being involved [227–229]. These conclusions are also in line with findings from other studies, including *in vitro* ones, pointing to the choroid and/or sclera as likely site(s) of action for the anti-myopic effects of antimuscarinic drugs, although underlying mechanisms remain poorly understood [217, 230, 231].

As a final aside, it should be noted that intravitreally-injected nAchR antagonists have been shown to influence eye growth in chicks [232]. As nAchRs have also been found in retina and RPE, they are plausible sites mediating the complex response patterns observed.

Glucagon and Vasoactive Intestinal Peptide (VIP)

Glucagon and vasoactive intestinal peptide (VIP) are part of a superfamily of secretin-glucagon peptides that function as neurotransmitters or neuromodulators in both central and peripheral nervous systems, acting through G-protein coupled receptors [233]. Both glucagon- and VIP-immunoreactive neurons have been described in chick retina [234–236]. Furthermore, the RPE also expresses glucagon receptor mRNA, and both glucagon and VIP have been shown to stimulate intracellular activities in RPE [237–240].

Evidence for roles of glucagon in eye growth regulation comes largely from studies in chicks. In the earliest of such studies, the expression of the immediate-early gene, ZENK, was reported to be decreased in glucagonergic amacrine cells in response to both form-deprivation and negative lens treatments and increased with positive lens treatments in chicks [241]. Later studies reported retinal glucagon mRNA to be also down-regulated with negative lens treatments and up-regulated with positive lens treatments [237, 242]. In addition, differential regulation of retinal mRNA levels of preproglucagon was found with form-deprivation and negative lens treatments [237, 243]. Finally, retinal glucagon peptide levels were found to be decreased after exposure to negative lenses [244]. That glucagon may act as a stop signal for eye growth, as suggested by these studies, is also consistent with results of pharmacological studies in which glucagon agonists, injected intravitreally, were found to inhibit experimentally induced myopia [244–246]. It is also plausible, but not conclusively established, that the RPE is the target for retinal and exogenous glucagon, serving as a signal relay for these ocular growth effects.

VIP has been the subject of far fewer studies, with one reporting levels of VIP to be significantly increased in the retinas of form-deprived monkeys and another reporting VIP gene expression to be up-regulated in tree shrew retina and retina-RPE, while down-regulated in RPE with negative lens wear [114, 247, 248]. VIP receptor antagonists, delivered by intravitreal injection, have also been reported to inhibit form-deprivation myopia in chicks [249]. However, neither the role of VIP nor the role of glucagon in form-deprivation myoia has been confirmed in the mouse model [250].

Ions, Ion Channels and Eye Growth Regulation

The RPE plays important roles in regulating the ion composition and volume of the subretinal space and choroid and thus the maintenance of tissue homeostasis. As already noted, the RPE comprises a monolayer of highly polarized cells interconnected with tight junctions, which restrict the paracellular movement of ions and fluid. That the paracellular resistance between RPE cells is ten times higher than the transcellular resistance is one measure of the effectiveness of these junctions. The polarized expression of ion channels and other functionally related molecules on RPE has been well documented and is consistent with the unidirectional fluid transport across the RPE, in an apical-to-basal direction, facilitated by the transport of ions [75, 80, 81, 251]. Thus Na^+-HCO_3^- and Na^+-K^+-$2Cl^-$ cotransporters, along with Na^+-K^+-ATPase, which are found on the apical membranes of the RPE, allow the intracellular uptake of Cl^- and regulation of intracellular pH. Cl^- ions along with K^+ ions are extruded into the choroid from ion channels on the basolateral membranes of the RPE, which also express the cystic fibrosis transmembrane conductance regulator (CFTR) [81, 252]. This movement of ions serves to drive the movement of water from the subretinal space into the choroid.

Investigations into the roles of ion channels in eye growth regulation and the possible involvement of RPE have been limited to the chick model [69, 72]. In eyes made myopic by form-deprivation, both retinal and choroidal tissues were found to have markedly raised Na^+ and Cl^- levels, with K^+ levels also elevated, albeit localized to the outer retina-RPE region [253]. In eyes allowed to recover from induced myopia, the levels of K^+, Na^+, and Cl^- normalized around the time of refractive error recovery, while during the recovery phase, the retina, RPE, and choroid all showed thickening and edema [253, 254]. These findings point to potential roles of ion and fluid movement across RPE in refractive error regulation, with more direct evidence contained in related pharmacological studies. Specifically, intravitreal injection of barium chloride, a nonspecific potassium channel inhibitor, was found to inhibit the compensatory ocular growth responses to imposed optical defocus, irrespective of its sign, while bumetanide, a selective Na^+-K^+-Cl^- cotransporter inhibitor, selectively inhibited the response to negative lenses [255]. In addition, an unrelated study reported differential regulation of several Cl^- transporters and channels in the RPE with negative lenses, with gene and protein expression being down-regulated after just one day of lens wear [256].

The identity of the signal molecules mediating the above changes in ion transport and fluid movement across the RPE during the development and recovery from myopia remains unresolved, although two *in vitro* studies point to dopamine and Ach as plausible candidates. In one of these studies, using retina-RPE-choroid preparations, dopamine was found to modulate basal membrane Cl^- conductance in chick RPE [202], and in the other study using human RPE cultures, mAchR agonists were found to induce rapid increases in intracellular calcium [213].

Morphological Changes in RPE in Experimental Myopia

In relation to myopic growth-related morphological changes in RPE, two studies of relevance include one involving chicks and another, quokka wallabies, which are a marsupial [257, 258]. As one of three layers lining the scleral cup, which undergoes substantial enlargement in myopia, the RPE must necessarily undergo substantial expansion of its surface area in parallel. In chicks made myopic by form-deprivation for 1–2 weeks, individual RPE cells were found to thin and stretch to maintain coverage of the expanding vitreous chamber, rather than dividing to add cell numbers; nonetheless, their hexagonal shapes were preserved [258]. Similarly in form-deprived quokkas, RPE cells were found to be enlarged in treated eyes, with their appearance being otherwise relatively unaffected, when compared against those of fellow, control eyes [257]. A unique finding of the latter study was the redistribution of multinucleated RPE cells in enlarged form-derived eyes, from the usual, mostly ventral location as seen in untreated (control) eyes, to more peripheral dorsal and nasal locations, around the retinal rim. However, it should also be noted that unlike most mammals and primates, the eyes of quokkas also grow throughout life, Nonetheless, these limited observations suggest that the RPE adapts to the expanding vitreous chamber in myopia, mostly through passive stretch, with possible implications for the long-term health of RPE cells and risk of pathology, especially in highly myopic eyes [45]. Finally, it is noteworthy that application of mechanical stress to cultured RPE cells has been reported to induce VEGF in rat RPE and MMP-2 activation in human RPE [259, 260]. These observations raise the possibility that the mechanical forces experienced by the RPE of growing eyes may themselves indirectly influence eye growth through effects on RPE activity.

Summary

In summary, the RPE likely plays an important role in local eye growth regulation and thus the development of myopia, reflecting in part its critical location, interposed between the retina and choroid. Observations of growth factor synthesis and secretion, neurotransmitter receptor expression and activation, ion exchanges and fluid movement across RPE, are also compatible with a role for the RPE in eye growth regulation. Further elucidation of the presumed eye growth modulatory signal pathways and the role of the RPE as a signal relay may lead to novel therapeutic interventions for myopia control. An improved understanding of the morphological and functional changes in RPE at various stages of disease development and the key mediating factors may also lead to improved management of the pathological complications of myopia, including myopic maculopathy.

Acknowledgments The authors thank Professor Kyoko Ohno-Matsui (Tokyo Medical and Dental University, Tokyo, Japan) for providing fundus and OCT images from a myopic patient with patchy chorioretinal atrophy, Sara Yasmin Azmoun (University of California, Berkeley, CA) for her assistance with manuscript preparation, and funding support from National Eye Institute Grants R01 EY012392 (C. F. W.), K08 EY023609 (Y. Z.), and K12 EY017269 (Y. Z.).

References

1. Bourne RR, Stevens GA, White RA, Smith JL, Flaxman SR, Price H, Jonas JB, Keeffe J, Leasher J, Naidoo K, Pesudovs K, Resnikoff S, Taylor HR. Causes of vision loss worldwide, 1990-2010: a systematic analysis. Lancet Glob Health. 2013;1(6):e339–49.
2. Ono K, Hiratsuka Y, Murakami A. Global inequality in eye health: country-level analysis from the Global Burden of Disease Study. Am J Public Health. 2010;100(9):1784–8.
3. Pascolini D, Mariotti SP. Global estimates of visual impairment: 2010. Br J Ophthalmol. 2012;96(5):614–8.
4. Curtin BJ, editor. The myopias: basic science and clinical management. Philadelphia: Harper & Row Publishers; 1985.
5. Whitmore WG. Congenital and developmental myopia. Eye (Lond). 1992;6(Pt 4):361–5.
6. McBrien NA, Millodot M. A biometric investigation of late onset myopic eyes. Acta Ophthalmol. 1987;65(4):461–8.
7. Flitcroft DI. The complex interactions of retinal, optical and environmental factors in myopia aetiology. Prog Retin Eye Res. 2012;31(6):622–60.
8. Holden BA, Jong M, Davis S, Wilson D, Fricke T, Resnikoff S. Nearly 1 billion myopes at risk of myopia-related sight-threatening conditions by 2050—time to act now. Clin Exp Optom. 2015;98(6):491–3.
9. Dolgin E. The myopia boom. Nature. 2015;519(7543):276–8.
10. Holden BA, Fricke TR, Wilson DA, Jong M, Naidoo KS, Sankaridurg P, Wong TY, Naduvilath TJ, Resnikoff S. Global prevalence of myopia and high myopia and temporal trends from 2000 through 2050. Ophthalmology. 2016;123(5):1036–42.
11. Jung SK, Lee JH, Kakizaki H, Jee D. Prevalence of myopia and its association with body stature and educational level in 19-year-old male conscripts in Seoul, South Korea. Invest Ophthalmol Vis Sci. 2012;53(9):5579–83.
12. Vitale S, Sperduto RD, Ferris FL 3rd. Increased prevalence of myopia in the United States between 1971-1972 and 1999-2004. Arch Ophthalmol. 2009;127(12):1632–9.
13. Pan CW, Ramamurthy D, Saw SM. Worldwide prevalence and risk factors for myopia. Ophthalmic Physiol Opt. 2012;32(1):3–16.
14. Wu PC, Huang HM, Yu HJ, Fang PC, Chen CT. Epidemiology of myopia. Asia Pac J Ophthalmol (Phila). 2016;5(6):386–93.
15. Rose K, Smith W, Morgan I, Mitchell P. The increasing prevalence of myopia: implications for Australia. Clin Exp Ophthalmol. 2001;29(3):116–20.
16. Fricke TR, Holden BA, Wilson DA, Schlenther G, Naidoo KS, Resnikoff S, Frick KD. Global cost of correcting vision impairment from uncorrected refractive error. Bull World Health Organ. 2012;90(10):728–38.
17. Holden B, Sankaridurg P, Smith E, Aller T, Jong M, He M. Myopia, an underrated global challenge to vision: where the current data takes us on myopia control. Eye (Lond). 2014;28(2):142–6.
18. Ramamurthy D, Lin Chua SY, Saw SM. A review of environmental risk factors for myopia during early life, childhood and adolescence. Clin Exp Optom. 2015;98(6):497–506.

19. Wallman J, Winawer J. Homeostasis of eye growth and the question of myopia. Neuron. 2004;43(4):447–68.
20. Wojciechowski R. Nature and nurture: the complex genetics of myopia and refractive error. Clin Genet. 2011;79(4):301–20.
21. Wojciechowski R, Cheng CY. Involvement of multiple molecular pathways in the genetics of ocular refraction and myopia. Retina. 2018;38(1):91–101.
22. Young TL, Metlapally R, Shay AE. Complex trait genetics of refractive error. Arch Ophthalmol. 2007;125(1):38–48.
23. Fan Q, Verhoeven VJ, Wojciechowski R, Barathi VA, Hysi PG, Guggenheim JA, Hohn R, Vitart V, Khawaja AP, Yamashiro K, Hosseini SM, Lehtimaki T, Lu Y, Haller T, Xie J, Delcourt C, Pirastu M, Wedenoja J, Gharahkhani P, Venturini C, Miyake M, Hewitt AW, Guo X, Mazur J, Huffman JE, Williams KM, Polasek O, Campbell H, Rudan I, Vatavuk Z, Wilson JF, Joshi PK, McMahon G, St Pourcain B, Evans DM, Simpson CL, Schwantes-An TH, Igo RP, Mirshahi A, Cougnard-Gregoire A, Bellenguez C, Blettner M, Raitakari O, Kahonen M, Seppala I, Zeller T, Meitinger T, Ried JS, Gieger C, Portas L, van Leeuwen EM, Amin N, Uitterlinden AG, Rivadeneira F, Hofman A, Vingerling JR, Wang YX, Wang X, Tai-Hui Boh E, Ikram MK, Sabanayagam C, Gupta P, Tan V, Zhou L, Ho CE, Lim W, Beuerman RW, Siantar R, Tai ES, Vithana E, Mihailov E, Khor CC, Hayward C, Luben RN, Foster PJ, Klein BE, Klein R, Wong HS, Mitchell P, Metspalu A, Aung T, Young TL, He M, Parssinen O, van Duijn CM, Jin Wang J, Williams C, Jonas JB, Teo YY, Mackey DA, Oexle K, Yoshimura N, Paterson AD, Pfeiffer N, Wong TY, Baird PN, Stambolian D, Wilson JE, Cheng CY, Hammond CJ, Klaver CC, Saw SM, Rahi JS, Korobelnik JF, Kemp JP, Timpson NJ, Smith GD, Craig JE, Burdon KP, Fogarty RD, Iyengar SK, Chew E, Janmahasatian S, Martin NG, MacGregor S, Xu L, Schache M, Nangia V, Panda-Jonas S, Wright AF, Fondran JR, Lass JH, Feng S, Zhao JH, Khaw KT, Wareham NJ, Rantanen T, Kaprio J, Pang CP, Chen LJ, Tam PO, Jhanji V, Young AL, Doring A, Raffel LJ, Cotch MF, Li X, Yip SP, Yap MK, Biino G, Vaccargiu S, Fossarello M, Fleck B, Yazar S, Tideman JW, Tedja M, Deangelis MM, Morrison M, Farrer L, Zhou X, Chen W, Mizuki N, Meguro A, Makela KM. Meta-analysis of gene-environment-wide association scans accounting for education level identifies additional loci for refractive error. Nat Commun. 2016;7:11008.
24. Hysi PG, Young TL, Mackey DA, Andrew T, Fernandez-Medarde A, Solouki AM, Hewitt AW, Macgregor S, Vingerling JR, Li YJ, Ikram MK, Fai LY, Sham PC, Manyes L, Porteros A, Lopes MC, Carbonaro F, Fahy SJ, Martin NG, van Duijn CM, Spector TD, Rahi JS, Santos E, Klaver CC, Hammond CJ. A genome-wide association study for myopia and refractive error identifies a susceptibility locus at 15q25. Nat Genet. 2010;42(10):902–5.
25. Verhoeven VJ, Hysi PG, Wojciechowski R, Fan Q, Guggenheim JA, Hohn R, MacGregor S, Hewitt AW, Nag A, Cheng CY, Yonova-Doing E, Zhou X, Ikram MK, Buitendijk GH, McMahon G, Kemp JP, Pourcain BS, Simpson CL, Makela KM, Lehtimaki T, Kahonen M, Paterson AD, Hosseini SM, Wong HS, Xu L, Jonas JB, Parssinen O, Wedenoja J, Yip SP, Ho DW, Pang CP, Chen LJ, Burdon KP, Craig JE, Klein BE, Klein R, Haller T, Metspalu A, Khor CC, Tai ES, Aung T, Vithana E, Tay WT, Barathi VA, Chen P, Li R, Liao J, Zheng Y, Ong RT, Doring A, Evans DM, Timpson NJ, Verkerk AJ, Meitinger T, Raitakari O, Hawthorne F, Spector TD, Karssen LC, Pirastu M, Murgia F, Ang W, Mishra A, Montgomery GW, Pennell CE, Cumberland PM, Cotlarciuc I, Mitchell P, Wang JJ, Schache M, Janmahasatian S, Igo RP Jr, Lass JH, Chew E, Iyengar SK, Gorgels TG, Rudan I, Hayward C, Wright AF, Polasek O, Vatavuk Z, Wilson JF, Fleck B, Zeller T, Mirshahi A, Muller C, Uitterlinden AG, Rivadeneira F, Vingerling JR, Hofman A, Oostra BA, Amin N, Bergen AA, Teo YY, Rahi JS, Vitart V, Williams C, Baird PN, Wong TY, Oexle K, Pfeiffer N, Mackey DA, Young TL, van Duijn CM, Saw SM, Bailey-Wilson JE, Stambolian D, Klaver CC, Hammond CJ. Genome-wide meta-analyses of multiancestry cohorts identify multiple new susceptibility loci for refractive error and myopia. Nat Genet. 2013;45(3):314–8.
26. Hysi PG, Wojciechowski R, Rahi JS, Hammond CJ. Genome-wide association studies of refractive error and myopia, lessons learned, and implications for the future. Invest Ophthalmol Vis Sci. 2014;55(5):3344–51.
27. He M, Xiang F, Zeng Y, Mai J, Chen Q, Zhang J, Smith W, Rose K, Morgan IG. Effect of time spent outdoors at school on the development of myopia among children in China: a randomized clinical trial. JAMA. 2015;314(11):1142–8.
28. Huang HM, Chang DS, Wu PC. The association between near work activities and myopia in children-a systematic review and meta-analysis. PLoS One. 2015;10(10):e0140419.
29. Rose KA, Morgan IG, Ip J, Kifley A, Huynh S, Smith W, Mitchell P. Outdoor activity reduces the prevalence of myopia in children. Ophthalmology. 2008;115(8):1279–85.
30. Sherwin JC, Reacher MH, Keogh RH, Khawaja AP, Mackey DA, Foster PJ. The association between time spent outdoors and myopia in children and adolescents: a systematic review and meta-analysis. Ophthalmology. 2012;119(10):2141–51.
31. Leo SW. Current approaches to myopia control. Curr Opin Ophthalmol. 2017;28(3):267–75.
32. Walline JJ, Lindsley K, Vedula SS, Cotter SA, Mutti DO, Twelker JD. Interventions to slow progression of myopia in children. Cochrane Database Syst Rev. 2011;(12):CD004916.
33. Aller TA, Liu M, Wildsoet CF. Myopia control with bifocal contact lenses: a randomized clinical trial. Optom Vis Sci. 2016;93(4):344–52.

34. Cheng D, Woo GC, Schmid KL. Bifocal lens control of myopic progression in children. Clin Exp Optom. 2011;94(1):24–32.
35. Cho P, Cheung SW. Protective role of orthokeratology in reducing risk of rapid axial elongation: a reanalysis of data from the ROMIO and TO-SEE studies. Invest Ophthalmol Vis Sci. 2017;58(3):1411–6.
36. Swarbrick HA, Alharbi A, Watt K, Lum E, Kang P. Myopia control during orthokeratology lens wear in children using a novel study design. Ophthalmology. 2015;122(3):620–30.
37. Walline JJ, Jones LA, Sinnott LT. Corneal reshaping and myopia progression. Br J Ophthalmol. 2009;93(9):1181–5.
38. Chia A, Chua WH, Cheung YB, Wong WL, Lingham A, Fong A, Tan D. Atropine for the treatment of childhood myopia: safety and efficacy of 0.5%, 0.1%, and 0.01% doses (Atropine for the Treatment of Myopia 2). Ophthalmology. 2012;119(2):347–54.
39. Siatkowski RM, Cotter SA, Crockett RS, Miller JM, Novack GD, Zadnik K. Two-year multicenter, randomized, double-masked, placebo-controlled, parallel safety and efficacy study of 2% pirenzepine ophthalmic gel in children with myopia. J AAPOS. 2008;12(4):332–9.
40. Tan DT, Lam DS, Chua WH, Shu-Ping DF, Crockett RS. One-year multicenter, double-masked, placebo-controlled, parallel safety and efficacy study of 2% pirenzepine ophthalmic gel in children with myopia. Ophthalmology. 2005;112(1):84–91.
41. Tran HDM, Tran YH, Tran TD, Jong M, Coroneo M, Sankaridurg P. A review of myopia control with atropine. J Ocul Pharmacol Ther. 2018;34(5):374–9.
42. Yam JC, Jiang Y, Tang SM, Law AKP, Chan JJ, Wong E, Ko ST, Young AL, Tham CC, Chen LJ, Pang CP. Low-concentration atropine for myopia progression (LAMP) study: a randomized, double-blinded, placebo-controlled trial of 0.05%, 0.025%, and 0.01% atropine eye drops in myopia control. Ophthalmology. 2019;126(1):113–24.
43. Trier K, Munk Ribel-Madsen S, Cui D, Brogger Christensen S. Systemic 7-methylxanthine in retarding axial eye growth and myopia progression: a 36-month pilot study. J Ocul Biol Dis Infor. 2008;1(2–4):85–93.
44. Liu HH, Xu L, Wang YX, Wang S, You QS, Jonas JB. Prevalence and progression of myopic retinopathy in Chinese adults: the Beijing Eye Study. Ophthalmology. 2010;117(9):1763–8.
45. Ohno-Matsui K, Lai TY, Lai CC, Cheung CM. Updates of pathologic myopia. Prog Retin Eye Res. 2016;52:156–87.
46. Vongphanit J, Mitchell P, Wang JJ. Prevalence and progression of myopic retinopathy in an older population. Ophthalmology. 2002;109(4):704–11.
47. Ohno-Matsui K, Jonas JB, Spaide RF. Macular Bruch membrane holes in highly myopic patchy chorioretinal atrophy. Am J Ophthalmol. 2016;166:22–8.
48. Jonas JB, Xu L. Histological changes of high axial myopia. Eye (Lond). 2014;28(2):113–7.
49. Jonas JB, Ohno-Matsui K, Holbach L, Panda-Jonas S. Retinal pigment epithelium cell density in relationship to axial length in human eyes. Acta Ophthalmol. 2017;95(1):e22–8.
50. Shin YJ, Nam WH, Park SE, Kim JH, Kim HK. Aqueous humor concentrations of vascular endothelial growth factor and pigment epithelium-derived factor in high myopic patients. Mol Vis. 2012;18:2265–70.
51. Zhuang H, Zhang R, Shu Q, Jiang R, Chang Q, Huang X, Jiang C, Xu G. Changes of TGF-beta2, MMP-2, and TIMP-2 levels in the vitreous of patients with high myopia. Graefes Arch Clin Exp Ophthalmol. 2014;252(11):1763–7.
52. Pardue MT, Faulkner AE, Fernandes A, Yin H, Schaeffel F, Williams RW, Pozdeyev N, Iuvone PM. High susceptibility to experimental myopia in a mouse model with a retinal on pathway defect. Invest Ophthalmol Vis Sci. 2008;49(2):706–12.
53. Schaeffel F, Burkhardt E, Howland HC, Williams RW. Measurement of refractive state and deprivation myopia in two strains of mice. Optom Vis Sci. 2004;81(2):99–110.
54. Sherman SM, Norton TT, Casagrande VA. Myopia in the lid-sutured tree shrew (Tupaia glis). Brain Res. 1977;124(1):154–7.
55. Troilo D, Judge SJ. Ocular development and visual deprivation myopia in the common marmoset (Callithrix jacchus). Vis Res. 1993;33(10):1311–24.
56. Troilo D, Wallman J. The regulation of eye growth and refractive state: an experimental study of emmetropization. Vis Res. 1991;31(7–8):1237–50.
57. Veth KN, Willer JR, Collery RF, Gray MP, Willer GB, Wagner DS, Mullins MC, Udvadia AJ, Smith RS, John SW, Gregg RG, Link BA. Mutations in zebrafish lrp2 result in adult-onset ocular pathogenesis that models myopia and other risk factors for glaucoma. PLoS Genet. 2011;7(2):e1001310.
58. Wiesel TN, Raviola E. Myopia and eye enlarge ment after neonatal lid fusion in monkeys. Nature. 1977;266(5597):66–8.
59. Wildsoet CF, Pettigrew JD. Kainic acid-induced eye enlargement in chickens: differential effects on anterior and posterior segments. Invest Ophthalmol Vis Sci. 1988;29(2):311–9.
60. Diether S, Schaeffel F. Local changes in eye growth induced by imposed local refractive error despite active accommodation. Vis Res. 1997;37(6):659–68.
61. Hodos W, Kuenzel WJ. Retinal-image degradation produces ocular enlargement in chicks. Invest Ophthalmol Vis Sci. 1984;25(6):652–9.
62. Norton TT, Essinger JA, McBrien NA. Lid-suture myopia in tree shrews with retinal ganglion cell blockade. Vis Neurosci. 1994;11(1):143–53.
63. Troilo D, Gottlieb MD, Wallman J. Visual deprivation causes myopia in chicks with optic nerve section. Curr Eye Res. 1987;6(8):993–9.
64. Wallman J, Gottlieb MD, Rajaram V, Fugate-Wentzek LA. Local retinal regions control local eye growth and myopia. Science. 1987;237(4810):73–7.

65. Wildsoet C. Neural pathways subserving negative lens-induced emmetropization in chicks—insights from selective lesions of the optic nerve and ciliary nerve. Curr Eye Res. 2003;27(6):371–85.
66. Wildsoet C, Wallman J. Choroidal and scleral mechanisms of compensation for spectacle lenses in chicks. Vis Res. 1995;35(9):1175–94.
67. Wildsoet CF, Pettigrew J. Experimental myopia and anomalous eye growth patterns unaffected by optic nerve section in chickens: evidence for local control of eye growth. Clin Vis Sci. 1988;3:99–107.
68. Smith EL 3rd, Hung LF, Huang J, Arumugam B. Effects of local myopic defocus on refractive development in monkeys. Optom Vis Sci. 2013;90(11):1176–86.
69. Crewther DP. The role of photoreceptors in the control of refractive state. Prog Retin Eye Res. 2000;19(4):421–57.
70. Nickla DL, Wallman J. The multifunctional choroid. Prog Retin Eye Res. 2010;29(2):144–68.
71. Rada JA, Shelton S, Norton TT. The sclera and myopia. Exp Eye Res. 2006;82(2):185–200.
72. Rymer J, Wildsoet CF. The role of the retinal pigment epithelium in eye growth regulation and myopia: a review. Vis Neurosci. 2005;22(3):251–61.
73. Stone RA, Khurana TS. Gene profiling in experimental models of eye growth: clues to myopia pathogenesis. Vis Res. 2010;50(23):2322–33.
74. Pfeffer BA, Flanders KC, Guerin CJ, Danielpour D, Anderson DH. Transforming growth factor beta 2 is the predominant isoform in the neural retina, retinal pigment epithelium-choroid and vitreous of the monkey eye. Exp Eye Res. 1994;59(3):323–33.
75. Reichhart N, Strauss O. Ion channels and transporters of the retinal pigment epithelium. Exp Eye Res. 2014;126:27–37.
76. Rizzolo LJ, Peng S, Luo Y, Xiao W. Integration of tight junctions and claudins with the barrier functions of the retinal pigment epithelium. Prog Retin Eye Res. 2011;30(5):296–323.
77. Saint-Geniez M, Kurihara T, Sekiyama E, Maldonado AE, D'Amore PA. An essential role for RPE-derived soluble VEGF in the maintenance of the choriocapillaris. Proc Natl Acad Sci U S A. 2009;106(44):18751–6.
78. Tanihara H, Inatani M, Honda Y. Growth factors and their receptors in the retina and pigment epithelium. Prog Retin Eye Res. 1997;16:271–301.
79. Blaauwgeers HG, Holtkamp GM, Rutten H, Witmer AN, Koolwijk P, Partanen TA, Alitalo K, Kroon ME, Kijlstra A, van Hinsbergh VW, Schlingemann RO. Polarized vascular endothelial growth factor secretion by human retinal pigment epithelium and localization of vascular endothelial growth factor receptors on the inner choriocapillaris. Evidence for a trophic paracrine relation. Am J Pathol. 1999;155(2):421–8.
80. Marmor M, Wolfensberger T, editors. The retinal pigment epithelium: function and disease. New York: Oxford University Press; 1998.
81. Strauss O. The retinal pigment epithelium in visual function. Physiol Rev. 2005;85(3):845–81.
82. Becerra SP, Fariss RN, Wu YQ, Montuenga LM, Wong P, Pfeffer BA. Pigment epithelium-derived factor in the monkey retinal pigment epithelium and interphotoreceptor matrix: apical secretion and distribution. Exp Eye Res. 2004;78(2):223–34.
83. Hirsch L, Nazari H, Sreekumar PG, Kannan R, Dustin L, Zhu D, Barron E, Hinton DR. TGF-beta2 secretion from RPE decreases with polarization and becomes apically oriented. Cytokine. 2015;71(2):394–6.
84. Wang Y, Subramanian P, Shen D, Tuo J, Becerra SP, Chan CC. Pigment epithelium-derived factor reduces apoptosis and pro-inflammatory cytokine gene expression in a murine model of focal retinal degeneration. ASN Neuro. 2013;5(5):e00126.
85. Byeon SH, Lee SC, Choi SH, Lee HK, Lee JH, Chu YK, Kwon OW. Vascular endothelial growth factor as an autocrine survival factor for retinal pigment epithelial cells under oxidative stress via the VEGF-R2/PI3K/Akt. Invest Ophthalmol Vis Sci. 2010;51(2):1190–7.
86. Campochiaro PA, Hackett SF, Vinores SA, Freund J, Csaky C, LaRochelle W, Henderer J, Johnson M, Rodriguez IR, Friedman Z, et al. Platelet-derived growth factor is an autocrine growth stimulator in retinal pigmented epithelial cells. J Cell Sci. 1994;107(Pt 9):2459–69.
87. Obata H, Kaji Y, Yamada H, Kato M, Tsuru T, Yamashita H. Expression of transforming growth factor-beta superfamily receptors in rat eyes. Acta Ophthalmol Scand. 1999;77(2):151–6.
88. Mathura JR Jr, Jafari N, Chang JT, Hackett SF, Wahlin KJ, Della NG, Okamoto N, Zack DJ, Campochiaro PA. Bone morphogenetic proteins-2 and -4: negative growth regulators in adult retinal pigmented epithelium. Invest Ophthalmol Vis Sci. 2000;41(2):592–600.
89. Matsumoto M, Yoshimura N, Honda Y. Increased production of transforming growth factor-beta 2 from cultured human retinal pigment epithelial cells by photocoagulation. Invest Ophthalmol Vis Sci. 1994;35(13):4245–52.
90. Akhurst RJ, Hata A. Targeting the TGFbeta signalling pathway in disease. Nat Rev Drug Discov. 2012;11(10):790–811.
91. Massague J. TGFbeta signalling in context. Nat Rev Mol Cell Biol. 2012;13(10):616–30.
92. Shi M, Zhu J, Wang R, Chen X, Mi L, Walz T, Springer TA. Latent TGF-beta structure and activation. Nature. 2011;474(7351):343–9.
93. Jenkins G. The role of proteases in transforming growth factor-beta activation. Int J Biochem Cell Biol. 2008;40(6–7):1068–78.
94. Munger JS, Huang X, Kawakatsu H, Griffiths MJ, Dalton SL, Wu J, Pittet JF, Kaminski N, Garat C, Matthay MA, Rifkin DB, Sheppard D. The integrin alpha v beta 6 binds and activates latent TGF beta 1:

a mechanism for regulating pulmonary inflammation and fibrosis. Cell. 1999;96(3):319–28.
95. Schultz-Cherry S, Ribeiro S, Gentry L, Murphy-Ullrich JE. Thrombospondin binds and activates the small and large forms of latent transforming growth factor-beta in a chemically defined system. J Biol Chem. 1994;269(43):26775–82.
96. Shi Y, Massague J. Mechanisms of TGF-beta signaling from cell membrane to the nucleus. Cell. 2003;113(6):685–700.
97. Gao H, Frost MR, Siegwart JT Jr, Norton TT. Patterns of mRNA and protein expression during minus-lens compensation and recovery in tree shrew sclera. Mol Vis. 2011;17:903–19.
98. Guo L, Frost MR, He L, Siegwart JT Jr, Norton TT. Gene expression signatures in tree shrew sclera in response to three myopiagenic conditions. Invest Ophthalmol Vis Sci. 2013;54(10):6806–19.
99. He L, Frost MR, Siegwart JT Jr, Norton TT. Gene expression signatures in tree shrew choroid in response to three myopiagenic conditions. Vis Res. 2014;102:52–63.
100. Honda S, Fujii S, Sekiya Y, Yamamoto M. Retinal control on the axial length mediated by transforming growth factor-beta in chick eye. Invest Ophthalmol Vis Sci. 1996;37(12):2519–26.
101. Jobling AI, Nguyen M, Gentle A, McBrien NA. Isoform-specific changes in scleral transforming growth factor-beta expression and the regulation of collagen synthesis during myopia progression. J Biol Chem. 2004;279(18):18121–6.
102. Jobling AI, Wan R, Gentle A, Bui BV, McBrien NA. Retinal and choroidal TGF-beta in the tree shrew model of myopia: isoform expression, activation and effects on function. Exp Eye Res. 2009;88(3):458–66.
103. Kusakari T, Sato T, Tokoro T. Visual deprivation stimulates the exchange of the fibrous sclera into the cartilaginous sclera in chicks. Exp Eye Res. 2001;73(4):533–46.
104. Mathis U, Schaeffel F. Transforming growth factor-beta in the chicken fundal layers: an immunohistochemical study. Exp Eye Res. 2010;90(6):780–90.
105. McBrien NA. Regulation of scleral metabolism in myopia and the role of transforming growth factor-beta. Exp Eye Res. 2013;114:128–40.
106. Schippert R, Brand C, Schaeffel F, Feldkaemper MP. Changes in scleral MMP-2, TIMP-2 and TGFbeta-2 mRNA expression after imposed myopic and hyperopic defocus in chickens. Exp Eye Res. 2006;82(4):710–9.
107. Seko Y, Shimokawa H, Tokoro T. Expression of bFGF and TGF-beta 2 in experimental myopia in chicks. Invest Ophthalmol Vis Sci. 1995;36(6):1183–7.
108. Simon P, Feldkaemper M, Bitzer M, Ohngemach S, Schaeffel F. Early transcriptional changes of retinal and choroidal TGFbeta-2, RALDH-2, and ZENK following imposed positive and negative defocus in chickens. Mol Vis. 2004;10:588–97.
109. Zhang Y, Raychaudhuri S, Wildsoet CF. Imposed optical defocus induces isoform-specific up-regulation of TGFbeta gene expression in chick retinal pigment epithelium and choroid but not neural retina. PLoS One. 2016;11(5):e0155356.
110. Chen BY, Wang CY, Chen WY, Ma JX. Altered TGF-beta2 and bFGF expression in scleral desmocytes from an experimentally-induced myopia guinea pig model. Graefes Arch Clin Exp Ophthalmol. 2013;251(4):1133–44.
111. Jobling AI, Gentle A, Metlapally R, McGowan BJ, McBrien NA. Regulation of scleral cell contraction by transforming growth factor-beta and stress: competing roles in myopic eye growth. J Biol Chem. 2009;284(4):2072–9.
112. Seko Y, Tanaka Y, Tokoro T. Influence of bFGF as a potent growth stimulator and TGF-beta as a growth regulator on scleral chondrocytes and scleral fibroblasts in vitro. Ophthalmic Res. 1995;27(3):144–52.
113. Rohrer B, Stell WK. Basic fibroblast growth factor (bFGF) and transforming growth factor beta (TGF-beta) act as stop and go signals to modulate postnatal ocular growth in the chick. Exp Eye Res. 1994;58(5):553–61.
114. He L, Frost MR, Siegwart JT Jr, Norton TT. Altered gene expression in tree shrew retina and retinal pigment epithelium produced by short periods of minus-lens wear. Exp Eye Res. 2018;168:77–88.
115. Shelton L, Troilo D, Lerner MR, Gusev Y, Brackett DJ, Rada JS. Microarray analysis of choroid/RPE gene expression in marmoset eyes undergoing changes in ocular growth and refraction. Mol Vis. 2008;14:1465–79.
116. Carreira AC, Alves GG, Zambuzzi WF, Sogayar MC, Granjeiro JM. Bone morphogenetic proteins: structure, biological function and therapeutic applications. Arch Biochem Biophys. 2014;561:64–73.
117. Kawabata M, Imamura T, Miyazono K. Signal transduction by bone morphogenetic proteins. Cytokine Growth Factor Rev. 1998;9(1):49–61.
118. Katagiri T, Watabe T. Bone morphogenetic proteins. Cold Spring Harb Perspect Biol. 2016;8(6):a021899.
119. Urist MR. Bone: formation by autoinduction. Science. 1965;150(3698):893–9.
120. Wagner DO, Sieber C, Bhushan R, Borgermann JH, Graf D, Knaus P. BMPs: from bone to body morphogenetic proteins. Sci Signal. 2010;3(107):mr1.
121. Wang RN, Green J, Wang Z, Deng Y, Qiao M, Peabody M, Zhang Q, Ye J, Yan Z, Denduluri S, Idowu O, Li M, Shen C, Hu A, Haydon RC, Kang R, Mok J, Lee MJ, Luu HL, Shi LL. Bone morphogenetic protein (BMP) signaling in development and human diseases. Genes Dis. 2014;1(1):87–105.
122. Xu J, Zhu D, Sonoda S, He S, Spee C, Ryan SJ, Hinton DR. Over-expression of BMP4 inhibits experimental choroidal neovascularization by modulating VEGF and MMP-9. Angiogenesis. 2012;15(2):213–27.
123. Zhang J, Li L. BMP signaling and stem cell regulation. Dev Biol. 2005;284(1):1–11.

124. Bragdon B, Moseychuk O, Saldanha S, King D, Julian J, Nohe A. Bone morphogenetic proteins: a critical review. Cell Signal. 2011;23(4):609–20.
125. Belecky-Adams T, Adler R. Developmental expression patterns of bone morphogenetic proteins, receptors, and binding proteins in the chick retina. J Comp Neurol. 2001;430(4):562–72.
126. Faber SC, Robinson ML, Makarenkova HP, Lang RA. Bmp signaling is required for development of primary lens fiber cells. Development. 2002;129(15):3727–37.
127. Fuhrmann S. Eye morphogenesis and patterning of the optic vesicle. Curr Top Dev Biol. 2010;93:61–84.
128. Furuta Y, Hogan BL. BMP4 is essential for lens induction in the mouse embryo. Genes Dev. 1998;12(23):3764–75.
129. Luo G, Hofmann C, Bronckers AL, Sohocki M, Bradley A, Karsenty G. BMP-7 is an inducer of nephrogenesis, and is also required for eye development and skeletal patterning. Genes Dev. 1995;9(22):2808–20.
130. Moshiri A, Close J, Reh TA. Retinal stem cells and regeneration. Int J Dev Biol. 2004;48(8–9):1003–14.
131. Sakuta H, Takahashi H, Shintani T, Etani K, Aoshima A, Noda M. Role of bone morphogenic protein 2 in retinal patterning and retinotectal projection. J Neurosci. 2006;26(42):10868–78.
132. Steinfeld J, Steinfeld I, Bausch A, Coronato N, Hampel ML, Depner H, Layer PG, Vogel-Hopker A. BMP-induced reprograming of the retina into RPE requires WNT signalling in the developing chick optic cup. Biol Open. 2017;6(7):979–92. https://doi.org/10.1242/bio.018739.
133. Steinfeld J, Steinfeld I, Coronato N, Hampel ML, Layer PG, Araki M, Vogel-Hopker A. RPE specification in the chick is mediated by surface ectoderm-derived BMP and Wnt signalling. Development. 2013;140(24):4959–69.
134. Ueki Y, Wilken MS, Cox KE, Chipman LB, Bermingham-McDonogh O, Reh TA. A transient wave of BMP signaling in the retina is necessary for Muller glial differentiation. Development. 2015;142(3):533–43.
135. Wordinger RJ, Clark AF. Bone morphogenetic proteins and their receptors in the eye. Exp Biol Med (Maywood). 2007;232(8):979–92.
136. Zhou S, Flamier A, Abdouh M, Tetreault N, Barabino A, Wadhwa S, Bernier G. Differentiation of human embryonic stem cells into cone photoreceptors through simultaneous inhibition of BMP, TGFbeta and Wnt signaling. Development. 2015;142(19):3294–306.
137. Zhou Y, Tanzie C, Yan Z, Chen S, Duncan M, Gaudenz K, Li H, Seidel C, Lewis B, Moran A, Libby RT, Kiernan AE, Xie T. Notch2 regulates BMP signaling and epithelial morphogenesis in the ciliary body of the mouse eye. Proc Natl Acad Sci U S A. 2013;110(22):8966–71.
138. Mohan RR, Kim WJ, Chen L, Wilson SE. Bone morphogenic proteins 2 and 4 and their receptors in the adult human cornea. Invest Ophthalmol Vis Sci. 1998;39(13):2626–36.
139. Shen W, Finnegan S, Lein P, Sullivan S, Slaughter M, Higgins D. Bone morphogenetic proteins regulate ionotropic glutamate receptors in human retina. Eur J Neurosci. 2004;20(8):2031–7.
140. Wordinger RJ, Agarwal R, Talati M, Fuller J, Lambert W, Clark AF. Expression of bone morphogenetic proteins (BMP), BMP receptors, and BMP associated proteins in human trabecular meshwork and optic nerve head cells and tissues. Mol Vis. 2002;8:241–50.
141. He L, Frost MR, Siegwart JT Jr, Norton TT. Gene expression signatures in tree shrew choroid during lens-induced myopia and recovery. Exp Eye Res. 2014;123:56–71.
142. Li H, Cui D, Zhao F, Huo L, Hu J, Zeng J. BMP-2 is involved in scleral remodeling in myopia development. PLoS One. 2015;10(5):e0125219.
143. McGlinn AM, Baldwin DA, Tobias JW, Budak MT, Khurana TS, Stone RA. Form-deprivation myopia in chick induces limited changes in retinal gene expression. Invest Ophthalmol Vis Sci. 2007; 48(8):3430–6.
144. Zhang Y, Liu Y, Hang A, Phan E, Wildsoet CF. Differential gene expression of BMP2 and BMP receptors in chick retina & choroid induced by imposed optical defocus. Vis Neurosci. 2016;33:E015.
145. Zhang Y, Liu Y, Ho C, Wildsoet CF. Effects of imposed defocus of opposite sign on temporal gene expression patterns of BMP4 and BMP7 in chick RPE. Exp Eye Res. 2013;109:98–106.
146. Zhang Y, Liu Y, Wildsoet CF. Bidirectional, optical sign-dependent regulation of BMP2 gene expression in chick retinal pigment epithelium. Invest Ophthalmol Vis Sci. 2012;53(10):6072–80.
147. Li H, Wu J, Cui D, Zeng J. Retinal and choroidal expression of BMP-2 in lens-induced myopia and recovery from myopia in guinea pigs. Mol Med Rep. 2016;13(3):2671–6.
148. Wang Q, Xue ML, Zhao GQ, Liu MG, Ma YN, Ma Y. Form-deprivation myopia induces decreased expression of bone morphogenetic protein-2, 5 in guinea pig sclera. Int J Ophthalmol. 2015;8(1):39–45.
149. Wang Q, Zhao G, Xing S, Zhang L, Yang X. Role of bone morphogenetic proteins in form-deprivation myopia sclera. Mol Vis. 2011;17:647–57.
150. Hu J, Cui D, Yang X, Wang S, Hu S, Li C, Zeng J. Bone morphogenetic protein-2: a potential regulator in scleral remodeling. Mol Vis. 2008;14:2373–80.
151. Li HH, Huo LJ, Gao ZY, Zhao F, Zeng JW. Regulation of scleral fibroblast differentiation by bone morphogenetic protein-2. Int J Ophthalmol. 2014;7(1):152–6.
152. Zhang Y, Yang W, Hang A, Zin E, Garcia M, Li M, Wildsoet CF. BMP2 protein increases the expression of genes for inhibitor of DNA binding proteins in cultured chick scleral fibroblasts. Invest Ophthalmol Vis Sci. 2017;58(8):5472.

153. Cui W, Bryant MR, Sweet PM, McDonnell PJ. Changes in gene expression in response to mechanical strain in human scleral fibroblasts. Exp Eye Res. 2004;78(2):275–84.
154. Riddell N, Giummarra L, Hall NE, Crewther SG. Bidirectional expression of metabolic, structural, and immune pathways in early myopia and hyperopia. Front Neurosci. 2016;10:390.
155. Stone RA, McGlinn AM, Baldwin DA, Tobias JW, Iuvone PM, Khurana TS. Image defocus and altered retinal gene expression in chick: clues to the pathogenesis of ametropia. Invest Ophthalmol Vis Sci. 2011;52(8):5765–77.
156. de Pablo F, Perez-Villamil B, Serna J, Gonzalez-Guerrero PR, Lopez-Carranza A, de la Rosa EJ, Alemany J, Caldes T. IGF-I and the IGF-I receptor in development of nonmammalian vertebrates. Mol Reprod Dev. 1993;35(4):427–32; discussion 423–432.
157. Denduluri SK, Idowu O, Wang Z, Liao Z, Yan Z, Mohammed MK, Ye J, Wei Q, Wang J, Zhao L, Luu HH. Insulin-like growth factor (IGF) signaling in tumorigenesis and the development of cancer drug resistance. Genes Dis. 2015;2(1):13–25.
158. Laviola L, Natalicchio A, Giorgino F. The IGF-I signaling pathway. Curr Pharm Des. 2007;13(7):663–9.
159. Danias J, Stylianopoulou F. Expression of IGF-I and IGF-II genes in the adult rat eye. Curr Eye Res. 1990;9(4):379–86.
160. Ocrant I, Valentino KL, King MG, Wimpy TH, Rosenfeld RG, Baskin DG. Localization and structural characterization of insulin-like growth factor receptors in mammalian retina. Endocrinology. 1989;125(5):2407–13.
161. Penha AM, Schaeffel F, Feldkaemper M. Insulin, insulin-like growth factor-1, insulin receptor, and insulin-like growth factor-1 receptor expression in the chick eye and their regulation with imposed myopic or hyperopic defocus. Mol Vis. 2011;17:1436–48.
162. Ritchey ER, Zelinka CP, Tang J, Liu J, Fischer AJ. The combination of IGF1 and FGF2 and the induction of excessive ocular growth and extreme myopia. Exp Eye Res. 2012;99:1–16.
163. Zhu X, Wallman J. Opposite effects of glucagon and insulin on compensation for spectacle lenses in chicks. Invest Ophthalmol Vis Sci. 2009;50(1):24–36.
164. Martin DM, Yee D, Feldman EL. Gene expression of the insulin-like growth factors and their receptors in cultured human retinal pigment epithelial cells. Brain Res Mol Brain Res. 1992;12(1–3):181–6.
165. Takagi H, Yoshimura N, Tanihara H, Honda Y. Insulin-like growth factor-related genes, receptors, and binding proteins in cultured human retinal pigment epithelial cells. Invest Ophthalmol Vis Sci. 1994;35(3):916–23.
166. Waldbillig RJ, Pfeffer BA, Schoen TJ, Adler AA, Shen-Orr Z, Scavo L, LeRoith D, Chader GJ. Evidence for an insulin-like growth factor autocrine-paracrine system in the retinal photoreceptor-pigment epithelial cell complex. J Neurochem. 1991;57(5):1522–33.
167. Sternfeld MD, Robertson JE, Shipley GD, Tsai J, Rosenbaum JT. Cultured human retinal pigment epithelial cells express basic fibroblast growth factor and its receptor. Curr Eye Res. 1989;8(10):1029–37.
168. Rohrer B, Tao J, Stell WK. Basic fibroblast growth factor, its high- and low-affinity receptors, and their relationship to form-deprivation myopia in the chick. Neuroscience. 1997;79(3):775–87.
169. Mao J, Liu S, Wen D, Tan X, Fu C. Basic fibroblast growth factor suppresses retinal neuronal apoptosis in form-deprivation myopia in chicks. Curr Eye Res. 2006;31(11):983–7.
170. Tian XD, Cheng YX, Liu GB, Guo SF, Fan CL, Zhan LH, Xu YC. Expressions of type I collagen, alpha2 integrin and beta1 integrin in sclera of guinea pig with defocus myopia and inhibitory effects of bFGF on the formation of myopia. Int J Ophthalmol. 2013;6(1):54–8.
171. Zhang Y, Wildsoet CF. RPE and choroid mechanisms underlying ocular growth and myopia. Prog Mol Biol Transl Sci. 2015;134:221–40.
172. Chakraborty R, Pardue MT. Molecular and biochemical aspects of the retina on refraction. Prog Mol Biol Transl Sci. 2015;134:249–67.
173. Feldkaemper M, Schaeffel F. An updated view on the role of dopamine in myopia. Exp Eye Res. 2013;114:106–19.
174. Zhou X, Pardue MT, Iuvone PM, Qu J. Dopamine signaling and myopia development: what are the key challenges. Prog Retin Eye Res. 2017;61:60–71.
175. Djamgoz MB, Wagner HJ. Localization and function of dopamine in the adult vertebrate retina. Neurochem Int. 1992;20(2):139–91.
176. Nguyen-Legros J, Versaux-Botteri C, Vernier P. Dopamine receptor localization in the mammalian retina. Mol Neurobiol. 1999;19(3):181–204.
177. Reis RA, Ventura AL, Kubrusly RC, de Mello MC, de Mello FG. Dopaminergic signaling in the developing retina. Brain Res Rev. 2007;54(1):181–8.
178. Vallone D, Picetti R, Borrelli E. Structure and function of dopamine receptors. Neurosci Biobehav Rev. 2000;24(1):125–32.
179. Bergen MA, Park HN, Chakraborty R, Landis EG, Sidhu C, He L, Iuvone PM, Pardue MT. Altered refractive development in mice with reduced levels of retinal dopamine. Invest Ophthalmol Vis Sci. 2016;57(10):4412–9.
180. Dong F, Zhi Z, Pan M, Xie R, Qin X, Lu R, Mao X, Chen JF, Willcox MD, Qu J, Zhou X. Inhibition of experimental myopia by a dopamine agonist: different effectiveness between form deprivation and hyperopic defocus in guinea pigs. Mol Vis. 2011;17:2824–34.
181. Guo SS, Sivak JG, Callender MG, Diehl-Jones B. Retinal dopamine and lens-induced refractive errors in chicks. Curr Eye Res. 1995;14(5):385–9.

182. Huang F, Zhang L, Wang Q, Yang Y, Li Q, Wu Y, Chen J, Qu J, Zhou X. Dopamine D1 receptors contribute critically to the apomorphine-induced inhibition of form-deprivation myopia in mice. Invest Ophthalmol Vis Sci. 2018;59(6):2623–34.
183. Iuvone PM, Tigges M, Fernandes A, Tigges J. Dopamine synthesis and metabolism in rhesus monkey retina: development, aging, and the effects of monocular visual deprivation. Vis Neurosci. 1989;2(5):465–71.
184. Iuvone PM, Tigges M, Stone RA, Lambert S, Laties AM. Effects of apomorphine, a dopamine receptor agonist, on ocular refraction and axial elongation in a primate model of myopia. Invest Ophthalmol Vis Sci. 1991;32(5):1674–7.
185. Jiang L, Long K, Schaeffel F, Zhou X, Zheng Y, Ying H, Lu F, Stell WK, Qu J. Effects of dopaminergic agents on progression of naturally occurring myopia in albino guinea pigs (Cavia porcellus). Invest Ophthalmol Vis Sci. 2014;55(11):7508–19.
186. Li XX, Schaeffel F, Kohler K, Zrenner E. Dose-dependent effects of 6-hydroxy dopamine on deprivation myopia, electroretinograms, and dopaminergic amacrine cells in chickens. Vis Neurosci. 1992;9(5):483–92.
187. Mao J, Liu S, Qin W, Li F, Wu X, Tan Q. Levodopa inhibits the development of form-deprivation myopia in guinea pigs. Optom Vis Sci. 2010;87(1):53–60.
188. McBrien NA, Cottriall CL, Annies R. Retinal acetylcholine content in normal and myopic eyes: a role in ocular growth control? Vis Neurosci. 2001;18(4):571–80.
189. McCarthy CS, Megaw P, Devadas M, Morgan IG. Dopaminergic agents affect the ability of brief periods of normal vision to prevent form-deprivation myopia. Exp Eye Res. 2007;84(1):100–7.
190. Nickla DL, Totonelly K. Dopamine antagonists and brief vision distinguish lens-induced- and form-deprivation-induced myopia. Exp Eye Res. 2011;93(5):782–5.
191. Nickla DL, Totonelly K, Dhillon B. Dopaminergic agonists that result in ocular growth inhibition also elicit transient increases in choroidal thickness in chicks. Exp Eye Res. 2010;91(5):715–20.
192. Rohrer B, Spira AW, Stell WK. Apomorphine blocks form-deprivation myopia in chickens by a dopamine D2-receptor mechanism acting in retina or pigmented epithelium. Vis Neurosci. 1993;10(3):447–53.
193. Schaeffel F, Bartmann M, Hagel G, Zrenner E. Studies on the role of the retinal dopamine/melatonin system in experimental refractive errors in chickens. Vis Res. 1995;35(9):1247–64.
194. Schaeffel F, Hagel G, Bartmann M, Kohler K, Zrenner E. 6-Hydroxy dopamine does not affect lens-induced refractive errors but suppresses deprivation myopia. Vis Res. 1994;34(2):143–9.
195. Schmid KL, Wildsoet CF. Inhibitory effects of apomorphine and atropine and their combination on myopia in chicks. Optom Vis Sci. 2004;81(2):137–47.
196. Stone RA, Lin T, Laties AM, Iuvone PM. Retinal dopamine and form-deprivation myopia. Proc Natl Acad Sci U S A. 1989;86(2):704–6.
197. Ward AH, Siegwart JT, Frost MR, Norton TT. Intravitreally-administered dopamine D2-like (and D4), but not D1-like, receptor agonists reduce form-deprivation myopia in tree shrews. Vis Neurosci. 2017;34:E003.
198. Pendrak K, Nguyen T, Lin T, Capehart C, Zhu X, Stone RA. Retinal dopamine in the recovery from experimental myopia. Curr Eye Res. 1997;16(2):152–7.
199. Cohen Y, Peleg E, Belkin M, Polat U, Solomon AS. Ambient illuminance, retinal dopamine release and refractive development in chicks. Exp Eye Res. 2012;103:33–40.
200. Rohrer B, Stell WK. Localization of putative dopamine D2-like receptors in the chick retina, using in situ hybridization and immunocytochemistry. Brain Res. 1995;695(2):110–6.
201. Versaux-Botteri C, Gibert JM, Nguyen-Legros J, Vernier P. Molecular identification of a dopamine D1b receptor in bovine retinal pigment epithelium. Neurosci Lett. 1997;237(1):9–12.
202. Gallemore RP, Steinberg RH. Effects of dopamine on the chick retinal pigment epithelium. Membrane potentials and light-evoked responses. Invest Ophthalmol Vis Sci. 1990;31(1):67–80.
203. Seko Y, Tanaka Y, Tokoro T. Apomorphine inhibits the growth-stimulating effect of retinal pigment epithelium on scleral cells in vitro. Cell Biochem Funct. 1997;15(3):191–6.
204. McKay BS, Goodman B, Falk T, Sherman SJ. Retinal pigment epithelial cell transplantation could provide trophic support in Parkinson's disease: results from an in vitro model system. Exp Neurol. 2006;201(1):234–43.
205. Ming M, Li X, Fan X, Yang D, Li L, Chen S, Gu Q, Le W. Retinal pigment epithelial cells secrete neurotrophic factors and synthesize dopamine: possible contribution to therapeutic effects of RPE cell transplantation in Parkinson's disease. J Transl Med. 2009;7:53.
206. Ford KJ, Feller MB. Assembly and disassembly of a retinal cholinergic network. Vis Neurosci. 2012;29(1):61–71.
207. Hutchins JB. Acetylcholine as a neurotransmitter in the vertebrate retina. Exp Eye Res. 1987;45(1):1–38.
208. Conley M, Fitzpatrick D, Lachica EA. Laminar asymmetry in the distribution of choline acetyltransferase-immunoreactive neurons in the retina of the tree shrew (Tupaia belangeri). Brain Res. 1986;399(2):332–8.
209. Millar TJ, Ishimoto I, Chubb IW, Epstein ML, Johnson CD, Morgan IG. Cholinergic amacrine cells of the chicken retina: a light and electron microscope immunocytochemical study. Neuroscience. 1987;21(3):725–43.
210. Schwahn HN, Kaymak H, Schaeffel F. Effects of atropine on refractive development, dopamine

release, and slow retinal potentials in the chick. Vis Neurosci. 2000;17(2):165–76.
211. Marritt AM, Cox BC, Yasuda RP, McIntosh JM, Xiao Y, Wolfe BB, Kellar KJ. Nicotinic cholinergic receptors in the rat retina: simple and mixed heteromeric subtypes. Mol Pharmacol. 2005;68(6):1656–68.
212. Mitchelson F. Muscarinic receptor agonists and antagonists: effects on ocular function. Handb Exp Pharmacol. 2012;208:263–98.
213. Friedman Z, Hackett SF, Campochiaro PA. Human retinal pigment epithelial cells possess muscarinic receptors coupled to calcium mobilization. Brain Res. 1988;446(1):11–6.
214. Matsumoto H, Shibasaki K, Uchigashima M, Koizumi A, Kurachi M, Moriwaki Y, Misawa H, Kawashima K, Watanabe M, Kishi S, Ishizaki Y. Localization of acetylcholine-related molecules in the retina: implication of the communication from photoreceptor to retinal pigment epithelium. PLoS One. 2012;7(8):e42841.
215. Osborne NN, FitzGibbon F, Schwartz G. Muscarinic acetylcholine receptor-mediated phosphoinositide turnover in cultured human retinal pigment epithelium cells. Vis Res. 1991;31(7–8):1119–27.
216. Salceda R. Muscarinic receptors binding in retinal pigment epithelium during rat development. Neurochem Res. 1994;19(9):1207–10.
217. Barathi VA, Beuerman RW. Molecular mechanisms of muscarinic receptors in mouse scleral fibroblasts: prior to and after induction of experimental myopia with atropine treatment. Mol Vis. 2011;17:680–92.
218. Bedrossian RH. The effect of atropine on myopia. Ophthalmology. 1979;86(5):713–9.
219. Chua WH, Balakrishnan V, Chan YH, Tong L, Ling Y, Quah BL, Tan D. Atropine for the treatment of childhood myopia. Ophthalmology. 2006;113(12):2285–91.
220. Cottriall CL, McBrien NA, Annies R, Leech EM. Prevention of form-deprivation myopia with pirenzepine: a study of drug delivery and distribution. Ophthalmic Physiol Opt. 1999;19(4):327–35.
221. Leech EM, Cottriall CL, McBrien NA. Pirenzepine prevents form deprivation myopia in a dose dependent manner. Ophthalmic Physiol Opt. 1995;15(5):351–6.
222. McBrien NA, Moghaddam HO, Reeder AP. Atropine reduces experimental myopia and eye enlargement via a nonaccommodative mechanism. Invest Ophthalmol Vis Sci. 1993;34(1):205–15.
223. Rickers M, Schaeffel F. Dose-dependent effects of intravitreal pirenzepine on deprivation myopia and lens-induced refractive errors in chickens. Exp Eye Res. 1995;61(4):509–16.
224. Stone RA, Lin T, Laties AM. Muscarinic antagonist effects on experimental chick myopia. Exp Eye Res. 1991;52(6):755–8.
225. Tong L, Huang XL, Koh AL, Zhang X, Tan DT, Chua WH. Atropine for the treatment of childhood myopia: effect on myopia progression after cessation of atropine. Ophthalmology. 2009;116(3):572–9.
226. Luft WA, Ming Y, Stell WK. Variable effects of previously untested muscarinic receptor antagonists on experimental myopia. Invest Ophthalmol Vis Sci. 2003;44(3):1330–8.
227. Carr BJ, Mihara K, Ramachandran R, Saifeddine M, Nathanson NM, Stell WK, Hollenberg MD. Myopia-inhibiting concentrations of muscarinic receptor antagonists block activation of alpha2A-adrenoceptors in vitro. Invest Ophthalmol Vis Sci. 2018;59(7):2778–91.
228. Carr BJ, Stell WK. Nitric oxide (NO) mediates the inhibition of form-deprivation myopia by atropine in chicks. Sci Rep. 2016;6(1):9.
229. McBrien NA, Stell WK, Carr B. How does atropine exert its anti-myopia effects? Ophthalmic Physiol Opt. 2013;33(3):373–8.
230. Lind GJ, Chew SJ, Marzani D, Wallman J. Muscarinic acetylcholine receptor antagonists inhibit chick scleral chondrocytes. Invest Ophthalmol Vis Sci. 1998;39(12):2217–31.
231. Nickla DL, Zhu X, Wallman J. Effects of muscarinic agents on chick choroids in intact eyes and eyecups: evidence for a muscarinic mechanism in choroidal thinning. Ophthalmic Physiol Opt. 2013;33(3):245–56.
232. Stone RA, Sugimoto R, Gill AS, Liu J, Capehart C, Lindstrom JM. Effects of nicotinic antagonists on ocular growth and experimental myopia. Invest Ophthalmol Vis Sci. 2001;42(3):557–65.
233. Bell GI. The glucagon superfamily: precursor structure and gene organization. Peptides. 1986;7(Suppl 1):27–36.
234. Ekman R, Tornqvist K. Glucagon and VIP in the retina. Invest Ophthalmol Vis Sci. 1985;26(10):1405–9.
235. Fischer AJ, Skorupa D, Schonberg DL, Walton NA. Characterization of glucagon-expressing neurons in the chicken retina. J Comp Neurol. 2006;496(4):479–94.
236. Fukuda M, Yeh HH, Puro DG. A vasoactive intestinal polypeptide system in retinal cell cultures: immunocytochemistry and physiology. Brain Res. 1987;414(1):177–81.
237. Buck C, Schaeffel F, Simon P, Feldkaemper M. Effects of positive and negative lens treatment on retinal and choroidal glucagon and glucagon receptor mRNA levels in the chicken. Invest Ophthalmol Vis Sci. 2004;45(2):402–9.
238. Koh SM. VIP enhances the differentiation of retinal pigment epithelium in culture: from cAMP and pp60(c-src) to melanogenesis and development of fluid transport capacity. Prog Retin Eye Res. 2000;19(6):669–88.
239. Koh SW. VIP stimulation of polarized macromolecule secretion in cultured chick embryonic retinal pigment epithelium. Exp Cell Res. 1991;197(1):1–7.
240. Koh SW, Chader GJ. Elevation of intracellular cyclic AMP and stimulation of adenylate cyclase activity by vasoactive intestinal peptide and glucagon in the retinal pigment epithelium. J Neurochem. 1984;43(6):1522–6.

241. Fischer AJ, McGuire JJ, Schaeffel F, Stell WK. Light- and focus-dependent expression of the transcription factor ZENK in the chick retina. Nat Neurosci. 1999;2(8):706–12.
242. Feldkaemper MP, Wang HY, Schaeffel F. Changes in retinal and choroidal gene expression during development of refractive errors in chicks. Invest Ophthalmol Vis Sci. 2000;41(7):1623–8.
243. Ashby R, Kozulin P, Megaw PL, Morgan IG. Alterations in ZENK and glucagon RNA transcript expression during increased ocular growth in chickens. Mol Vis. 2010;16:639–49.
244. Feldkaemper MP, Schaeffel F. Evidence for a potential role of glucagon during eye growth regulation in chicks. Vis Neurosci. 2002;19(6):755–66.
245. Vessey KA, Lencses KA, Rushforth DA, Hruby VJ, Stell WK. Glucagon receptor agonists and antagonists affect the growth of the chick eye: a role for glucagonergic regulation of emmetropization? Invest Ophthalmol Vis Sci. 2005;46(11):3922–31.
246. Vessey KA, Rushforth DA, Stell WK. Glucagon- and secretin-related peptides differentially alter ocular growth and the development of form-deprivation myopia in chicks. Invest Ophthalmol Vis Sci. 2005;46(11):3932–42.
247. Stone RA, Laties AM, Raviola E, Wiesel TN. Increase in retinal vasoactive intestinal polypeptide after eyelid fusion in primates. Proc Natl Acad Sci U S A. 1988;85(1):257–60.
248. Tkatchenko AV, Walsh PA, Tkatchenko TV, Gustincich S, Raviola E. Form deprivation modulates retinal neurogenesis in primate experimental myopia. Proc Natl Acad Sci U S A. 2006;103(12):4681–6.
249. Seltner RL, Stell WK. The effect of vasoactive intestinal peptide on development of form deprivation myopia in the chick: a pharmacological and immunocytochemical study. Vis Res. 1995;35(9):1265–70.
250. Mathis U, Schaeffel F. Glucagon-related peptides in the mouse retina and the effects of deprivation of form vision. Graefes Arch Clin Exp Ophthalmol. 2007;245(2):267–75.
251. Marmor MF. Control of subretinal fluid: experimental and clinical studies. Eye (Lond). 1990;4(Pt 2):340–4.
252. Wimmers S, Karl MO, Strauss O. Ion channels in the RPE. Prog Retin Eye Res. 2007;26(3):263–301.
253. Crewther SG, Liang H, Junghans BM, Crewther DP. Ionic control of ocular growth and refractive change. Proc Natl Acad Sci U S A. 2006;103(42):15663–8.
254. Liang H, Crewther SG, Crewther DP, Junghans BM. Structural and elemental evidence for edema in the retina, retinal pigment epithelium, and choroid during recovery from experimentally induced myopia. Invest Ophthalmol Vis Sci. 2004;45(8):2463–74.
255. Crewther SG, Murphy MJ, Crewther DP. Potassium channel and NKCC cotransporter involvement in ocular refractive control mechanisms. PLoS One. 2008;3(7):e2839.
256. Zhang H, Wong CL, Shan SW, Li KK, Cheng AK, Lee KL, Ge J, To CH, Do CW. Characterisation of Cl(−) transporter and channels in experimentally induced myopic chick eyes. Clin Exp Optom. 2011;94(6):528–35.
257. Harman AM, Hoskins R, Beazley LD. Experimental eye enlargement in mature animals changes the retinal pigment epithelium. Vis Neurosci. 1999;16(4):619–28.
258. Lin T, Grimes PA, Stone RA. Expansion of the retinal pigment epithelium in experimental myopia. Vis Res. 1993;33(14):1881–5.
259. Hou X, Han QH, Hu D, Tian L, Guo CM, Du HJ, Zhang P, Wang YS, Hui YN. Mechanical force enhances MMP-2 activation via p38 signaling pathway in human retinal pigment epithelial cells. Graefes Arch Clin Exp Ophthalmol. 2009;247(11):1477–86.
260. Seko Y, Fujikura H, Pang J, Tokoro T, Shimokawa H. Induction of vascular endothelial growth factor after application of mechanical stress to retinal pigment epithelium of the rat in vitro. Invest Ophthalmol Vis Sci. 1999;40(13):3287–91.

Retinal Pigment Epithelium in Proliferative Disorders

8

Willem A. Dik, Jeroen Bastiaans, and Jan C. van Meurs

Introduction

Proliferative vitreoretinopathy (PVR), proliferative diabetic retinopathy (PDR) and age-related macular degeneration (AMD) are diseases that, despite a different initiating cause, share several common pathological features, including a (disturbed) healing response and inflammation. Neovascularization represents an additional component in PDR and AMD. However, the newly formed vessels appear weak and are prone to haemorrhage leading to further activation of the healing response. Ultimately these diseases are typically characterized by the formation of fibrotic retinal membranes or may lead to fibrotic changes in the retina itself [1].

Retinal membranes are fibrocellular proliferations located at the retinal surfaces. Based on their location the membranes can be divided into two main groups, (1) epiretinal membranes (ERMs) that are located on the inner surface of the retina, and (2) subretinal membranes that are typically formed between the outer neuroretina and the retinal pigment epithelial monolayer, although intraretinal membranes have also been described [2, 3]. Besides location, retinal membranes can also be divided on the basis of histopathological features, more specifically avascular membranes as occur in PVR or those that display a prominent vascular component as is seen in PDR and AMD [2].

Several different cell types, including astrocytes, Müller cells, myofibroblasts and inflammatory cells can be present in these membranes, and in case of fibrovascular membranes also endothelial cells are abundant. In addition to the afore mentioned cell types retinal membranes often contain numerous retinal pigment epithelial (RPE) cells [3–5]. These RPE cells contribute significantly to the local fibrotic, inflammatory and pro-angiogenic responses (Fig. 8.1). In this chapter we will discuss various aspects of RPE cell function and regulation in relation to its regulatory role in fibrosis, inflammation and angiogenesis in retinal proliferative disease.

W. A. Dik (✉)
Department of Immunology, Laboratory Medical Immunology, Erasmus MC, University Medical Center Rotterdam, Rotterdam, The Netherlands
e-mail: w.dik@erasmusmc.nl

J. Bastiaans
Departments of Ophthalmology, Pathology and Cell Biology, Columbia University, New York, NY, USA
e-mail: jeb2068@med.cornell.edu

J. C. van Meurs
The Rotterdam Eye Hospital, Rotterdam, The Netherlands

Department of Ophthalmology, Erasmus MC, University Medical Center, Rotterdam, The Netherlands
e-mail: J.vanMeurs@oogziekenhuis.nl

A. K. Klettner, S. Dithmar (eds.), *Retinal Pigment Epithelium in Health and Disease*,
https://doi.org/10.1007/978-3-030-28384-1_8

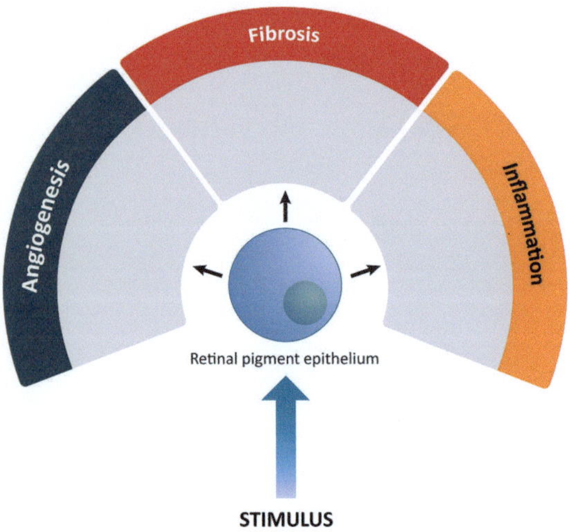

Fig. 8.1 Fibrosis, inflammation and angiogenesis represent important pathologic characteristics of retinal proliferative disease. Activation of the retinal pigment epithelium (RPE) that can occur by different types of stimuli contributes to the pathogenesis of these pathologic features

Retinal Pigment Epithelium and Retinal Proliferative Disease

RPE cells are mitotically quiescent, differentiated and polarized cells residing as a monolayer between the photoreceptors and Bruch's membrane. The main functions of the RPE are (1) transport of nutrients, ions and water, (2) absorption of light and protection against photo-oxidation, (3) re-isomerization of all-trans-retinal into 11-cis-retinal, which is a key element of the visual cycle, (4) phagocytosis of shed photoreceptor membranes, and (5) secretion of various essential factors for structural integrity of the retina. Moreover, the RPE constitutes the outer blood-retinal barrier which requires specialized tight junction molecules between the RPE cells to provide them with their barrier function. However, RPE can be become activated for instance in response to injury associated with breakdown of the blood-retinal barrier and subsequent exposure to plasma proteins, but also by high glucose levels, drusen-components or hypoxia [6–10]. In addition RPE cells can be activated by cytokines/chemokines and growth factors, for instance derived from infiltrating immune cells [11]. Activated RPE are considered key cellular elements in the development of fibrovascular membranes where they can augment the pro-fibrotic, pro-inflammatory and pro-angiogenic responses in the retinal tissue.

RPE and Fibrosis

Fibrosis is often considered to result from a dysregulated healing attempt through continual local injury or impaired control over repair mechanisms and is characterized by excessive deposition of extracellular matrix (ECM) components associated with loss of normal tissue architecture and function [12]. Retinal membranes also contain abundant ECM proteins, mainly the fibrillary collagen subtypes-I and -III, but also subtypes II, IV, and V. Besides collagen, also other ECM components can be present in retinal membranes, including elastin, laminin, fibronectin, tenascin and vitronectin [13–16]. The ECM composition of retinal membranes may however vary in the course of disease. For instance fibronectin may be more abundant in membranes of short clinical duration while the collagen content increases over time [14, 17, 18].

Regardless of the initiating insult or the organ affected, accumulation of fibroblasts and especially myofibroblasts along with excessive ECM deposition and tissue contraction represent key events in the formation of fibrotic tissue. Myofibroblasts are specialized fibroblast-like cells characterized by the expression of α-smooth muscle actin (αSMA), enhanced contractility, migratory and proliferative potential and an increased synthesis of the above mentioned ECM components (present in retinal membranes) when compared to normal fibroblasts, especially when stimulated with growth factors such as transforming growth factor (TGF)-β and platelet-derived growth factor (PDGF) [19–22]. During normal tissue repair myofibroblasts appear and eventually disappear by apoptosis. In contrast, chronic presence and activity of myofibroblasts characterize many fibrotic pathologies. In fibrotic disease myofibroblasts can originate from several sources including resident tissue fibroblasts, for instance upon stimulation with TGF-β or PDGF, but also from other precursor cell types including keratocytes in the eye and perivascular mesenchymal stem cells and circulating CD34 expressing fibrocytes [23–25]. In addition myofibroblasts may develop through endothelial mesenchymal transition (EndoMT) or epithelial mesenchymal transition (EMT) [19, 20, 26].

EMT is associated with loss of typical epithelial features (e.g. tight junction molecules like zonula occludens and E-cadherin) while mesenchymal features (e.g. αSMA, collagen and fibronectin expression) that promote migratory capacity, invasiveness and traction forces are acquired. Essentially EMT represents a normal physiological tissue response to injury to promote wound closure and tissue repair. EMT is normally tightly controlled by various factors and key transcription factors, including SNAIL family members, zinc-finger E-box-binding (ZEB) and basic helix-loop-helix (bHLH) transcription factors that typically repress expression of epithelial proteins while they enhance expression of mesenchymal proteins [27]. Yet, in fibrotic situations EMT programs are not attenuated, resulting in persistent myofibroblast formation and excessive ECM accumulation [27, 28]. Myofibroblasts have been detected in retinal fibrovascular membranes [5, 29, 30] where they are considered as important cellular source of ECM accumulation and membrane contraction. Immunohistochemical analysis of membranes have identified RPE cells as source of myofibroblasts, for instance based on co-localization of cytokeratin-18 as an RPE marker with αSMA as myofibroblastic marker [31].

Retinal Pigment Epithelial Cells and Epithelial Mesenchymal Transition

A variety of growth factors, their receptors and signaling pathways have been found elevated in vitreous and membranes from patients with fibroproliferative retinal diseases and are considered to contribute to RPE EMT in these diseases. Some of the most well examined growth factors and signaling cascades involved in RPE EMT are discussed in more detail hereunder.

Transforming-Growth Factor-β

TGF-β contains three isoforms, TGF-β1, TGF-β2 and TGF-β3. TGF-β molecules are dimeric and initially secreted by the producing cells as a large latent complex that also contains two latency associated peptide (LAP) chains and a latent TGF-β binding protein (LTBP) [32]. After secretion active TGF-β is released from the latent complex, mainly via the action of proteases for instance plasmin, matrix metalloproteases (MMP)-2, and -9, bone morphogenetic protein (BMP)-1, but also other molecules such as thrombospondin-1, retinoic acid, αV integrins as wells as by reactive oxygen species and an acidic environment [33–37]. After formation the active TGF-β molecules interact with a receptor complex containing two type-I TGF-β receptors (TGF-βR-I) and two TGF-βR-II subunits with resultant activation of intracellular signaling processes [38].

TGF-β signaling is generally considered to represent a major regulator of fibrosis and is a very potent inducer of EMT [38, 39]. Increased TGF-β and TGF-βR expression has been observed in retinal membranes [40]. In line with this, TGF-β1 and TGF-β2 induce dedifferentiation of cultured RPE cells into myofibroblasts [41–45]. TGF-β-induced EMT in RPE involves the canonical Smad signaling pathway, which requires phosphorylation of Smad2 and Smad3 and formation of a complex with Smad4 that subsequently translocates into the nucleus regulating transcription of TGF-β responsive genes [38, 46, 47]. Smad7 is an inhibitory Smad which recruits Smurf to TGF-β receptors for polyubiquitination and degradation [38]. Smad7 overexpression abolished TGF-β2/Smad2/3/4 signaling and expression of collagen type-1 in ARPE-19 cells. Also in an in vivo retinal detachment-induced PVR model Smad7 overexpression was found to suppress Smad2/3 signaling and EMT by RPE [48]. Although TGF-β signals mainly via Smads, upon receptor binding TGF-β can also activate other signaling pathways, referred to as "non-canonical" TGF-β signaling, including the MAPK and PI3K signaling pathways [38]. These non-canonical TGF-β pathways, involving molecules as TAK1, p38MAPK, PI3K/Akt [49–53] also contribute to TGF-β induced EMT in RPE. Yet, cross-talk between the canonical TGF-β-Smad signaling pathways, the non-canonical signaling pathways and jagged-notch signaling are likely involved in EMT in RPE [51, 54]. Moreover, these pathways induce the expression of Snail and ZEB, transcription factors that are fundamental in EMT by repressing epithelial proteins including E-cadherin and ZO-1 and enhancing expression of mesenchymal proteins such as αSMA, fibronectin and collagen and are involved in TGF-β-induced EMT in RPE [27, 55, 56].

Platelet-Derived Growth Factor

PDGF is a family of growth stimulating polypeptides that exert broad functions in health and disease. The PDGF family comprises of four genes that encode the peptide chains PDGF-A, PDGF-B, PDGF-C and PDGF-D, which by disulfide bridging can form the homodimeric molecules PDGF-AA, PDGF-BB, PDGF-CC and PDGF-DD or the heterodimeric PDGF-AB molecule [57]. Pro-peptide chains of PDGF-A and PDGF-B dimerize intracellulary, and intracellular removal of the N-terminal pro-domains is required for secretion and activity. In contrast, PDGF-CC and PDGF-DD are secreted as latent molecules that become activated in the extracellular space by proteolytic removal of the N-terminal CUB domain, for instance by proteases as plasmin and tissue plasminogen activator [57]. PDGF dimers exert their activity via binding to specific receptors consisting of two PDGF-receptor (PDGF-R) chains (αα, αβ or ββ chains). PDGF-A and PDGF-C chains are ligands for PDGF-Rα, the PDGF-D chain binds PDGF-Rβ, while the PDGF-B chain can bind both PDGF-Rα and PDGF-Rβ, yet with a higher affinity for PDGF-Rβ [57]. Thus depending on the PDGF isoform that binds, PDGF-R chains dimerize in either one of three dimeric forms; αα, αβ, ββ. PDGF-R belongs to the receptor tyrosine kinase (RTK) family and PDGF binding is followed by autophosphorylation of crucial tyrosine residues within the receptor chain, with subsequent activation of downstream signaling pathways, including RAS-MAPK, PI3K/Akt and PLC [57]. PDGF molecules are generally considered as key driving forces in fibrosis. They promote fibroblast proliferation and chemotaxis, increase the production of ECM components and inflammatory cytokines by fibroblasts and stimulate EMT [57, 58].

Increased PDGF and PDGF-R activity has been observed in human PVR and PDR vitreous and membranes and the PDGF molecules can be blood borne or locally produced, for instance by glial cells, RPE cells, and macrophages. PDGF is a strong stimulator of EMT in RPE, as reflected by increased αSMA and collagen production and decreased expression of ZO-1 [59–64]. Moreover, PDGF-receptor inhibition prevents EMT in vitro and in vivo as well as PVR development in experimental animal models [63–66]. RPE cells express the PDGF-Rβ chain at far higher levels than the PDGF-Rα chain [62, 64]. Yet, despite its low expression by RPE, activation of PDGF-Rα is considered as important determinant to elicit cellular responses, including cellular contraction in RPE [67]. Whether this is related to a specific PDGF isoform, PDGF-Rαα homodimer or PDGF-Rαβ heterodimer formation is unclear so far. Also trans-activation of PDGF-Rα via other growth factor receptors activated by their own ligand (e.g. fibroblasts growth factor (FGF), epidermal growth factor (EGF) or hepatocyte growth factor (HGF)) can occur and result in the dedifferentiation of RPE into the contractile myofibroblast phenotype [68].

PDGF-induced EMT is associated with increased proliferation, migration and cellular contraction, and involves activation of signaling molecules including ERK1/2, p38 and Akt [63, 65, 69, 70]. Presumably these signaling cascades result in induction of Snail of which overexpression in ARPE-19 induces EMT characterized by loss of the epithelial markers E-cadherin and ZO-1 and upregulation of the mesenchymal

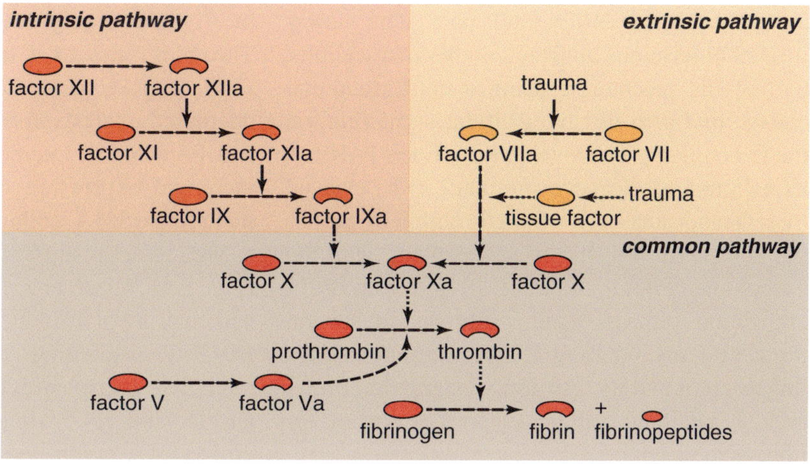

Fig. 8.2 Simplified scheme of the coagulation cascade. Indicated is the stepwise activation of serine proteases by the extrinsic and intrinsic pathways. At the point of convergence of these two pathways, factor Xa converts prothrombin into active thrombin. Thrombin subsequently converts soluble fibrinogen into insoluble fibrin

markers αSMA and fibronectin [27, 71, 72]. Moreover, overexpression of Snail significantly enhanced motility and migration (typical features of myofibroblasts) by RPE [72].

Coagulation Cascade

Tissue injury associated with vascular damage/dysfunction results in activation of the coagulation cascade and is crucial to facilitate the healing process [73]. Stepwise activation of coagulation serine proteases present in the plasma results, at a certain point, in the conversion of factor X into activated factor X (FXa). FXa subsequently cleaves pro-thrombin into active thrombin, which converts soluble plasma fibrinogen into an insoluble fibrin clot along with aggregation and degranulation of platelets [74]. The main function of the fibrin clot is to re-establish blood vessel integrity, to act as a reservoir of growth factors and cytokines, and to provide a scaffold to promote migration, activation, proliferation and differentiation of leukocytes and mesenchymal cells in order to restore tissue homeostasis [73]. Two pathways of coagulation cascade activation are recognized, the extrinsic pathway and the intrinsic pathway. Extrinsic coagulation is driven by tissue factor and directly initiated upon tissue injury (vascular injury) and critical for the initial fibrin formation. Amplification and maintenance of coagulation is subsequently controlled through feed-forward regulation via the intrinsic pathway (Fig. 8.2) [73].

Uncontrolled activation of the coagulation cascade has been recognized to contribute to fibrosis in several organ systems [73]. Classically the fibrin clot was thought to influence a fibrotic response by acting as a provisional structural matrix for fibroblasts, endothelial cells and inflammatory cells to migrate and to proliferate on, and by acting as a reservoir of growth factors and fibrogenic cytokines [75]. Damage to the blood vessels associated with breakdown of the blood retinal barrier is an important pathological event in PVR, PDR and AMD. Along this line, fibrin deposits have been found in the eyes of patients with retinal proliferative disease and it has been reported that RPE can use fibrin as scaffold supporting myofibroblastic de-differentiation and migration [76–80]. However studies in lung fibrosis clearly revealed that fibrin generation *per se* may not be required for a fibrotic response, and that thrombin and FXa directly contribute to the fibrotic response by regulating cellular activity [81–83].

FXa and thrombin can directly activate cell surface expressed proteinase-activated receptors (PARs), thereby initiating cellular processes associated with tissue healing, including cellular migration, proliferation and myofibroblast differentiation [73]. Four different PAR types (PAR1–4) exist. PARs are G-coupled proteins of which signalling is initiated via proteolytic cleavage of the extracellular N-terminal part. The newly formed N-terminus binds to another extracellular part of the receptor, causing a conformational change that activates intracellular signalling via the G-coupled proteins (Fig. 8.3). Each PAR has its own unique cleavage site that can be cleaved by several proteases of which thrombin by far has the highest affinity for these receptors, with the exception of PAR2 (Table 8.1) [84]. Indeed PAR1 abrogation protects against fibrosis in several organ systems, pointing at an important role for this receptor and its activating coagulation proteases in eliciting cellular responses crucial for fibrosis to develop [73].

Besides fibrin, increased thrombin activity and elevated levels of coagulation proteins have been found in vitreous from patients with PVR, PDR and AMD [85–90]. RPE cells express PARs, mostly abundantly PAR1 and PAR3 [91, 92]. Thrombin, and to a lesser extent FXa, induce EMT in RPE cells, which is associated with decreased expression of epithelial markers ZO-1 and E-cadherin, intercellular gap formation and increased expression of mesenchymal markers including αSMA, collagen type-1 and N-cadherin as well as actin stress fiber assembly [64, 92–95] (Fig. 8.4). These processes are PAR1 dependent and may involve induction of autocrine PDGF-PDGF-R signalling and signalling cascades including phosphatidylinositol 3-kinase (PI3K) and inositol 1,4,5-triphosphate (IP3)/diacylglycerol (DAG) controlled protein kinase C (PKC) activation followed by phosphorylation of PKC-potentiated inhibitory protein of 17 kDa (CPI-17) and subsequent myosin light chain phosphorylation as well as Snail induction [64, 91, 94–96].

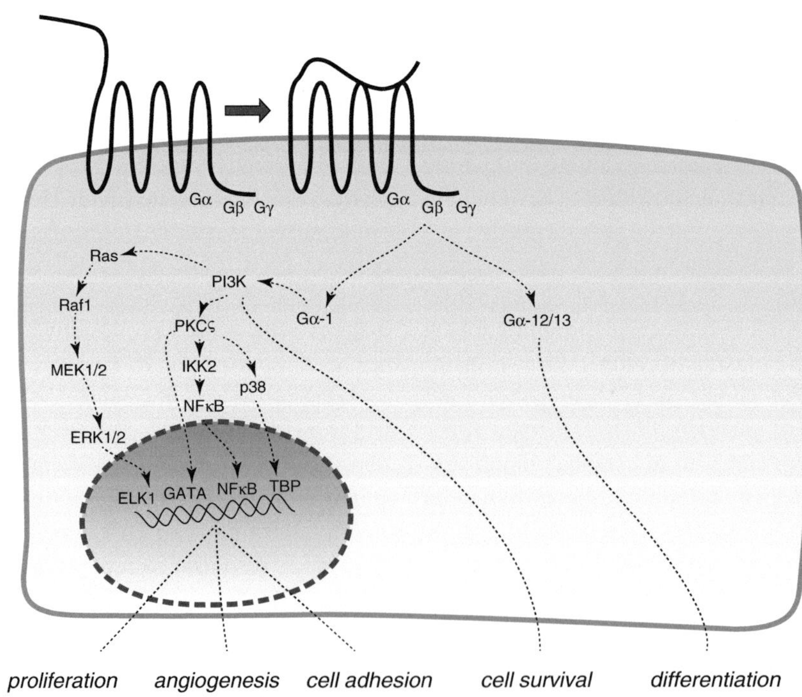

Fig. 8.3 Activation of proteinase-activated receptors (PARs). PARs are seven transmembrane domain receptors which activation involves proteolytic cleavage of the N-terminus. This leads to unmasking of a tethered ligand, which then binds to the second extracellular loop. This then results in a conformational change at the C-terminus, recruitment of heterotrimeric G-proteins and subsequent activation of signaling pathways that elicit cellular effects, including proliferative, pro-angiogenic, pro-inflammatory and differentiation responses. (Figure source: J. Bastiaans, Thesis 2015, Erasmus University, ISBN/EAN 978–94–6233-054-2)

Table 8.1 Agonists of protease activated receptors

PAR1	PAR2
Activated protein C Cathepsin G *Factor Xa* Granzyme A Kallikrein 1, 4, 5, 6, 14 Matrix metalloprotease 1 Meziothrombin (desF1) Penicillium citrinum 13 Plasmin Proatherocytin *Thrombin* Trypsin IV	Acrosin Bacterial gingipains Chitinase Granzyme A Kallikrein 2, 4, 5, 6, 14 Mast cell tryptase Matriptase/membrane-type serine protease 1 Penicillium citrinum 13 Peptidase 1, 2, 3 Tissue factor:*Factor Xa*:Factor VIIa Transmembrane protease serine 2 Transmembrane protease serine 11D Trypsin Trypsin IV
PAR3	**PAR4**
Thrombin	Bacterial gingipains Cathepsin G *Factor Xa* Kallikrein1, 14 Mannon binding lectin serine peptidase 1 Plasmin *Thrombin* Trypsin Trypsin IV

Hypoxia and Glucose

Retinal hypoxia is an important determinant in the pathogenesis of AMD and PDR, where it results from drusen deposition and thickening of Bruch's membrane or retinal microvasculopathy, respectively [97, 98]. Hypoxic culture conditions induce EMT in ARPE-19 as evidenced by enhanced αSMA expression. This involves hypoxia-induced TGF-β2 production and Snail induction [99]. Moreover, prolonged hyperglycemia is involved in diabetes and may influence EMT by RPE in PDR. It was observed that high glucose level further increased RPE barrier breakdown under in vitro hypoxic conditions, which involved p38 MAPK activation [100]. Moreover, high glucose induces RPE EMT in vitro, which is associated with increased Snail activity, cellular migration, fibronectin and collagen production, PI3K/AKT signaling and induction of connective tissue growth factor [7, 101].

RPE Monolayer Disruption

Although it has been observed that several different stimuli can be involved in EMT induction in RPE, it seems that disruption of RPE cell-cell contact and dissociation from Bruch's membrane may represent absolute prerequisites for EMT [102, 103]. For instance it was observed that RPE cells in the center of cultured porcine RPE sheets maintained cell-cell contact and retained a differentiated epithelial phenotype, while RPE cells at the edge of the sheet migrated away from the sheet, lost their epithelial morphology and pigment and dedifferentiated into fibroblast-like cells. Moreover, disruption of the RPE cell cell contact in the center of the sheets was associated with EMT, as evidenced by the acquirement of vimentin and N-cadherin expression while P-cadherin expression diminished, which was also associated with enhanced cellular proliferation [103]. Importantly, in vitro studies revealed that TGF-β1 and TGF-β2 induced dedifferentiation of cultured RPE cells into myofibroblasts [42–44]. Yet, TGF-β2 did not induce αSMA expression in differentiated RPE cells in the central region of cultured porcine RPE sheets, while it did enhance αSMA expression in those cells that already had undergone EMT [103].

Maintenance of RPE layer integrity is controlled by junctional complexes (adherens junctions and tight junctions) that typically sequester EMT signaling molecules. Cadherins, which form part of the adherens junctions, sequester β-catenin at the plasma membrane/cytoplasm. In RPE cells undergoing EMT, β-catenin translocates to the nucleus while inhibition of β-catenin signaling prevents EMT and the associated proliferation [27, 104, 105]. Hepatocyte growth factor (HGF), a factor that induces disruption of cell layers, induces β-catenin release from adherens junctions and enhances EMT, proliferation and migration by RPE [106–110]. Also ZO-1 as part of the tight junction links transcription molecules crucial for maintenance of epithelial layer integrity. ZO-1-associated nucleic-acid-binding protein (ZONAB) binds to ZO-1 and knock-down of ZO-1 or overexpression of ZONAB results in RPE monolayer breaks, EMT and associated proliferation, both in vivo and in vitro [111].

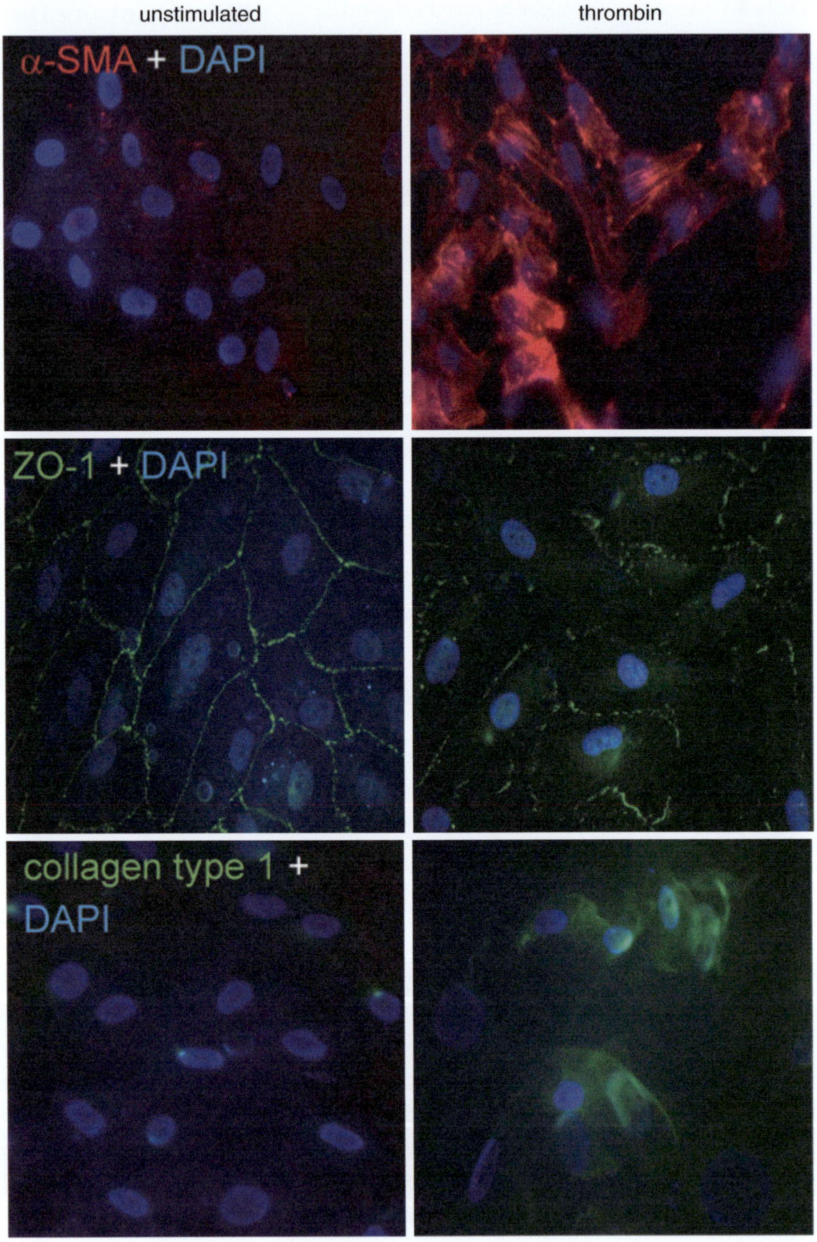

Fig. 8.4 Thrombin induces epithelial mesenchymal transition by RPE cells. ARPE-19 cells were cultured under standard conditions (left column) or stimulated for 48 h with thrombin (5 U/mL) and the cells were fixed and stained for the myofibroblast marker alpha smooth muscle actin (α-SMA, red: top row), the tight junction protein zonula occludens-1 (ZO-1, green: middle row) and collagen type-1 (green: lower row). The nuclei were counterstained with DAPI (blue). Thrombin enhances the expression of αSMA fibers and collagen type-1 in ARPE-19 and reduces expression of ZO-1. (Figure modified from [64])

MicroRNA Regulation

MicroRNAs (miRNAs) are small noncoding RNAs that selectively bind mRNA, thereby inhibiting their translation or promoting their degradation and, in addition to the direct effect of transcription factors on gene expression, miRNAs also regulate the epithelial phenotype and EMT [27]. In RPE miRNA-204 and miRNA-211 are abundantly expressed and target TGF-βR2 and Snail mRNA while reduced expression of miRNA-204/211 results in diminished expression of tight junction associated claudin molecules, increased TGF-βR2, PDGF-B, Snail1/2 expression, decreased trans-epithelial resistance and increased proliferation. This all points at a critical role for these miRNAs in maintaining retinal epithelial integrity and barrier function

[112]. Differential expression of miRNAs occurs upon TGF-β2-induced EMT in RPE [113]. This includes miRNA downregulation of miRNA-29b that is associated with increased collagen production [113]. TGF-β1-induced EMT in RPE is also associated with downregulation of miRNA-29b and overexpression of miRNA-29b inhibits TGF-β1-induced EMT by RPE as it prevented downregulation of ZO-1 and E-cadherin and upregulation of αSMA [53]. In addition, TGF-β1-induced EMT in RPE has been found to be associated with downregulation of miRNA-124, while miRNA-124 overexpression upregulated the levels of ZO-1 and occludin and downregulated αSMA, fibronectin and vimentin expression in RPE and reduced RPE mediated collagen-gel contraction [114]. This involved the inhibitory effect of miRNA-124 on RHOG (Ras homology Growth-related) expression, a protein that controls RAC1 (Ras-related C3 botulinum toxin substrate 1), which is a regulator of EMT in RPE [114, 115]. RPE differentiation is promoted by miRNA-184 via suppression of AKT2/mTOR signaling. Decreased miRNA-184 expression has been observed in RPE from AMD along with increased AKT2 levels while in RPE miRNA-184 was found to block AKT/mTOR signaling and to suppress proliferation and migration [116]. All together this illustrates that miRNAs fulfill an important regulatory effect on pathways crucial in EMT in RPE, which warrants further studies into this regulatory mechanism.

RPE and Myofibroblast Dedifferentiation by Other Cell Types

Müller cells may represent another important source for myofibroblasts in retinal membranes [31, 117]. This can be induced by growth factors including, insulin-like growth factor-I (IGF-I), IGF-II and PDGF, which facilitate tractional potential of these cells [118, 119]. Activated and dedifferentiated RPE have been identified as source of such growth factors and culture medium obtained from RPE that have undergone myofibroblastic differentiation induces a myofibroblastic phenotype in Müller cells [64, 91, 120]. In addition thrombin-induced myofibroblast differentiation of RPE can be associated with the production of IGFBP-3, a factor that may reduce IGF-I and IGF-II induced Müller cell contraction [64, 91, 119]. This illustrates that in retinal fibrosis the RPE may thus represent a source of mediators that modulate myofibroblastic dedifferentiation of other retinal cell types in a paracrine manner.

RPE and Inflammation

Inflammation is an important pathologic component in proliferative retinal disease. Infiltration of the vitreous, retina, fibroproliferative retinal membranes and choroid by leukocytes, including neutrophils, monocytes, macrophages as well as T- and B-lymphocytes, is observed in PVR, PDR and AMD [5, 121–128].

Cytokines/Chemokines Produced by RPE

Chemokines are chemotactic cytokines that regulate the recruitment of leukocytes to sites of injury and elevated levels of chemokines, including chemokine (C-C motif) ligand (CCL)2, CCL14, chemokine (C-X-C motif) ligand (CXCL)7, CXCL8, CXCL10, CXCL12, CXCL16, IL-6 and macrophage-colony stimulating factor (M-CSF), have been detected in vitreous from patients with PVR, PDR and AMD [30, 127, 129–134].

RPE cells may represent an important source of chemokines upon activation by different types of stimuli. Several inflammatory cytokines, including IFN-γ, IL-1β, and TNF-α, induce the production of for instance CCL2, CCL5, CCL7, CXCL8, CXCL9, CXCL10, CXCL11, CXCL16 and CX3CL1 by RPE, which may be further enhanced upon costimulation with combinations of these cytokines [135, 136]. IL-4 typically induces production of the eotaxins CCL11 and CCL26, and while not by itself affecting CCL5 and CCL7 production by RPE, it does enhance the effect of TNFα on the production of these chemokines [136]. In addition, RPE can increase their production of other pro-inflammatory cytokines, including IL-1α, IL-1β and IL-6, for instance upon activation with IL-1, TNF-α or LPS [11].

The cytokines that activate chemokine/cytokine production by RPE may derive from infiltrating leukocytes as it was found that for instance activated T-lymphocytes stimulate the production of CCL2, CCL5, CCL7, CCL8, CXCL1, CXCL2, CXCL3, CXCL8, CXCL9, CXCL10 and CXCL11 by RPE via secretion of TNFα and IFN-γ [135]. However since RPE cells express receptors for cytokines they produce themselves, autocrine or paracrine effects induced by these cytokines might be involved as well.

TLRs (toll-like receptors) are a family of evolutionary conserved innate immune receptors which can either be expressed at the cell membrane (e.g. TLRs 1, 2, 4, 5 and 6) or intracellularly (e.g. TLRs 3, 7 and 9) and recognize and respond to microbial pathogen-associated molecular patterns (PAMPs) as well as endogenous ligands for instance derived from damaged cells (damage-associated molecular patterns: (DAMPs)). TLRs are thus crucial components of innate immunity that participate in host defense against infection, tissue damage, repair and regeneration [137]. Well known PAMPs are bacterial lipopolysaccharides for TLR4, bacterial lipoproteins and lipotechoic acid and fungal zymosan for TLR1, TLR2 and TLR6 and bacterial flagellin for TLR5, while double stranded RNA typically binds to TLR3, single stranded RNA to TLR7 and bacterial unmethylated CpG DNA to TLR9 [137, 138]. Endogenous ligands (DAMPs) that may activate TLRs, in particular TLR2 and TLR4, comprise amongst others heat shock proteins, HMGB1, but also extracellular matrix molecules including fibronectin, fibrinogen, hyaluronan, or breakdown products thereof, while mRNA molecules exhibit the capacity to activate TLR3 [137, 138]. RPE cells abundantly express TLRs and especially TLR1 and 3 are most highly expressed and expression of such TLR molecules is even further enhanced by inflammatory stimuli [139].

Although the contribution of TLRs to proliferative retinal disease has not been studied in great depth so far, TLR activation on RPE likely contributes to these diseases, for instance by contributing to the generation of a local pro-angiogenic and inflammatory environment. For instance amyloid-β enhances cytokine production by RPE cells, including CXCL2, CXCL8, CX3CL1, IL-1β, IL-6, IL-18, IL-33 and TNF-α, which may involve TLR4 mediated activation of the MyD88-NF-κB signaling pathway and NLRP3 inflammasome activation [140–142]. But possibly also TLR 3 and TLR4 activation in RPE cells through RNA released from damaged cells or HMGB1, respectively, is involved in shaping the local inflammatory/pro-fibrotic milieu as this enhances the release of cytokines and growth factors by the RPE [139, 143–148]. In addition, histones, which are DNA binding proteins essential to chromatin remodeling and gene expression, can also be released after retinal tissue injury and exhibit the ability to stimulate cytokine production by RPE in a TLR4 dependent manner [149].

The coagulation and complement systems may also be involved in shaping the inflammatory environment in retinal proliferative disease. Thrombin, FXa as well as complement components can induce production of several different cytokines/chemokines by RPE, including CCL2, CCL7, CXCL8, GM-CSF and IL-6 [85, 91, 150, 151]. Furthermore, hyperglycemic and hypoxic conditions can trigger inflammatory cytokine production, including CXCL8, CXCL12, IL-1β, IL-6 and IL-18, by RPE cells [152, 153].

Altogether, these data illustrate that RPE cells can produce cytokines/chemokines in response to a variety of stimuli associated with proliferative retinal diseases. These cytokines and chemokines are involved in recruitment, activation and differentiation of immune cells (Table 8.2), but also in the activation of other retinal resident cells.

Adhesion Molecule Expression by RPE

Transmigration of immune cells across the vascular endothelium into tissue not only depends on local chemokine/cytokine gradients, but also

Table 8.2 Chemokines produced by RPE cells

Chemokine	Chemotactic for
CCL2 (MCP-1)	Monocytes, basophils
CCL5 (RANTES)	T-lymphocytes, monocytes, eosinophils
CCL7 (MCP-3)	Monocytes, eosinophils
CCL8 (MCP-2)	Monocytes, lymphocytes, basophils, eosinophils
CCL11 (eotaxin-1)	Eosinophils
CCL26 (eotaxin-3)	Basophils, eosinophils
CXCL1 (GRO-α)	Neutrophils
CXCL2 (MIP-2α)	Neutrophils
CXCL3 (MIP-2β)	Neutrophils
CXCL8 (IL-8)	Neutrophils, basophils, T-lymphocytes
CXCL9 (MIG)	T-lymphocytes
CXCL10 (IP-10)	T-lymhpocytes, monocytes
CXCL11 (I-TAC)	T-lymphocytes, neutrophils, monocytes
CXCL16 (SR-PSOX)	T-lymphocytes
CX3CL1 (fractalkine)	T-lymphocytes, monocytes

Chemokines are indicated by their official nomenclature, in between brackets common aliases used

requires expression of adhesion molecules, not only on the immune cells and endothelial cells, but also tissue resident cells [154].

Intercellular adhesion molecule-1 (ICAM-1: CD54) interacts with other adhesion molecules, including lymphocyte function associated antigen-1 (LFA-1: CD11a/CD18), macrophage adhesion ligand-1 (MAC-1: CD11b/CD18), and the integrin p150,95 (CD11c/CD18: type-4 complement receptor), which are expressed by immune cells and are required for adhesion and chemotaxis. Adhesion molecule expression by RPE cells is crucial for immune cell adhesion and migration. RPE cells have been found to express ICAM-1 and binding of leukocytes, including neutrophils and activated (T-) lymphocytes, hugely depends on this ICAM-1 expression [155, 156]. Several inflammatory stimuli, including IL-1β, TNF-α, or IFN-γ upregulate ICAM-1 expression by RPE and significantly enhance ICAM-1 dependent leukocyte binding to RPE cells [155]. Yet, under strong inflammatory conditions also ICAM-1 independent mechanisms may be involved in adhesion of leukocytes to RPE, while leukocyte activation associated with integrin/adhesion molecule activation appears crucial as well [156, 157]. Migration of lymphocytes through RPE monolayers involves ICAM-1 and LFA-1 as antibodies against these adhesion molecules abrogated the migration of T-lymphocytes across an RPE monolayer [158]. Also other adhesion molecules expressed by (activated) RPE cells, including VCAM-1, facilitate T-lymphocyte migration across RPE monolayers [159].

It has been described that thrombin stimulates ICAM-1 expression by RPE cells and strengthens the physical interaction between RPE cells and monocytes when co-cultured [91, 160]. Moreover, stimulation of monocyte-RPE (ARPE-19) co-cultures with thrombin significantly enhances monocyte to macrophage differentiation, which is blocked by neutralizing antibodies directed against ICAM-1 (CD54) or integrin-β2 (CD18) and thus indicating the importance of the ICAM-1-LFA-1/MAC-1 system in RPE driven macrophage differentiation (Fig. 8.5). Yet whether such macrophages are of the so-called M2 type (CD163 positive) that are typically associated with tissue repair, angiogenesis and fibrosis, also in fibro(vascular) retinal membranes [133, 161], is unclear so far. M2 macrophages secrete huge amounts of pro-fibrotic/angiogenic mediators (including TGF-β, PDGF and VEGF) that drive for instance EMT and ECM production, while M1 macrophages typically produce pro-inflammatory mediators, which may however (for instance CCL2) also be involved in the recruitment of fibrocytes that, once infiltrated into the tissue, can adopt a pro-fibrotic phenotype and have been observed in vitreous and retinal membranes [12, 162–165]. Nevertheless these data demonstrate that adhesion molecules expressed by RPE are involved in immune cell recruitment, activation as well as differentiation and thereby thus modulate the local inflammatory/pro-angiogenic/pro-fibrotic milieu in the retina/vitreous.

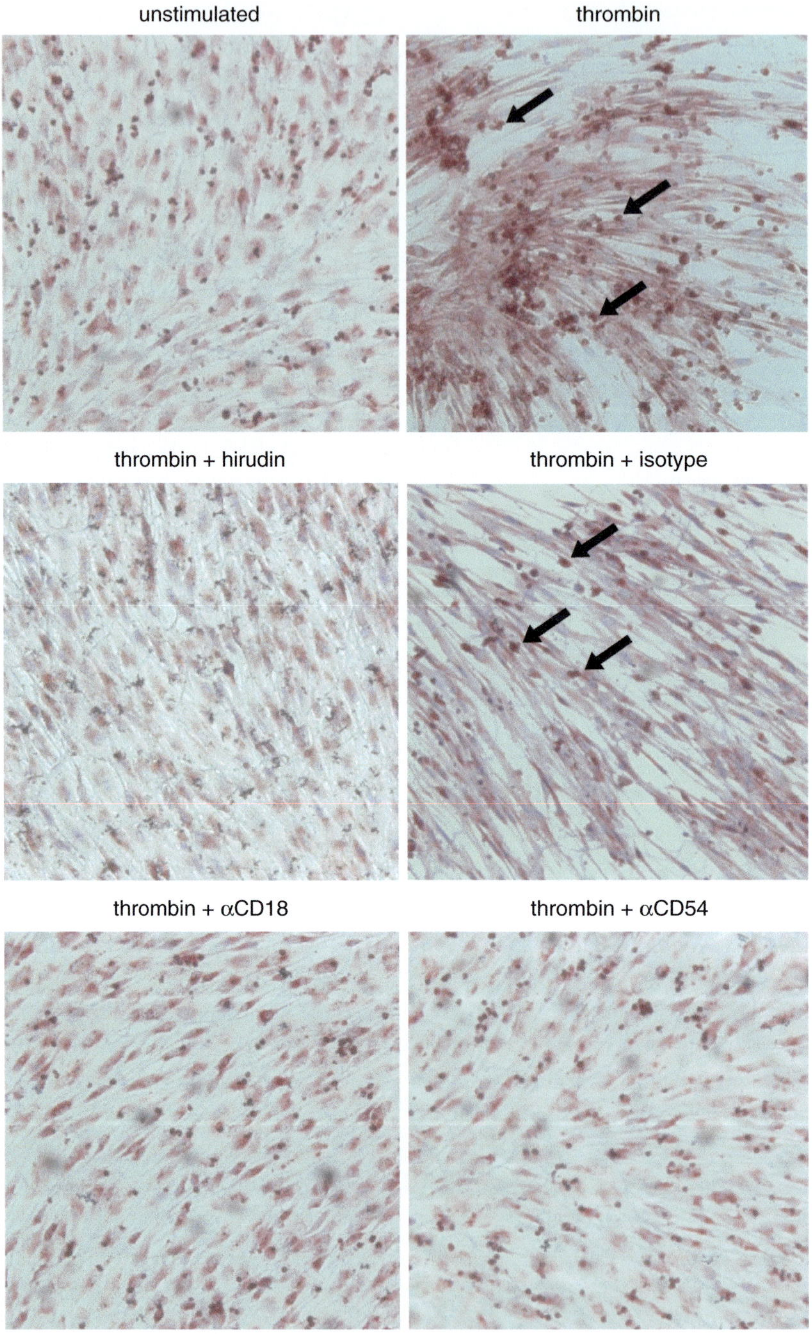

Fig. 8.5 Thrombin facilitates ICAM-1-LFA-1/MAC-1 interactions between RPE and monocytes that are involved in RPE-induced monocyte to macrophage differentiation. CD14+ monocytes isolated from peripheral blood mononuclear cell fraction and ARPE-19 cells were co-cultured on glass slides for 72 hours. The cells remained unstimulated, were stimulated with thrombin (5 U/mL), stimulated with thrombin (5 U/mL) in the presence of the direct thrombin inhibitor hirudin (7.5 U/mL), neutralizing antibodies against CD18 (αCD18; LFA-1/MAC-1), CD54 (αCD54; ICAM-1) or an isotype control (each antibody at 1 μg/mL). Non-adherent cells were washed away and adherent cells were stained with CD68 to identify macrophages (dark red staining). Thrombin stimulation is associated with (myo)fibroblastic dedifferentiation of the RPE cells as evidenced by the spindle shaped morphology they adopt. Moreover this stimulation is clearly associated with the differentiation of monocytes into macrophages (top right panel, some macrophages are indicated by arrows), which was inhibited by hirudin as well as neutralizing antibodies directed against CD18 and CD54, but not the isotype control. (Figure adapted from: J. Bastiaans, Thesis 2015, Erasmus University, ISBN/EAN 978–94–6233-054-2)

RPE and Angiogenesis

Choroidal and retinal neovascularization as seen in wet AMD and PDR, respectively, is highly dependent on local growth factor activity. Vascular endothelial growth factor (VEGF) is considered a key growth factor in stimulating neovascularization that, in order to establish its full pro-angiogenic action, does depend on the additive or synergistic help from other angiogenic factors, including for instance PDGF, IGF-I, placental growth factor (PlGF) and bFGF [166–168].

RPE cells within the direct vicinity of endothelial cells likely contribute to pathological neovascularization through production of pro-angiogenic factors [169, 170]. Studies with transwell co-culture of choroidal endothelial cells (CEC) with RPE cells (ARPE-19) clearly revealed that RPE cells release VEGF that facilitates CEC transmigration, yet VEGF by itself was not able to induce proliferation which required additional factors produced by the RPE [171]. Increased production of pro-angiogenic factors by RPE can occur upon different types of stimuli. Hypoxia induces VEGF and PDGF expression in RPE which involves PKC-signaling and hypoxia-inducible factor 1-α (HIF-1α) transcriptional activity and may be further enhanced by alterations in ECM composition [9, 10, 172–175]. Moreover, hyperglycemic conditions upregulate VEGF production by RPE, which involves activation of the transcription factors specificity protein 1 (Sp1) and HIF-1α [173, 176–178]. In contrast, bFGF production by RPE may be reduced under hyperglycemic conditions [179].

Pigment epithelium-derived factor (PEDF) is under normal conditions secreted by the RPE and retains retinal and choriocapillaris structure by inhibition of endothelial cell proliferation [180, 181]. However, decreased PEDF expression by RPE can occur under hyperglycemic and hypoxic conditions [182].

Activation of innate immune receptors on RPE may also promote neovascularization. For instance activation of receptor for advanced glycation end products (RAGE), a pattern recognition receptor abundantly expressed by RPE, by accumulated glycation end products but also amyloid-β present in drusen, or high mobility group box 1 protein (HMGB1) and calcium-binding S100 proteins, released from dying cells, stimulate VEGF secretion by RPE cells [141, 183–191]. Besides RAGE, amyloid-β can activate TLR4 signaling in RPE and thereby promotes VEGF and bFGF production [142]. In addition, amyloid-β may cause decreased PEDF production by RPE cells and conditioned media from amyloid-β exposed RPE cells was found to cause a steep increase in tubule formation by human umbilical vein endothelial cells. This clearly indicates that drusen components may stimulate retinal neovascularization by altering the balance between pro-angiogenic and anti-angiogenic factors produced by RPE cells [184].

Inflammatory mediators and growth factors, for instance IL-1β, TNF-α, IFN-γ and TGF-β1, TGF-β 2 and TGF-β3 that can be elevated in fibroproliferative retinal disorders also induce VEGF production by RPE [192–195]. The complement system may also promote the creation of a pro-angiogeninic environment by RPE as C3a stimulates VEGF production by RPE while it decreases PEDF production [196]. In addition, coagulation cascade activity may drive pro-angiogenic mediator production by RPE as FXa and thrombin stimulate expression and release of VEGF, PDGF and bFGF by RPE cells [64, 91, 92, 193, 197]. The effect of FXa and thrombin on VEGF production likely involves autocrine/paracrine TGF-β signaling and comprises activation of MAPK, ERK1/2, p38, PI3K and Akt signaling molecules [92, 193, 197]. The effect of thrombin on VEGF production by RPE can by further amplified, either in an additive or synergistic manner, by other pro-angiogenic factors like TNF-α and TGF-β2 as well as monocytes [193].

These data point at the existence of a direct link between, inflammation, coagulation, a pro-angiogenic RPE phenotype, and retinal neovascularization.

Conclusion

Studies conducted over the last decades revealed that RPE cells play an essential role in several pathologic characteristics of retinal proliferative

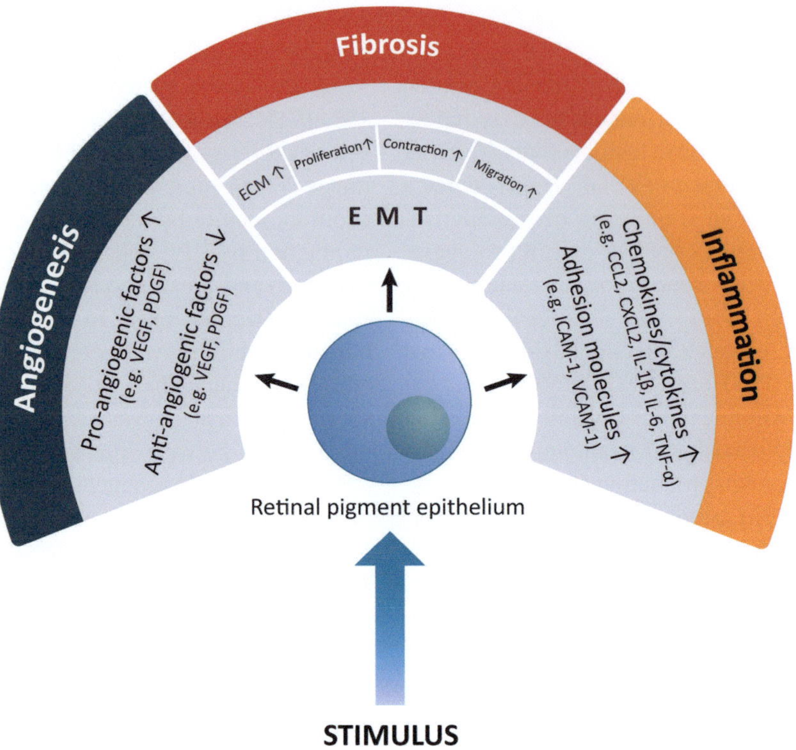

Fig. 8.6 Fibrosis, inflammation and angiogenesis represent important pathologic characteristics of retinal proliferative disease. Retinal pigment epithelium (RPE) cells play an important role in the pathogenesis of these characteristics. RPE cells contribute to fibrosis via the process of epithelial mesenchymal transition (EMT) in which they lose typical epithelial characteristics and dedifferentiate into myofibroblast-like cells. Myofibroblasts are specialized cells and represent the main effector cells in fibrosis. They exhibit migratory capacity that promotes invasiveness, proliferate and resist apoptosis, facilitating excessive cell accumulation. Importantly myofibroblasts exhibit strong capacity to produce extracellular matrix (ECM) components and display contractile properties thereby contributing to excessive ECM deposition and tissue distortion, respectively. RPE cells contribute to inflammation via the production of a plethora of chemokines and cytokines that regulate immune cell recruitment, activation and differentiation within the ocular tissue. In addition, the RPE cells enhance their expression of adhesion molecules, thereby facilitating cellular interaction with immune cells required for immune cell infiltration and activation. The RPE contributes to angiogenesis via enhanced production of pro-angiogenic factors and diminished production of anti-angiogenic factors, which promotes the creation of a local pro-angiogenic growth factor environment. To adopt these effector functions the RPE cells need to be activated by a stimulus. The nature of the stimulus can be diverse (e.g. cytokines, growth factors, coagulation proteins, drusen, hypoxia, hyperglycemia, loss of junctional integrity, damage-associated molecular patterns; for details see text)

diseases. This includes at least (1) the formation of fibro(vascular)membranes by undergoing EMT, associated with migration, proliferation, ECM production and cellular contraction, (2) inflammation via the production of cytokines/chemokines and adhesion molecules that facilitate leukocyte recruitment and differentiation which further shapes the local pro-fibrotic and pro-angiogenic environment, and (3) angiogenesis by creating a pro-angiogenic environment which typically involves the production of pro-angiogenic factors along with diminished production of anti-angiogenic factors (Fig. 8.6). A challenge for the future is to further unravel the molecular mechanisms involved in these processes as such knowledge may serve as the basis for improved or novel therapeutic approaches.

References

1. Charteris DG, Downie J, Aylward GW, Sethi C, Luthert P. Intraretinal and periretinal pathology in anterior proliferative vitreoretinopathy. Graefes Arch Clin Exp Ophthalmol. 2007;245(1):93–100.
2. Hiscott P, Hagan S, Heathcote L, Sheridan CM, Groenewald CP, Grierson I, et al. Pathobiology of epiretinal and subretinal membranes: possible roles for the matricellular proteins thrombospondin 1 and osteonectin (SPARC). Eye (Lond). 2002;16(4):393–403.
3. Pastor JC, de la Rua ER, Martin F. Proliferative vitreoretinopathy: risk factors and pathobiology. Prog Retin Eye Res. 2002;21(1):127–44.
4. Oberstein SY, Byun J, Herrera D, Chapin EA, Fisher SK, Lewis GP. Cell proliferation in human epiretinal membranes: characterization of cell types and correlation with disease condition and duration. Mol Vis. 2011;17:1794–805.
5. Seregard S, Algvere PV, Berglin L. Immunohistochemical characterization of surgically removed subfoveal fibrovascular membranes. Graefes Arch Clin Exp Ophthalmol. 1994;232(6):325–9.
6. Cao L, Wang H, Wang F, Xu D, Liu F, Liu C. Abeta-induced senescent retinal pigment epithelial cells create a proinflammatory microenvironment in AMD. Invest Ophthalmol Vis Sci. 2013;54(5):3738–50.
7. Che D, Zhou T, Lan Y, Xie J, Gong H, Li C, et al. High glucose-induced epithelial-mesenchymal transition contributes to the upregulation of fibrogenic factors in retinal pigment epithelial cells. Int J Mol Med. 2016;38(6):1815–22.
8. Yoshida A, Elner SG, Bian ZM, Elner VM. Induction of interleukin-8 in human retinal pigment epithelial cells after denuding injury. Br J Ophthalmol. 2001;85(7):872–6.
9. Mousa SA, Lorelli W, Campochiaro PA. Role of hypoxia and extracellular matrix-integrin binding in the modulation of angiogenic growth factors secretion by retinal pigmented epithelial cells. J Cell Biochem. 1999;74(1):135–43.
10. Forooghian F, Razavi R, Timms L. Hypoxia-inducible factor expression in human RPE cells. Br J Ophthalmol. 2007;91(10):1406–10.
11. Holtkamp GM, Kijlstra A, Peek R, de Vos AF. Retinal pigment epithelium-immune system interactions: cytokine production and cytokine-induced changes. Prog Retin Eye Res. 2001;20(1):29–48.
12. Dik WA. Acute lung injury: can the fibrocyte of today turn into the fibroguide of the future? Crit Care Med. 2012;40(1):300–1.
13. Casaroli Marano RP, Vilaro S. The role of fibronectin, laminin, vitronectin and their receptors on cellular adhesion in proliferative vitreoretinopathy. Invest Ophthalmol Vis Sci. 1994;35(6):2791–803.
14. Hiscott P, Sheridan C, Magee RM, Grierson I. Matrix and the retinal pigment epithelium in proliferative retinal disease. Prog Retin Eye Res. 1999;18(2):167–90.
15. Jerdan JA, Pepose JS, Michels RG, Hayashi H, de Bustros S, Sebag M, et al. Proliferative vitreoretinopathy membranes. An immunohistochemical study. Ophthalmology. 1989;96(6):801–10.
16. Ioachim E, Stefaniotou M, Gorezis S, Tsanou E, Psilas K, Agnantis NJ. Immunohistochemical study of extracellular matrix components in epiretinal membranes of vitreoproliferative retinopathy and proliferative diabetic retinopathy. Eur J Ophthalmol. 2005;15(3):384–91.
17. Hiscott PS, Grierson I, McLeod D. Natural history of fibrocellular epiretinal membranes: a quantitative, autoradiographic, and immunohistochemical study. Br J Ophthalmol. 1985;69(11):810–23.
18. Morino I, Hiscott P, McKechnie N, Grierson I. Variation in epiretinal membrane components with clinical duration of the proliferative tissue. Br J Ophthalmol. 1990;74(7):393–9.
19. Kalluri R, Neilson EG. Epithelial-mesenchymal transition and its implications for fibrosis. J Clin Invest. 2003;112(12):1776–84.
20. Kalluri R, Weinberg RA. The basics of epithelial-mesenchymal transition. J Clin Invest. 2009;119(6):1420–8.
21. Hinz B, Phan SH, Thannickal VJ, Prunotto M, Desmouliere A, Varga J, et al. Recent developments in myofibroblast biology: paradigms for connective tissue remodeling. Am J Pathol. 2012;180(4):1340–55.
22. Darby IA, Zakuan N, Billet F, Desmouliere A. The myofibroblast, a key cell in normal and pathological tissue repair. Cell Mol Life Sci. 2016;73(6):1145–57.
23. Kramann R, Schneider RK, DiRocco DP, Machado F, Fleig S, Bondzie PA, et al. Perivascular Gli1+ progenitors are key contributors to injury-induced organ fibrosis. Cell Stem Cell. 2015;16(1):51–66.
24. Reilkoff RA, Bucala R, Herzog EL. Fibrocytes: emerging effector cells in chronic inflammation. Nat Rev Immunol. 2011;11(6):427–35.
25. Torricelli AA, Santhanam A, Wu J, Singh V, Wilson SE. The corneal fibrosis response to epithelial-stromal injury. Exp Eye Res. 2016;142:110–8.
26. Piera-Velazquez S, Li Z, Jimenez SA. Role of endothelial-mesenchymal transition (EndoMT) in the pathogenesis of fibrotic disorders. Am J Pathol. 2011;179(3):1074–80.
27. Lamouille S, Xu J, Derynck R. Molecular mechanisms of epithelial-mesenchymal transition. Nat Rev Mol Cell Biol. 2014;15(3):178–96.
28. Duffield JS, Lupher M, Thannickal VJ, Wynn TA. Host responses in tissue repair and fibrosis. Annu Rev Pathol. 2013;8:241–76.
29. Abu El-Asrar AM, Alam K, Siddiquei MM, Van den Eynde K, Mohammad G, Hertogh G, et al. Myeloid-related protein-14/MRP-14/S100A9/calgranulin B is associated with inflammation in prolif-

erative diabetic retinopathy. Ocul Immunol Inflamm. 2018;26(4):615–24.
30. Abu El-Asrar AM, Struyf S, Kangave D, Geboes K, Van Damme J. Chemokines in proliferative diabetic retinopathy and proliferative vitreoretinopathy. Eur Cytokine Netw. 2006;17(3):155–65.
31. Feist RM Jr, King JL, Morris R, Witherspoon CD, Guidry C. Myofibroblast and extracellular matrix origins in proliferative vitreoretinopathy. Graefes Arch Clin Exp Ophthalmol. 2014;252(2):347–57.
32. Hyytiainen M, Penttinen C, Keski-Oja J. Latent TGF-beta binding proteins: extracellular matrix association and roles in TGF-beta activation. Crit Rev Clin Lab Sci. 2004;41(3):233–64.
33. Khalil N. Post translational activation of latent transforming growth factor beta (L-TGF-beta): clinical implications. Histol Histopathol. 2001;16(2):541–51.
34. Munger JS, Harpel JG, Gleizes PE, Mazzieri R, Nunes I, Rifkin DB. Latent transforming growth factor-beta: structural features and mechanisms of activation. Kidney Int. 1997;51(5):1376–82.
35. Sakai K, Sumi Y, Muramatsu H, Hata K, Muramatsu T, Ueda M. Thrombospondin-1 promotes fibroblast-mediated collagen gel contraction caused by activation of latent transforming growth factor beta-1. J Dermatol Sci. 2003;31(2):99–109.
36. Stetler-Stevenson WG, Aznavoorian S, Liotta LA. Tumor cell interactions with the extracellular matrix during invasion and metastasis. Annu Rev Cell Biol. 1993;9:541–73.
37. Wipff PJ, Hinz B. Integrins and the activation of latent transforming growth factor beta1—an intimate relationship. Eur J Cell Biol. 2008;87(8–9):601–15.
38. Massague J. TGFbeta signalling in context. Nat Rev Mol Cell Biol. 2012;13(10):616–30.
39. Wynn TA. Cellular and molecular mechanisms of fibrosis. J Pathol. 2008;214(2):199–210.
40. Bochaton-Piallat ML, Kapetanios AD, Donati G, Redard M, Gabbiani G, Pournaras CJ. TGF-beta1, TGF-beta receptor II and ED-A fibronectin expression in myofibroblast of vitreoretinopathy. Invest Ophthalmol Vis Sci. 2000;41(8):2336–42.
41. Stocks SZ, Taylor SM, Shiels IA. Transforming growth factor-beta1 induces alpha-smooth muscle actin expression and fibronectin synthesis in cultured human retinal pigment epithelial cells. Clin Exp Ophthalmol. 2001;29(1):33–7.
42. Lee SC, Kwon OW, Seong GJ, Kim SH, Ahn JE, Kay ED. Epitheliomesenchymal transdifferentiation of cultured RPE cells. Ophthalmic Res. 2001;33(2):80–6.
43. Gamulescu MA, Chen Y, He S, Spee C, Jin M, Ryan SJ, et al. Transforming growth factor beta2-induced myofibroblastic differentiation of human retinal pigment epithelial cells: regulation by extracellular matrix proteins and hepatocyte growth factor. Exp Eye Res. 2006;83(1):212–22.
44. Lee H, O'Meara SJ, O'Brien C, Kane R. The role of gremlin, a BMP antagonist, and epithelial-to-mesenchymal transition in proliferative vitreoretinopathy. Invest Ophthalmol Vis Sci. 2007;48(9):4291–9.
45. Parapuram SK, Chang B, Li L, Hartung RA, Chalam KV, Nair-Menon JU, et al. Differential effects of TGFbeta and vitreous on the transformation of retinal pigment epithelial cells. Invest Ophthalmol Vis Sci. 2009;50(12):5965–74.
46. Choi K, Lee K, Ryu SW, Im M, Kook KH, Choi C. Pirfenidone inhibits transforming growth factor-beta1-induced fibrogenesis by blocking nuclear translocation of Smads in human retinal pigment epithelial cell line ARPE-19. Mol Vis. 2012;18:1010–20.
47. Saika S, Kono-Saika S, Tanaka T, Yamanaka O, Ohnishi Y, Sato M, et al. Smad3 is required for dedifferentiation of retinal pigment epithelium following retinal detachment in mice. Lab Investig. 2004;84(10):1245–58.
48. Saika S, Yamanaka O, Nishikawa-Ishida I, Kitano A, Flanders KC, Okada Y, et al. Effect of Smad7 gene overexpression on transforming growth factor beta-induced retinal pigment fibrosis in a proliferative vitreoretinopathy mouse model. Arch Ophthalmol. 2007;125(5):647–54.
49. Dvashi Z, Goldberg M, Adir O, Shapira M, Pollack A. TGF-beta1 induced transdifferentiation of rpe cells is mediated by TAK1. PLoS One. 2015;10(4):e0122229.
50. Kimoto K, Nakatsuka K, Matsuo N, Yoshioka H. p38 MAPK mediates the expression of type I collagen induced by TGF-beta 2 in human retinal pigment epithelial cells ARPE-19. Invest Ophthalmol Vis Sci. 2004;45(7):2431–7.
51. Saika S, Yamanaka O, Ikeda K, Kim-Mitsuyama S, Flanders KC, Yoo J, et al. Inhibition of p38MAP kinase suppresses fibrotic reaction of retinal pigment epithelial cells. Lab Investig. 2005;85(7):838–50.
52. Yokoyama K, Kimoto K, Itoh Y, Nakatsuka K, Matsuo N, Yoshioka H, et al. The PI3K/Akt pathway mediates the expression of type I collagen induced by TGF-beta2 in human retinal pigment epithelial cells. Graefes Arch Clin Exp Ophthalmol. 2012;250(1):15–23.
53. Li M, Li H, Liu X, Xu D, Wang F. MicroRNA-29b regulates TGF-beta1-mediated epithelial-mesenchymal transition of retinal pigment epithelial cells by targeting AKT2. Exp Cell Res. 2016;345(2):115–24.
54. Chen X, Xiao W, Wang W, Luo L, Ye S, Liu Y. The complex interplay between ERK1/2, TGFbeta/Smad, and Jagged/Notch signaling pathways in the regulation of epithelial-mesenchymal transition in retinal pigment epithelium cells. PLoS One. 2014;9(5):e96365.
55. Li H, Wang H, Wang F, Gu Q, Xu X. Snail involves in the transforming growth factor beta1-mediated epithelial-mesenchymal transition of retinal pigment epithelial cells. PLoS One. 2011;6(8):e23322.
56. Chen X, Xiao W, Liu X, Zeng M, Luo L, Wu M, et al. Blockade of Jagged/Notch pathway abrogates

transforming growth factor beta2-induced epithelial-mesenchymal transition in human retinal pigment epithelium cells. Curr Mol Med. 2014;14(4):523–34.
57. Virakul S, van Steensel L, Dalm VA, Paridaens D, van Hagen PM, Dik WA. Platelet-derived growth factor: a key factor in the pathogenesis of graves' ophthalmopathy and potential target for treatment. Eur Thyroid J. 2014;3(4):217–26.
58. Bonner JC. Regulation of PDGF and its receptors in fibrotic diseases. Cytokine Growth Factor Rev. 2004;15(4):255–73.
59. Cui J, Lei H, Samad A, Basavanthappa S, Maberley D, Matsubara J, et al. PDGF receptors are activated in human epiretinal membranes. Exp Eye Res. 2009;88(3):438–44.
60. Cui JZ, Chiu A, Maberley D, Ma P, Samad A, Matsubara JA. Stage specificity of novel growth factor expression during development of proliferative vitreoretinopathy. Eye (Lond). 2007;21(2):200–8.
61. Lei H, Rheaume MA, Kazlauskas A. Recent developments in our understanding of how platelet-derived growth factor (PDGF) and its receptors contribute to proliferative vitreoretinopathy. Exp Eye Res. 2010;90(3):376–81.
62. Robbins SG, Mixon RN, Wilson DJ, Hart CE, Robertson JE, Westra I, et al. Platelet-derived growth factor ligands and receptors immunolocalized in proliferative retinal diseases. Invest Ophthalmol Vis Sci. 1994;35(10):3649–63.
63. Si Y, Wang J, Guan J, Han Q, Hui Y. Platelet-derived growth factor induced alpha-smooth muscle actin expression by human retinal pigment epithelium cell. J Ocul Pharmacol Ther. 2013;29(3):310–8.
64. Bastiaans J, van Meurs JC, van Holten-Neelen C, Nagtzaam NM, van Hagen PM, Chambers RC, et al. Thrombin induces epithelial-mesenchymal transition and collagen production by retinal pigment epithelial cells via autocrine PDGF-receptor signaling. Invest Ophthalmol Vis Sci. 2013;54(13):8306–14.
65. Chan CM, Chang HH, Wang VC, Huang CL, Hung CF. Inhibitory effects of resveratrol on PDGF-BB-induced retinal pigment epithelial cell migration via PDGFRbeta, PI3K/Akt and MAPK pathways. PLoS One. 2013;8(2):e56819.
66. Umazume K, Liu L, Scott PA, de Castro JP, McDonald K, Kaplan HJ, et al. Inhibition of PVR with a tyrosine kinase inhibitor, dasatinib, in the swine. Invest Ophthalmol Vis Sci. 2013;54(2):1150–9.
67. Lei H, Rheaume MA, Velez G, Mukai S, Kazlauskas A. Expression of PDGFRalpha is a determinant of the PVR potential of ARPE19 cells. Invest Ophthalmol Vis Sci. 2011;52(9):5016–21.
68. Lei H, Velez G, Hovland P, Hirose T, Gilbertson D, Kazlauskas A. Growth factors outside the PDGF family drive experimental PVR. Invest Ophthalmol Vis Sci. 2009;50(7):3394–403.
69. Hollborn M, Bringmann A, Faude F, Wiedemann P, Kohen L. Signaling pathways involved in PDGF-evoked cellular responses in human RPE cells. Biochem Biophys Res Commun. 2006;344(3):912–9.
70. Bando H, Ikuno Y, Hori Y, Sayanagi K, Tano Y. Mitogen-activated protein kinase (MAPK) and phosphatidylinositol-3 kinase (PI3K) pathways differently regulate retinal pigment epithelial cell-mediated collagen gel contraction. Exp Eye Res. 2006;82(3):529–37.
71. Xu W, Yang Z, Lu N. A new role for the PI3K/Akt signaling pathway in the epithelial-mesenchymal transition. Cell Adhes Migr. 2015;9(4):317–24.
72. Li H, Li M, Xu D, Zhao C, Liu G, Wang F. Overexpression of Snail in retinal pigment epithelial triggered epithelial-mesenchymal transition. Biochem Biophys Res Commun. 2014;446(1):347–51.
73. Mercer PF, Chambers RC. Coagulation and coagulation signalling in fibrosis. Biochim Biophys Acta. 2013;1832(7):1018–27.
74. Davie EW. Biochemical and molecular aspects of the coagulation cascade. Thromb Haemost. 1995;74(1):1–6.
75. Chambers RC, Laurent GJ. Coagulation cascade proteases and tissue fibrosis. Biochem Soc Trans. 2002;30(2):194–200.
76. Schwartz D, de la Cruz ZC, Green WR, Michels RG. Proliferative vitreoretinopathy. Ultrastructural study of 20 retroretinal membranes removed by vitreous surgery. Retina. 1988;8(4):275–81.
77. Vidaurri-Leal JS, Glaser BM. Effect of fibrin on morphologic characteristics of retinal pigment epithelial cells. Arch Ophthalmol. 1984;102(9):1376–9.
78. Weller M, Wiedemann P, Bresgen M, Heimann K. Giant preretinal membrane formation behind a silicone oil bubble in a hypotensive eye. Retina. 1990;10(1):86–91.
79. Murata T, Ishibashi T, Inomata H. Immunohistochemical detection of extravasated fibrinogen (fibrin) in human diabetic retina. Graefes Arch Clin Exp Ophthalmol. 1992;230(5):428–31.
80. Sarks JP, Sarks SH, Killingsworth MC. Morphology of early choroidal neovascularisation in age-related macular degeneration: correlation with activity. Eye (Lond). 1997;11(Pt 4):515–22.
81. Hattori N, Degen JL, Sisson TH, Liu H, Moore BB, Pandrangi RG, et al. Bleomycin-induced pulmonary fibrosis in fibrinogen-null mice. J Clin Invest. 2000;106(11):1341–50.
82. Howell DC, Goldsack NR, Marshall RP, McAnulty RJ, Starke R, Purdy G, et al. Direct thrombin inhibition reduces lung collagen, accumulation, and connective tissue growth factor mRNA levels in bleomycin-induced pulmonary fibrosis. Am J Pathol. 2001;159(4):1383–95.
83. Scotton CJ, Krupiczojc MA, Konigshoff M, Mercer PF, Lee YC, Kaminski N, et al. Increased local expression of coagulation factor X contributes to the fibrotic response in human and murine lung injury. J Clin Invest. 2009;119(9):2550–63.
84. Adams MN, Ramachandran R, Yau MK, Suen JY, Fairlie DP, Hollenberg MD, et al. Structure, function

and pathophysiology of protease activated receptors. Pharmacol Ther. 2011;130(3):248–82.

85. Bastiaans J, van Meurs JC, Mulder VC, Nagtzaam NM, Smits-te Nijenhuis M, Dufour-van den Goorbergh DC, et al. The role of thrombin in proliferative vitreoretinopathy. Invest Ophthalmol Vis Sci. 2014;55(7):4659–66.
86. Koss MJ, Hoffmann J, Nguyen N, Pfister M, Mischak H, Mullen W, et al. Proteomics of vitreous humor of patients with exudative age-related macular degeneration. PLoS One. 2014;9(5):e96895.
87. Murthy KR, Goel R, Subbannayya Y, Jacob HK, Murthy PR, Manda SS, et al. Proteomic analysis of human vitreous humor. Clin Proteomics. 2014;11(1):29.
88. Shitama T, Hayashi H, Noge S, Uchio E, Oshima K, Haniu H, et al. Proteome profiling of vitreoretinal diseases by cluster analysis. Proteomics Clin Appl. 2008;2(9):1265–80.
89. Walia S, Clermont AC, Gao BB, Aiello LP, Feener EP. Vitreous proteomics and diabetic retinopathy. Semin Ophthalmol. 2010;25(5–6):289–94.
90. Wang H, Feng L, Hu JW, Xie CL, Wang F. Characterisation of the vitreous proteome in proliferative diabetic retinopathy. Proteome Sci. 2012;10(1):15.
91. Bastiaans J, van Meurs JC, van Holten-Neelen C, Nijenhuis MS, Kolijn-Couwenberg MJ, van Hagen PM, et al. Factor Xa and thrombin stimulate proinflammatory and profibrotic mediator production by retinal pigment epithelial cells: a role in vitreoretinal disorders? Graefes Arch Clin Exp Ophthalmol. 2013;251(7):1723–33.
92. Hollborn M, Petto C, Steffen A, Trettner S, Bendig A, Wiedemann P, et al. Effects of thrombin on RPE cells are mediated by transactivation of growth factor receptors. Invest Ophthalmol Vis Sci. 2009;50(9):4452–9.
93. Sakamoto T, Sakamoto H, Sheu SJ, Gabrielian K, Ryan SJ, Hinton DR. Intercellular gap formation induced by thrombin in confluent cultured bovine retinal pigment epithelial cells. Invest Ophthalmol Vis Sci. 1994;35(2):720–9.
94. Ruiz-Loredo AY, Lopez E, Lopez-Colome AM. Thrombin promotes actin stress fiber formation in RPE through Rho/ROCK-mediated MLC phosphorylation. J Cell Physiol. 2011;226(2):414–23.
95. Ruiz-Loredo AY, Lopez E, Lopez-Colome AM. Thrombin stimulates stress fiber assembly in RPE cells by PKC/CPI-17-mediated MLCP inactivation. Exp Eye Res. 2012;96(1):13–23.
96. Palma-Nicolas JP, Lopez-Colome AM. Thrombin induces slug-mediated E-cadherin transcriptional repression and the parallel up-regulation of N-cadherin by a transcription-independent mechanism in RPE cells. J Cell Physiol. 2013;228(3):581–9.
97. Blasiak J, Petrovski G, Vereb Z, Facsko A, Kaarniranta K. Oxidative stress, hypoxia, and autophagy in the neovascular processes of age-related macular degeneration. Biomed Res Int. 2014;2014:768026.
98. Harding S. Diabetic retinopathy. Clin Evid. 2006;15:900–7.
99. Feng Z, Li R, Shi H, Bi W, Hou W, Zhang X. Combined silencing of TGF-beta2 and Snail genes inhibit epithelial-mesenchymal transition of retinal pigment epithelial cells under hypoxia. Graefes Arch Clin Exp Ophthalmol. 2015;253(6):875–84.
100. Wang S, Du S, Wu Q, Hu J, Li T. Decorin prevents retinal pigment epithelial barrier breakdown under diabetic conditions by suppressing p38 MAPK activation. Invest Ophthalmol Vis Sci. 2015;56(5):2971–9.
101. Qin D, Zhang GM, Xu X, Wang LY. The PI3K/Akt signaling pathway mediates the high glucose-induced expression of extracellular matrix molecules in human retinal pigment epithelial cells. J Diabetes Res. 2015;2015:920280.
102. Grisanti S, Guidry C. Transdifferentiation of retinal pigment epithelial cells from epithelial to mesenchymal phenotype. Invest Ophthalmol Vis Sci. 1995;36(2):391–405.
103. Tamiya S, Liu L, Kaplan HJ. Epithelial-mesenchymal transition and proliferation of retinal pigment epithelial cells initiated upon loss of cell-cell contact. Invest Ophthalmol Vis Sci. 2010;51(5):2755–63.
104. Chen HC, Zhu YT, Chen SY, Tseng SC. Wnt signaling induces epithelial-mesenchymal transition with proliferation in ARPE-19 cells upon loss of contact inhibition. Lab Investig. 2012;92(5):676–87.
105. Umazume K, Tsukahara R, Liu L, Fernandez de Castro JP, McDonald K, Kaplan HJ, et al. Role of retinal pigment epithelial cell beta-catenin signaling in experimental proliferative vitreoretinopathy. Am J Pathol. 2014;184(5):1419–28.
106. Jun EJ, Kim HS, Kim YH. Role of HGF/c-Met in serum-starved ARPE-19 cells. Korean J Ophthalmol. 2007;21(4):244–50.
107. Lashkari K, Rahimi N, Kazlauskas A. Hepatocyte growth factor receptor in human RPE cells: implications in proliferative vitreoretinopathy. Invest Ophthalmol Vis Sci. 1999;40(1):149–56.
108. Liou GI, Matragoon S, Samuel S, Behzadian MA, Tsai NT, Gu X, et al. MAP kinase and beta-catenin signaling in HGF induced RPE migration. Mol Vis. 2002;8:483–93.
109. Jin M, Chen Y, He S, Ryan SJ, Hinton DR. Hepatocyte growth factor and its role in the pathogenesis of retinal detachment. Invest Ophthalmol Vis Sci. 2004;45(1):323–9.
110. Grierson I, Heathcote L, Hiscott P, Hogg P, Briggs M, Hagan S. Hepatocyte growth factor/scatter factor in the eye. Prog Retin Eye Res. 2000;19(6):779–802.
111. Georgiadis A, Tschernutter M, Bainbridge JW, Balaggan KS, Mowat F, West EL, et al. The tight junction associated signalling proteins ZO-1 and ZONAB regulate retinal pigment epithelium homeostasis in mice. PLoS One. 2010;5(12):e15730.

112. Wang FE, Zhang C, Maminishkis A, Dong L, Zhi C, Li R, et al. MicroRNA-204/211 alters epithelial physiology. FASEB J. 2010;24(5):1552–71.
113. Chen X, Ye S, Xiao W, Luo L, Liu Y. Differentially expressed microRNAs in TGFbeta2-induced epithelial-mesenchymal transition in retinal pigment epithelium cells. Int J Mol Med. 2014;33(5):1195–200.
114. Jun JH, Joo CK. MicroRNA-124 controls transforming growth factor beta1-induced epithelial-mesenchymal transition in the retinal pigment epithelium by targeting RHOG. Invest Ophthalmol Vis Sci. 2016;57(1):12–22.
115. Huang X, Wei Y, Ma H, Zhang S. Vitreous-induced cytoskeletal rearrangements via the Rac1 GTPase-dependent signaling pathway in human retinal pigment epithelial cells. Biochem Biophys Res Commun. 2012;419(2):395–400.
116. Jiang C, Qin B, Liu G, Sun X, Shi H, Ding S, et al. MicroRNA-184 promotes differentiation of the retinal pigment epithelium by targeting the AKT2/mTOR signaling pathway. Oncotarget. 2016;7(32):52340–53.
117. Guidry C, King JL, Mason JO 3rd. Fibrocontractive Muller cell phenotypes in proliferative diabetic retinopathy. Invest Ophthalmol Vis Sci. 2009;50(4):1929–39.
118. Guidry C. Tractional force generation by porcine Muller cells. Development and differential stimulation by growth factors. Invest Ophthalmol Vis Sci. 1997;38(2):456–68.
119. King JL, Guidry C. Vitreous IGFBP-3 effects on Muller cell proliferation and tractional force generation. Invest Ophthalmol Vis Sci. 2012;53(1):93–9.
120. Mamballikalathil I, Mann C, Guidry C. Tractional force generation by porcine Muller cells: paracrine stimulation by retinal pigment epithelium. Invest Ophthalmol Vis Sci. 2000;41(2):529–36.
121. Baudouin C, Fredj-Reygrobellet D, Gordon WC, Baudouin F, Peyman G, Lapalus P, et al. Immunohistologic study of epiretinal membranes in proliferative vitreoretinopathy. Am J Ophthalmol. 1990;110(6):593–8.
122. Baudouin C, Gordon WC, Fredj-Reygrobellet D, Baudouin F, Peyman G, Gastaud P, et al. Class II antigen expression in diabetic preretinal membranes. Am J Ophthalmol. 1990;109(1):70–4.
123. Charteris DG, Hiscott P, Grierson I, Lightman SL. Proliferative vitreoretinopathy. Lymphocytes in epiretinal membranes. Ophthalmology. 1992;99(9):1364–7.
124. Tang S, Le-Ruppert KC. Activated T lymphocytes in epiretinal membranes from eyes of patients with proliferative diabetic retinopathy. Graefes Arch Clin Exp Ophthalmol. 1995;233(1):21–5.
125. Tang S, Scheiffarth OF, Wildner G, Thurau SR, Lund OE. Lymphocytes, macrophages and HLA-DR expression in vitreal and epiretinal membranes of proliferative vitreoretinopathy. An immunohistochemical study. Ger J Ophthalmol. 1992;1(3–4):176–9.
126. Tang S, Scheiffarth OF, Thurau SR, Wildner G. Cells of the immune system and their cytokines in epiretinal membranes and in the vitreous of patients with proliferative diabetic retinopathy. Ophthalmic Res. 1993;25(3):177–85.
127. Canataroglu H, Varinli I, Ozcan AA, Canataroglu A, Doran F, Varinli S. Interleukin (IL)-6, interleukin (IL)-8 levels and cellular composition of the vitreous humor in proliferative diabetic retinopathy, proliferative vitreoretinopathy, and traumatic proliferative vitreoretinopathy. Ocul Immunol Inflamm. 2005;13(5):375–81.
128. Canton A, Martinez-Caceres EM, Hernandez C, Espejo C, Garcia-Arumi J, Simo R. CD4-CD8 and CD28 expression in T cells infiltrating the vitreous fluid in patients with proliferative diabetic retinopathy: a flow cytometric analysis. Arch Ophthalmol. 2004;122(5):743–9.
129. Elner SG, Elner VM, Jaffe GJ, Stuart A, Kunkel SL, Strieter RM. Cytokines in proliferative diabetic retinopathy and proliferative vitreoretinopathy. Curr Eye Res. 1995;14(11):1045–53.
130. El-Ghrably IA, Dua HS, Orr GM, Fischer D, Tighe PJ. Intravitreal invading cells contribute to vitreal cytokine milieu in proliferative vitreoretinopathy. Br J Ophthalmol. 2001;85(4):461–70.
131. Mitamura Y, Takeuchi S, Yamamoto S, Yamamoto T, Tsukahara I, Matsuda A, et al. Monocyte chemotactic protein-1 levels in the vitreous of patients with proliferative vitreoretinopathy. Jpn J Ophthalmol. 2002;46(2):218–21.
132. Yoshimura T, Sonoda KH, Sugahara M, Mochizuki Y, Enaida H, Oshima Y, et al. Comprehensive analysis of inflammatory immune mediators in vitreoretinal diseases. PLoS One. 2009;4(12):e8158.
133. Yoshida S, Kubo Y, Kobayashi Y, Zhou Y, Nakama T, Yamaguchi M, et al. Increased vitreous concentrations of MCP-1 and IL-6 after vitrectomy in patients with proliferative diabetic retinopathy: possible association with postoperative macular oedema. Br J Ophthalmol. 2015;99(7):960–6.
134. Liu F, Ding X, Yang Y, Li J, Tang M, Yuan M, et al. Aqueous humor cytokine profiling in patients with wet AMD. Mol Vis. 2016;22:352–61.
135. Juel HB, Faber C, Udsen MS, Folkersen L, Nissen MH. Chemokine expression in retinal pigment epithelial ARPE-19 cells in response to coculture with activated T cells. Invest Ophthalmol Vis Sci. 2012;53(13):8472–80.
136. Nagineni CN, Kommineni VK, Ganjbaksh N, Nagineni KK, Hooks JJ, Detrick B. Inflammatory cytokines induce expression of chemokines by human retinal cells: role in chemokine receptor mediated age-related macular degeneration. Aging Dis. 2015;6(6):444–55.
137. Rakoff-Nahoum S, Medzhitov R. Toll-like receptors and cancer. Nat Rev Cancer. 2009;9(1):57–63.
138. Achek A, Yesudhas D, Choi S. Toll-like receptors: promising therapeutic targets for inflammatory diseases. Arch Pharm Res. 2016;39(8):1032–49.

139. Kumar MV, Nagineni CN, Chin MS, Hooks JJ, Detrick B. Innate immunity in the retina: toll-like receptor (TLR) signaling in human retinal pigment epithelial cells. J Neuroimmunol. 2004;153(1–2):7–15.
140. Kurji KH, Cui JZ, Lin T, Harriman D, Prasad SS, Kojic L, et al. Microarray analysis identifies changes in inflammatory gene expression in response to amyloid-beta stimulation of cultured human retinal pigment epithelial cells. Invest Ophthalmol Vis Sci. 2010;51(2):1151–63.
141. Liu RT, Gao J, Cao S, Sandhu N, Cui JZ, Chou CL, et al. Inflammatory mediators induced by amyloid-beta in the retina and RPE in vivo: implications for inflammasome activation in age-related macular degeneration. Invest Ophthalmol Vis Sci. 2013;54(3):2225–37.
142. Chen L, Bai Y, Zhao M, Jiang Y. TLR4 inhibitor attenuates amyloid-beta-induced angiogenic and inflammatory factors in ARPE-19 cells: implications for age-related macular degeneration. Mol Med Rep. 2016;13(4):3249–56.
143. Arimura N, Ki-i Y, Hashiguchi T, Kawahara K, Biswas KK, Nakamura M, et al. Intraocular expression and release of high-mobility group box 1 protein in retinal detachment. Lab Investig. 2009;89(3):278–89.
144. Chen XL, Zhang XD, Li YY, Chen XM, Tang DR, Ran RJ. Involvement of HMGB1 mediated signalling pathway in diabetic retinopathy: evidence from type 2 diabetic rats and ARPE-19 cells under diabetic condition. Br J Ophthalmol. 2013;97(12):1598–603.
145. Murakami Y, Matsumoto H, Roh M, Giani A, Kataoka K, Morizane Y, et al. Programmed necrosis, not apoptosis, is a key mediator of cell loss and DAMP-mediated inflammation in dsRNA-induced retinal degeneration. Cell Death Differ. 2014;21(2):270–7.
146. Wornle M, Merkle M, Wolf A, Ribeiro A, Himmelein S, Kernt M, et al. Inhibition of TLR3-mediated proinflammatory effects by alkylphosphocholines in human retinal pigment epithelial cells. Invest Ophthalmol Vis Sci. 2011;52(9):6536–44.
147. Zhang YF, Wei W, Li L, Tu G, Zhang Y, Yang J, et al. Sirt1 and HMGB1 regulate the AGE-induced pro-inflammatory cytokines in human retinal cells. Clin Lab. 2015;61(8):999–1008.
148. Xu WQ, Wang YS. The role of Toll-like receptors in retinal ischemic diseases. Int J Ophthalmol. 2016;9(9):1343–51.
149. Kawano H, Ito T, Yamada S, Hashiguchi T, Maruyama I, Hisatomi T, et al. Toxic effects of extracellular histones and their neutralization by vitreous in retinal detachment. Lab Investig. 2014;94(5):569–85.
150. Lueck K, Wasmuth S, Williams J, Hughes TR, Morgan BP, Lommatzsch A, et al. Sub-lytic C5b-9 induces functional changes in retinal pigment epithelial cells consistent with age-related macular degeneration. Eye (Lond). 2011;25(8):1074–82.
151. Lueck K, Busch M, Moss SE, Greenwood J, Kasper M, Lommatzsch A, et al. Complement stimulates retinal pigment epithelial cells to undergo pro-inflammatory changes. Ophthalmic Res. 2015;54(4):195–203.
152. Losso JN, Truax RE, Richard G. Trans-resveratrol inhibits hyperglycemia-induced inflammation and connexin downregulation in retinal pigment epithelial cells. J Agric Food Chem. 2010;58(14):8246–52.
153. Zhang J, Zhao J, Bai Y, Huang L, Yu W, Li X. Effects of p75 neurotrophin receptor on regulating hypoxia-induced angiogenic factors in retinal pigment epithelial cells. Mol Cell Biochem. 2015;398(1–2):123–34.
154. Dik WA, Virakul S, van Steensel L. Current perspectives on the role of orbital fibroblasts in the pathogenesis of Graves' ophthalmopathy. Exp Eye Res. 2016;142:83–91.
155. Elner SG, Elner VM, Pavilack MA, Todd RF 3rd, Mayo-Bond L, Franklin WA, et al. Modulation and function of intercellular adhesion molecule-1 (CD54) on human retinal pigment epithelial cells. Lab Investig. 1992;66(2):200–11.
156. Liversidge J, Sewell HF, Forrester JV. Interactions between lymphocytes and cells of the blood-retina barrier: mechanisms of T lymphocyte adhesion to human retinal capillary endothelial cells and retinal pigment epithelial cells in vitro. Immunology. 1990;71(3):390–6.
157. Mesri M, Liversidge J, Forrester JV. ICAM-1/LFA-1 interactions in T-lymphocyte activation and adhesion to cells of the blood-retina barrier in the rat. Immunology. 1994;83(1):52–7.
158. Devine L, Lightman S, Greenwood J. Lymphocyte migration across the anterior and posterior blood-retinal barrier in vitro. Cell Immunol. 1996;168(2):267–75.
159. Devine L, Lightman SL, Greenwood J. Role of LFA-1, ICAM-1, VLA-4 and VCAM-1 in lymphocyte migration across retinal pigment epithelial monolayers in vitro. Immunology. 1996;88(3):456–62.
160. Yoshida A, Elner SG, Bian ZM, Kunkel SL, Lukacs NW, Elner VM. Thrombin regulates chemokine induction during human retinal pigment epithelial cell/monocyte interaction. Am J Pathol. 2001;159(3):1171–80.
161. Kobayashi Y, Yoshida S, Nakama T, Zhou Y, Ishikawa K, Arita R, et al. Overexpression of CD163 in vitreous and fibrovascular membranes of patients with proliferative diabetic retinopathy: possible involvement of periostin. Br J Ophthalmol. 2015;99(4):451–6.
162. Braga TT, Agudelo JS, Camara NO. Macrophages during the fibrotic process: M2 as friend and foe. Front Immunol. 2015;6:602.
163. Abu El-Asrar AM, Struyf S, Van Damme J, Geboes K. Circulating fibrocytes contribute to the myofibroblast population in proliferative vitreoretinopathy epiretinal membranes. Br J Ophthalmol. 2008;92(5):699–704.

164. Abu El-Asrar AM, De Hertogh G, van den Eynde K, Alam K, Van Raemdonck K, Opdenakker G, et al. Myofibroblasts in proliferative diabetic retinopathy can originate from infiltrating fibrocytes and through endothelial-to-mesenchymal transition (EndoMT). Exp Eye Res. 2015;132:179–89.
165. Tamaki K, Usui-Ouchi A, Murakami A, Ebihara N. Fibrocytes and fibrovascular membrane formation in proliferative diabetic retinopathy. Invest Ophthalmol Vis Sci. 2016;57(11):4999–5005.
166. Castellon R, Hamdi HK, Sacerio I, Aoki AM, Kenney MC, Ljubimov AV. Effects of angiogenic growth factor combinations on retinal endothelial cells. Exp Eye Res. 2002;74(4):523–35.
167. Jo N, Mailhos C, Ju M, Cheung E, Bradley J, Nishijima K, et al. Inhibition of platelet-derived growth factor B signaling enhances the efficacy of anti-vascular endothelial growth factor therapy in multiple models of ocular neovascularization. Am J Pathol. 2006;168(6):2036–53.
168. Oshima Y, Oshima S, Nambu H, Kachi S, Hackett SF, Melia M, et al. Increased expression of VEGF in retinal pigmented epithelial cells is not sufficient to cause choroidal neovascularization. J Cell Physiol. 2004;201(3):393–400.
169. Kvanta A, Algvere PV, Berglin L, Seregard S. Subfoveal fibrovascular membranes in age-related macular degeneration express vascular endothelial growth factor. Invest Ophthalmol Vis Sci. 1996;37(9):1929–34.
170. Lopez PF, Sippy BD, Lambert HM, Thach AB, Hinton DR. Transdifferentiated retinal pigment epithelial cells are immunoreactive for vascular endothelial growth factor in surgically excised age-related macular degeneration-related choroidal neovascular membranes. Invest Ophthalmol Vis Sci. 1996;37(5):855–68.
171. Geisen P, McColm JR, Hartnett ME. Choroidal endothelial cells transmigrate across the retinal pigment epithelium but do not proliferate in response to soluble vascular endothelial growth factor. Exp Eye Res. 2006;82(4):608–19.
172. Blaauwgeers HG, Holtkamp GM, Rutten H, Witmer AN, Koolwijk P, Partanen TA, et al. Polarized vascular endothelial growth factor secretion by human retinal pigment epithelium and localization of vascular endothelial growth factor receptors on the inner choriocapillaris. Evidence for a trophic paracrine relation. Am J Pathol. 1999;155(2):421–8.
173. Young TA, Wang H, Munk S, Hammoudi DS, Young DS, Mandelcorn MS, et al. Vascular endothelial growth factor expression and secretion by retinal pigment epithelial cells in high glucose and hypoxia is protein kinase C-dependent. Exp Eye Res. 2005;80(5):651–62.
174. Kernt M, Thiele S, Liegl RG, Kernt B, Eibl K, Haritoglou C, et al. Axitinib modulates hypoxia-induced blood-retina barrier permeability and expression of growth factors. Growth Factors. 2012;30(1):49–61.
175. Zheng F, Jang WC, Fung FK, Lo AC, Wong IY. Up-regulation of ENO1 by HIF-1alpha in retinal pigment epithelial cells after hypoxic challenge is not involved in the regulation of VEGF secretion. PLoS One. 2016;11(2):e0147961.
176. Donovan K, Alekseev O, Qi X, Cho W, Azizkhan-Clifford J. O-GlcNAc modification of transcription factor Sp1 mediates hyperglycemia-induced VEGF-A upregulation in retinal cells. Invest Ophthalmol Vis Sci. 2014;55(12):7862–73.
177. Chang ML, Chiu CJ, Shang F, Taylor A. High glucose activates ChREBP-mediated HIF-1alpha and VEGF expression in human RPE cells under normoxia. Adv Exp Med Biol. 2014;801:609–21.
178. Cai Y, Li X, Wang YS, Shi YY, Ye Z, Yang GD, et al. Hyperglycemia promotes vasculogenesis in choroidal neovascularization in diabetic mice by stimulating VEGF and SDF-1 expression in retinal pigment epithelial cells. Exp Eye Res. 2014;123:87–96.
179. Layton CJ, Becker S, Osborne NN. The effect of insulin and glucose levels on retinal glial cell activation and pigment epithelium-derived fibroblast growth factor-2. Mol Vis. 2006;12:43–54.
180. Becerra SP, Fariss RN, Wu YQ, Montuenga LM, Wong P, Pfeffer BA. Pigment epithelium-derived factor in the monkey retinal pigment epithelium and interphotoreceptor matrix: apical secretion and distribution. Exp Eye Res. 2004;78(2):223–34.
181. Dawson DW, Volpert OV, Gillis P, Crawford SE, Xu H, Benedict W, et al. Pigment epithelium-derived factor: a potent inhibitor of angiogenesis. Science. 1999;285(5425):245–8.
182. Yao Y, Guan M, Zhao XQ, Huang YF. Downregulation of the pigment epithelium derived factor by hypoxia and elevated glucose concentration in cultured human retinal pigment epithelial cells. Zhonghua Yi Xue Za Zhi. 2003;83(22):1989–92.
183. Handa JT, Verzijl N, Matsunaga H, Aotaki-Keen A, Lutty GA, te Koppele JM, et al. Increase in the advanced glycation end product pentosidine in Bruch's membrane with age. Invest Ophthalmol Vis Sci. 1999;40(3):775–9.
184. Yoshida T, Ohno-Matsui K, Ichinose S, Sato T, Iwata N, Saido TC, et al. The potential role of amyloid beta in the pathogenesis of age-related macular degeneration. J Clin Invest. 2005;115(10):2793–800.
185. Kaarniranta K, Salminen A, Haapasalo A, Soininen H, Hiltunen M. Age-related macular degeneration (AMD): Alzheimer's disease in the eye? J Alzheimers Dis. 2011;24(4):615–31.
186. Ma W, Lee SE, Guo J, Qu W, Hudson BI, Schmidt AM, et al. RAGE ligand upregulation of VEGF secretion in ARPE-19 cells. Invest Ophthalmol Vis Sci. 2007;48(3):1355–61.
187. Pachydaki SI, Tari SR, Lee SE, Ma W, Tseng JJ, Sosunov AA, et al. Upregulation of RAGE and its ligands in proliferative retinal disease. Exp Eye Res. 2006;82(5):807–15.
188. Abu El-Asrar AM, Mohammad G, Nawaz MI, Siddiquei MM. High-mobility group box-1 modu-

lates the expression of inflammatory and angiogenic signaling pathways in diabetic retina. Curr Eye Res. 2015;40(11):1141–52.
189. Abu El-Asrar AM, Nawaz MI, De Hertogh G, Alam K, Siddiquei MM, Van den Eynde K, et al. S100A4 is upregulated in proliferative diabetic retinopathy and correlates with markers of angiogenesis and fibrogenesis. Mol Vis. 2014;20:1209–24.
190. El-Asrar AM, Nawaz MI, Kangave D, Geboes K, Ola MS, Ahmad S, et al. High-mobility group box-1 and biomarkers of inflammation in the vitreous from patients with proliferative diabetic retinopathy. Mol Vis. 2011;17:1829–38.
191. Fu D, Tian X. Effect of high mobility group box 1 on the human retinal pigment epithelial cell in high-glucose condition. Int J Clin Exp Med. 2015;8(10):17796–803.
192. Oh H, Takagi H, Takagi C, Suzuma K, Otani A, Ishida K, et al. The potential angiogenic role of macrophages in the formation of choroidal neovascular membranes. Invest Ophthalmol Vis Sci. 1999;40(9):1891–8.
193. Bian ZM, Elner SG, Elner VM. Thrombin-induced VEGF expression in human retinal pigment epithelial cells. Invest Ophthalmol Vis Sci. 2007;48(6):2738–46.
194. Nagineni CN, Kommineni VK, William A, Detrick B, Hooks JJ. Regulation of VEGF expression in human retinal cells by cytokines: implications for the role of inflammation in age-related macular degeneration. J Cell Physiol. 2012;227(1):116–26.
195. Nagineni CN, Samuel W, Nagineni S, Pardhasaradhi K, Wiggert B, Detrick B, et al. Transforming growth factor-beta induces expression of vascular endothelial growth factor in human retinal pigment epithelial cells: involvement of mitogen-activated protein kinases. J Cell Physiol. 2003;197(3):453–62.
196. Long Q, Cao X, Bian A, Li Y. C3a increases VEGF and decreases PEDF mRNA levels in human retinal pigment epithelial cells. Biomed Res Int. 2016;2016:6958752.
197. Hollborn M, Kohen L, Werschnik C, Tietz L, Wiedemann P, Bringmann A. Activated blood coagulation factor X (FXa) induces angiogenic growth factor expression in human retinal pigment epithelial cells. Invest Ophthalmol Vis Sci. 2012;53(9):5930–9.

Retinal Pigment Epithelium in Age-Related Macular Degeneration

9

Kai Kaarniranta, Antero Salminen, and Anu Kauppinen

RPE in the Pathology of AMD

Age-related macular degeneration (AMD) is a complex eye disease with multifactorial aetiology [1]. Its development is associated with aging, genetics and many cardiovascular risk factors. In AMD straight lines appear wavy, objects look smaller than normal, and colours are less bright. Peripheric vision usually remains unchanged. Rod and cone photoreceptors, retinal pigment epithelial cells (RPE) and the underlying choroid perform degenerative changes in AMD. Chronic oxidative stress, impaired protein clearance, mitochondrial dysfunction, endoplasmic reticulum stress and inflammation are strongly linked to AMD (Fig. 9.1; [2, 3]). Clinically, RPE mottling and drusen accumulation are the primary hallmarks of degenerative cellular processes in AMD (Fig. 9.2). The RPE degeneration secondarily leads to damage and cell death of photoreceptor cells and thereby to the loss of vision. Decreased RPE functionality usually occurs gradually during several years and decades with high individual variability. Lipofuscin accumulates into lysosomes and the extracellular protein/lipid deposits drusen between the basal lamina of the RPE and the inner collagenous layer of the Bruch's membrane (Fig. 9.1). Since both lipofuscin and drusen are highly autofluorescent, they are easy to detect with fundus imaging (Fig. 9.3). AMD is subdivided mainly to dry and wet forms with 80% and 20% prevalences, respectively [1]. Choroidal neovascularization sprouting into retina is a clinical sign of wet AMD. There are no effective therapy options for dry AMD, while intraocular injections of antibodies against vascular endothelial growth factor (VEGF) are used for wet AMD [4]. RPE cells have a central role in the production of VEGF and thereby in the development of wet AMD [5].

K. Kaarniranta (✉)
Department of Ophthalmology, Institute of Clinical Medicine, University of Eastern Finland, Kuopio, Finland

Department of Ophthalmology, Kuopio University Hospital, Kuopio, Finland
e-mail: kai.kaarniranta@uef.fi

A. Salminen
Department of Neurology, Institute of Clinical Medicine, University of Eastern Finland, Kuopio, Finland

A. Kauppinen
Faculty of Health Sciences, School of Pharmacy, University of Eastern Finland, Kuopio, Finland

Functions of RPE Cells

Highly pigmented RPE cells grow as a hexagonal monolayer that extends anteriorly from the optic disc to the *ora serrata* where neurosensory retina ends. From *ora serrata*, the RPE layer continues

A. K. Klettner, S. Dithmar (eds.), *Retinal Pigment Epithelium in Health and Disease*,
https://doi.org/10.1007/978-3-030-28384-1_9

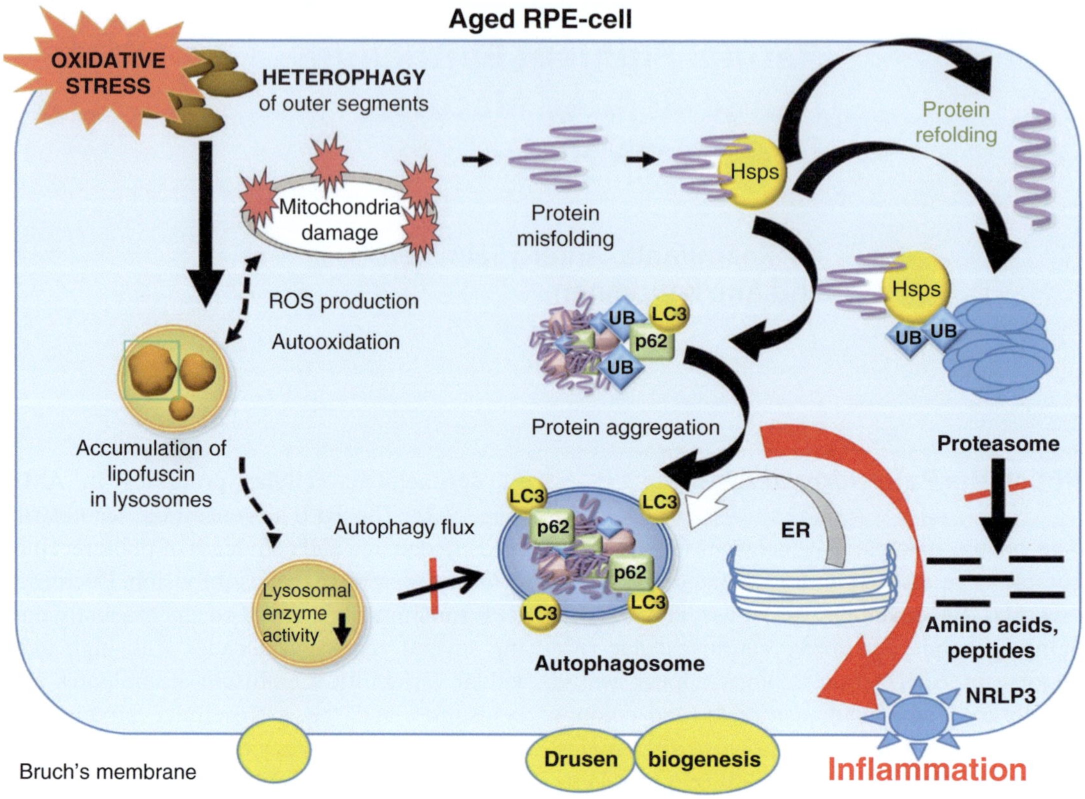

Fig. 9.1 Schematic presentation of retinal pigment epithelium (RPE)-derived age-related macular degeneration development. Constant oxidative stress induces protein misfolding and aggregation once the refolding capacity of heat shock proteins (Hsps) is exceeded. Decline in lysosomal clearance system including autophagy evokes lipofuscin accumulation, increases oxidative stress, mitochondrial damage, endoplasmic reticulum stress (ER), protein aggregation and NLRP3 inflammasome activation. Damaged and aggregated proteins undergo exocytosis process that is estimated to be involved in drusen biogenesis. Ubiquitin (Ub) regulates primarily proteasomal clearance, but is also involved autophagy due to its binding sites with autophagy receptors LC3 and p62

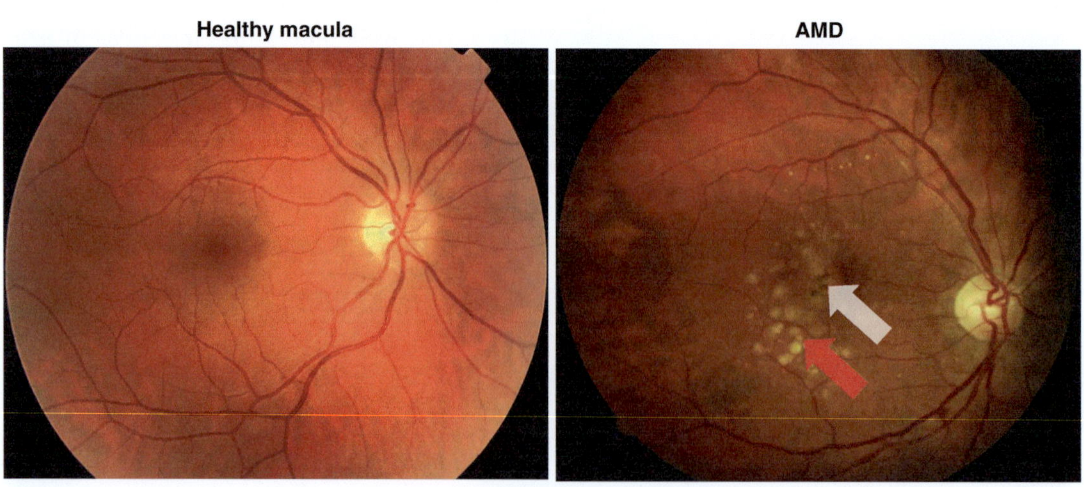

Fig. 9.2 Fundus photographs of healthy retina and dry age-related macular degeneration (AMD). Red arrow indicates drusen and white arrow retinal pigment epithelium mottling

Fundus autofluorescence in AMD

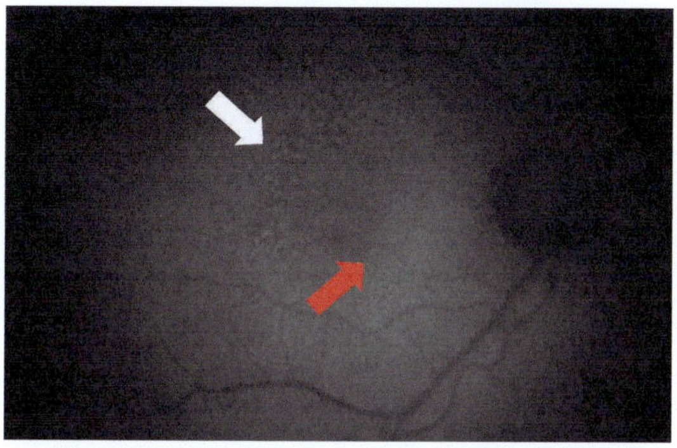

Fig. 9.3 Fundus autofluorescence photographs of dry age-related macular degeneration (AMD). Red arrow indicates autofluorescence coming mainly from lysosomal lipofuscin, while white arrow reveals drusen autofluorescence

as a membrane passing over the ciliary body and covers the posterior part of the iris. The apical side of the RPE faces the light-sensitive outer segments of rod and cone photoreceptors, while the basal membrane of the RPE is in contact with the fenestrated capillaries of the choroid. RPE cells have a symbiotic relationship with photoreceptors through the apical microvilli that surround the outer segments of the neural cells. The Bruch's membrane between the RPE layer and choroidal endothelial cells regulates the exchange of nutrients and signalling molecules. RPE cells regulate the vitamin A metabolism, heat exchange, ion balance, light absorption, production of various growth factors, and active transport of molecules in and out of the RPE [6]. RPE cells also function as nonprofessional phagocytes by degrading retinal outer segments [7]. Major functions of the RPE also include the establishment of the blood–retina barrier and maintenance of the immune privilege of the eye [6, 8]. In addition, RPE cells have a crucial role in the production of various growth factors including VEGF [9, 10].

Oxidative Stress in the RPE

The retina is the most prominent oxygen consumer among human tissues [11]. Its photo-oxidative activity is increased by the load of mitochondria-driven short-lived reactive oxygen species (ROS). They are produced due to diurnal phagocytosis of lipid-rich photoreceptor outer segments (Fig. 9.1; heterophagy), high retinal oxygen concentration, constant need of energy, and constant light exposure [2]. In addition to elevated ROS levels, lipid peroxidation may lead to the accumulation of long-lived 4-hydroxynonenal (HNE), malondialdehyde (MDA), and glycation end (AGE) products [12]. These lipid peroxidation end-products tend to concentrate around the macular area and evoke additional and chronic oxidative stress to RPE cells.

High cellular pigmentation is a central character of RPE. The pigmentation of postmitotic RPE cells mainly results from melanosomal melanin [13, 14], which acts as a ROS scavenger and thus protects the neural retina [15, 16]. The majority of light is absorbed via melanin that is located in the melanosomes of RPE cells [17]. In addition to melanin, photoreceptors and their pigments, such as carotenoids, lutein, zeaxanthin, and meso-zeaxanthin, absorb light [18]. All those macular pigments prevent auto-oxidation and the subsequent generation of ROS in RPE cells. Due to persistent oxidative stress, RPE cells also contain high amounts of anti-oxidative enzymes, such as superoxide dismutase and catalase [19].

During the aging process, RPE cells experience increased oxidative stress, altered melanin content, and decreased antioxidant production [20–23]. Elevated melanosomal oxygen consumption and ROS production contribute to increased oxidative stress, which in turn is estimated to occur due to auto-oxidative melanosomal lipofuscin accumulation onto the surface of melanosomes in RPE cells [20]. In young RPE, melanosomes and melanin are cytoprotective while in aged cells, lipofuscin shifts them into toxic organelles [22, 24, 25]. In contrast to melanosomal lipofuscin, lysosomal lipofuscin is better characterized and known to play a role in the pathology of AMD. Once oxidated polyunsaturated fatty acids (PUFAs) from retinal outer segments are not efficiently digested in the lysosomes of aged RPE cells, they start to accumulate in the form of lipofuscin (Fig. 9.1).

Lipofuscin is a chromophore, serving as the major RPE photosensitizer [26]. It contains vitamin A-derived fluorophores that have been shown to suppress mitochondrial functionality and increase the RPE cell damage [27, 28]. In line with melanolipofuscin, lysosomal lipofuscin absorbs high-energy photons, especially from blue light, and undergoes a variety of photochemical reactions involving ROS formation and secondary photochemical damage in the retina and RPE cells [26]. The accumulating free radicals also damage the lysosomes of RPE cells resulting in the further loss of their capacity to degrade the photoreceptor outer segment material, which again accelerates the lipofuscin formation [27, 28]. In addition to the ability of lipofuscin to decline the lysosomal enzyme activity and mitochondria respiration, it promotes the misfolding of intracellular proteins, which evokes additional oxidative stress in RPE cells.

It is widely accepted that RPE degeneration is associated with detrimental events in cellular functions, such as increased oxidative stress, decreased capacity to repair DNA, and protein damages (Fig. 9.1; [2, 29]). This then leads to protein misfolding and aggregation, and in certain circumstances even to cell death [30].

Proteasomes and Lysosomal Autophagy in AMD

Maintenance of the cellular balance of proteins or protein homeostasis, also referred to as proteostasis, comprises the regulation of protein synthesis, folding, location, and degradation [27, 28]. Molecular chaperones, ubiquitin-proteasome degradation, autophagy-lysosomal pathway, and endoplasmic reticulum (ER) are central systems to regulate the proteostasis in cells (Fig. 9.1). Heat shock proteins (Hsps) are molecular chaperones that have a capacity to refold misfolded proteins. This is a unique system in cells to repair damaged proteins. Heat shock proteins protect RPE cells against oxidative stress, but it seems that the protective mechanism become weakened during the AMD process [31, 32].

Once Hsps' repair capacity becomes exceeded, misfolded proteins have a tendency to gather into detrimental aggregates. Prior to protein aggregation, soluble proteins are tagged with small ubiquitin moieties that target damaged proteins to degradation in the large enzyme complexes called proteasomes. If proteasomes are not able to remove damaged proteins, and aggregation occurs, autophagy system tries to compensate the proteasomal response (Fig. 9.1; [27, 28]).

Autophagy, sometimes called self-eating, directs the degradation of unnecessary cellular molecules and organelles by delivering them to lysosomes where they become broken down by hydrolytic enzymes. Three basic types of autophagy are distinguished: macroautophagy, chaperone-mediated autophagy (CMA), and microautophagy [33]. Macroautophagy is mediated by the formation of autophagosome, a double-membrane vacuole that includes materials to be degraded. An autophagosome fuses with a lysosome, resulting in a structure called autolysosome, in which the final degradation of the cellular material occurs (Fig. 9.1). Microautophagy is conceptually the simplest mechanism of autophagy as it involves the direct uptake of cytoplasmic material thorough invaginated lysosomal membrane. Heat shock proteins Hsp90, Hsc70, or Hsp40 regulate the CMA process. The role of microautophagy or CMA in AMD is little known. Macroautophagy is considered as the major autophagic pathway and has been the most extensively studied in AMD research. It involves combined activity of autophagosomes and lysosomes where the hydrolysis by lysosomal enzymes is supported by several autophagy-related proteins (Atgs) [34]. In addition to basal regulation, autophagy is a host defence response to stress. The autophagic process is mainly regulated via the mechanistic target of rapamysin (mTOR) and adenosine monophosphatekinase (AMPK)-controlled signaling. Both of them are responsible for monitoring the nutritional status of the cell. Oxidative stress activates via AMPK host defence autophagy [35, 36].

There is mounting evidence showing that decreased autophagy in RPE cells is associated with the development of AMD [37–39]. One indication of that is the upregulation of the autophagy receptor SQSTM1/p62, a protein shuttling between autophagy and proteasome-mediated proteolysis, and clearly present in the macula of AMD donor samples [39]. Circulating autoantibodies in AMD recognize human macular tissue antigens implicated in autophagy [40]. Moreover, autophagy proteins, autophagosomes, and autophagy flux are significantly reduced in tissue from human donor AMD eyes [38].

Cross-Talk Between Endoplasmic Reticulum, Mitochondria, and Lysosomes

Autophagosomes originate at the contact point of endoplasmic reticulum (ER) and mitochondria, called mitochondria-associated membranes (MAM) (Fig. 9.1; [41]). That forms one link between mitochondria and ER in the regulation of protein clearance in RPE cells [42]. ER is a large cellular organelle containing a machinery for protein production, post-translational modification, folding, and secretion to extracellular space via the Golgi apparatus processing [41]. Moreover, the ER participates in drug detoxification, and regulates calcium balance, carbohydrate metabolism, and lipid biosynthesis. ER is rich of heat shock proteins that control the protein folding with calcium [43]. Oxidative stress and excessive ROS production in mitochondria result in the calcium efflux from the ER and the formation of misfolded protein aggregates. In order to maintain proteostasis and cellular functionality, the ER activates an adaptive quality control system, which is called the unfolded protein response (UPR). The UPR is initiated by three independent transmembrane stress transducers; (1) inositol-requiring kinase-1 (IRE1), (2) RNA-activated protein kinase-like ER kinase (PERK), and (3) activating transcription factor-6 (ATF6). The UPR activation evokes increased levels of ER-derived heat shock proteins, such as glucose-regulated protein-78 (GRP78), that prevent protein aggregation by refolding of misfolded proteins. However, prolonged and excessive stress will induce caspase activation, mitochondrial dysfunction, and cell death [30].

Mitochondrial dysfunction for excessive ROS and DNA damage may lead to mitophagy, which is the selective autophagy degradation of mitochondria [27, 28, 35, 44]. Generally, this process involves the elimination of damaged and depolarized mitochondria via the PINK1-Parkin pathway that is regulated by SQSTM1/p62 and proteasomes [35]. Role of mitophagy in AMD is little known. However, dysfunctional proteasomal and autophagy clearance systems, excessive ROS production by damaged mitochondria, and ER stress induce inflammation in AMD (Fig. 9.1; [38, 39, 43, 45, 46]).

Compromized Functionality of Lysosomes Predisposes RPE Cells to Inflammasome Activation

The activation of NLRP3 inflammasome has been associated with aged RPE and the pathogenesis of AMD (Fig. 9.1; [3, 47, 48]). NLRP3 is an intracellular pattern recognition receptor (PRR) that forms a large protein complex upon a two-phase activation process. In the priming phase, a signal activating the transcription factor nuclear factor kappa B (NF-κB) e.g. through Toll-like receptors (TLRs) or cytokine receptors results in the production of NLRP3 protein as well as the pro-forms of inflammatory cytokines IL-1β and IL-18 [49, 50]. The second signal becomes recognized by NLRP3 that gets activated and initiates the assembly of an inflammasome where a small adaptor protein, apoptosis-associated speck-like protein containing a CARD (ASC), connects NLRP3 to the executing enzyme, caspase-1. Activated caspase-1 cleaves IL-1β and IL-18 into their mature forms that can be secreted out of the cell [51, 52]. Caspase-1 activation is also capable of driving cell death called pyroptosis, which probably contributes also to the RPE atrophy [47]. For example, blue light-induced oxidative stress in lipofuscin-loaded RPE cells resulted in apoptotic cell death until the cells received a priming signal for the inflammasome activation [53]. A pre-treatment of RPE cells with IL-1α, complement component C5a, or conditioned medium of pyroptotic cells, promoted lipofuscin-mediated photo-oxidative stress to switch the cell death mechanism from apoptosis to pyroptosis along with the inflammasome activation and IL-1β release [53].

NLRP3 senses numerous activators ranging from biological and chemical to physical and particulate stressors [54]. Lysosomal rupture [55–57] as well as the major lipofuscin fluorophore N-retinylidene-N-retinylethanolamine (A2E; [58]) are known to activate the NLRP3 inflammasome. Similarly, dysfunctionality of proteasomes and/or autophagy along with the accumulating waste material induced the inflammasome signaling in human RPE cells [59, 60]. It has been suggested that insufficient intracellular clearance forces RPE cells to exocytose the waste material, which could then participate the formation of drusen, another type of deposits found as the clinical marks of AMD (Fig. 9.1; [61, 62]). Drusen material isolated from AMD patients [63] as well as its components, such as amyloid β (Aβ; [64–66]) and complement components [63, 66], are also well-known activators of inflammasome signaling in RPE cells or activated macrophages in the retina of dry AMD model mice. C1Q-mediated inflammasome activation was observed to result from the release of cathepsin B from lysosomes to the cytosol [63]. Excessive complement activity plays a role in the pathogenesis of AMD especially through the deficiency the complement factor H (CFH) that normally inhibits the complement cascade [67–70]. Also deficiency in pentraxin 3 (PTX3), an upstream regulator of CFH, has been linked to increased inflammasome activation in RPE cells [65].

Oxidative Stress Drives and Mediates Inflammasome Activation in the RPE

The activation of NLRP3 differs from that of many traditional PRRs that recognize evolutionarily conserved structures in their ligands. The NLRP3 activation is more complex and in many cases an indirect process. Cathepsin B escaping from lysosomes to the cytosol along with potassium efflux and oxidative stress comprise the three major models suggested to promote the NLRP3 activation [71]. Those events also overlap and contribute to each other, making it challenging to define the ultimate activating mechanism. For example, both oxidative stress [72, 73] and potassium efflux [74] have been suggested to function as the final activator for several independent activating factors.

Oxidative stress can contribute both to priming and the activation of AMD-related inflammasome signaling. Reactive oxygen species damage cellular macromolecules, such as proteins, lipids, and DNA. The oxidative stress-induced protein modification carboxyethylpyrrole (CEP) primed macrophages for the inflammasome activation with drusen components [63], whereas the lipid peroxidation end product 4-hydroxynonenal provided the activating signal in LPS-primed human RPE cells [75]. HNE and another lipid peroxidation end product malondealdehyde (MDA) have also been used experimentally to stabilize isolated porcine photoreceptor outer segments (POS) against autophagy for creating lipofuscin-loaded RPE cells [76]. In another study, the uptake of oxidized but not native lipoprotein activated the NLRP3 inflammasome in human RPE cells [77]. Oxidative stress also reduces the expression of DICER1, a cytoplasmic RNase III-type endoribonuclease responsible for cleaving *Alu* RNA into non-toxic fragments [78, 79]. In addition to DICER1 loss, iron accumulation is another AMD-related event resulting in the increased levels of *Alu* RNA [80]. *Alu* RNA can both prime and activate NLRP3 and it also induces mitochondrial ROS production in human RPE cells [81]. Besides the probable role of oxidative stress, the ATP receptor P_2X_7 has been observed important in *Alu* RNA-induced retinal degeneration [82], alluding that changes in ionic balance may neither be excluded in this process [83].

Zhou et al. showed that autophagy/mitophagy decline activates NLRP3 through mitochondria-derived ROS production in macrophages [84]. Similar findings were observed also in another study where ammonium pyrrolidinedithiocarbamate (APDC) prevented the inflammasome signaling in addition to a mitochondrial ROS scavenger, suggesting that NADPH oxidase may also participate the ROS-mediated inflammasome activation in RPE cells with dysfunctional intracellular clearance (Piippo et al. unpublished data). In any case, the role of dysfunctional mitochondria is prominent in aged RPE. In addition to increased ROS release and reduced energy production, mitochondrial (mt)DNA functions as a danger factor when released from mitochondria to the cytosol. NLRP3 inflammasome activation can promote the relocation of mtDNA [85], and oxidized mtDNA is further capable of activating NLRP3 by direct contact with the receptor [86]. In human RPE cells, mtDNA primed NLRP3 along with the induction of other pro-inflammatory cytokines, such as IL-6 and IL-8 [87]. AMD patients with the high-risk allele for CFH were shown also to possess significantly higher mtDNA damage when compared to subjects having wild-type genes [27, 28]. AMD retinas have also been shown to contain higher levels of more oxidized mtDNA and more single nucleotide polymorphism (SNPs) when compared to age-matched controls [88].

Interestingly, MAMs have been shown to provide a platform also to the inflammasome activation [84, 89]. In macrophages upon the inflammasome activation, NLRP3 translocated to MAMs and attracted also ASC there [84]. The idea of MAMs for bringing mitochondria, ER, autophagy, and inflammasomes into very close contact is attractive in AMD but more studies on RPE cells are needed on this topic.

Conclusions

RPE degeneration is one of the primary clinical sign in AMD development. It has been known for a long time that oxidative stress, protein aggregation and inflammation coincide with AMD pathogenesis. Recent findings indicate that lysosomal autophagy has a key role in the suppression of oxidative stress induced protein aggregation and inflammasome mediated inflammation in RPE cells. Currently, there are no effective therapies for treatment of dry AMD, while different formulations of intravitreal anti-VEGF are increasing for wet AMD treatment. All clinical trials that have targeted to suppress inflammation in AMD have been failed. Since AMD is complex disease, drug development will be challenging especially taking account of personalized medicine demands. Based on the existing data, RPE at a cellular level is a central therapy target to develop novel AMD treatments. The prevention of protein aggregation and acceleration of clearance might have an important place in the slowing of AMD progression.

References

1. Kaarniranta K, Sinha D, Blasiak J, Kauppinen A, Vereb Z, Salminen A, Boulton ME, Petrovski G. Autophagy and heterophagy dysregulation leads to retinal pigment epithelium dysfunction and development of age-related macular degeneration. Autophagy. 2013;9:973–84.
2. Blasiak J, Petrovski G, Veréb Z, Facskó A, Kaarniranta K. Oxidative stress, hypoxia, and autophagy in the neovascular processes of age-related macular degeneration. Biomed Res Int. 2014;2014:768026.
3. Kauppinen A, Paterno JJ, Blasiak J, Salminen A, Kaarniranta K. Inflammation and its role in age-related macular degeneration. Cell Mol Life Sci. 2016;73:1765–86.
4. Kaarniranta K, Xu H, Kauppinen A. Mechanistical retinal drug targets and challenges. Adv Drug Deliv Rev. 2018;126:177–84.
5. Klettner A, Kauppinen A, Blasiak J, Roider J, Salminen A, Kaarniranta K. Cellular and molecular mechanisms of age-related macular degeneration: from impaired autophagy to neovascularization. Int J Biochem Cell Biol. 2013;45:1457–67.
6. Strauss O. The retinal pigment epithelium in visual function. Physiol Rev. 2005;85:845–81.
7. Szatmári-Tóth M, Kristóf E, Veréb Z, Akhtar S, Facskó A, Fésüs L, Kauppinen A, Kaarniranta K, Petrovski G. Clearance of autophagy-associated dying retinal pigment epithelial cells—a possible source for inflammation in age-related macular degeneration. Cell Death Dis. 2016;7:e2367.
8. Chen M, Xu H. Parainflammation, chronic inflammation, and age-related macular degeneration. J Leukoc Biol. 2015;98:713–25.
9. Klettner A, Kaya L, Flach J, Lassen J, Treumer F, Roider J. Basal and apical regulation of VEGF-A and placenta growth factor in the RPE/choroid and primary RPE. Mol Vis. 2015;21:736–48.
10. Klettner A, Roider J. Constitutive and oxidative-stress-induced expression of VEGF in the RPE are differently regulated by different mitogen-activated protein kinases. Graefes Arch Clin Exp Ophthalmol. 2009;247:1487–92.
11. Yu DY, Cringle SJ. Oxygen distribution and consumption within the retina in vascularised and avascular retinas and in animal models of retinal disease. Prog Retin Eye Res. 2001;20:175–208.

12. Schutt F, Bergmann M, Holz FG, Kopitz J. Proteins modified by malondialdehyde, 4-hydroxynonenal, or advanced glycation end products in lipofuscin of human retinal pigment epithelium. Invest Ophthalmol Vis Sci. 2003;44:3663–8.
13. Juuti-Uusitalo K, Koskela A, Kivinen N, Viiri J, Hyttinen JMT, Reinisalo M, Koistinen A, Uusitalo H, Sinha D, Skottman H, Kaarniranta K. Autophagy regulates proteasome inhibitor-induced pigmentation in human embryonic stem cell-derived retinal pigment epithelial cells. Int J Mol Sci. 2017;18(5):E1089.
14. Simon JD, Hong L, Peles DN. Insights into melanosomes and melanin from some interesting spatial and temporal properties. J Phys Chem B. 2008;112:13201–17.
15. Peters S, Lamah T, Kokkinou D, Bartz-Schmidt KU, Schraermeyer U. Melanin protects choroidal blood vessels against light toxicity. Z Naturforsch. 2006;61:427–33.
16. Wang Z, Dillon J, Gaillard ER. Antioxidant properties of melanin in retinal pigment epithelial cells. Photochem Photobiol. 2006;82:474–9.
17. Schraermeyer U, Heimann K. Current understanding on the role of retinal pigment epithelium and its pigmentation. Pigment Cell Res. 1999;12:219–36.
18. Landrum JT, Bone RA. Lutein, zeaxanthin, and the macular pigment. Arch Biochem Biophys. 2001;385:28–40.
19. Tokarz P, Kaarniranta K, Blasiak J. Role of antioxidant enzymes and small molecular weight antioxidants in the pathogenesis of age-related macular degeneration (AMD). Biogerontology. 2013;14:461–82.
20. Biesemeier A, Yoeruek E, Eibl O, Schraermeyer U. Iron accumulation in Bruch's membrane and melanosomes of donor eyes with age-related macular degeneration. Exp Eye Res. 2015;137:39–49.
21. He Y, Tombran-Tink J. Mitochondrial decay and impairment of antioxidant defenses in aging RPE cells. Adv Exp Med Biol. 2010;664:165–83.
22. Rozankowski B, Burke JM, Boulton ME, Sarna T, Rozanowska M. Human RPE melanosomes protect from photosensitized and iron-mediated oxidation but become pro-oxidant in the presence of iron upon photodegradation. Invest Ophthalmol Vis Sci. 2008;49:2838–47.
23. Sarna T, Burke JM, Korytowski W, Rózanowska M, Skumatz CM, Zareba A, Zareba M. Loss ofmelanin from human RPE with aging: possible role of melanin photooxidation. Exp Eye Res. 2003;76:89–98.
24. Warburton S, Davis WE, Southwick K, Xin H, Woolley AT, Burton GF, Thulin CD. Proteomic and phototoxic characterization of melanolipofuscin: correlation to disease and model for its origin. Mol Vis. 2007;13:318–29.
25. Wihlmark U, Wrigstad A, Roberg K, Nilsson SE, Brunk UT. Lipofuscin accumulation in cultured retinal pigment epithelial cells causes enhanced sensitivity to blue light irradiation. Free Radic Biol Med. 1997;22:1229–34.
26. Dontsov AE, Glickman RD, Ostrovsky MA. Retinal pigment epithelium pigment granules stimulate the photo-oxidation of unsaturated fatty acids. Free Radic Biol Med. 1999;26:1436–46.
27. Ferrington DA, Kapphahn RJ, Leary MM, Atilano SR, Terluk MR, Karunadharma P, Chen GK, Ratnapriya R, Swaroop A, Montezuma SR, Kenney MC. Increased retinal mtDNA damage in the CFH variant associated with age-related macular degeneration. Exp Eye Res. 2016;145:269–77.
28. Ferrington DA, Sinha D, Kaarniranta K. Defects in retinal pigment epithelial cell proteolysis and the pathology associated with age-related macular degeneration. Prog Retin Eye Res. 2016;51:69–89.
29. Klettner A. Oxidative stress induced cellular signalling in RPE cells. Front Biosci (Schol Ed). 2012;4:392–411.
30. Kaarniranta K, Tokarz P, Koskela A, Patero J, Blasiak J. Autophagy regulates death of retinal pigment epithelium cells in age-related macular degeneration. Cell Biol Toxicol. 2017;33:113–28.
31. Decanini A, Nordgaard CL, Feng X, Ferrington DA, Olsen TW. Changes in select redox proteins of the retinal pigment epithelium in age-related macular degeneration. Am J Ophthalmol. 2007;143:607–15.
32. Subrizi A, Toropainen E, Ramsay E, Airaksinen AJ, Kaarniranta K, Urtti A. Oxidative stress protection by exogenous delivery of rhHsp70 chaperone to the retinal pigment epithelium (RPE), a possible therapeutic strategy against RPE degeneration. Pharm Res. 2015;32:211–21.
33. Galluzzi L, Bravo-San Pedro JM, Levine B, Green DR, Kroemer G. Pharmacological modulation of autophagy: therapeutic potential and persisting obstacles. Nat Rev Drug Discov. 2017;16(7):487–511. https://doi.org/10.1038/nrd.2017.22.
34. Tsukada M, Ohsumi Y. Isolation and characterization of autophagy-defective mutants of Saccharomyces cerevisiae. FEBS Lett. 1993;333:169–74.
35. Boya P, Esteban-Martínez L, Serrano-Puebla A, Gómez-Sintes R, Villarejo-Zori B. Autophagy in the eye: development, degeneration, and aging. Prog Retin Eye Res. 2016;55:206–45.
36. Hyttinen JM, Petrovski G, Salminen A, Kaarniranta K. 5′-Adenosine monophosphate-activated protein kinase—mammalian target of rapamycin axis as therapeutic target for age-related macular degeneration. Rejuvenation Res. 2011;14:651–60.
37. Kim JY, Zhao H, Martinez J, Doggett TA, Kolesnikov AV, Tang PH, Ablonczy Z, Chan CC, Zhou Z, Green DR, Ferguson TA. Noncanonical autophagy promotes the visual cycle. Cell. 2013;154:365–76.
38. Mitter SK, Song C, Qi X, Mao H, Rao H, Akin D, Lewin A, Grant M, Dunn W Jr, Ding J, Bowes Rickman C, Boulton M. Dysregulated autophagy in the RPE is associated with increased susceptibility to oxidative stress and AMD. Autophagy. 2014;10:1989–2005.
39. Viiri J, Amadio M, Marchesi N, Hyttinen JM, Kivinen N, Sironen R, Rilla K, Akhtar S, Provenzani A, D'Agostino VG, Govoni S, Pascale A, Agostini H, Petrovski G, Salminen A, Kaarniranta K. Autophagy activation clears ELAVL1/HuR-mediated accumula-

tion of SQSTM1/p62 during proteasomal inhibition in human retinal pigment epithelial cells. PLoS One. 2013;8(7):e69563.

40. Iannaccone A, Giorgianni F, New DD, Hollingsworth TJ, Umfress A, Alhatem AH, Neeli I, Lenchik NI, Jennings BJ, Calzada JI, Satterfield S, Mathews D, Diaz RI, Harris T, Johnson KC, Charles S, Kritchevsky SB, Gerling IC, Beranova-Giorgianni S, Radic MZ, Health ABC study. Circulating autoantibodies in age-related macular degeneration recognize human macular tissue antigens implicated in autophagy, immunomodulation, and protection from oxidative stress and apoptosis. PLoS One. 2015;10:e0145323.
41. Nascimbeni AC, Giordano F, Dupont N, Grasso D, Vaccaro MI, Codogno P, Morel E. ER-plasma membrane contact sites contribute to autophagosome biogenesis by regulation of local PI3P synthesis. EMBO J. 2017;36(14):2018–33. https://doi.org/10.15252/embj.201797006. pii: e201797006.
42. Sreekumar PG, Hinton DR, Kannan R. Endoplasmic reticulum-mitochondrial crosstalk: a novel role for the mitochondrial peptide humanin. Neural Regen Res. 2017;12:35–8.
43. Salminen A, Kauppinen A, Hyttinen JM, Toropainen E, Kaarniranta K. Endoplasmic reticulum stress in age-related macular degeneration: trigger for neovascularization. Mol Med. 2010;16:535–42.
44. Lee SY, Oh JS, Rho JH, Jeong NY, Kwon YH, Jeong WJ, Ryu WY, Ahn HB, Park WC, Rho SH, Yoon YG, Jeong SY, Choi YH, Kim HY, Yoo YH. Retinal pigment epithelial cells undergoing mitotic catastrophe are vulnerable to autophagy inhibition. Cell Death Dis. 2014;5:e1303.
45. Kheitan S, Minuchehr Z, Soheili ZS. Exploring the cross talk between ER stress and inflammation in age-related macular degeneration. PLoS One. 2017;12:e0181667.
46. Terluk MR, Kapphahn RJ, Soukup LM, Gong H, Gallardo C, Montezuma SR, Ferrington DA. Investigating mitochondria as a target for treating age-related macular degeneration. J Neurosci. 2015;35:7304–11.
47. Celkova LS, Doyle L, Campbell M. NLRP3 inflammasome and pathobiology in AMD. J Clin Med. 2015;4:172–92.
48. Gao J, Liu RT, Cao S, Cui JZ, Wang A, To A, Matsubara JA. NLRP3 inflammasome: activation and regulation in age-related macular degeneration. Mediat Inflamm. 2015;2015:690243.
49. Bauernfeind F, Horvath GG, Stutz A, Alnemri ES, MacDonald K, Speert D, Fernandes-Alnemri T, Wu J, Monks BK, Fitzgerald KA, Hornung V, Latz E. Cutting edge: NF-kappaB activating pattern recognition and cytokine receptors license NLRP3 inflammasome activation by regulating NLRP3 expression. J Immunol. 2009;183:787–91.
50. Hornung V, Latz E. Critical functions of priming and lysosomal damage for NLRP3 activation. Eur J Immunol. 2010;40:620–3.
51. Martinon F, Gaide O, Petrilli V, Mayor A, Tschopp J. NALP inflammasomes: a central role in innate immunity. Semin Immunopathol. 2007;29:213–29.
52. Petrilli V, Dostert C, Muruve DA, Tschopp J. The inflammasome: a danger sensing complex triggering innate immunity. Curr Opin Immunol. 2007;19:615–22.
53. Brandstetter C, Patt J, Holz FG, Krohne U. Inflammasome priming increases retinal pigment epithelial cell susceptibility to lipofuscin phototoxicity by changing the cell death mechanism from apoptosis to pyroptosis. J Photochem Photobiol B. 2016;161:177–83.
54. Schroder K, Zhou R, Tschopp. The NLRP3 inflammasome: a sensor for metabolic danger? Science. 2010;327:296–300.
55. Mohr LK, Hoffmann AV, Brandstetter C, Holz FG, Krohne TU. Effects of inflammasome activation on secretion of inflammatory cytokines and vascular endothelial growth factor by retinal pigment epithelial cells. Invest Ophthalmol Vis Sci. 2015;56:6404–13.
56. Nebel C, Aslanidis A, Rashid K, Langmann T. Activated microglia trigger inflammasome activation and lysosomal destabilization in human RPE cells. Biochem Biophys Res Commun. 2017;484:681–6.
57. Tseng WA, Thein T, Kinnunen K, Lashkari K, Gregory MS, D'Amore PA, Ksander BR. NLRP3 inflammasome activation in retinal pigment epithelial cells by lysosomal destabilization: implications for age-related macular degeneration. Invest Ophthalmol Vis Sci. 2013;54:110–20.
58. Anderson OA, Finkelstein A, Shima DT. A2E induces IL-1ss production in retinal pigment epithelial cells via the NLRP3 inflammasome. PLos One. 2013;8:e67263.
59. Piippo N, Korkmaz A, Hytti M, Kinnunen K, Salminen A, Atalay M, Kaarniranta K, Kauppinen A. Decline in cellular clearance systems induces inflammasome signaling in human ARPE-19 cells. Biochim Biophys Acta. 2014;1843:3038–46.
60. Shi H, Zhang Z, Wang X, Li R, Hou W, Bi W, Zhang X. Inhibition of autophagy induces IL-1beta release from ARPE-19 cells via ROS mediated NLRP3 inflammasome activation under high glucose stress. Biochem Biophys Res Commun. 2015;463:1071–6.
61. Kinnunen K, Petrovski G, Moe MC, Berta A, Kaarniranta K. Molecular mechanisms of retinal pigment epithelium damage and development of age-related macular degeneration. Acta Ophthalmol. 2012;90:299–309.
62. Wang AL, Lukas TJ, Yuan M, Du N, Tso MO, Neufeld AH. Autophagy and exosomes in the aged retinal pigment epithelium: possible relevance to drusen formation and age-related macular degeneration. PLoS One. 2009;4:e4160.
63. Doyle SL, Campbell M, Ozaki E, Salomon RG, Mori A, Kenna PF, Farrar GJ, Kiang AS, Humphries MM, Lavelle EC, O'Neill LA, Hollyfield JG, Humphries P. NLRP3 has a protective role in age-related macular

degeneration through the induction of IL-18 by drusen components. Nat Med. 2012;18:791–8.
64. Liu RT, Gao J, Cao S, Sandhu N, Cui JZ, Chou CL, Fang E, Matsubara JA. Inflammatory mediators induced by amyloid-beta in the retina and RPE in vivo: implications for inflammasome activation in age-related macular degeneration. Invest Ophthalmol Vis Sci. 2013;54:2225–37.
65. Wang K, Yao Y, Zhu X, Zhang K, Zhou F, Zhu L. Amyloid beta induces NLRP3 inflammasome activation in retinal pigment epithelial cells via NADPH oxidase- and mitochondria-dependent ROS production. J Biochem Mol Toxicol. 2017;31. https://doi.org/10.1002/jbt.21887. Epub 2016 Dec 22.
66. Zhao T, Gao J, Van J, To E, Wang A, Cao S, Cui JZ, Guo JP, Lee M, McGeer PL, Matsubara JA. Age-related increases in amyloid beta and membrane attack complex: evidence of inflammasome activation in the rodent eye. J Neuroinflammation. 2015;12:121.
67. Bhutto IA, Baba T, Merges C, Juriasinghani V, McLeod DS, Lutty GA. C-reactive protein and complement factor H in aged human eyes and eyes with age-related macular degeneration. Br J Ophthalmol. 2011;95:1323–30.
68. Chen M, Forrester JV, Xu H. Synthesis of complement factor H by retinal pigment epithelial cells is down-regulated by oxidized photoreceptor outer segments. Exp Eye Res. 2007;84:635–45.
69. Holliday EG, Smith AV, Cornes BK, Buitendijk GH, Jensen RA, Sim X, Aspelund T, Aung T, Baird PN, Boerwinkle E, Cheng CY, van Duijn CM, Eiriksdottir G, Gudnason V, Harris T, Hewitt AW, Inouye M, Jonasson F, Klein BE, Launer L, Li X, Liew G, Lumley T, McElduff P, McKnight B, Mitchell P, Psaty BM, Rochtchina E, Rotter JI, Scott RJ, Tay W, Taylor K, Teo YY, Uitterlinden AG, Viswanathan A, Xie S, Wellcome Trust Case Control Consortium 2, Vingerling JR, Klaver CC, Tai ES, Siscovick D, Klein R, Cotch MF, Wong TY, Attia J, Wang JJ. Insights into the genetic architecture of early stage age-related macular degeneration: a genome-wide association study meta-analysis. PLoS One. 2013;8:e53830.
70. Johnson PT, Betts KE, Radeke MJ, Hageman GS, Anderson DH, Johnson LV. Individuals homozygous for the age-related macular degeneration risk-conferring variant of complement factor H have elevated levels of CRP in the choroid. Proc Natl Acad Sci U S A. 2006;103:17456–61.
71. Jin C, Flavell RA. Molecular mechanism of NLRP3 inflammasome activation. J Clin Immunol. 2010;30:628–31.
72. Martinon F. Signaling by ROS drives inflammasome activation. Eur J Immunol. 2010;40:616–9.
73. Tschopp J, Schroder K. NLRP3 inflammasome activation: the convergence of multiple signalling pathways on ROS production? Nat Rev Immunol. 2010;10:210–5.
74. Munoz-Planillo R, Kuffa P, Martinez-Colon G, Smith BL, Rajendiran TM, Nunez G. K(+) efflux is the common trigger of NLRP3 inflammasome activation by bacterial toxins and particulate matter. Immunity. 2013;38:1142–53.
75. Kauppinen A, Niskanen H, Suuronen T, Kinnunen K, Salminen A, Kaarniranta K. Oxidative stress activates NLRP3 inflammasomes in ARPE-19 cells-implications for age-related macular degeneration (AMD). Immunol Lett. 2012;147:29–33.
76. Brandstetter C, Mohr LK, Latz E, Holz FG, Krohne TU. Light induces NLRP3 inflammasome activation in retinal pigment epithelial cells via lipofuscin-mediated photooxidative damage. J Mol Med (Berl). 2015;93:905–16.
77. Gnanaguru G, Choi AR, Amarnani D, D'Amore PA. Oxidized lipoprotein uptake through the CD36 receptor activates the NLRP3 inflammasome in human retinal pigment epithelial cells. Invest Ophthalmol Vis Sci. 2016;57:4704–12.
78. Bernstein E, Caudy AA, Hammond SM, Hannon GJ. Role for a bidentate ribonuclease in the initiation step of RNA interference. Nature. 2001;409:363–6.
79. Kaneko H, Dridi S, Tarallo V, Gelfand BD, Fowler BJ, Cho WG, Kleinman ME, Ponicsan SL, Hauswirth WW, Chiodo VA, Karikó K, Yoo JW, Lee DK, Hadziahmetovic M, Song Y, Misra S, Chaudhuri G, Buaas FW, Braun RE, Hinton DR, Zhang Q, Grossniklaus HE, Provis JM, Madigan MC, Milam AH, Justice NL, Albuquerque RJ, Blandford AD, Bogdanovich S, Hirano Y, Witta J, Fuchs E, Littman DR, Ambati BK, Rudin CM, Chong MM, Provost P, Kugel JF, Goodrich JA, Dunaief JL, Baffi JZ, Ambati J. DICER1 deficit induces Alu RNA toxicity in age-related macular degeneration. Nature. 2011;471:325–30.
80. Gelfand BD, Wright CB, Kim Y, Yasuma T, Yasuma R, Li S, Fowler BJ, Bastos-Carvalho A, Kerur N, Uittenbogaard A, Han YS, Lou D, Kleinman ME, McDonald WH, Núñez G, Georgel P, Dunaief JL, Ambati J. Iron toxicity in the retina requires alu RNA and the NLRP3 inflammasome. Cell Rep. 2015;11:1686–93.
81. Tarallo V, Hirano Y, Gelfand BD, Dridi S, Kerur N, Kim Y, Cho WG, Kaneko H, Fowler BJ, Bogdanovich S, Albuquerque RJ, Hauswirth WW, Chiodo VA, Kugel JF, Goodrich JA, Ponicsan SL, Chaudhuri G, Murphy MP, Dunaief JL, Ambati BK, Ogura Y, Yoo JW, Lee DK, Provost P, Hinton DR, Núñez G, Baffi JZ, Kleinman ME, Ambati J. DICER1 loss and Alu RNA induce age-related macular degeneration via the NLRP3 inflammasome and MyD88. Cell. 2012;149:847–59.
82. Kerur N, Hirano Y, Tarallo V, Fowler BJ, Bastos-Carvalho A, Yasuma T, Yasuma R, Kim Y, Hinton DR, Kirschning CJ, Gelfand BD, Ambati J. TLR-independent and P2X7-dependent signaling mediate Alu RNA-induced NLRP3 inflammasome activation in geographic atrophy. Invest Ophthalmol Vis Sci. 2013;54:7395–401.
83. Mao X, Fang W, Liu Q. An emerging role of Alu RNA in geographic atrophy pathogenesis: the impli-

cation for novel therapeutic strategies. Discov Med. 2016;22:337–49.

84. Zhou R, Yazdi AS, Menu P, Tschopp J. A role for mitochondria in NLRP3 inflammasome activation. Nature. 2011;469:221–5.
85. Nakahira K, Haspel JA, Rathinam VA, Lee SJ, Dolinay T, Lam HC, Englert JA, Rabinovitch M, Cernadas M, Kim HP, Fitzgerald KA, Ryter SW, Choi AM. Autophagy proteins regulate innate immune responses by inhibiting the release of mitochondrial DNA mediated by the NALP3 inflammasome. Nat Immunol. 2011;12:222–30.
86. Shimada K, Crother TR, Karlin J, Dagvadorj J, Chiba N, Chen S, Ramanujan VK, Wolf AJ, Vergnes L, Ojcius DM, Rentsendorj A, Vargas M, Guerrero C, Wang Y, Fitzgerald KA, Underhill DM, Town T, Arditi M. Oxidized mitochondrial DNA activates the NLRP3 inflammasome during apoptosis. Immunity. 2012;36:401–14.
87. Dib B, Lin H, Maidana DE, Tian B, Miller JB, Bouzika B, Miller JW, Vavvas DG. Mitochondrial DNA has a pro-inflammatory role in AMD. Biochim Biophys Acta. 2015;1853:2897–906.
88. Udar N, Atilano SR, Memarzadeh M, Boyer DS, Chwa M, Lu S, Maguen B, Langberg J, Coskun P, Wallace DC, Nesburn AB, Khatibi N, Hertzog D, Le K, Hwang D, Kenney MC. Mitochondrial DNA haplogroups associated with age-related macular degeneration. Invest Ophthalmol Vis Sci. 2009;50:2966–74.
89. Thoudam T, Jeon JH, Ha CM, Lee IK. Role of mitochondria-associated endoplasmic reticulum membrane in inflammation-mediated metabolic diseases. Mediat Inflamm. 2016;2016:1851420.

10 Retinal Pigment Epithelium in Health and Disease: Maturation, Aging and Age-Related Macular Degeneration

Thomas Ach, Ioana-Sandra Tarau, and Christine A. Curcio

Introduction

Human retinal pigment epithelium (RPE) development starts early in embryogenesis. At birth, RPE cells already show pigmentation (melanosomes) and with further maturation a significant increase of other intracellular granule types (lipofuscin and melanolipofuscin) will lead to the characteristic (healthy) RPE phenotype: a cell monolayer embedded between the photoreceptor outer segments and Bruch membrane, filled with different types of granules.

Knowledge on the principles of RPE development is a necessary first step in order to separate aging processes and, henceforward, age-related changes. This chapter will summarize the current knowledge in RPE development. Furthermore, findings from recent systematic and unbiased histological studies emphasize normal age-related changes to discriminate diseased RPE in age-related macular degeneration (AMD).

T. Ach (✉) · I.-S. Tarau
Department of Ophthalmology, University Hospital Würzburg, Würzburg, Germany
e-mail: ach_t@ukw.de; tarau_i@ukw.de

C. A. Curcio
Department of Ophthalmology, University of Alabama at Birmingham, Birmingham, AL, USA
e-mail: christinecurcio@uabmc.edu

RPE Development

As a preliminary remark, most of our knowledge on RPE development arises from multiple studies in animal models which helped to elucidate molecules, proteins, and cells involved in these complex processes. These findings in molecules and proteins functions can serve as a basis for studies in human RPE development.

The evolution of the vertebrate eye starts in a region of the ventral forebrain by an evagination of the neuroepithelium towards the surface ectoderm. The distal optical vesicle, as a part of the "eye field", will develop into pigmented (iris, ciliary body, and RPE) and unpigmented (neuroretinal) structures of the eye [1], regulated by multiple eye field transcription factors, EFTFs, like Rx, Pax6, Six3, Six6, Lhx2, and others [2, 3].

Also, close relationship between ectoderm and optical vesicle leads to optic cup formation. RPE, though in developmental stage itself, is a required partner and has significant influence in further eye development (control of the closure of the optic fissure) and retinal differentiation [1, 4–9]. With the closure of the optic fissure, RPE covers the complete outer wall of the optic cup [1].

In the embryonic mouse, the development of the RPE starts as early as day 13, and few days later first pigmented granules (melanosomes) are visible [10]. At this time point, RPE cells also show epithelial character arranged in a monolayer. In humans, pigment granules are usually observed very early within the first weeks of foetal development [11].

A. K. Klettner, S. Dithmar (eds.), *Retinal Pigment Epithelium in Health and Disease*,
https://doi.org/10.1007/978-3-030-28384-1_10

For an optimal epithelial development several cell-cell interactions have been described: actin microfilament—intermediate filament and cell surface—cell surface connections [12–14].

RPE Differentiation

For agonistic and/or antagonistic properties on RPE differentiation an extensive number of intrinsic and extrinsic proteins and factors (inter alia retinoids, FGF/MAP kinase, FGF, notch signal, IGF-1, hedgehog, Sox2, Rx, Pax2, Pax6, Gas1, hedgehog, BMP) are necessary which originate from the adjacent tissue and extracellular matrix [1, 5, 15–29]. In addition, several signaling pathways maintain RPE differentiation.

Especially, two pathways seem to be important for RPE differentiation and pigmentation, and, therefore, impact on RPE phenotype: Wnt and Mitf pathways.

Wingless-Related Integration Site "Wnt"-Expression

Wnt/β-catenin signaling has major impact on the conversion of retinal progenitor cells into RPE and subsequent RPE differentiation in several animal models [28, 30, 31]. Wnt/β-catenin is regulated by Otx2 [28, 31–33], suppressed by Six3 [31, 33], while overstimulation of the Wnt/β-catenin pathway leads to RPE development of the whole optic vesicle [33–37]. β-catenin activation is also reported in epithelial–mesenchymal transitions (EMT) during embryogenesis and cancer progression [4, 34, 38], but also in RPE EMT, a process with clinical relevance in which RPE loses epithelial phenotype and exhibits migratory properties (e.g., in proliferative retinopathy) [12, 39–43].

Mitf (Microphthalmia Associated Transcription Factor)

Mitf [44] is important at the early stages of eye formation, especially in melanin-producing cells: for the transition from eye field into optic cup and for RPE cell transformation [5, 33, 45, 46]. In this context, Mitf activates several genes for RPE pigment differentiation, especially in melanosomes (inter alia tyrosinase and tyrosinase-related protein) [47–49]. Absence or loss of Mitf activity results in altered melanin/melanosome content and affected RPE pigmentation [4, 6, 9], and might also result in RPE transdifferentiation [6, 50]. Mitf activity itself is regulated by a number of proteins (e.g., Vsx2, FGF, Sox2, and Lhx2) [6, 51–53].

It is still under investigation at which time point the RPE differentiation process stops (and whether it stops at all, or can be re-initiated at a later time point). Histological studies hint that RPE differentiation is not finished at birth but might continue postnatally (e.g., spatial organization, pigmentation) [54–57].

RPE Proliferation and Transdifferentiation

It is believed that the mitotic ability of RPE cells decreases significantly with further development, in utero and postnatal. However, there is still ongoing debate whether RPE is capable of cell division under physiological circumstances or not. Kokkinopoulos et al. found that peripheral RPE cells show proliferative properties, distinguishable from central RPE in which proliferative behavior is considerably less [58]. A few reports indicate that some cells remain in a proliferative status throughout life. In early studies, human RPE cells were reported to be post-mitotic, non-dividing cells [56, 59]. However, in a study examining monkey RPE, Rapaport et al. [60] found 3H-thymidine-labeled RPE more than 200 days postnatal. This could be evidence that some (probably not all) post-mitotic RPE cells carry cell regenerating capabilities (mitotic stem or progenitor cells) under physiological conditions to maintain cell repair and regeneration [61, 62]. Similar effects can also be observed under pathologic conditions, e.g., after laser treatment and in cell culture experiments [63].

A related and distinctive feature of RPE cells is the presence of multinucleate cells which are common in rodents, but reported only sporadically in humans [59]. A recent systematic analysis of macular RPE cells provided evidence that multinucleated RPE cells are nearly completely absent at the human fovea, while perifovea showed around 10% multinucleated cells [64]. The differences may reflect the regional differences in photoreceptor topography [65] and the different needs of RPE cells in the photoreceptor supporting system.

Transdifferentiation (conversion of one differentiated cell type to another, with or without an intervening cell division) [66] is a phenomenon observable in RPE cells. Since mature RPE also has capabilities of retinal gene expression, there might exist (mostly unknown) mechanisms which control and suppress intrinsic RPE transdifferentiation in the healthy retina/RPE. In diseased retina/RPE, these protective and inhibitory effects might be repealed to initiate transdifferentiation cascades. Once transdifferentiation has started, a return to properties of native RPE-cell seems to be not possible. In age-related macular degeneration, dissociated RPE cells from the monolayer ("sloughed cells" [67]) have not only lost direct cell contact but also apical-basal polarity [68–70]. These cells have migratory capabilities and may migrate between basal laminar deposits and inner collagenous layer of Bruch's membrane ("subducted cells") or across the subretinal space and into the retina (see below, changes in diseased RPE).

RPE Postnatal and in Adolescence

A key feature of maturation of RPE cells is the accumulation of different intracellular granule types (melanosomes, lipofuscin, melanolipofuscin, Fig. 10.1).

Pre-melanosomes and melanosomes are generated in utero [11]. At birth, the human RPE contains only melanosomes. About 8% of the total cell volume is occupied by melanin in the first two decades of life, decreasing to 6% in the subsequent two decades and to 3.5% at age 60 and higher [54].

In a histological RPE study examining human donor eyes, Feeney reported precursors of lipofuscin and lipofuscin granules in the first decade [72]. She and others also provided evidence that a significant increase in lipofuscin accumulation occurs in adolescence, followed by a lesser increase between 20 and 40 years and a second significant increase after age 40 [72, 73]. Feeney was the first who reported number of granules per cell profile. Recent high resolution structured illumination autofluorescence microscopy and 3D electron microscopy studies showed that RPE cells contain hundreds (up to 500!) of granules (Fig. 10.1) [74, 75].

Granule content per cell differs not only by regional location (fovea vs. perifovea vs.

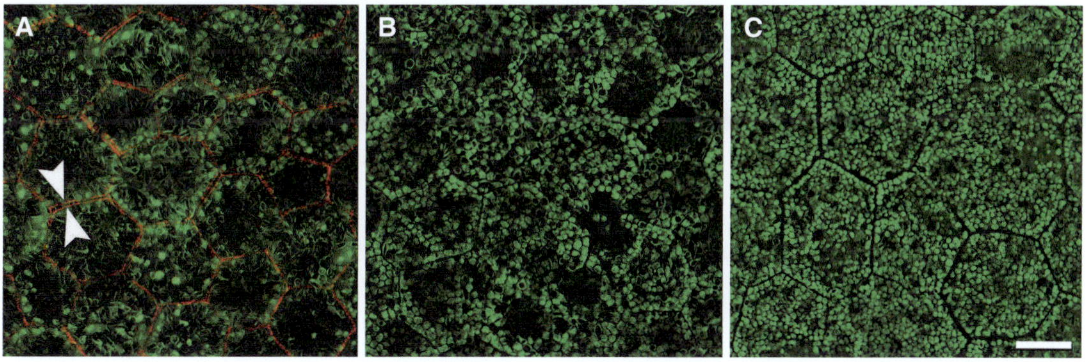

Fig. 10.1 RPE granule abundance depends on retinal location. Normal RPE granule distribution and F-actin cytoskeleton. High-resolution structured illumination microscopy enables delineation of individual intracellular autofluorescent lipofuscin and melanolipofuscin granules. Melanosomes, which are only minimally autofluorescent, are visible only by blocking signal from underlying autofluorescent granules, and non-autofluorescent cell nuclei create dark areas within the cells (**a** fovea; **b** perifovea). At near-periphery (out to 10-mm eccentricity), granule ratio changes and RPE cells contain fewer melanosomes and more lipofuscin/melanolipofuscin granules (**c**). The normal polygonal shape of RPE cells is highlighted by the stained circumferential F-actin bundle of the RPE cytoskeleton (*red* in **a**). Adjacent cells have parallel cytoskeletons (*arrowheads* in **a**). Donor: 83 years, female. F-actin labeled with AlexaFluor647-Phalloidin. *Scale bar*: 10 μm. (Reprinted from Ach et al. [71] with permission from the Association for Research in Vision and Ophthalmology)

periphery) but also within a location which leads to phenotypic heterogeneity of the monolayer [71, 76]. Despite this massive intracellular deposition of granules RPE cells still look healthy with regular actin cytoskeleton and exhibiting a polygonal geometry (Fig. 10.2) [77].

The total number of RPE cells varies between 4.2 and 6.1 million per eye [59]. Whether RPE cell density at the macula changes with age is dis-

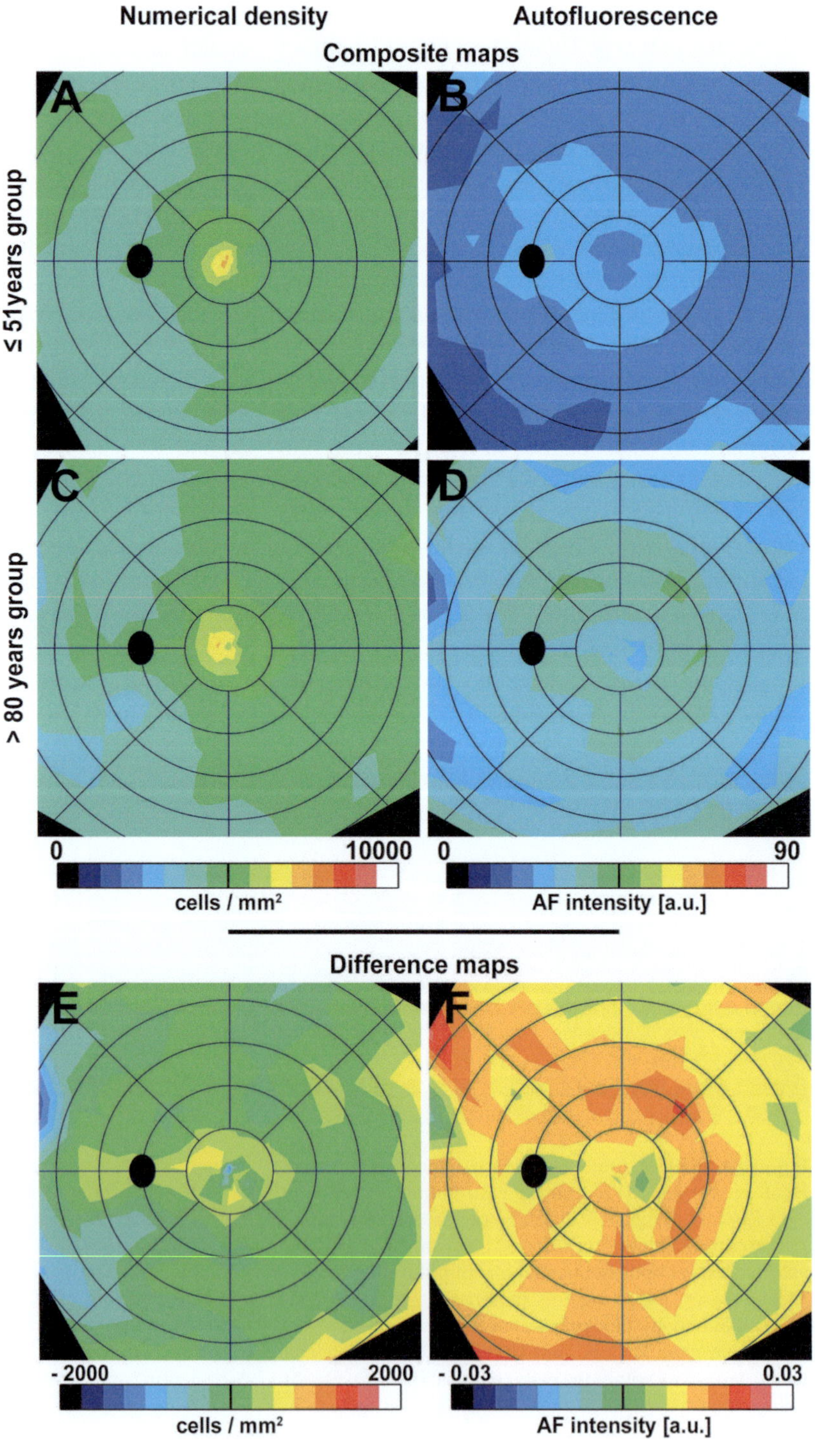

Fig. 10.2 Composite and difference maps of RPE numerical density and AF in two different age groups: <51 years versus >80 years. (**a–d**) RPE numerical density peaks at the fovea (≤51 years old: 6520 ± 946 cells/mm^2; >80 years old: 6405 ± 1323 cells/mm^2) and decreases with eccentricity in both age groups. Cell numbers were determined in flat-mounts of RPE-Bruch's membrane in short post-mortem human eyes. (**e**, **f**) Warm colors indicate higher values, and cool colors indicate lower values in the older group. Green indicates minimal differences between groups. The numerical density difference map shows no significant age change at fovea and periphery and a significant increase in cell density with age at the perifovea. The AF difference map shows significantly increased intensity in all regions with age, especially at 2–4 mm from the foveal center (corresponds with a ring of highest density of rods). Color bar for differences in numerical density ranges between −2000 and +2000 cells in increments of 250 cells/mm^2. Color bar for differences in AF intensity ranges between −0.3 and +0.3 in increments of 0.0375 arbitrary units. (Reprinted with permission from the Association for Research in Vision and Ophthalmology from Ach et al. [77])

cussed controversially. Previous reports showed RPE cell loss with aging [78–80]. These studies have been plagued by long post-mortem delay to preservation, vertical sections without appropriate correction factors, tangential sections through a limited number of retinal locations, or insufficient and biased sampling schemes underlying the steep gradients of neuroretinal cell density in the fovea.

A recent histologic study using a systematic and unbiased sampling scheme shows stability of macular RPE in humans with aging [77], consistent with findings of studies with the largest series of eyes [81, 82]. It is unclear whether changes in cell number are dominant in the periphery and near the ora serrata.

Another feature of the aging RPE are changes in the monolayer's geometry. The RPE shows polygonal cell structure when viewed en face. Predominantly hexagonal cells are found at the fovea; however, with increasing distance from the fovea, hexagonal predominance gets lost and RPE cells show more or less than six neighbors.

In addition, several reports demonstrate a decrease of hexagonal cells with aging, showing a life-long re-arrangement (Fig. 10.3) [77, 83]. A histological study found cells with 3–13 neighbors, and, of interest, cells with more than six neighbors fitted perfectly into the polygonal monolayer geometry, suggesting that they are healthy [77]. Reasons for the cell re-arrangement could include cell division (though controversially discussed), compensatory enlargement after focal cell loss, and fusion of neighboring cells. Whether the decreased regularity in RPE cell geometry actually results in a reduced functionality of the cells remains unclear.

Oxidative stress which leads to alterations in the cytoskeleton might be the cause for cellular de-organization [84]. In AMD affected RPE cells, stress fibers and massive alterations in the filamentous action cytoskeleton are detectable (Fig. 10.4) [71, 84–86]. It is widely accepted that intracellular microfilaments and microtubules are involved in many cellular functions and structures like membranes and organelles. In addition, in RPE cells microfilaments are also necessary for pigment transport (melanosomes) to and from the apical processes [87–89] and altered cytoskeleton function might lead to de- or hyperpigmentation in AMD [90], known as risk factors for AMD progression.

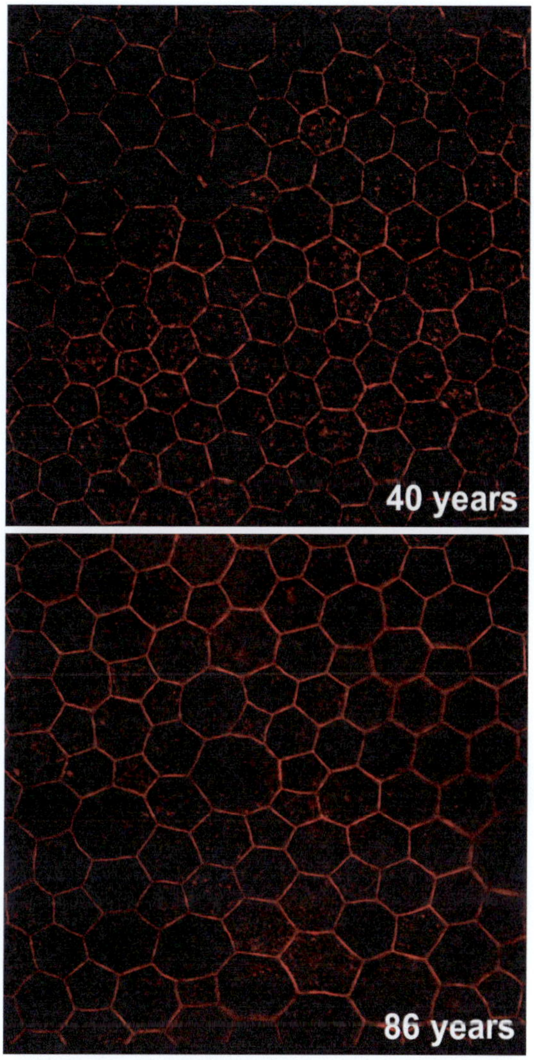

Fig. 10.3 RPE geometry changes with age. Cytoskeleton of retinal pigment epithelium (RPE) in an RPE–BrM flat-mount from two donors (40 years and 86 years) labeled with Phalloidin for filamentous actin (F-actin). While RPE cell density remains stable with aging, the monolayer geometry changes. The number of hexagonal cell decreases and there are more cells with <5 and >7 neighbors. Of note: all cells of the 86 years old donor have a regular shape and cytoskeleton, suggesting a healthy cell state. (Reprinted with permission in part from Ach et al. [77])

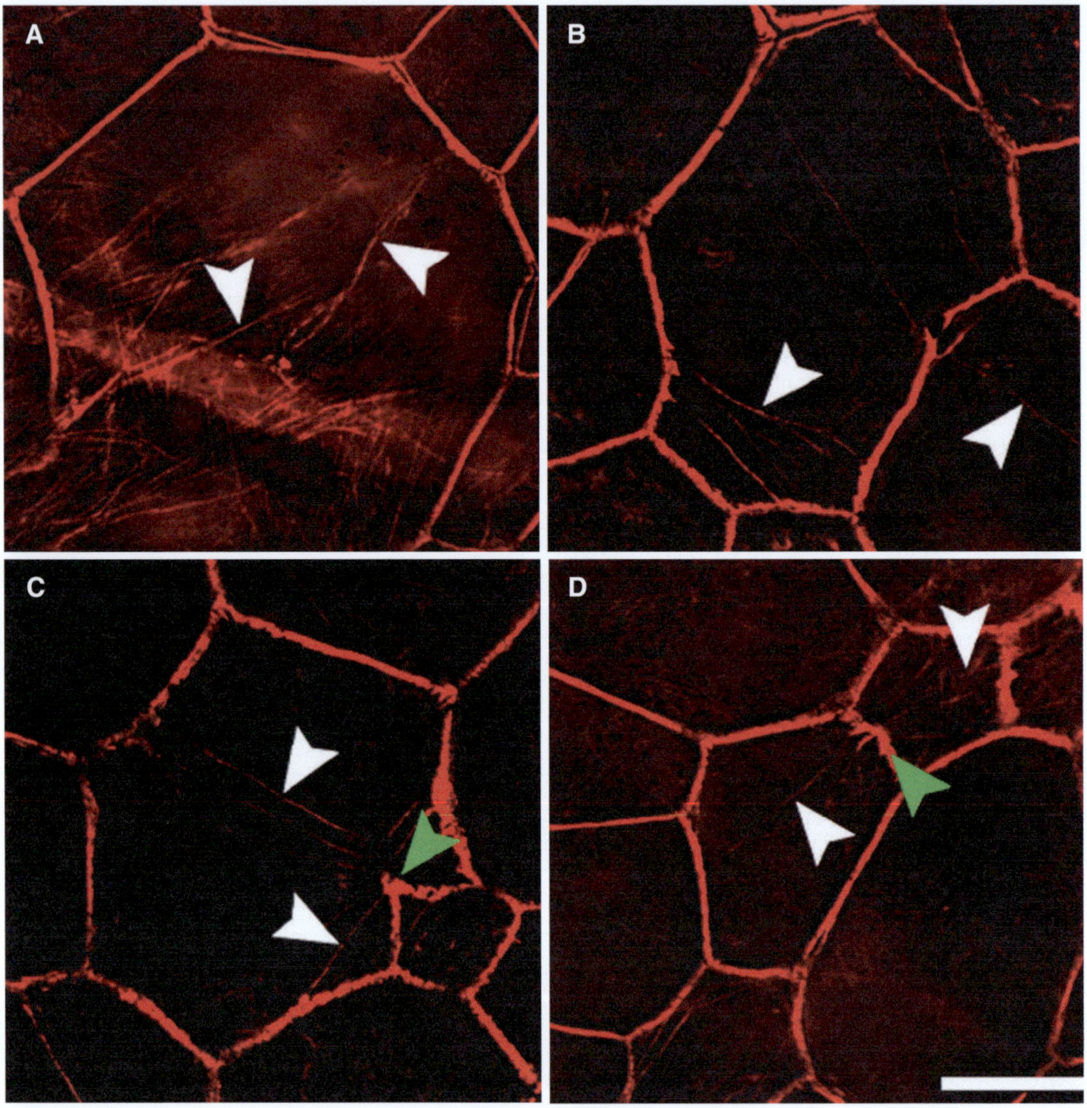

Fig. 10.4 Affected RPE cytoskeleton in AMD. Retinal pigment epithelial cells show stress fibers in AMD-affected eyes. Multiple intracellular stress fibers (*white arrowheads*) arbitrarily cross RPE cells (**a**–**d**). Also, all RPE cells are enlarged. At sites where stress fibers insert, the cytoskeleton appears frayed and thickened (**c**, **d** *green arrowheads*). Although scattered RPE cells are found within atrophic areas, only those outside the atrophic area had recognizable actin cytoskeleton and thus stress fibers. Donors: (**a**, **d**) 94 years, female, incipient AMD; (**b**, **c**) 81 years, male, geographic atrophy. F-actin labeled with AlexaFluor647-Phalloidin. *Scale bar*: 20 μm. (Reprinted with permission from the Association for Research in Vision and Ophthalmology from Ach et al. [71])

Interestingly, in higher age and intermediate AMD, fundus autofluorescence shows a decrease in overall autofluorescence intensity [91, 92] confirmed by histology demonstrating a loss of lipofuscin/melanolipofuscin granules from RPE cells [71].

From Aged to Diseased RPE

As mentioned earlier, RPE cells have the capability of transdifferentiation and, remarkably, phenotype transformation. These phenomena can clearly be observed in age-related diseases like

AMD, both in histology and in vivo using spectral domain optical coherence tomography (SD-OCT) [93]. Histologically, RPE cells in AMD eyes show enlargement and formation of stress fibers, also in areas which are not affected by RPE cell transformation or cell loss.

Currently, 15 different histological RPE phenotypes, including epithelial and non-epithelial morphologies, have been described varying from normal to complete absence in atrophic areas (Fig. 10.5) [94]. These phenotype changes and presumed transdifferentiation in AMD occur in a chronological and predictable order from epithelial to non-epithelial and to atrophy at late stage AMD [93–95]. This survey suggested two main pathways of RPE fate in AMD, an apoptotic path-

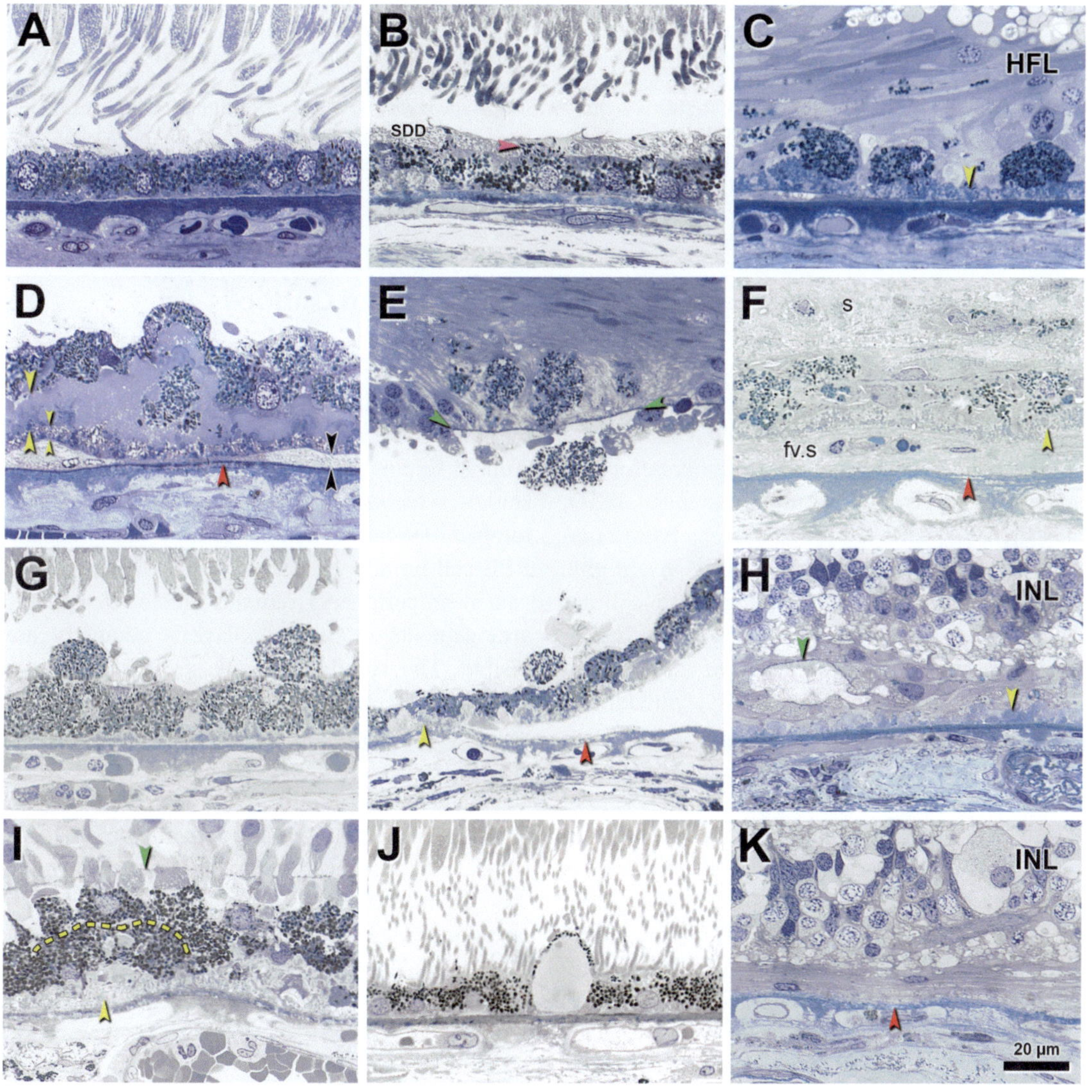

Fig. 10.5 RPE changes its phenotype in age-related macular degeneration. Grades of RPE morphology in late AMD. Submicrometer epoxy resin sections were stained with toluidine blue. Epithelial RPE and RPE morphologies with epithelial components (**a**, **b**, **d**, **e**, **g**, **i**, **j**); nonepithelial (noncontinuous) morphologies (**c**, **f**); atrophic RPE (**h**, **k**). *BLamD* basal laminar deposits, *BLinD* basal linear deposits, *ELM* external limiting membrane, *HFL* Henle fiber layer, *INL* inner nuclear layer, *RPE* retinal pigment epithelium. (**a**) 'Non-uniform' RPE: slightly 'Non-

(continued)

Fig. 10.5 (continued)

uniform' morphology and pigmentation with small patches of early BLamD. (**b**) 'Very Nonuniform' RPE: more nonuniformity in shape and pigmentation; melanosomes within apical processes (*pink arrowhead*). Subretinal drusenoid deposits (SDD) localize to RPE apical aspect. (**c**) 'Dissociated' RPE: individual RPE cells with or without nuclei in atrophic area, adherent to early BLamD. Some RPE granules are translocated among HFL fibers. (**d**) 'Shedding' RPE: basal translocation of shed RPE fragments into a thick continuous layer of BLamD (late and early forms shown by *large* and *small yellow arrowheads*, respectively); BLinD (*black arrowheads*). (**e**) 'Intraretinal' RPE: anterior migration through ELM. Epithelial component remains atop BLamD (*bottom*), which in turn overlies an artifactually empty soft druse. Photoreceptors have degenerated. Retina is artifactually detached. (**f**) Cells 'Entombed' by a subretinal scar(s) together with non-pigmented cells, in neovascular AMD. Persistent BLamD divides subretinal fibrocellular scar in the subretinal space from fibrovascular scar (fv.s) in sub-RPE space. (**g**) 'Sloughed' RPE: release of spherical cells into the subretinal space; the epithelial component overlies BLamD (*blue*) and BLinD (*gray*). (**h**) 'Atrophy with BLamD': absent RPE and persistent BLamD. Photoreceptors have atrophied. ELM delimits end-stage outer retinal tubulation. (**i**) 'Bilaminar': double layers of epithelial RPE (delimited by *dotted line*) adherent to BLamD, a minority phenotype. (**j**) 'Vacuolated' RPE: cells with a single large vacuole delimited apically by extremely effaced cytoplasm, a minority phenotype. (**k**) 'Atrophy without BLamD': absent RPE, absent BLamD. Photoreceptors have atrophied. *Yellow arrowheads*: BLamD; *red arrowheads*: calcification in BrM; *green arrowheads*: ELM. (Reprinted with permission from the Association for Research in Vision and Ophthalmology from Zanzottera et al. [94])

way and an anterior migratory pathway, both of which were visible in clinical optical coherence tomography.

Early RPE changes include "non-uniform" and "very non-uniform" RPE cells which lose regularity in size, shape, and pigmentation. At advanced stages of non-neovascular AMD, "Dissociated" cells are the final steps before dissolution of the RPE layer, resulting in atrophy. "Dissociated" cells likely give rise to cellular fragments and loose granules seen in the neurosensory retina. Predecessors of "Dissociated" are "Sloughed"/"Intraretinal" and "Shedding". "Sloughed" cells leave the monolayer and are released into the subretinal space, still carrying autofluorescent granules similar to the original RPE cells. The "Sloughed" phenotype is sometimes seen as "Intraretinal" RPE. "Intraretinal" is migrating RPE which crosses external limiting membrane and is found in the inner retina. "Shedding" RPE is a form of cellular fragmentation. These cells contain intracellular granule aggregations (i.e., lipofuscin and melanolipofuscin) [71], which are then released basolaterally into basal laminar deposits, where they can be seen clinically by optical coherence tomography.

Of note, most of these putatively transformed RPE cells retain their pigment, even when "Subducted".

Summary and Outlook

Many pathways of RPE development have been explored over the last decades. The development in detail, however, is not completely understood. Animal studies provide a good basis for in human studies, which need further exploration. New histological studies of human tissues show that the RPE cell number at central retina (fovea, perifovea, near periphery) remains stable, though rearrangements in the monolayer's geometry are visible. The significant increase of intracellular granules (lipofuscin and melanolipofuscin) seems to reflect maturation in healthy eyes. At higher age and in age-related macular degeneration, RPE cells tend to lose granules. Also, in diseased eyes, RPE cells show dramatic phenotype changes (from non-uniform to complete absence), which, now, can be tracked *in vivo* thanks to optical coherence tomography.FundingIZKF Würzburg, N-304 (T. A.); Dr. Werner Jackstädt-Foundation (T. A.).

References

1. Bharti K, Nguyen MT, Skuntz S, et al. The other pigment cell: specification and development of the pigmented epithelium of the vertebrate eye. Pigment Cell Res. 2006;19:380–94.

2. Bailey TJ, El-Hodiri H, Zhang L, et al. Regulation of vertebrate eye development by Rx genes. Int J Dev Biol. 2004;48:761–70.
3. Zuber ME, Gestri G, Viczian AS, et al. Specification of the vertebrate eye by a network of eye field transcription factors. Development. 2003;130:5155–67.
4. Fuhrmann S, Zou C, Levine EM. Retinal pigment epithelium development, plasticity, and tissue homeostasis. Exp Eye Res. 2014;123:141–50.
5. Martinez-Morales JR, Rodrigo I, Bovolenta P. Eye development: a view from the retina pigmented epithelium. Bioessays. 2004;26:766–77.
6. Nguyen M, Arnheiter H. Signaling and transcriptional regulation in early mammalian eye development: a link between FGF and MITF. Development. 2000;127:3581–91.
7. Pearson RA, Dale N, Llaudet E, et al. ATP released via gap junction hemichannels from the pigment epithelium regulates neural retinal progenitor proliferation. Neuron. 2005;46:731–44.
8. Raymond SM, Jackson IJ. The retinal pigmented epithelium is required for development and maintenance of the mouse neural retina. Curr Biol. 1995;5:1286–95.
9. Strauss O. The retinal pigment epithelium in visual function. Physiol Rev. 2005;85:845–81.
10. Pei YF, Rhodin JA. The prenatal development of the mouse eye. Anat Rec. 1970;168:105–25.
11. Breathnah AS, Wyllie LM. Ultrastructure of retinal pigment epithelium of the human fetus. J Ultrastruct Res. 1966;16:584–97.
12. Burke JM. Epithelial phenotype and the RPE: is the answer blowing in the Wnt? Prog Retin Eye Res. 2008;27:579–95.
13. Hitt AL, Luna EJ. Membrane interactions with the actin cytoskeleton. Curr Opin Cell Biol. 1994;6:120–30.
14. Rodriguez-Boulan E, Nelson WJ. Morphogenesis of the polarized epithelial cell phenotype. Science. 1989;245:718 25.
15. Araki M. Regeneration of the amphibian retina: role of tissue interaction and related signaling molecules on RPE transdifferentiation. Develop Growth Differ. 2007;49:109–20.
16. Arresta E, Bernardini S, Bernardini E, et al. Pigmented epithelium to retinal transdifferentiation and Pax6 expression in larval Xenopus laevis. J Exp Zool A Comp Exp Biol. 2005;303:958–67.
17. Azuma N, Tadokoro K, Asaka A, et al. Transdifferentiation of the retinal pigment epithelia to the neural retina by transfer of the Pax6 transcriptional factor. Hum Mol Genet. 2005;14:1059–68.
18. Barbosa-Sabanero K, Hoffmann A, Judge C, et al. Lens and retina regeneration: new perspectives from model organisms. Biochem J. 2012;447:321–34.
19. Fuhrmann S. Eye morphogenesis and patterning of the optic vesicle. Curr Top Dev Biol. 2010;93:61–84.
20. Ishii Y, Weinberg K, Oda-Ishii I, et al. Morphogenesis and cytodifferentiation of the avian retinal pigmented epithelium require downregulation of group B1 sox genes. Development. 2009;136:2579–89.
21. Kuriyama F, Ueda Y, Araki M. Complete reconstruction of the retinal laminar structure from a cultured retinal pigment epithelium is triggered by altered tissue interaction and promoted by overlaid extracellular matrices. Dev Neurobiol. 2009;69:950–8.
22. Martinez-De Luna RI, Kelly LE, El-Hodiri HM. The retinal Homeobox (Rx) gene is necessary for retinal regeneration. Dev Biol. 2011;353:10–8.
23. Mitsuda S, Yoshii C, Ikegami Y, et al. Tissue interaction between the retinal pigment epithelium and the choroid triggers retinal regeneration of the newt Cynops pyrrhogaster. Dev Biol. 2005;280:122–32.
24. Nabeshima A, Nishibayashi C, Ueda Y, et al. Loss of cell-extracellular matrix interaction triggers retinal regeneration accompanied by Rax and Pax6 activation. Genesis. 2013;51:410–9.
25. Reh TA, Nagy T, Gretton H. Retinal pigmented epithelial cells induced to transdifferentiate to neurons by laminin. Nature. 1987;330:68–71.
26. Sakami S, Etter P, Reh TA. Activin signaling limits the competence for retinal regeneration from the pigmented epithelium. Mech Dev. 2008;125:106–16.
27. Spence JR, Madhavan M, Ewing JD, et al. The hedgehog pathway is a modulator of retina regeneration. Development. 2004;131:4607–21.
28. Westenskow PD, Mckean JB, Kubo F, et al. Ectopic Mitf in the embryonic chick retina by co-transfection of beta-catenin and Otx2. Invest Ophthalmol Vis Sci. 2010;51:5328–35.
29. Zhao S, Rizzolo LJ, Barnstable CJ. Differentiation and transdifferentiation of the retinal pigment epithelium. In: Kwang WJ, editor. International review of cytology. London: Academic; 1997. p. 225–66.
30. Agathocleous M, Iordanova I, Willardsen MI, et al. A directional Wnt/beta-catenin-Sox2-proneural pathway regulates the transition from proliferation to differentiation in the Xenopus retina. Development. 2009;136:3289–99.
31. Fujimura N, Taketo MM, Mori M, et al. Spatial and temporal regulation of Wnt/beta-catenin signaling is essential for development of the retinal pigment epithelium. Dev Biol. 2009;334:31–45.
32. Fuhrmann S. Wnt signaling in eye organogenesis. Organogenesis. 2008;4:60–7.
33. Liu W, Lagutin O, Swindell E, et al. Neuroretina specification in mouse embryos requires Six3-mediated suppression of Wnt8b in the anterior neural plate. J Clin Invest. 2010;120:3568–77.
34. Doble BW, Patel S, Wood GA, et al. Functional redundancy of GSK-3alpha and GSK-3beta in Wnt/beta-catenin signaling shown by using an allelic series of embryonic stem cell lines. Dev Cell. 2007;12:957–71.
35. Kim CH, Oda T, Itoh M, et al. Repressor activity of headless/Tcf3 is essential for vertebrate head formation. Nature. 2000;407:913–6.
36. Lagutin OV, Zhu CC, Kobayashi D, et al. Six3 repression of Wnt signaling in the anterior neuroectoderm is essential for vertebrate forebrain development. Genes Dev. 2003;17:368–79.

37. Meyers JR, Hu L, Moses A, et al. Beta-catenin/Wnt signaling controls progenitor fate in the developing and regenerating zebrafish retina. Neural Dev. 2012;7:30.
38. Moustakas A, Heldin CH. Signaling networks guiding epithelial-mesenchymal transitions during embryogenesis and cancer progression. Cancer Sci. 2007;98:1512–20.
39. Casaroli-Marano RP, Pagan R, Vilaro S. Epithelial-mesenchymal transition in proliferative vitreoretinopathy: intermediate filament protein expression in retinal pigment epithelial cells. Invest Ophthalmol Vis Sci. 1999;40:2062–72.
40. Chen HC, Zhu YT, Chen SY, et al. Wnt signaling induces epithelial-mesenchymal transition with proliferation in ARPE-19 cells upon loss of contact inhibition. Lab Investig. 2012;92:676–87.
41. Han JW, Lyu J, Park YJ, et al. Wnt/beta-catenin signaling mediates regeneration of retinal pigment epithelium after laser photocoagulation in mouse eye. Invest Ophthalmol Vis Sci. 2015;56:8314–24.
42. Tamiya S, Kaplan HJ. Role of epithelial-mesenchymal transition in proliferative vitreoretinopathy. Exp Eye Res. 2016;142:26–31.
43. Tamiya S, Liu L, Kaplan HJ. Epithelial-mesenchymal transition and proliferation of retinal pigment epithelial cells initiated upon loss of cell-cell contact. Invest Ophthalmol Vis Sci. 2010;51:2755–63.
44. Hodgkinson CA, Moore KJ, Nakayama A, et al. Mutations at the mouse microphthalmia locus are associated with defects in a gene encoding a novel basic-helix-loop-helix-zipper protein. Cell. 1993;74:395–404.
45. Tachibana M. MITF: a stream flowing for pigment cells. Pigment Cell Res. 2000;13:230–40.
46. Yun S, Saijoh Y, Hirokawa KE, et al. Lhx2 links the intrinsic and extrinsic factors that control optic cup formation. Development. 2009;136:3895–906.
47. Li WB, Zhang YS, Lu ZY, et al. Development of retinal pigment epithelium from human parthenogenetic embryonic stem cells and microRNA signature. Invest Ophthalmol Vis Sci. 2012;53:5334–43.
48. Shibahara S, Takeda K, Yasumoto K, et al. Microphthalmia-associated transcription factor (MITF): multiplicity in structure, function, and regulation. J Investig Dermatol Symp Proc. 2001;6:99–104.
49. Yasumoto K, Yokoyama K, Takahashi K, et al. Functional analysis of microphthalmia-associated transcription factor in pigment cell-specific transcription of the human tyrosinase family genes. J Biol Chem. 1997;272:503–9.
50. Bharti K, Gasper M, Ou J, et al. A regulatory loop involving PAX6, MITF, and WNT signaling controls retinal pigment epithelium development. PLoS Genet. 2012;8:e1002757.
51. Cai Z, Feng GS, Zhang X. Temporal requirement of the protein tyrosine phosphatase Shp2 in establishing the neuronal fate in early retinal development. J Neurosci. 2010;30:4110–9.
52. Cimadamore F, Shah M, Amador-Arjona A, et al. SOX2 modulates levels of MITF in normal human melanocytes, and melanoma lines in vitro. Pigment Cell Melanoma Res. 2012;25:533–6.
53. Zou C, Levine EM. Vsx2 controls eye organogenesis and retinal progenitor identity via homeodomain and non-homeodomain residues required for high affinity DNA binding. PLoS Genet. 2012;8:e1002924.
54. Boulton M, Docchio F, Dayhaw-Barker P, et al. Age-related changes in the morphology, absorption and fluorescence of melanosomes and lipofuscin granules of the retinal pigment epithelium. Vis Res. 1990;30:1291–303.
55. Marmorstein AD. The polarity of the retinal pigment epithelium. Traffic. 2001;2:867–72.
56. Robb RM. Regional changes in retinal pigment epithelial cell density during ocular development. Invest Ophthalmol Vis Sci. 1985;26:614–20.
57. Streeten BW. Development of the human retinal pigment epithelium and the posterior segment. Arch Ophthalmol. 1969;81:383–94.
58. Kokkinopoulos I, Shahabi G, Colman A, et al. Mature peripheral RPE cells have an intrinsic capacity to proliferate; a potential regulatory mechanism for age-related cell loss. PLoS One. 2011;6:e18921.
59. Ts'o MO, Friedman E. The retinal pigment epithelium. 3. Growth and development. Arch Ophthalmol. 1968;80:214–6.
60. Rapaport DH, Rakic P, Yasamura D, et al. Genesis of the retinal pigment epithelium in the macaque monkey. J Comp Neurol. 1995;363:359–76.
61. Campisi J, D'adda Di Fagagna F. Cellular senescence: when bad things happen to good cells. Nat Rev Mol Cell Biol. 2007;8:729–40.
62. Romanov SR, Kozakiewicz BK, Holst CR, et al. Normal human mammary epithelial cells spontaneously escape senescence and acquire genomic changes. Nature. 2001;409:633–7.
63. Roider J, Michaud NA, Flotte TJ, et al. Response of the retinal pigment epithelium to selective photocoagulation. Arch Ophthalmol. 1992;110:1786–92.
64. Starnes AC, Huisingh C, Mcgwin G Jr, et al. Multinucleate retinal pigment epithelium cells of the human macula exhibit a characteristic and highly specific distribution. Vis Neurosci. 2016;33:e001.
65. Curcio CA, Sloan KR, Kalina RE, et al. Human photoreceptor topography. J Comp Neurol. 1990;292:497–523.
66. Tosh D, Slack JM. How cells change their phenotype. Nat Rev Mol Cell Biol. 2002;3:187–94.
67. Zanzottera EC, Messinger JD, Ach T, et al. Subducted and melanotic cells in advanced age-related macular degeneration are derived from retinal pigment epithelium. Invest Ophthalmol Vis Sci. 2015;56:3269–78.
68. Nelson WJ. Cytoskeleton functions in membrane traffic in polarized epithelial cells. Semin Cell Biol. 1991;2:375–85.
69. Wollner DA, Krzeminski KA, Nelson WJ. Remodeling the cell surface distribution of membrane proteins

during the development of epithelial cell polarity. J Cell Biol. 1992;116:889–99.
70. Wollner DA, Nelson WJ. Establishing and maintaining epithelial cell polarity. Roles of protein sorting, delivery and retention. J Cell Sci. 1992;102(Pt 2):185–90.
71. Ach T, Tolstik E, Messinger JD, et al. Lipofuscin redistribution and loss accompanied by cytoskeletal stress in retinal pigment epithelium of eyes with age-related macular degeneration. Invest Ophthalmol Vis Sci. 2015;56:3242–52.
72. Feeney-Burns L, Hilderbrand ES, Eldridge S. Aging human RPE: morphometric analysis of macular, equatorial, and peripheral cells. Invest Ophthalmol Vis Sci. 1984;25:195–200.
73. Wing GL, Blanchard GC, Weiter JJ. The topography and age relationship of lipofuscin concentration in the retinal pigment epithelium. Invest Ophthalmol Vis Sci. 1978;17:601–7.
74. Ach T. Retinales Pigmentepithel im Alter: Umbauprozesse: ja; Abnahme der Zelldichte: nein. Der Ophthalmologe. 2017;114(7):670.
75. Pollreisz A, Messinger JD, Sloan KR, et al. Visualizing melanosomes, lipofuscin, and melanolipofuscin in human retinal pigment epithelium using serial block face scanning electron microscopy. Exp Eye Res. 2018; 166:131–9
76. Burke JM, Hjelmeland LM. Mosaicism of the retinal pigment epitheliums. Mol Interv. 2005;5:9.
77. Ach T, Huisingh C, Mcgwin G Jr, et al. Quantitative autofluorescence and cell density maps of the human retinal pigment epithelium. Invest Ophthalmol Vis Sci. 2014;55:4832–41.
78. Dorey CK, Wu G, Ebenstein D, et al. Cell loss in the aging retina. Relationship to lipofuscin accumulation and macular degeneration. Invest Ophthalmol Vis Sci. 1989;30:1691–9.
79. Feeney-Burns L, Burns RP, Gao CL. Age-related macular changes in humans over 90 years old. Am J Ophthalmol. 1990;109:265–78.
80. Panda-Jonas S, Jonas JB, Jakobczyk-Zmija M. Retinal pigment epithelial cell count, distribution, and correlations in normal human eyes. Am J Ophthalmol. 1996;121:181–9.
81. Del Priore LV, Kuo YH, Tezel TH. Age-related changes in human RPE cell density and apoptosis proportion in situ. Invest Ophthalmol Vis Sci. 2002;43:3312–8.
82. Gao H, Hollyfield JG. Aging of the human retina. Differential loss of neurons and retinal pigment epithelial cells. Invest Ophthalmol Vis Sci. 1992;33: 1–17.
83. Watzke RC, Soldevilla JD, Trune DR. Morphometric analysis of human retinal pigment epithelium: correlation with age and location. Curr Eye Res. 1993;12:133–42.
84. Bailey TA, Kanuga N, Romero IA, et al. Oxidative stress affects the junctional integrity of retinal pigment epithelial cells. Invest Ophthalmol Vis Sci. 2004;45:675–84.
85. Akeo K, Hiramitsu T, Yorifuji H, et al. Membranes of retinal pigment epithelial cells in vitro are damaged in the phagocytotic process of the photoreceptor outer segment discs peroxidized by ferrous ions. Pigment Cell Res. 2002;15:341–7.
86. Garg TK, Chang JY. Oxidative stress causes ERK phosphorylation and cell death in cultured retinal pigment epithelium: prevention of cell death by AG126 and 15-deoxy-delta 12, 14-PGJ2. BMC Ophthalmol. 2003;3:5.
87. Barral DC, Seabra MC. The melanosome as a model to study organelle motility in mammals. Pigment Cell Res. 2004;17:111–8.
88. Coudrier E. Myosins in melanocytes: to move or not to move? Pigment Cell Res. 2007;20:153–60.
89. Futter CE. The molecular regulation of organelle transport in mammalian retinal pigment epithelial cells. Pigment Cell Res. 2006;19:104–11.
90. Bhardwaj G, Chowdhury V, Jacobs MB, et al. A systematic review of the diagnostic accuracy of ocular signs in pediatric abusive head trauma. Ophthalmology. 2010;117:983–992 e917.
91. Delori FC. Age-related accumulation and spatial distribution of lipofuscin in RPE of normal subjects. Investig Ophthalmol. 2001;42:1855–66.
92. Gliem M, Muller PL, Finger RP, et al. Quantitative fundus autofluorescence in early and intermediate age-related macular degeneration. JAMA Ophthalmol. 2016;134:817–24.
93. Curcio CA, Zanzottera EC, Ach T, et al. Activated retinal pigment epithelium, an optical coherence tomography biomarker for progression in age-related macular degeneration. Invest Ophthalmol Vis Sci. 2017;58:BIO211–26.
94. Zanzottera EC, Messinger JD, Ach T, et al. The project MACULA retinal pigment epithelium grading system for histology and optical coherence tomography in age-related macular degeneration. Invest Ophthalmol Vis Sci. 2015;56:3253–68.
95. Zanzottera EC, Ach T, Huisingh C, et al. Visualizing retinal pigment epithelium phenotypes in the transition to atrophy in neovascular age-related macular degeneration. Retina. 2016;36(Suppl 1):S26–39.

11 Sex Related Differences in Retinal Pigment Epithelium and Retinal Disease

Gloriane Schnabolk, Elisabeth Obert, and Bärbel Rohrer

Gender and Sex Based Differences in Retinal Disease

From cardiovascular to neurological diseases, differences have been observed in disease occurrence between males and females [1–4]. These sex-based differences are largely attributed to hormone variation, which in females fluctuate at various stages of life such as puberty, pregnancy, menstrual cycles, and menopause [3]. While we know that sex-based differences in disease penetrance and severity exist between females and males, there is still much we do not understand about the factors underlying sex and gender-based differences in disease pathogenesis. Our lack of understanding is largely due to the previous practice in which clinical studies were mainly restricted to male test subjects. By excluding pre-menopausal women from research, it reduced the risk of harm to a fetus in the event of pregnancy, and by excluding women of all ages it was found to reduce experimental deviation brought about by hormone oscillation. This practice also extended into basic science research, with male animals being used primarily for rodent studies. Unfortunately, excluding women from research studies made it impossible to investigate sex and gender differences in disease progression, treatment response, pharmacokinetics, and multiple other critical areas. The NIH Revitalization Act of 1993 established guidelines requiring the inclusion of women and minorities in clinical research. Over two decades later, the NIH has started to implement policies requiring the use of male and female animal and cell-based models in pre-clinical trials as well. These new guidelines have helped to strengthen our understanding of the role that gender and sex-differences play in health and disease. In this chapter, we will explore what is known about sex-differences in ocular diseases, specifically diseases affecting the retina and retinal pigment epithelium (RPE). A greater understanding of sex differences in ocular disease pathogenesis will allow for the development of advanced therapeutics for these diseases. Both gender and sex play a role in women's health. Gender, which refers to social and cultural differences between men and women, can have a large impact on women's ocular health. Women have been reported to make up 60% of blindness worldwide [5], with socioeconomical factors believed to play a role. In many parts of the world women are less educated, and have less financial stability than males,

G. Schnabolk (✉) · E. Obert
Department of Ophthalmology, Medical University of South Carolina, Charleston, SC, USA
e-mail: faith@musc.edu; obert@musc.edu

B. Rohrer (✉)
Department of Ophthalmology, Medical University of South Carolina, Charleston, SC, USA

Division of Research, Ralph H. Johnson VA Medical Center, Charleston, SC, USA
e-mail: rohrer@musc.edu

A. K. Klettner, S. Dithmar (eds.), *Retinal Pigment Epithelium in Health and Disease*,
https://doi.org/10.1007/978-3-030-28384-1_11

resulting in impeded access to healthcare [6, 7]. As ocular trauma due to domestic abuse is more prevalent in women, it may also be considered a gender-based difference [8, 9]. In contrast to gender differences, sex differences refer to biological variables that are different between male and females, such as reproductive organs, encoded DNA, and hormones. Males and females produce different sex-specific hormones (SSH). For women, estrogen and progesterone are produced and released predominantly by the ovaries, while in men, the testes are the main source of androgen production, primarily testosterone. Testosterone in both sexes is also secreted in small amounts by the adrenal glands [10]. Hormone levels fluctuate at different stages of the female menstrual cycle, where estrogen levels peak during the ovulatory phase, and progesterone levels increase during the luteal phase. During pregnancy, estrogen levels remain low, but increase dramatically during the final trimester. In addition, both estrogen and progesterone levels dramatically decrease following menopause. These fluctuations in female hormone levels have been found to correlate with various ocular complications. Intraocular pressure (IOP) is found to be lower during pregnancy [11–15]. However, after menopause when estrogen levels decrease, IOP levels increase [11–16]. Differences to the cornea have also been documented with pregnancy, resulting in increased thickness [17, 18], steepening [19] and reduction in cornea sensitivity [20, 21]. In the retina, central serous chorioretinopathy [22] and diabetic retinopathy [23–26] are associated with pregnancy [22]. Dry age-related macular degeneration (AMD) incident is associated with the start of menopause at an increased age [27]. In general, females are known to have increased risk for dry eye [28], certain forms of glaucoma (although open-angle glaucoma has a lower prevalence in women [29–31]), and cataracts [32, 33]. Diseases such as Leber's Hereditary Optic Neuropathy (LHON) and Coat's disease, however, are more common in males [34–36]. Unlike estrogen, which can fluctuate drastically at different stages of a woman's life, testosterone levels appear to remain fairly level in men following puberty. Overall, testosterone production is ~20 times greater in males than in females, with plasma clearance of testosterone being approximately twice the amount in females [37, 38]. Progesterone levels between males and females are similar, except during the luteal phase of a woman's cycle, when levels rise ~3-fold. Based on these sex-specific findings, it is no surprise that hormone regulation can occur in the eye and hormone receptors have been identified throughout the eye.

Retina/RPE Function and Sex Differences

As estrogen levels fluctuate throughout the lifespan of healthy women, effects of these changes on visual function should be examined. Eisner and colleagues measured visual sensitivity through a series of test-wavelengths at different stages of the menstrual cycle [39]. This study observed modulation of short-wavelength sensitive (SWS)-cone mediated sensitivities for one individual out of six that peaked near ovulation, indicating that in some individuals menstrual-related changes in retinal function may occur.

Differences in spatial acuity and contrast sensitivity can be analyzed in rodents using optokinetic reflex (OKR) analyses [40]. Van Alphen and colleagues determined that 4-month old female C57BL/6J mice had no difference in absolute spatial acuity [41]. Our unpublished results, observing the optomoter response to moving sine-wave gratings (OptoMotry), confirm the observation on spatial acuity; with absolute thresholds recorded at 100% contrast, being indistinguishable between 3-month old C57BL/6J males and females (Fig. 11.1a; $P = 0.2663$). Interestingly in the same study performed by van Alphen, it was determined that 4 month old female C57BL/6J mice had a lower OKR gain when compared to males [41]. This finding further indicates the importance of providing sex-matched controls when studying animals for visual sensitivity.

Advances in optical coherence tomography (OCT) technology allows for specific retinal layer thickness and volume to be analyzed in order to monitor healthy and diseased eyes. In

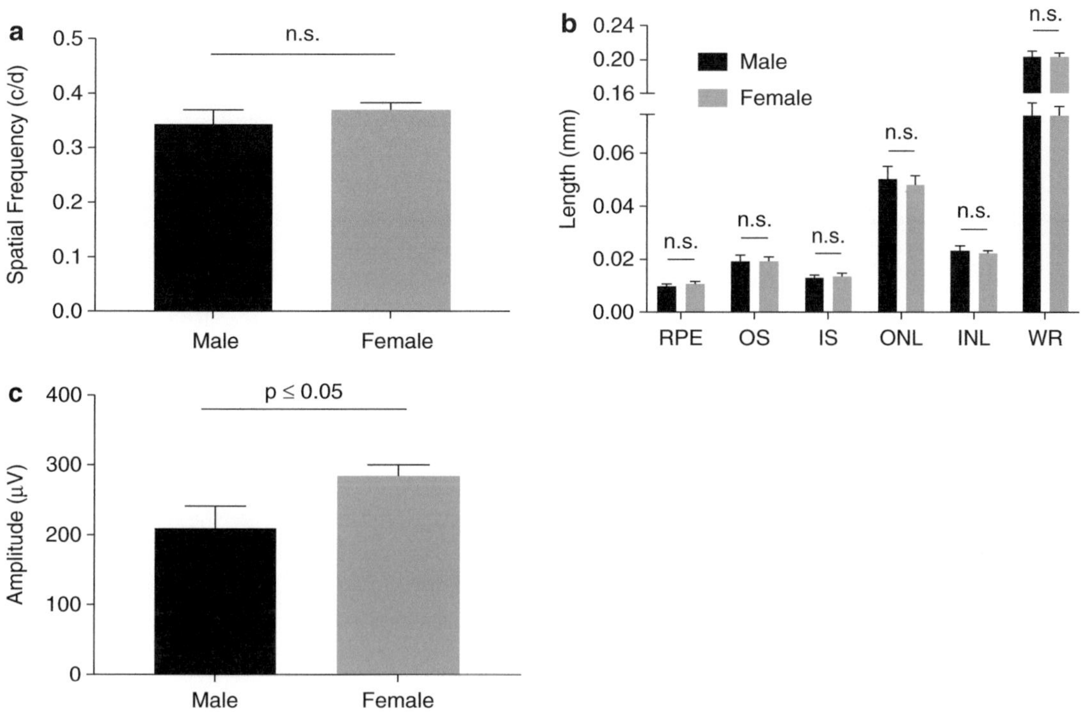

Fig. 11.1 Sex-differences in C57BL/6J mice RPE response. (**a**) Optomoter responses were measured for 3 month old male and female C57BL/6J mice. Spatial frequency threshold at a constant speed (12 deg/s) and contrast (100%) was used to measure visual acuity. Here we observed no significant difference in spatial frequency between male and female mice (n = 6–9 mice/group; $P = 0.27$). (**b**) Optical coherence tomography (Bioptigen) analysis indicated no significant difference between males and females for RPE ($P = 0.64$), outer segments (OS; $P = 0.97$), inner segments (IS; $P = 0.72$), outer nuclear layer (ONL; $P = 0.68$), inner nuclear layer (INL; $P = 0.42$), or whole retina (WR, $P = 0.91$). (**c**) Prior to recording fullfield ERG response, mice were dark-adapted overnight. Mice were anesthetized using xylazine (20 mg/kg) and ketamine (80 mg/kg) before pupils were dilated with 2.5% phenylephrine and 1% atropine. Goniovisc (Rancho Cucamonga, CA) was dropped onto the eye to create an electrical contact between the electrode and the cornea, as well as keep the eyes hydrated. The UTAS E-4000 System (LKC Technologies, Gaithersburg, MD) was used to record c-waves in response to 4 s flashes of 100 cd s mm^{-2}. In order to analyze response, the baseline to peak of the c-wave was measured (n = 4 mice/8 eyes per group; $P < 0.05$). Data are all expressed mean ± SEM

a recent study, comparisons between males and females demonstrated significant differences in mean retinal layer thickness, with men having significantly thicker retinal nerve fiber layer, ganglion cell layer, inner plexiform layer, inner retina, inner nuclear layer and outer plexiform layer in the fovea, and outer plexiform layer in the pericentral ring [42]. In contrast, women were shown to have a greater mean thickness of the outer nuclear layer than men [42]. This difference appears to be specific for the human retina, as no sex-specific differences in overall thickness have been observed in 3-month-old C57BL/6J mice, analyzing retina structure by OCT (Bioptigen; Fig. 11.1b).

Electroretinogram (ERG) recordings have also demonstrated varying results between male and females. Females have demonstrated larger amplitudes than males from single flash illumination under scotopic conditions [43–45]. In addition, photopic multifocal electroretinogram (mfERG) recording of neuroretinal function have demonstrated shorter implicit times in females than males subjects <50 years of age [46]. In a study of sex differences in Sprague-Dawley rats, female rats from 60 to 200 days old had a significant increase in scotopic a and b-wave response when compared to age-matched males [47]. It has been noted previously that estrus cycle levels reach a maximum by day 240 in mice [48]. Therefore, the time period of 60–200 days old may coincide with an increase of estrogen levels for the female rats during this period [47]. In our laboratory, we have also found a significant difference between male and female mice in RPE electrical response (c-waves) using full field ERG. In this experiment healthy 3-month old C57BL/6J mice were dark adapted overnight before recording of c-waves in response to 4 s flashes of 100 cd s mm^{-2} using the UTAS E-4000 System (LKC Technologies, Gaithersburg, MD). Measurement of baseline to peak of each c-wave illustrated a significant increase in RPE response in female mice when compared to age-matched males (Fig. 11.1c; $P < 0.05$). This study however, did not take into account estrous levels, which however, may additionally affect the c-wave results.

Hormone Regulation and Ocular Health

Natural Hormones

There are three types of estrogen: estrone (E1), estradiol (E2 or 17-β-estradiol), and estriol (E3). Estrone is produced primarily in the ovaries and is converted from testosterone by way of estradiol or directly from androstenedione. In addition to the ovaries, estrone can be produced in the placenta and in adipose tissue in men and postmenopausal women. As the ovaries of postmenopausal women continue to produce androstenedione and testosterone, a significant amount of estrone is produced in older women. Estriol, a metabolite of estradiol or estrone, is only found in significant amounts during pregnancy when it is produced by the placenta [49]. Estradiol, the most abundant estrogen, is needed for the development of the female reproductive system. In men, estradiol is produced in the testes to prevent sperm cell apoptosis [50]. Estradiol also plays a key role in promoting bone [51], brain [52], skin health [53], and is important in eye health [54]. Estradiol is able to bind to estrogen receptor α (ERα) and estrogen receptor β (ERβ). These two types of nuclear estrogen receptors are present throughout the human eye tissue including cornea [55, 56], lens [56, 57], lacrimal gland [56], meibonian gland [58], iris and ciliary body [56, 57] conjunctiva [56, 59], and retina [13, 57, 60]. In the retina, ERα is expressed in neuronal cells and localized to the outer synaptic layer (outer plexiform layer, OPL) [61]. ERβ is expressed to a lesser extent in the neuronal cells of the retina and more predominately in the inner synaptic layer (inner plexiform layer, IPL) [5]. Estrogen hormone signaling can be activated through genomic or non-genomic pathways. In the genomic pathway, hormone binding to the receptor allows for the receptor to translocate from the cytosol into the nucleus [62]. In the nucleus, the receptor forms homodimers or heterodimers before binding to the hormone response element (HRE) [63]. Once bound to the HRE, transcription of the different response genes is regulated. The non-genomic pathway varies from the genomic pathway in that steroid activation takes place rapidly [64]. This pathway often involves secondary messenger and signal-transduction cascades, which can alter protein kinase pathways, ion flux, and cyclic AMP [64].

In addition to estrogen receptors, androgen and progesterone receptors are also present throughout the eye, where they too have been found in the cornea [55, 56, 65], lens [56, 65, 66], iris [55, 56], lacrimal gland [56, 67], meibomian gland [56, 65], conjunctiva [56, 65], retina [56, 65, 66, 68], as well as the RPE [65]. The androgen receptor (AR) is also known as the nuclear receptor subfamily 3, group C, member 4 (NR3C4). Like the estrogen receptors, the AR is a nuclear receptor that is activated in the cytoplasm before being translocated into the nucleus [69]. The AR is activated by binding of testosterone or dihydrotestosterone (DHT). DHT, also known as 5α-DHT, acts as potent agonist for the AR [70, 71], which, based on its impact on the expression of lipid and keratin related genes, has been suggested to potentially play a therapeutic role in the alleviation of dry eye disease [72]. Dry eye, which can affect both males and females,

Table 11.1 Sex hormone receptors in the retina and RPE

Ocular tissue	Receptor	Species
Retina	ER (unspecified)	Human mRNA [56], rat mRNA and protein [163], bovine mRNA and protein [163]
	ERα	Human mRNA [57, 164]
	ERβ	Human mRNA [164]
	AR	Human [56], rabbit mRNA [56], rat mRNA [56], mouse
	PR	Human mRNA [56], rabbit mRNA [56], rat mRNA [56]
RPE	ERα	Human mRNA [57, 60], mouse cultured cells [95]
	ERβ	Human mRNA [60]
	PR	Mouse cultured cells [95], human mRNA [56]
	AR	Human protein [65], human mRNA [56]

ER estrogen receptor, *AR* androgen receptor, *PR* androgen receptor

results from dysfunction of the meibomian gland [73, 74], a target site for androgens [75]. Finally, androgens have also been found to play a role in wound healing [76], stimulation of mitosis [77] and suppression of angiogenesis [78]. Sex Hormone receptors identified in the retina and RPE are summarized in Table 11.1.

The protective effects of progesterone have also been investigated for the treatment of retinal neurodegenerative diseases, specifically retinitis pigmentosa [79, 80]. Norgestrel, a synthetic progesterone has been acknowledged to provide a protective effect against photoreceptor cell death in both the light damage model of retinal degeneration as well as the rd10 mouse (Pde6b mutation) [80]. In a study by Jackson and colleagues, the specific progesterone receptors A and B, progesterone receptor membrane complex 1 and 2 (PGRMC1, PGRMC2) and membrane progesterone receptor isoforms α, β, and γ have been identified in adult mouse retina using QRT-PCR [79]. Of note, PGRMC1 knockdown in 661w photoreceptors or pharmacological inhibition of PGRMC1 in rd10 retinal explants cultures reduced the effects of Norgestrel, indicating the importance of this receptor in retinal photoreceptor neuroprotection [79]. Recent studies have suggested that in addition to activation through the classical genomic pathway, these receptors may also be activated through the non-genomic pathway [81, 82].

Hormone Regulation and RPE/Retinal Health

Dysfunction of the RPE and retina are associated with many ocular diseases such as retinitis pigmentosa, diabetic retinopathy, Stargardt disease, and age-related macular degeneration. As part of the retina, the RPE's basolateral membrane sits on top of Bruch's membrane, with the RPE's apical membrane being in contact with the photoreceptor outer segments. The RPE plays a vital role in maintaining retina health by forming tight junctions with neighboring endothelial cells, thereby constituting the outer blood-retinal barrier. These tight junctions allow for the RPE to help facilitate the fluctuation of various ions and nutrients required by the retina. Bruch's membrane, which is an extracellular matrix (ECM) deposited by the RPE, choroidal endothelial cells as well as fibroblast during development and beyond, also assists in controlling the diffusion of nutrients and molecules [83–86]. When RPE homeostasis is impaired, the structural elements of the ECM may get damaged, leading to the accumulation of deposits under the RPE layer [87]. More specifically, deregulation of matrix metalloproteinases (MMP)-2, an enzyme needed for collagen IV digestion, can lead to an increase of collagen IV and concomitant thickening of Bruch's membrane [87], leading to a decrease in fluid movement and transport of metabolites [88, 89]. Interestingly, estrogen has been found to correlate with MMP activity and subretinal deposit formation. In a study performed by Cousin's and colleagues, older female mice (16 month) compared to age-matched male mice, and ovariectomized middle-aged mice (9 months) compared to ovary intact age-matched females had increased sub-RPE deposits [90]. Sub-retinal deposits formation was also increased in estrogen deficient mice [91]. As deposit formation was not decreased with the addition of hormone replacement therapy alone, it is believed that loss of MMP-2 activity, which participates in ECM homeostasis [92], and dysregulation of matrix turnover played a role [90]. Using primary RPE cells from either ERα or ERβ deficient mice, it was identified that ERβ alone is able to promote higher MMP-2 baseline activity and therefore promote a positive regulatory effect within RPE cells [93]. In addition to MMP-2, MMP-14, and TIMP-2 (tissue inhibitors of metalloproteinase-2) are also found to play an important role in allowing for activation of MMP-2 and ERβ in the presence of 17β-estradiol [93].

Proliferative vitreoretinopathy (PVR), like AMD, is affected by local inflammation in the eye [94]. In this disease, proliferative fibrocellular tissue formed by RPE cells differentiate into fibroblast-like cells and thereby produce extracellular matrix leading to collagen contraction and retinal detachment [95]. However, 17β-estradiol and, to a lesser extent, progesterone were found to inhibit this collagen contraction through inhibition of TGF-β2 [95]. The DNA transcription factor NF-κB has also been associated with estrogen receptor signaling. Studies show that estrogen receptors are able to inhibit NF-κB DNA binding, therefore suppressing interleukin 6 (IL-6) production [96, 97], a pro-inflammatory cytokine found to be elevated in the eyes of PVR [98] as well as serum of AMD patients [99].

Supplemented Hormones

Synthetic forms of progesterone and estrogen introduced into the body through oral contraceptives or hormone replacement therapy can also affect ocular health. By decreasing the release of follicle-stimulating hormone and thereby inhibiting the surge in luteinizing hormone that results in ovulation, synthetic progesterone taken through contraceptive use are able to prevent pregnancy [100]. Oral contraceptives combining both progesterone and estrogen are often prescribed in the United States and Western Europe [101] with low doses of estrogen used to inhibit follicular development and stabilize the endometrium [102]. A report published in 2014 by the Center for Disease Control and the U.S. Department of Health and Human Services, stated that approximately 16% of women between the ages of 15 and 44 use oral contraception [103]. Investigation into the role that oral contraceptives might have on ocular disease has revealed an increase in self-reported glaucoma or ocular hypertension in subjects on birth control [104]. Use of oral contraceptives has also been documented to result in rare cases of retinal vascular occlusion [105–107], pigmentary retinopathy [108], and acute macular retinopathy [109, 110]. While uncommon, if not treated, retinal vein occlusion can lead to macular edema, neovascularization, increased eye pressure, and even blindness.

In addition to hormones used for contraception, hormone replacement therapy (HRT) taken during menopause is also linked to eye health. Prescribed to alleviate the symptoms of menopause as the result of diminished estrogen and progesterone levels, HRT involves synthetic use of estrogen (estradiol) and progesterone. Women currently using postmenopausal hormones consisting of estrogen only or estrogen-plus progesterone for a period of 3 or more years had a significantly higher risk of early AMD compared to women never using postmenopausal hormones [111]; in contrast, their risk for advanced neovascular AMD was significantly reduced [111, 112].

The effect of synthetic hormones on ocular health may also be classified as gender-based differences. With primarily women receiving oral contraceptives to prevent pregnancy or hormone replacement therapy to treat menopause, they are more likely to be affected by the role that synthetic hormones play in ocular disease. In addition, as the majority of synthetic hormones are prescribed in the United States and Western Europe, these gender-based differences are more likely to occur in these geographical regions where the use of synthetic hormones are readily accessible and socially accepted.

Preclinical Studies

The role of estradiol in the retina has been a subject of interest in recent years, sparking further basic science research. Estradiol, also referred to as 17β-estradiol or 17β-E2, is the most abundant estrogen and is biosynthesized from cholesterol. In the retina, cholesterol can be either taken up from the circulation, or synthesized de novo in the RPE [113, 114], the latter expressing various lipoproteins and scavenger receptors [114]. Recent studies indicate that estradiol provides a protective effect against inflammation [97, 115]. In addition, Elliot and colleagues have shown that female estrogen receptor β knockout (ERβKO) mice have increased accumulation of subretinal deposits and thickening of Bruch's membrane [116]. Experiments performed by our laboratory have identified neuroprotective effects of ERβ activation. Using light-induced retinal degeneration as a model for dry AMD, female 3-month-old Balb/C mice were exposed to constant fluorescent light (~1500 lux) for 10 days as previously described [117]. To determine the effects of estrogen, mice received either 0.2 mg/kg dosage of 17β-E2 each day, 25 μg/kg every 2 days of the selective estrogen ERβ receptor antagonist 4-[2-Phenyl-5,7-*bis*(trifluoromethyl)pyrazolo[1,5-*a*]pyrimidin-3-yl]phenol (PHTPP), a combination of both, or a vehicle control by intraperitoneal injections. Histological analyses of retina sections stained with 0.1% toluene blue [118] revealed that animals receiving estrogen treatment contained significantly more photoreceptors following light damage compared to animals receiving vehicle alone (Fig. 11.2a; $P < 0.001$; n = 5–10 per condition). While the administration of PHTPP alone did not alter the rate of photoreceptor cell death, it eliminated the protective effect of estrogen when co-administered. Better rod survival was found to result in improved rod-photoreceptor-driven ERG responses. Estrogen supplementation led to improved scotopic photoreceptor function across all three light intensities tested when compared to the vehicle control group (Fig. 11.2b; $P < 0.01$), whereas ERG amplitudes in PHTTP−, or estrogen + PHTTP-treated animals did not differ from vehicle control animals (Fig. 11.2c, d; $P > 0.05$). Cones on the other hand, are more resistant to cell death induced by light damage [119]. Nevertheless, immunohistochemical analyses using an antibody against the predominant form of mouse cone opsin (UV cone opsin) (acc # 16186377) showed that following 10 days of light damage significant shortening of the cone outer segments had occurred (Fig. 11.3b, g), whereas long cone outer segments were observed in age-matched control mice reared under cyclic light (Fig. 11.3a). This effect was ameliorated in mice treated with estrogen (Fig. 11.3c, g). Again, the protective effect of estrogen was reversed in the presence of estrogen + PHTPP (Fig. 11.3e, g), whereas no effect was observed with PHTPP alone (Fig. 11.3d, g). As a secondary control, no cone staining was present in the absence of a primary antibody (Fig. 11.3f). Estradiol has also been found to reduce light damage in Sprague-Dawley rats by modulating antioxidant activity [120]. In a study by Wang and colleagues, it was determined that female ovariectomized rats had a reduction in superoxide dismutase (SOD) 1 and 2, glutathione peroxidase (GPx) 2 and 4, whereas male rats had an increase in GPx1, Gpx2, GPx4, and Nrf2 following light damage [120]. Interestingly, in both male as well as ovariectomized female rats, exogenous application of estradiol upregulated all of the antioxidant genes [120]. These results suggest that further research is warranted to explore the therapeutic effects of estrogen in retinal degenerative disorders.

Autoimmune Disease and Retinal/RPE Health

As previously mentioned, fluctuations in a woman's estrogen levels can have significant effects in the eye. This is true also in relation to autoimmune disease and the role that estrogen levels play in disease severity. Diagnosis of autoimmune disease, such as systemic lupus

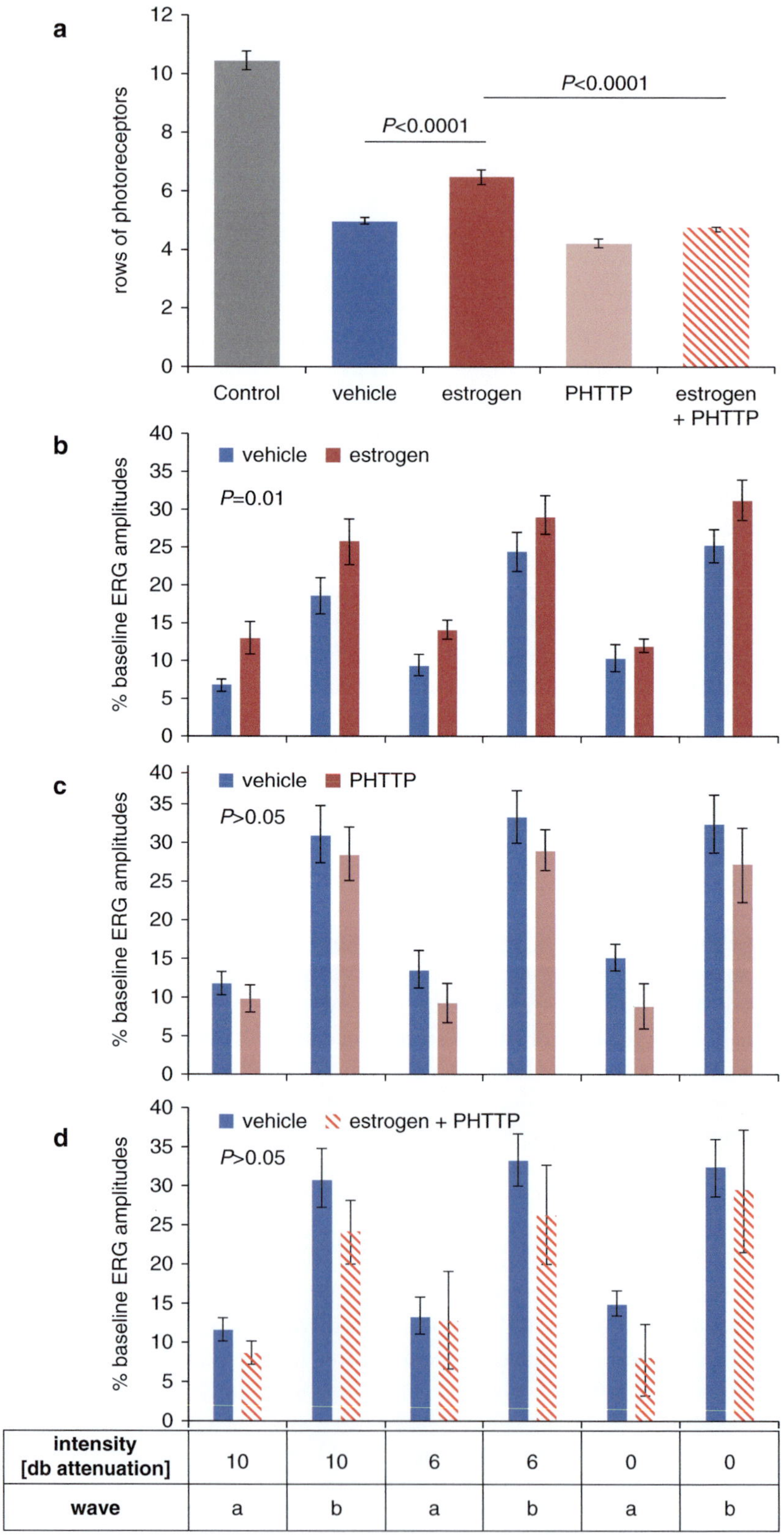

Fig. 11.2 Estrogen reduces light-induced rod photoreceptor cell death and function. (**a**) Rows of photoreceptors were counted in ten different locations across the retina from ventral to dorsal to obtain an average row count per retina. After 10 days of constant light, vehicle-treated Balb/c mice had ~4.5 rows of photoreceptors. Animals treated with estrogen (17β-ED) contained an additional ~1.5 rows ($P < 0.001$). While PHTPP (ERβ-antagonist) did not increase cell death due to light damage, it negated the protective effect of estrogen (estrogen + PHTTP; $P < 0.0001$) (n = 5–10 per condition). (**b–d**) Photoreceptor cell function was determined using electroretinography. Dark-adapted scotopic conditions were used to measure rod function (3 light intensities using white light; 10, 6 and 0 dB of attenuation; max intensity 2.48 photopic cd s/m^2). Here, averaged % baseline ERG amplitudes are presented for the individual animals. (**b**) Mice treated daily with estrogen showed a significant increase in scotopic ERG amplitudes. Similar to the results obtained in the histological studies, (**c**) PHTPP by itself did not lead to further deterioration of function; but blunted the protective effects of estrogen when co-administered (**d**) (n = 5–10 animals per condition)

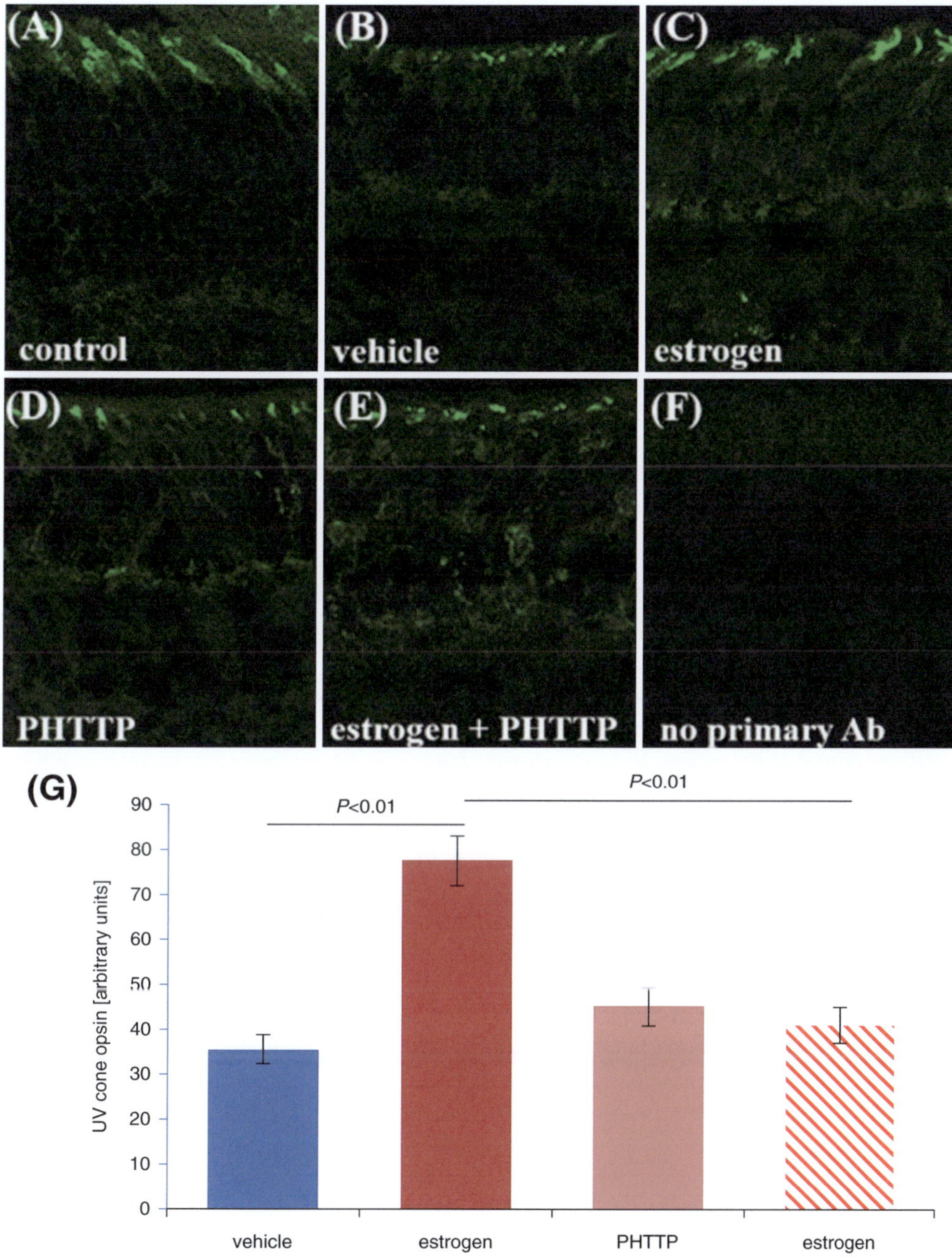

Fig. 11.3 Estrogen prevents light-induced UV cone opsin loss. Retina sections were labeled with an antibody against UV-opsin to evaluate the presence of cone outer segments. (**a**) Long cone outer segments can be demonstrated in control, cyclic light reared age-matched controls. (**b**) Vehicle-treated animals have very short outer segments; whereas UV cone opsin immunoreactivity levels were increased in LD mice after estrogen treatment (**c**). ERβ inhibitor (PHTTP) treatment did not alter cone OS structure when compared to controls (**d**), but PHTTP treatment coadministered with estrogen reversed the protective effect of estrogen alone (**e**). No primary antibody was used as a control (**f**). (**g**) UV opsin protein levels were quantified from binarized and thresholded images normalized to a fixed size using Image J software. Estrogen treatment significantly elevated UV opsin level in light damaged mice ($P < 0.01$), an effect that reversed by co-administration with PHTTP ($P < 0.01$). No difference was observed between vehicle control, PHTPP and PHTPP and estrogen co-treated groups

erythematosus (SLE), scleroderma, rheumatoid arthritis (RA), hyperthyroidism, and multiple sclerosis (MS) are all more common in women than men. Women diagnosed with RA prior to menopause, when levels of estradiol are higher, exhibited decreased severity of symptoms compared to woman over the age of 50 [121, 122]. Disease severity for women at this age is comparable to men and interestingly, men with RA have higher levels of serum estradiol compared to men who do not have RA [123]. During pregnancy when estriol levels are increased, many women with RA experience a decrease in RA symptoms [124]. Patients with MS also experience relief from symptoms when levels of estriol are at pregnancy levels [125]. Still, Jorgensen and colleagues found that with increased numbers of pregnancies, women are more likely to experience greater severity in disease symptoms [126]. Like RA, SLE is also diagnosed in a higher percentage of women. However, while RA symptoms seem to be exacerbated following menopause, women with SLE have more severe symptoms during their reproductive years. In addition to RA and SLE, patients with other rheumatological conditions such as Wegener's granulomatosis, relapsing polychronditis, polyarteritis nodosa, seronegative spondyloathropathies, Behecet's disease, plymyagia, rheumatic, sarcoidosis, and systemic sclerosis have increased risk of ocular disorders including corneal melt, retinitis, glaucoma, cataract scleritis, and uveitis [7]. When RA patients were examined for ocular manifestations dry eye, episcleritis, scleritis, peripheral ulceratie karatitis and sclerosing keratitis were identified [127]. For patients with SLE, 10% suffer from retinal disease [128]. Retinal conditions such as severe vaso-occlusive retinopathy, central retinal vein occlusion branch retinal vein occlusion, central retinal arteriole occlusion, branch retinal arteriole occlusion, and exudative retinal detachment can all lead to vision loss in SLE patients [128]. As with retina and RPE dysfunction, estrogen receptors have been found to play a role in autoimmune disorders. Synovial tissue from RA patients has been found to be positive for ERα and ERβ [129, 130]. In SLE patients, ERα levels are decreased while ERβ levels are increased, suggesting an ERβ-mediated effect on inflammation [14]. Oxidative stress, which can affect many inflammatory diseases as well as ocular diseases, is shown to increase the expression of ERβ [131].

In some cases secondary ocular disorders in autoimmune diseases can result from medications given to treat the autoimmune diseases; however, for these reports, no data is available that stratifies the results based on sex. With an increased prevalence for autoimmune diseases diagnosis in women, it is important to be aware of the role that these prescriptions play in ocular disorders in women's health. Hydroxychloroquine (HCQ) is commonly used to treat autoimmune disorders including RA and SLE. This drug inhibits the immune response through a variety of mechanisms and is being investigated as a therapeutic for other diseases. Currently HCQ is being investigated as a drug to use in high dose in combination with various chemotherapy drugs [132–135]. While this drug serves as a potent immunosuppressor, there is still concern over its ability to induce retinal toxicity. The mechanism of retinal toxicity by HCQ is still being investigated, however research has shown that it is able to bind in the RPE as well as the retina [136]. As an inhibitor of all-*trans*-retinol in primary human RPE cells [137], HCQ may have an adverse effect on the visual cycle. Indomethacin, a non-steroidal inflammatory drug (NSAIDs), has also been linked to retinopathy with pigmentary scattering of the RPE observed [138]. The use of biologics has also been associated with ocular side effects. Rituximab, a monoclonal antibody used for the treatment of RA, was found in a small percentage of patients to result in loss of visual function [139]. Recombinant interferon (IFNs), an anti-viral medication used in the treatment of MS has reported ophthalmic side effects that include retinal vascular abnormalities [140–142]. Methotrexate is an antifolate that serves as an effective immunosuppressant for diseases such as RA and lupus. However, in the absence of folate supplementation, use of methotrexate can result in ocular side effects. In one reported case, b-wave amplitudes in full-field ERG was reduced after prolonged methotrexate use [143]. Interestingly, folate is transported by

RPE cells by folate receptors found in the RPE and retina [144]. Studies have also linked the use of folic acid in AMD prevention [145]. Therefore it may be especially important for individuals with AMD to use caution when using methotrexate. High doses of corticosteroid use among MS patients can result in retinal detachment due to central serous chorioretinopathy [146].

General modifications to lifestyle such as diet, exercise, and cessation of smoking are noted as beneficial for both autoimmune and ocular diseases such as AMD. Though not accounting for sex differences, dietary sodium has recently been linked as a risk factor for MS, with mouse studies showing an increase of Th17 cells and experimental autoimmune encephyalomyelitis (EAE) in the presence of a high sodium diet [147, 148]. Using the SJL mouse strain, it was observed that dietary sodium exacerbated the effects of EAE in females but not males [149]. Conversely to dietary sodium, current studies are investigating the protective effect of vitamin D in AMD [150] and rheumatic diseases [151]. It has been found that higher levels of 25-hydroxyvitamin D resulted in a lower incidence in female patients with MS, indicating a sex-specific difference in vitamin D benefits [152, 153].

Secondary ocular disorders may also be increased in autoimmune patients even in the absence of harmful medications, and for some of these reports, effects of estradiol is presented. Patients with RA have an increased diagnosis of Sjorgen's Syndrome, a disease which results in chronic dry eye. Studies have investigated the correlation between RA and AMD. One study concluded that RA patients had a reduced risk for AMD diagnosis, which they believed was most likely the result of long-term NSAID use [154]. Using a much larger cohort, however, Keenan and colleagues determined that patients with RA are at a higher risk of developing AMD and this risk is highest after first hospital admission with RA [155]. As many inflammatory cytokines are present in both autoimmune disease and AMD, it is interesting to note that estradiol is able to downregulate pro-inflammatory cytokines including interleukin-6 (IL-6) and monocyte chemotactic protein 1 (MCP-1) [156]. Inflammation in various autoimmune diseases as well as in AMD has been shown to be regulated, in part, by the complement pathway. While it is still unknown how exactly sex differences may affect complement activity, studies have shown that classical and alternative complement pathway activity is weaker in female mice [157–161]. This has been confirmed more recently when terminal pathway component C9 was found to have 4- to 7-times less activity in female mouse serum when compared to males [162]. Sex differences in the human complement system await further analysis.

Summary

The purpose of this chapter has been to review some of the previous and current literature exploring the role that sex plays in the pathogenesis of retinal/RPE dysfunction and disease. As discussed, estrogens play an important role in inflammation whether it is in a systemic autoimmune disease or locally within the eye. It is important to continue to investigate the role of sex-related hormones in disease in order to develop more effective therapeutics and be more proactive in preventative care. In the future, estrogen screenings may prove to be valuable in assessment of drug treatment plans for women suffering from one or more inflammatory disease. In addition, we may be able to better identify women at risk for ocular disorders and regularly monitor their eye health with ophthalmology tools such as OCT. As new treatments are developed to fight systemic inflammation, it is important that the effects of these drugs on ocular health be monitored. As discussed, biological differences in retinal layer thickness and visual responses between men and women make it essential to compare sex-differences when monitoring disease. In addition, a woman's hormonal status also must be accounted for in the analysis. The use of oral contraceptives and hormone replacement therapies may also result in ocular gender-based differences. Taken together, current research demonstrates a significant role of sex hormones in multiple ocular tissues, including retina and RPE. Therefore, we further emphasize the importance of accounting for sex-differences in RPE and retinal disease pathogenesis and function.

Acknowledgements We thank Mausumi Bandyopadhyay for her expertise and effort in data generated in Figs. 11.1 and 11.2, as well as her overall intellectual expertise, Lara Seidman for her technical assistance with Figs. 11.1 and 11.2, and Kathleen Brady for critical review.

The authors' responsibilities were as follows: E.O. and G.S. conducted research and analyzed data; G.S wrote manuscript; B.R. assisted with research design and manuscript edits; and all authors read and approved the final manuscript.

This work was sponsored in part by the National Institutes of Health (NIH) K12HD055885 Building Interdisciplinary Research Careers in Women's Health (BIRCWH) fellowship. Additional research was supported by the National Institutes of Health (NIH) (R01EY019320), Department of Veterans Affairs (I01 RX000444), and the South Carolina SmartState Endowment. All animal experiments were performed in accordance with the ARVO Statement for the Use of Animals in Ophthalmic and Vision Research, and were approved by the University Animal Care and Use Committee.

References

1. Popkov VA, Plotnikov EY, Silachev DN, Zorova LD, Pevzner IB, Jankauskas SS, et al. Diseases and aging: gender matters. Biochem Biokhim. 2015;80(12):1560–70.
2. Podcasy JL, Epperson CN. Considering sex and gender in Alzheimer disease and other dementias. Dialogues Clin Neurosci. 2016;18(4):437–46.
3. Ober C, Loisel DA, Gilad Y. Sex-specific genetic architecture of human disease. Nat Rev Genet. 2008;9(12):911–22.
4. Arain FA, Kuniyoshi FH, Abdalrhim AD, Miller VM. Sex/gender medicine. The biological basis for personalized care in cardiovascular medicine. Circ J. 2009;73(10):1774–82.
5. Stevens GA, White RA, Flaxman SR, Price H, Jonas JB, Keeffe J, et al. Global prevalence of vision impairment and blindness: magnitude and temporal trends, 1990-2010. Ophthalmology. 2013;120(12):2377–84.
6. Wagner H, Fink BA, Zadnik K. Sex- and gender-based differences in healthy and diseased eyes. Optometry (St Louis, MO). 2008;79(11):636–52.
7. Clayton JA, Davis AF. Sex/gender disparities and women's eye health. Curr Eye Res. 2015;40(2):102–9.
8. Beck SR, Freitag SL, Singer N. Ocular injuries in battered women. Ophthalmology. 1996;103(1):148–51.
9. Hartzell KN, Botek AA, Goldberg SH. Orbital fractures in women due to sexual assault and domestic violence. Ophthalmology. 1996;103(6):953–7.
10. Longcope C. Adrenal and gonadal androgen secretion in normal females. Clin Endocrinol Metab. 1986;15(2):213–28.
11. Akar Y, Yucel I, Akar ME, Zorlu G, Ari ES. Effect of pregnancy on intraobserver and intertechnique agreement in intraocular pressure measurements. Ophthalmologica. 2005;219(1):36–42.
12. Qureshi IA. Intraocular pressure: association with menstrual cycle, pregnancy and menopause in apparently healthy women. Chin J Physiol. 1995;38(4):229–34.
13. Qureshi IA, Xi XR, Wu XD. Intraocular pressure trends in pregnancy and in the third trimester hypertensive patients. Acta Obstet Gynecol Scand. 1996;75(9):816–9.
14. Qureshi IA. Measurements of intraocular pressure throughout the pregnancy in Pakistani women. Chin Med Sci J. 1997;12(1):53–6.
15. Phillips CI, Gore SM. Ocular hypotensive effect of late pregnancy with and without high blood pressure. Br J Ophthalmol. 1985;69(2):117–9.
16. Qureshi IA. Ocular hypertensive effect of menopause with and without systemic hypertension. Acta Obstet Gynecol Scand. 1996;75(3):266–9.
17. Weinreb RN, Lu A, Beeson C. Maternal corneal thickness during pregnancy. Am J Ophthalmol. 1988;105(3):258–60.
18. Ziai N, Ory SJ, Khan AR, Brubaker RF. Beta-human chorionic gonadotropin, progesterone, and aqueous dynamics during pregnancy. Arch Ophthalmol. 1994;112(6):801–6.
19. Park SB, Lindahl KJ, Temnycky GO, Aquavella JV. The effect of pregnancy on corneal curvature. CLAO J. 1992;18(4):256–9.
20. Millodot M. The influence of pregnancy on the sensitivity of the cornea. Br J Ophthalmol. 1977;61(10):646–9.
21. Riss B, Riss P. Corneal sensitivity in pregnancy. Ophthalmologica. 1981;183(2):57–62.
22. Gass JD. Central serous chorioretinopathy and white subretinal exudation during pregnancy. Arch Ophthalmol. 1991;109(5):677–81.
23. Klein BE, Moss SE, Klein R. Effect of pregnancy on progression of diabetic retinopathy. Diabetes Care. 1990;13(1):34–40.
24. Chan WC, Lim LT, Quinn MJ, Knox FA, McCance D, Best RM. Management and outcome of sight-threatening diabetic retinopathy in pregnancy. Eye (London, England). 2004;18(8):826–32.
25. Dinn RB, Harris A, Marcus PS. Ocular changes in pregnancy. Obstet Gynecol Surv. 2003;58(2):137–44.
26. Ohrt V. The influence of pregnancy on diabetic retinopathy with special regard to the reversible changes shown in 100 pregnancies. Acta Ophthalmol. 1984;62(4):603–16.
27. Smith W, Mitchell P, Wang JJ. Gender, oestrogen, hormone replacement and age-related macular degeneration: results from the Blue Mountains eye study. Aust N Z J Ophthalmol. 1997;25(Suppl 1):S13–5.

28. Schaumberg DA, Sullivan DA, Dana MR. Epidemiology of dry eye syndrome. Adv Exp Med Biol. 2002;506(Pt B):989–98.
29. Wolfs RC, Borger PH, Ramrattan RS, Klaver CC, Hulsman CA, Hofman A, et al. Changing views on open-angle glaucoma: definitions and prevalences--the Rotterdam study. Invest Ophthalmol Vis Sci. 2000;41(11):3309–21.
30. Leske MC, Connell AM, Wu SY, Nemesure B, Li X, Schachat A, et al. Incidence of open-angle glaucoma: the Barbados eye studies. The Barbados Eye Studies Group. Arch Ophthalmol. 2001;119(1):89–95.
31. Leske MC, Wu SY, Hennis A, Honkanen R, Nemesure B, Group BES. Risk factors for incident open-angle glaucoma: the Barbados eye studies. Ophthalmology. 2008;115(1):85–93.
32. Mukesh BN, Le A, Dimitrov PN, Ahmed S, Taylor HR, McCarty CA. Development of cataract and associated risk factors: the visual impairment project. Arch Ophthalmol. 2006;124(1):79–85.
33. Klein BE, Klein R, Lee KE. Incidence of age-related cataract: the Beaver Dam Eye Study. Arch Ophthalmol. 1998;116(2):219–25.
34. Cahill M, O'Keefe M, Acheson R, Mulvihill A, Wallace D, Mooney D. Classification of the spectrum of Coats' disease as subtypes of idiopathic retinal telangiectasis with exudation. Acta Ophthalmol Scand. 2001;79(6):596–602.
35. Shields JA, Shields CL, Honavar SG, Demirci H. Clinical variations and complications of coats disease in 150 cases: the 2000 Sanford Gifford Memorial Lecture. Am J Ophthalmol. 2001;131(5):561–71.
36. Smithen LM, Brown GC, Brucker AJ, Yannuzzi LA, Klais CM, Spaide RF. Coats' disease diagnosed in adulthood. Ophthalmology. 2005;112(6):1072–8.
37. Southren AL, Gordon GG, Tochimoto S, Pinzon G, Lane DR, Stypulkowski W. Mean plasma concentration, metabolic clearance and basal plasma production rates of testosterone in normal young men and women using a constant infusion procedure: effect of time of day and plasma concentration on the metabolic clearance rate of testosterone. J Clin Endocrinol Metab. 1967;27(5):686–94.
38. Southren AL, Tochimoto S, Carmody NC, Isurugi K. Plasma production rates of testosterone in normal adult men and women and in patients with the syndrome of feminizing testes. J Clin Endocrinol Metab. 1965;25(11):1441–50.
39. Eisner A, Burke SN, Toomey MD. Visual sensitivity across the menstrual cycle. Vis Neurosci. 2004;21(4):513–31.
40. Prusky GT, Alam NM, Beekman S, Douglas RM. Rapid quantification of adult and developing mouse spatial vision using a virtual optomotor system. Invest Ophthalmol Vis Sci. 2004;45(12):4611–6.
41. van Alphen B, Winkelman BH, Frens MA. Age- and sex-related differences in contrast sensitivity in C57BL/6 mice. Invest Ophthalmol Vis Sci. 2009;50(5):2451–8.
42. Won JY, Kim SE, Park YH. Effect of age and sex on retinal layer thickness and volume in normal eyes. Medicine. 2016;95(46):e5441.
43. Birch DG, Anderson JL. Standardized full-field electroretinography. Normal values and their variation with age. Arch Ophthalmol. 1992;110(11):1571–6.
44. Vainio-Mattila B. The clinical electroretinogram; II. The difference between the electroretinogram in men and in women. Acta Ophthalmol. 1951;29(1):25–32.
45. Zeidler I. The clinical electroretinogram. IX. The normal electroretinogram. Value of the b-potential in different age groups and its differences in men and women. Acta Ophthalmol. 1959;37:294–301.
46. Ozawa GY, Bearse MA Jr, Harrison WW, Bronson-Castain KW, Schneck ME, Barez S, et al. Differences in neuroretinal function between adult males and females. Optom Vis Sci. 2014;91(6):602–7.
47. Chaychi S, Polosa A, Lachapelle P. Differences in retinal structure and function between aging male and female Sprague-Dawley rats are strongly influenced by the Estrus Cycle. PLoS One. 2015;10(8):e0136056.
48. Nelson JF, Felicio LS. Hormonal influences on reproductive aging in mice. Ann N Y Acad Sci. 1990;592:8–12; discussion 44–51.
49. Tulchinsky D, Hobel CJ. Plasma human chorionic gonadotropin, estrone, estradiol, estriol, progesterone, and 17 alpha-hydroxyprogesterone in human pregnancy. 3. Early normal pregnancy. Am J Obstet Gynecol. 1973;117(7):884–93.
50. Pentikainen V, Erkkila K, Suomalainen L, Parvinen M, Dunkel L. Estradiol acts as a germ cell survival factor in the human testis in vitro. J Clin Endocrinol Metab. 2000;85(5):2057–67.
51. Wang Q, Nicholson PH, Suuriniemi M, Lyytikainen A, Helkala E, Alen M, et al. Relationship of sex hormones to bone geometric properties and mineral density in early pubertal girls. J Clin Endocrinol Metab. 2004;89(4):1698–703.
52. Pansiot J, Mairesse J, Baud O. Protecting the developing brain by 17beta-estradiol. Oncotarget. 2017;8(6):9011–2.
53. Rittie L, Kang S, Voorhees JJ, Fisher GJ. Induction of collagen by estradiol: difference between sun-protected and photodamaged human skin in vivo. Arch Dermatol. 2008;144(9):1129–40.
54. Freeman EE, Munoz B, Schein OD, West SK. Hormone replacement therapy and lens opacities: the Salisbury Eye Evaluation project. Arch Ophthalmol. 2001;119(11):1687–92.
55. Suzuki T, Kinoshita Y, Tachibana M, Matsushima Y, Kobayashi Y, Adachi W, et al. Expression of sex steroid hormone receptors in human cornea. Curr Eye Res. 2001;22(1):28–33.
56. Wickham LA, Gao J, Toda I, Rocha EM, Ono M, Sullivan DA. Identification of androgen, estrogen and progesterone receptor mRNAs in the eye. Acta Ophthalmol Scand. 2000;78(2):146–53.

57. Ogueta SB, Schwartz SD, Yamashita CK, Farber DB. Estrogen receptor in the human eye: influence of gender and age on gene expression. Invest Ophthalmol Vis Sci. 1999;40(9):1906–11.
58. Auw-Haedrich C, Feltgen N. Estrogen receptor expression in meibomian glands and its correlation with age and dry-eye parameters. Graefes Arch Clin Exp Ophthalmol. 2003;241(9):705–9.
59. Fuchsjager-Mayrl G, Nepp J, Schneeberger C, Sator M, Dietrich W, Wedrich A, et al. Identification of estrogen and progesterone receptor mRNA expression in the conjunctiva of premenopausal women. Invest Ophthalmol Vis Sci. 2002;43(9):2841–4.
60. Marin-Castano ME, Elliot SJ, Potier M, Karl M, Striker LJ, Striker GE, et al. Regulation of estrogen receptors and MMP-2 expression by estrogens in human retinal pigment epithelium. Invest Ophthalmol Vis Sci. 2003;44(1):50–9.
61. Cascio C, Russo D, Drago G, Galizzi G, Passantino R, Guarneri R, et al. 17beta-estradiol synthesis in the adult male rat retina. Exp Eye Res. 2007;85(1):166–72.
62. Chan L, O'Malley BW. Mechanism of action of the sex steroid hormones (first of three parts). N Engl J Med. 1976;294(24):1322–8.
63. Singh S, Gupta PD. Induction of phosphoinositide-mediated signal transduction pathway by 17 beta-oestradiol in rat vaginal epithelial cells. J Mol Endocrinol. 1997;19(3):249–57.
64. Simoncini T, Mannella P, Fornari L, Caruso A, Varone G, Genazzani AR. Genomic and non-genomic effects of estrogens on endothelial cells. Steroids. 2004;69(8–9):537–42.
65. Rocha EM, Wickham LA, da Silveira LA, Krenzer KL, Yu FS, Toda I, et al. Identification of androgen receptor protein and 5alpha-reductase mRNA in human ocular tissues. Br J Ophthalmol. 2000;84(1):76–84.
66. Tachibana M, Kobayashi Y, Kasukabe T, Kawajiri K, Matsushima Y. Expression of androgen receptor in mouse eye tissues. Invest Ophthalmol Vis Sci. 2000;41(1):64–6.
67. Rocha FJ, Wickham LA, Pena JD, Gao J, Ono M, Lambert RW, et al. Influence of gender and the endocrine environment on the distribution of androgen receptors in the lacrimal gland. J Steroid Biochem Mol Biol. 1993;46(6):737–49.
68. Bigsby RM, Cardenas H, Caperell-Grant A, Grubbs CJ. Protective effects of estrogen in a rat model of age-related cataracts. Proc Natl Acad Sci U S A. 1999;96(16):9328–32.
69. Lu NZ, Wardell SE, Burnstein KL, Defranco D, Fuller PJ, Giguere V, et al. International Union of Pharmacology. LXV. The pharmacology and classification of the nuclear receptor superfamily: glucocorticoid, mineralocorticoid, progesterone, and androgen receptors. Pharmacol Rev. 2006;58(4):782–97.
70. Saartok T, Dahlberg E, Gustafsson JA. Relative binding affinity of anabolic-androgenic steroids: comparison of the binding to the androgen receptors in skeletal muscle and in prostate, as well as to sex hormone-binding globulin. Endocrinology. 1984;114(6):2100–6.
71. Purushottamachar P, Njar VC. A new simple and high-yield synthesis of 5alpha-dihydrotestosterone (DHT), a potent androgen receptor agonist. Steroids. 2012;77(14):1530–4.
72. Khandelwal P, Liu S, Sullivan DA. Androgen regulation of gene expression in human meibomian gland and conjunctival epithelial cells. Mol Vis. 2012;18:1055–67.
73. Knop E, Knop N, Millar T, Obata H, Sullivan DA. The international workshop on meibomian gland dysfunction: report of the subcommittee on anatomy, physiology, and pathophysiology of the meibomian gland. Invest Ophthalmol Vis Sci. 2011;52(4):1938–78.
74. Kang YS, Lee HS, Li Y, Choi W, Yoon KC. Manifestation of meibomian gland dysfunction in patients with Sjogren's syndrome, non-Sjogren's dry eye, and non-dry eye controls. Int Ophthalmol. 2018;38(3):1161–7.
75. Sullivan DA, Sullivan BD, Ullman MD, Rocha EM, Krenzer KL, Cermak JM, et al. Androgen influence on the meibomian gland. Invest Ophthalmol Vis Sci. 2000;41(12):3732–42.
76. Schumacher H, Machemer R. [Experimental studies on the therapy of corneal lesions due to cortisone]. Klin Monbl Augenheilkd. 1966;148(1):121–6.
77. Tsai TH, Scheving LE, Scheving LA, Pauly JE. Sex differences in circadian rhythms of several variables in lymphoreticular organs, liver, kidney, and corneal epithelium in adult CD2F1 mice. Anat Rec. 1985;211(3):263–70.
78. Yamamoto T, Terada N, Nishizawa Y, Petrow V. Angiostatic activities of medroxyprogesterone acetate and its analogues. Int J Cancer. 1994;56(3):393–9.
79. Jackson AC, Roche SL, Byrne AM, Ruiz-Lopez AM, Cotter TG. Progesterone receptor signalling in retinal photoreceptor neuroprotection. J Neurochem. 2016;136(1):63–77.
80. Doonan F, O'Driscoll C, Kenna P, Cotter TG. Enhancing survival of photoreceptor cells in vivo using the synthetic progestin Norgestrel. J Neurochem. 2011;118(5):915–27.
81. Moussatche P, Lyons TJ. Non-genomic progesterone signalling and its non-canonical receptor. Biochem Soc Trans. 2012;40(1):200–4.
82. Petersen SL, Intlekofer KA, Moura-Conlon PJ, Brewer DN, Del Pino SJ, Lopez JA. Nonclassical progesterone signalling molecules in the nervous system. J Neuroendocrinol. 2013;25(11):991–1001.
83. Liotta LA, Steeg PS, Stetler-Stevenson WG. Cancer metastasis and angiogenesis: an imbalance of positive and negative regulation. Cell. 1991;64(2):327–36.
84. Van Agtmael T, Bruckner-Tuderman L. Basement membranes and human disease. Cell Tissue Res. 2010;339(1):167–88.
85. Bai X, Dilworth DJ, Weng YC, Gould DB. Developmental distribution of collagen IV isoforms and relevance to ocular diseases. Matrix Biol. 2009;28(4):194–201.

86. Schittny JC, Yurchenco PD. Basement membranes: molecular organization and function in development and disease. Curr Opin Cell Biol. 1989;1(5):983–8.
87. Leu ST, Batni S, Radeke MJ, Johnson LV, Anderson DH, Clegg DO. Drusen are cold spots for proteolysis: expression of matrix metalloproteinases and their tissue inhibitor proteins in age-related macular degeneration. Exp Eye Res. 2002;74(1):141–54.
88. Booij JC, Baas DC, Beisekeeva J, Gorgels TG, Bergen AA. The dynamic nature of Bruch's membrane. Prog Retin Eye Res. 2010;29(1):1–18.
89. Nita M, Strzalka-Mrozik B, Grzybowski A, Mazurek U, Romaniuk W. Age-related macular degeneration and changes in the extracellular matrix. Med Sci Monitor. 2014;20:1003–16.
90. Cousins SW, Marin-Castano ME, Espinosa-Heidmann DG, Alexandridou A, Striker L, Elliot S. Female gender, estrogen loss, and sub-RPE deposit formation in aged mice. Invest Ophthalmol Vis Sci. 2003;44(3):1221–9.
91. Espinosa-Heidmann DG, Marin-Castano ME, Pereira-Simon S, Hernandez EP, Elliot S, Cousins SW. Gender and estrogen supplementation increases severity of experimental choroidal neovascularization. Exp Eye Res. 2005;80(3):413–23.
92. Nagase H, Visse R, Murphy G. Structure and function of matrix metalloproteinases and TIMPs. Cardiovasc Res. 2006;69(3):562–73.
93. Elliot S, Catanuto P, Fernandez P, Espinosa-Heidmann D, Karl M, Korach K, et al. Subtype specific estrogen receptor action protects against changes in MMP-2 activation in mouse retinal pigmented epithelial cells. Exp Eye Res. 2008;86(4):653–60.
94. Limb GA, Little BC, Meager A, Ogilvie JA, Wolstencroft RA, Franks WA, et al. Cytokines in proliferative vitreoretinopathy. Eye (London, England). 1991;5(Pt 6):686–93.
95. Kimura K, Orita T, Fujitsu Y, Liu Y, Wakuta M, Morishige N, et al. Inhibition by female sex hormones of collagen gel contraction mediated by retinal pigment epithelial cells. Invest Ophthalmol Vis Sci. 2014;55(4):2621–30.
96. Stein B, Yang MX. Repression of the interleukin-6 promoter by estrogen receptor is mediated by NF-kappa B and C/EBP beta. Mol Cell Biol. 1995;15(9):4971–9.
97. Paimela T, Ryhanen T, Mannermaa E, Ojala J, Kalesnykas G, Salminen A, et al. The effect of 17beta-estradiol on IL-6 secretion and NF-kappaB DNA-binding activity in human retinal pigment epithelial cells. Immunol Lett. 2007;110(2):139–44.
98. Kauffmann DJ, van Meurs JC, Mertens DA, Peperkamp E, Master C, Gerritsen ME. Cytokines in vitreous humor: interleukin-6 is elevated in proliferative vitreoretinopathy. Invest Ophthalmol Vis Sci. 1994;35(3):900–6.
99. Ambreen F, Ismail M, Qureshi, IZ. Association of gene polymorphism with serum levels of inflammatory and angiogenic factors in Pakistani patients with age-related macular degeneration. Mol. Vis. 2015; 21:985–99.
100. Ahn RS, Choi JH, Choi BC, Kim JH, Lee SH, Sung SS. Cortisol, estradiol-17beta, and progesterone secretion within the first hour after awakening in women with regular menstrual cycles. J Endocrinol. 2011;211(3):285–95.
101. Brynhildsen J. Combined hormonal contraceptives: prescribing patterns, compliance, and benefits versus risks. Ther Adv Drug Safety. 2014;5(5):201–13.
102. Sech LA, Mishell DR Jr. Oral steroid contraception. Womens Health (London, England). 2015;11(6):743–8.
103. Daniels K, Daugherty J, Jones J, Mosher W. Current contraceptive use and variation by selected characteristics among women aged 15–44: United States, 2011-2013. Natl Health Stat Rep. 2015(86):1–14.
104. Wang YE, Kakigi C, Barbosa D, Porco T, Chen R, Wang S, et al. Oral contraceptive use and prevalence of self-reported glaucoma or ocular hypertension in the United States. Ophthalmology. 2016;123(4):729–36.
105. Thapa R, Paudyal G. Central retinal vein occlusion in young women: rare cases with oral contraceptive pills as a risk factor. Nepal Med Coll J. 2009;11(3):209–11.
106. Klein R, Klein BE, Knudtson MD, Meuer SM, Swift M, Gangnon RE. Fifteen-year cumulative incidence of age-related macular degeneration: the Beaver Dam Eye Study. Ophthalmology. 2007;114(2):253–62.
107. Aggarwal RS, Mishra VV, Aggarwal SV. Oral contraceptive pills: a risk factor for retinal vascular occlusion in in-vitro fertilization patients. J Hum Reprod Sci. 2013;6(1):79–81.
108. Giovannini A, Consolani A. Contraceptive-induced unilateral retinopathy. Ophthalmologica. 1979;179(5):302–5.
109. Pellegrini F, Interlandi E, Pavesio C, Ferreyra HA. We cannot see what she cannot ignore. Surv Ophthalmol. 2017;62:882–5.
110. Rush JA. Acute macular neuroretinopathy. Am J Ophthalmol. 1977;83(4):490–4.
111. Feskanich D, Cho E, Schaumberg DA, Colditz GA, Hankinson SE. Menopausal and reproductive factors and risk of age-related macular degeneration. Arch Ophthalmol. 2008;126(4):519–24.
112. Edwards DR, Gallins P, Polk M, Ayala-Haedo J, Schwartz SG, Kovach JL, et al. Inverse association of female hormone replacement therapy with age-related macular degeneration and interactions with ARMS2 polymorphisms. Invest Ophthalmol Vis Sci. 2010;51(4):1873–9.
113. Cascio C, Deidda I, Russo D, Guarneri P. The estrogenic retina: the potential contribution to healthy aging and age-related neurodegenerative diseases of the retina. Steroids. 2015;103:31–41.
114. Fliesler SJ, Bretillon L. The ins and outs of cholesterol in the vertebrate retina. J Lipid Res. 2010;51(12):3399–413.

115. Stork S, von Schacky C, Angerer P. The effect of 17beta-estradiol on endothelial and inflammatory markers in postmenopausal women: a randomized, controlled trial. Atherosclerosis. 2002;165(2):301–7.
116. Elliot SJ, Catanuto P, Espinosa-Heidmann DG, Fernandez P, Hernandez E, Saloupis P, et al. Estrogen receptor beta protects against in vivo injury in RPE cells. Exp Eye Res. 2010;90(1):10–6.
117. Lohr HR, Kuntchithapautham K, Sharma AK, Rohrer B. Multiple, parallel cellular suicide mechanisms participate in photoreceptor cell death. Exp Eye Res. 2006;83(2):380–9.
118. Rohrer B, Matthes MT, LaVail MM, Reichardt LF. Lack of p75 receptor does not protect photoreceptors from light-induced cell death. Exp Eye Res. 2003;76(1):125–9.
119. Organisciak DT, Vaughan DK. Retinal light damage: mechanisms and protection. Prog Retin Eye Res. 2010;29(2):113–34.
120. Wang S, Wang B, Feng Y, Mo M, Du F, Li H, et al. 17beta-estradiol ameliorates light-induced retinal damage in Sprague-Dawley rats by reducing oxidative stress. J Mol Neurosci. 2015;55(1):141–51.
121. Tengstrand B, Ahlmen M, Hafstrom I. The influence of sex on rheumatoid arthritis: a prospective study of onset and outcome after 2 years. J Rheumatol. 2004;31(2):214–22.
122. Seriolo B, Cutolo M, Garnero A, Accardo S. Relationships between serum 17 beta-oestradiol and anticardiolipin antibody concentrations in female patients with rheumatoid arthritis. Rheumatology (Oxford, England). 1999;38(11):1159–61.
123. Tengstrand B, Carlstrom K, Fellander-Tsai L, Hafstrom I. Abnormal levels of serum dehydroepiandrosterone, estrone, and estradiol in men with rheumatoid arthritis: high correlation between serum estradiol and current degree of inflammation. J Rheumatol. 2003;30(11):2338–43.
124. Nelson JL, Ostensen M. Pregnancy and rheumatoid arthritis. Rheum Dis Clin N Am. 1997;23(1):195–212.
125. Sicotte NL, Liva SM, Klutch R, Pfeiffer P, Bouvier S, Odesa S, et al. Treatment of multiple sclerosis with the pregnancy hormone estriol. Ann Neurol. 2002;52(4):421–8.
126. Jorgensen C, Picot MC, Bologna C, Sany J. Oral contraception, parity, breast feeding, and severity of rheumatoid arthritis. Ann Rheum Dis. 1996;55(2):94–8.
127. Vignesh AP, Srinivasan R. Ocular manifestations of rheumatoid arthritis and their correlation with anti-cyclic citrullinated peptide antibodies. Clin Ophthalmol (Auckland, NZ). 2015;9:393–7.
128. Sivaraj RR, Durrani OM, Denniston AK, Murray PI, Gordon C. Ocular manifestations of systemic lupus erythematosus. Rheumatology (Oxford, England). 2007;46(12):1757–62.
129. Ushiyama T, Inoue K, Nishioka J. Expression of estrogen receptor related protein (p29) and estradiol binding in human arthritic synovium. J Rheumatol. 1995;22(3):421–6.
130. Ishizuka M, Hatori M, Suzuki T, Miki Y, Darnel AD, Tazawa C, et al. Sex steroid receptors in rheumatoid arthritis. Clin Sci (London, England: 1979). 2004;106(3):293–300.
131. Tamir S, Izrael S, Vaya J. The effect of oxidative stress on ERalpha and ERbeta expression. J Steroid Biochem Mol Biol. 2002;81(4–5):327–32.
132. Goldberg SB, Supko JG, Neal JW, Muzikansky A, Digumarthy S, Fidias P, et al. A phase I study of erlotinib and hydroxychloroquine in advanced non-small-cell lung cancer. J Thorac Oncol. 2012;7(10):1602–8.
133. Mahalingam D, Mita M, Sarantopoulos J, Wood L, Amaravadi RK, Davis LE, et al. Combined autophagy and HDAC inhibition: a phase I safety, tolerability, pharmacokinetic, and pharmacodynamic analysis of hydroxychloroquine in combination with the HDAC inhibitor vorinostat in patients with advanced solid tumors. Autophagy. 2014;10(8):1403–14.
134. Rangwala R, Chang YC, Hu J, Algazy KM, Evans TL, Fecher LA, et al. Combined MTOR and autophagy inhibition: phase I trial of hydroxychloroquine and temsirolimus in patients with advanced solid tumors and melanoma. Autophagy. 2014;10(8):1391–402.
135. Rangwala R, Leone R, Chang YC, Fecher LA, Schuchter LM, Kramer A, et al. Phase I trial of hydroxychloroquine with dose-intense temozolomide in patients with advanced solid tumors and melanoma. Autophagy. 2014;10(8):1369–79.
136. Rosenthal AR, Kolb H, Bergsma D, Huxsoll D, Hopkins JL. Chloroquine retinopathy in the rhesus monkey. Invest Ophthalmol Vis Sci. 1978;17(12):1158–75.
137. Xu C, Zhu L, Chan T, Lu X, Shen W, Madigan MC, et al. Chloroquine and hydroxychloroquine are novel inhibitors of human organic anion transporting polypeptide 1A2. J Pharm Sci. 2016;105(2):884–90.
138. Graham CM, Blach RK. Indomethacin retinopathy: case report and review. Br J Ophthalmol. 1988;72(6):434–8.
139. Foran JM, Rohatiner AZ, Cunningham D, Popescu RA, Solal-Celigny P, Ghielmini M, et al. European phase II study of rituximab (chimeric anti-CD20 monoclonal antibody) for patients with newly diagnosed mantle-cell lymphoma and previously treated mantle-cell lymphoma, immunocytoma, and small B-cell lymphocytic lymphoma. J Clin Oncol. 2000;18(2):317–24.
140. Tokai R, Ikeda T, Miyaura T, Sato K. Interferon-associated retinopathy and cystoid macular edema. Arch Ophthalmol. 2001;119(7):1077–9.
141. Perez-Alvarez AF, Jimenez-Alonso J, Reche-Molina I, Leon-Ruiz L, Hidalgo-Tenorio C, Sabio JM. Retinal vasculitis and vitreitis in a patient with chronic hepatitis C virus. Arch Intern Med. 2001;161(18):2262.
142. Jain K, Lam WC, Waheeb S, Thai Q, Heathcote J. Retinopathy in chronic hepatitis C patients during interferon treatment with ribavirin. Br J Ophthalmol. 2001;85(10):1171–3.

143. Ponjavic V, Granse L, Stigmar EB, Andreasson S. Reduced full-field electroretinogram (ERG) in a patient treated with methotrexate. Acta Ophthalmol Scand. 2004;82(1):96–9.
144. Bridges CC, El-Sherbeny A, Ola MS, Ganapathy V, Smith SB. Transcellular transfer of folate across the retinal pigment epithelium. Curr Eye Res. 2002;24(2):129–38.
145. Christen WG, Glynn RJ, Chew EY, Albert CM, Manson JE. Folic acid, pyridoxine, and cyanocobalamin combination treatment and age-related macular degeneration in women: the Women's Antioxidant and Folic Acid Cardiovascular Study. Arch Intern Med. 2009;169(4):335–41.
146. Sharma T, Shah N, Rao M, Gopal L, Shanmugam MP, Gopalakrishnan M, et al. Visual outcome after discontinuation of corticosteroids in atypical severe central serous chorioretinopathy. Ophthalmology. 2004;111(9):1708–14.
147. Kleinewietfeld M, Manzel A, Titze J, Kvakan H, Yosef N, Linker RA, et al. Sodium chloride drives autoimmune disease by the induction of pathogenic TH17 cells. Nature. 2013;496(7446):518–22.
148. Wu C, Yosef N, Thalhamer T, Zhu C, Xiao S, Kishi Y, et al. Induction of pathogenic TH17 cells by inducible salt-sensing kinase SGK1. Nature. 2013;496(7446):513–7.
149. Krementsov DN, Case LK, Hickey WF, Teuscher C. Exacerbation of autoimmune neuroinflammation by dietary sodium is genetically controlled and sex specific. FASEB J. 2015;29(8):3446–57.
150. Annweiler C, Drouet M, Duval GT, Pare PY, Leruez S, Dinomais M, et al. Circulating vitamin D concentration and age-related macular degeneration: systematic review and meta-analysis. Maturitas. 2016;88:101–12.
151. Cutolo M. Further emergent evidence for the vitamin D endocrine system involvement in autoimmune rheumatic disease risk and prognosis. Ann Rheum Dis. 2013;72(4):473–5.
152. Kragt J, van Amerongen B, Killestein J, Dijkstra C, Uitdehaag B, Polman C, et al. Higher levels of 25-hydroxyvitamin D are associated with a lower incidence of multiple sclerosis only in women. Mult Scler. 2009;15(1):9–15.
153. Vasile M, Corinaldesi C, Antinozzi C, Crescioli C. Vitamin D in autoimmune rheumatic diseases: a view inside gender differences. Pharmacol Res. 2017;117:228–41.
154. McGeer PL, Sibley J. Sparing of age-related macular degeneration in rheumatoid arthritis. Neurobiol Aging. 2005;26(8):1199–203.
155. Keenan TD, Goldacre R, Goldacre MJ. Associations between age-related macular degeneration, osteoarthritis and rheumatoid arthritis: record linkage study. Retina (Philadelphia, PA). 2015;35(12):2613–8.
156. Stubelius A, Andersson A, Islander U, Carlsten H. Ovarian hormones in innate inflammation. Immunobiology. 2017;222(8–9):878–83.
157. Churchill WH Jr, Weintraub RM, Borsos T, Rapp HJ. Mouse complement: the effect of sex hormones and castration on two of the late-acting components. J Exp Med. 1967;125(4):657–72.
158. Beurskens FJ, Kuenen JD, Hofhuis F, Fluit AC, Robins DM, Van Dijk H. Sex-limited protein: in vitro and in vivo functions. Clin Exp Immunol. 1999;116(3):395–400.
159. Buras JA, Rice L, Orlow D, Pavlides S, Reenstra WR, Ceonzo K, et al. Inhibition of C5 or absence of C6 protects from sepsis mortality. Immunobiology. 2004;209(8):629–35.
160. Ong GL, Mattes MJ. Mouse strains with typical mammalian levels of complement activity. J Immunol Methods. 1989;125(1–2):147–58.
161. Ong GL, Baker AE, Mattes MJ. Analysis of high complement levels in Mus hortulanus and BUB mice. J Immunol Methods. 1992;154(1):37–45.
162. Kotimaa J, Klar-Mohammad N, Gueler F, Schilders G, Jansen A, Rutjes H, et al. Sex matters: systemic complement activity of female C57BL/6J and BALB/cJ mice is limited by serum terminal pathway components. Mol Immunol. 2016;76:13–21.
163. Kobayashi K, Kobayashi H, Ueda M, Honda Y. Estrogen receptor expression in bovine and rat retinas. Invest Ophthalmol Vis Sci. 1998;39(11):2105–10.
164. Munaut C, Lambert V, Noel A, Frankenne F, Deprez M, Foidart JM, et al. Presence of oestrogen receptor type beta in human retina. Br J Ophthalmol. 2001;85(7):877–82.

Part III

The RPE in Diagnostics

RPE in SD-OCT

12

Andrea Hassenstein and Carsten Grohmann

Introduction

Optical coherence tomography (OCT) was developed in 1991 by Huang, Swanson, and Fujimoto [1, 2]. One of the first OCT prototypes arrived in 1997 in Boston and Hamburg for the first application OCT started with the time-domain technique (TD-OCT) and switched to the faster application of the spectral-domain OCT (SD-OCT) or swept-source OCT (SS-OCT) (Fig. 12.1). The new OCT-angiography (OCT-A) method has been under development since 2015, and provides non-invasive angiography of the retinal and chorioretinal vessels (Fig. 12.1a–f). Since 2001, OCT has been an important component of among macular diagnostic tools due to its capacity for higher resolution and precision.

OCT Technology

OCT offers cross-sectional or tomographic images with micron resolution in eye tissue. The physical basis of OCT imaging depends on the contrast of optical reflectivity between different microstructures of the eye tissue. The light beam is either transmitted, absorbed, or scattered. In most tissue, light scattering outweighs absorption. OCT works in the same way as B-mode ultrasound imaging, except that it uses laser light rather than acoustic waves. The principle of OCT is called low coherence interferometry. The resolution of a typical ultrasound device for eye diagnostics is approximately 150 µm at 10 MHz. A higher resolution of the ultrasound is possible, but attenuates strongly in eye tissue of only 4–5 mm. Therefore, high-resolution ultrasound is limited to the anterior segment of the eye and is not suitable for macular diseases.

OCT is primarily a diagnostic tool for the macula and not for peripheral fundus imaging. Restrictions of OCT are pathologies in the retinal periphery, opacified optical media such as cataract or vitreous hemorrhage, and the absence of fixation. The scanning speed has increased in recent years and therefore OCT images are also now possible in nystagmus patients. Due to its greater wavelengths, OCT images are also available in turbid media. The contralateral eye can be fixed to show the mid-periphery of the fundus. However, imaging of the retinal periphery through the 3-mirror glass is not possible due to the complete backscattering of the light beam.

Time Domain OCT

The first OCT imaging technologies (Time Domain OCT = TD OCT) deliver images

A. Hassenstein (✉) · C. Grohmann
Department of Ophthalmology, University Hospital Hamburg, Hamburg, Germany
e-mail: hassenstein@uke.de; c.grohmann@uke.de

A. K. Klettner, S. Dithmar (eds.), *Retinal Pigment Epithelium in Health and Disease*,
https://doi.org/10.1007/978-3-030-28384-1_12

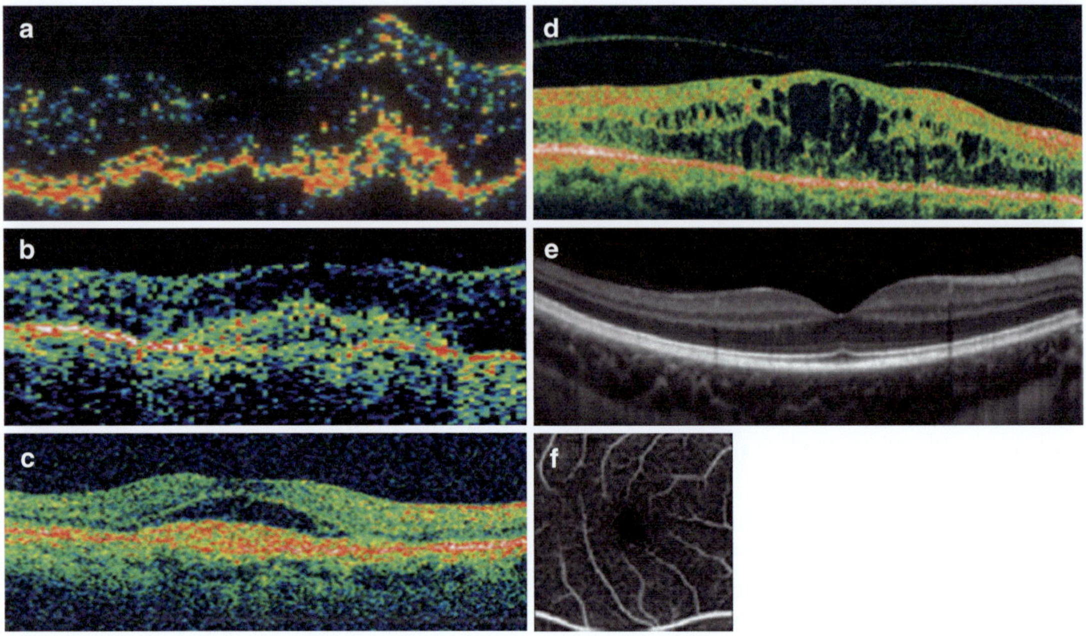

Fig. 12.1 Development of the OCTs from 1997 to 2009 (evolution): OCT started with Time Domain OCT and reached the SD-OCT and SS-OCT generation with improved resolution. Since 2015, OCT angiography has been a new tool for non-invasive angiography through OCT. (**a**) Prototype OCT1, 1997; (**b**) OCT 2, 1998; (**c**) OCT 3 TD Stratus, 2001; (**d**) OCT 4 SD Cirrus, 2007; (**e**) OCT SD, 2009; (**f**) OCT angiography, 2015

with a resolution about ten times higher than conventional ultrasonic B-mode images. The reasons for this are different wave velocities: acoustic wave velocity of 1530 m/s and light wave velocity of 300,000 km/s and different speed of the A-scan application. The resolution of the first TD-OCT components was 10 μm axial and 15 μm transverse. In the next generation of Spectral Domain OCT (SD-OCT), the axial resolution was 3.5 μm.

Ultrasound has a lower resolution of 150 μm but visualizes intransparent structures such as globe boundaries. Due to the light waves, the resolution of the OCT is very high (axial up to 5 μm), but this depends on good transmission (cornea, lens, vitreous hemorrhage).

The light source for the interferometer is a superluminescent laser diode. The interferometer can measure the time delay of optical echoes by comparing the reflected light beam with a reference beam. The reference beam contains a mechanically movable mirror. In TD-OCT, 820 nm wavelength was generally used (1998–2007). The operating wavelength of the SD-OCT probe beam is near infrared (~800 nm), and therefore only minimally visible to the patient. SD-OCT uses either 840 or 870 nm (since 2007) (Table 12.1).

The light from a source is directed onto a partially reflecting mirror and divided into a reference beam and a measuring beam. The measuring beam is reflected by a sample with different time delays.

The light of the sample and the light of the reference mirror are combined and detected. Different reflectivity in the sample leads to different time delays of the reflectivity and leads to a tissue image with reflective properties.

During the generation of TD-OCT, motion artifacts of the eye were also visible due to a longer scanning time through the movable mirror in the reference beam. Patients suffering from poor fixation and lens opacity may not achieve good OCT image quality. In TD generation, TD-OCT can be successfully performed as long as the fundus is visible.

Table 12.1 Overview of the TD OCT, SD-OCT, and SS-OCT and characteristic parameters

	TD-OCT	SD-OCT	SS-OCT
Wavelength	820 nm	840 nm	1050 nm
		870 nm	
Axial resolution	10–20	5	3.5
Transverse resolution	20	15	10
Measurements per A/scan	500	1024	1024
A-scans per B-scan	512	4096	4096
A-scans/s	400	40,000	100,000
Pupil size	4 mm	3 mm	3 mm

The scanning patterns in TD-OCT are radial lines, single or multiple horizontal lines. The macula could never be fully scanned because the areas between the radial lines were interpolated. This was a problem for the interpretation of macular disease, as a pathology could be overlooked due to the absence of a scan position. This problem was solved in the next generation of SD-OCT. The movable mirror in the reference beam is the limiting element which makes TD-OCT unable to provide a higher resolution. The greatest step towards higher resolution was made by SD-OCT by replacing the movable mirror in the reference beam.

Spectral Domain OCT

In contrast to TD-OCT, SD-OCT does not have a mechanically movable mirror in the reference beam, so that significantly higher repetition rates for the A-scan are currently possible (Table 12.1), with more than 40,000 scans per second. An A-scan is generated using an inverse Fourier transformation on the simultaneously acquired data. This results in a higher resolution in axial (currently up to less than 1 μm) and lateral (currently less than 15 μm) direction, with the scan speed also compensating for motion artifacts—which minimizes the likelihood of eye movement during capture, especially in patients with poor fixation. The modern OCT devices have a live eye tracker so that the exact location of the fovea can be guaranteed for follow-up. This was previously a problem for interpretation in TD-OCT.

Another advantage is an improved signal-to-noise ratio by using Fourier transformation of the entire spectrum in SD-OCT and repeated scans for averaging. The spectral interference pattern between the reference beam and the sample beam is dispersed by a spectrometer and collected simultaneously by an array detector. SD-OCT uses either 840 or 870 nm (since 2007). In 840 nm OCT devices, the retinal pigment epithelium (RPE) attenuates the laser beam. This effect increases in RPE thickening/lump formation and drusen and is important for diagnosis.

In addition, SD-OCT generation offers new scanning protocols, i.e. the macular cube protocol of 6 × 6 mm. Here, the entire macular area can be captured with the OCT without missing any pathology. This was made possible by the higher acquisition speed of OCT images and the higher resolution. A high-resolution 5-line horizontal scan is also available depending on the macular pathology.

The difference between TD-OCT (400 scans per second) performed by a mechanical reference mirror and SD-OCT (40,000 scans per second) performed by multiple wavelengths is a factor of 100.

The advantages of higher resolution, scanning speed and macular cube led to the integration of OCT as the macular diagnostic standard specifically for age-related macular degeneration (AMD) and other macular diseases.

Swept Source OCT

In OCT scanning with swept source (SS-OCT, optical frequency range), the light source is rapidly swept in wavelength and the spectral interference pattern is captured on a single or small number of receivers as a function of time. Higher scanning speeds enable denser scanning and better registration. The swept source OCT also has a lower depth sensitivity, which allows better visualization of structures in the depth of the retina. The reason for this is that SS-OCT has a longer wavelength (infrared) than SD-OCT, so there may be less scattering of optical opacity (i.e. lens or vitreous exchange) and the imaging of deeper retinal structures has fewer signal-to-noise patterns. Faster acquisition speeds also mean a higher scanning density of the macula, minimizing the risk of missing pathology and enabling three-dimensional OCT scans (100,000 A-scans per second). The SS-OCT (1050 nm) offers slightly better penetration of the RPE and thus better visualization of the underlying choroid (enhanced depth imaging). The invisible infrared laser does not distract the patient during the scan (Table 12.1).

OCT Angiography

High-resolution OCT images and fast image acquisition led to the development of OCT angiography. The presentation of OCT images in the z-axis (en-face visualization) became increasingly important in SD-OCT generation. This technique enabled the en-face visualization of retinal and choroidal vascular supply by OCT.

The current gold standard for the diagnosis of vascular diseases of the retina or choroid vessels is fluorescence angiography (FLA) or ICG angiography (ICG). However, other diagnostic methods have been developed for significant contraindications (renal dysfunction in the FLA or hyperthyroidism on ICG allergies).

Rapidly repeated OCT scans track the movement of intravascular corpuscular parts of the blood and subtract it from the static topographic OCT image. This allows the detection of blood vessels and the monitoring of blood flow without invasive methods such as digital subtraction angiography (DSA for cardiovascular imaging).

The common SD-OCT is usually used in two dimensions and mainly as tomography. Nevertheless, 3D animation is possible in the viewer of the devices. In OCT-A, B-scans are used en-face and a three-dimensional image is created. If the blood flow is slower than the time between the B-scans of the OCT device, the OCTA interprets this as a lack of blood flow and no vascular system becomes visible. Therefore, OCT-A does not detect any leakage or blockage. This is important for the interpretation of OCT-A images. With the 3 × 3 mm retinal scan cube, the images are high-resolution, and they are of poorer quality in larger cubes (6 × 6 mm).

The lowest flow velocity detectable with OCT-A is called the "slowest detectable flow (SDF)". This depends on the interscan time of the OCT-A device. OCT-A devices with slow intermediate scan speed detect slower flow rates.

The most common four layers of retinal vascular structures are represented by the OCT-A: The superficial retinal plexus, the deep retinal plexus, the outer retinal layer and the choriocapillaris. Neovascularizations penetrating the RPE can be visualized with this technology. Today (2019) there is a common nomenclature, but due to different algorithms and visualization possibilities a comparison between images of different providers is still a challenge. The OCT-A can be performed with SD-OCT or SS-OCT technology. The axial resolution for small capillaries is less than 5 μm and laterally less than 15 μm. Infrared lasers that are not visible to the patient are usually used. Due to the longer scanning times, eye tracking and averaging technologies are used. The main problem with OCT-A is the different standards of the layers in the different devices. A comparison between OCT-A devices is not possible.

SD-OCT and RPE Absorption Spectrum

The laser light of the OCT (central wavelengths, e.g. 840 nm) reaches the melanin of the RPE where absorption takes place. In the laser beam, three pigments are highlighted, which lead to absorption—and thus to an impairment of image resolution: The hemoglobin in the blood vessels (especially in visible light absorbing yellow/green and especially blue, Fig. 12.2), the xan-

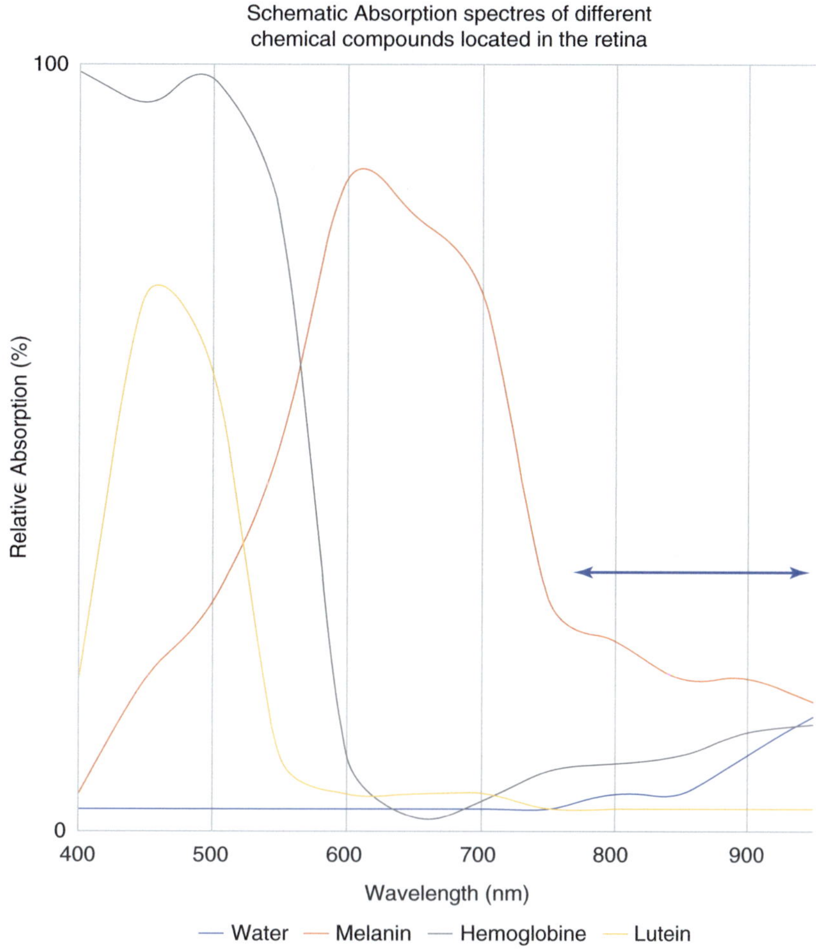

Fig. 12.2 Schematic absorption of light from melanin, lutein, hemoglobin and water depending on different wavelengths. The blue line with two arrows marks the optical window for OCT imaging. It is also clearly visible that lutein absorbs at shorter wavelengths (like "natural sunglasses")

thophyll and lutein in the macula lutea region (absorption maxima in the blue spectral range, "natural sunglasses", Fig. 12.2) and the melanin of the RPE (visible light, 400–1400 nm) [3, 4]. With increasing wavelength, the absorption of the retinal pigment epithelium decreases, so that OCT lasers with a higher wavelength are more advantageous for the visualization of pathologies in the RPE and sub-RPE structures (Fig. 12.2). The best optical window for SD-OCT imaging of the macula is therefore in the near infrared range from a wavelength of approx. 800 nm (Fig. 12.2).

Indocyanine green (ICG) is used for the fluorescence angiographic examination of choroidal pathologies. The emission and absorption spectrum of tissue is solvent-dependent and lies in the optically transparent range of the RPE (fluorescence maximum around 800 nm). Fluorescein, on the other hand, has its emission maxima at about 510 nm, so that it cannot be used as a means of imaging sub-RPE structures. An exception are pathologies without RPE, i.e. geographic atrophy or RPE rips [5].

Scan Pattern

TD-OCT began with radial scans consisting of 6–12 high-resolution line scans passing through the macula. The disadvantage of radial scanning is that the device interpolates between scans. The TD-OCT scan patterns were not suitable for the follow-up of wet AMD. The risk of overlooking an intraretinal cyst was too high without the macular cube.

In SD-OCT generation (and SS-OCT), the macular cube scan and various line scans are most common. The macular cube scan consists of a square area of 6 × 6 mm centered on the fovea. The scans are usually of relatively lower resolution due to time gain. Raster scanning is the technique used to obtain cube scans of the macula. Other scanning protocols improve the size of the scanned area.

In order to scan the entire macula, a cube scan is essential, especially for the detection of fluid in wet age-related macular degeneration (AMD). The highest resolution is achieved with three or five high-resolution linear scans. For the follow-up of macular pathologies, it is very important that the devices can reliably scan the same position for each examination. The same OCT device should always be used for tracking, as the software of different devices defines different reference lines for segmentation. The macular cube scan is probably the safest way to ensure that no pathologies are overlooked. Although the scanning protocols of different manufacturers differ, the standard protocol is a 6 mm macular cube [6–8].

It is very important to define the segmentation lines in OCT-A to make diseases and research comparable. Segmentation lines for automated segmentation must be clearly distinguishable: "for the RPE-Bruch's membrane (BM) complex), the highly reflective edges of the ellipsoid zone and the RPE-BM complex are suitable [9]".

With DICOM import and export as the target, registration and tracking by various devices and vendors will be possible. Eye tracking is established in SD-OCT generation. Tracking should only be performed with the same device. With the OCT-A, the standard level descriptions between the devices are different, therefore standardization is very difficult.

Interpretation of the OCT

Qualitative Assessment

The qualitative interpretation of OCT images in macular diseases is clinically more important than quantitative evaluation. Typical qualitative diagnostics using OCT are macular holes and epiretinal membranes as well as cystoid macular edema.

Linear scans with high resolution are used for the interpretation of RPE. For control examinations of e.g. wet AMD, it is absolutely necessary to scroll through the entire macular cube. It is not sufficient to interpret only one high-resolution scan for one treatment indication. The RPE and the choriocapillaris are difficult to distinguish due to the similar reflection pattern. The RPE layers can be clearly distinguished by the higher resolution of SD-OCT (Fig. 12.3). The RPE layer is highly reflective and leads to a backscattering of the light beam of the OCT (shading of the light beam below the RPE). The atrophy of the highly reflective RPE leads to a reverse shadowing [10–12].

The most important for perfect visualization of individual retinal layers is the different reflectivity of the merging structures, e.g. in the retinal nerve fiber layer (high reflectivity) and in the vitreous body (no reflectivity).

Figure 12.3 shows a detailed description of each retinal layer in SD-OCT. The outer segments of the photoreceptor contact the RPE located on the BM as a single cubic layer. Below the BM, the choriocapillaris and the larger choroid vessels appear in the OCT.

The high-resolution SD-OCT image increasingly resembles a histological tomogram. For the interpretation of OCT images, however, it is important to note that OCT is still an image of reflectivity and not a true histology. Therefore, OCT may show several reflectivity lines of a cell structure such as the photoreceptors (outer segments and the connection to the inner segments), but also vice versa. In Best's disease, highly reflective deposits within the outer retina simulate a lack of highly reflective photoreceptors and RPE, although they are present but not visible to the light beam.

Quantitative Assessment

Quantitative evaluation is particularly helpful for the measurement of the optic disc and the retinal nerve fiber layer (RNFL) for glaucoma diagnostics. The thickness of macular edema can be easily measured using topographic maps. Quantitative

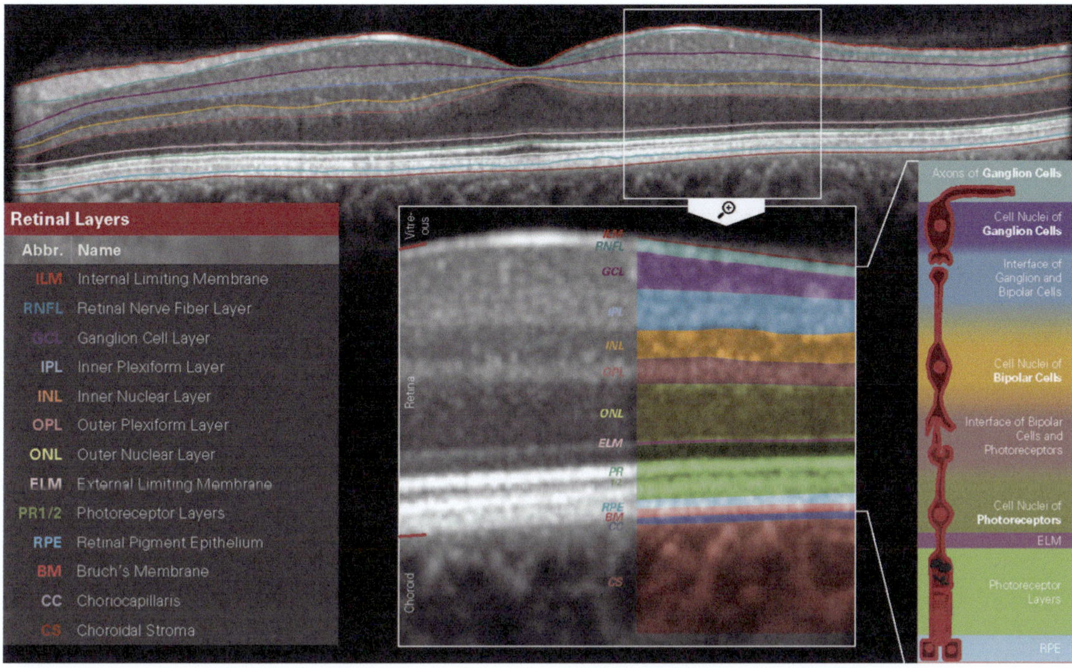

Fig. 12.3 A detailed colored representation of each layer of the retina in SD-OCT (image courtesy of Heidelberg Engineering GmbH, Heidelberg)

OCT interpretation is based on the OCT device's ability to distinguish between different retinal layers with different reflectivities, which requires specific segmentation. The RPE is a very important baseline for manual and automated segmentation together with the retinal nerve fiber layer.

OCT Characteristics of RPE and Bruch's membrane (BM)

Modern SD-OCT has enabled a deeper understanding of RPE and its function in pathology. The RPE and the underlying Bruch's membrane (BM), which can be considered as a coherent region, have an average thickness of about 18–25 μm. BM represents a boundary between the choroid and the RPE. Histologically, it is surrounded by the basement membranes of the choroid vessels on one side and the RPE cells on the other. It consists of elastic fibers and collagens. The retinal pigment epithelium is histologically cubic with nuclei that are essentially close to BM. On the apical side, RPE cells are filled with melanin granules, numerous mitochondria and lipofuscin. Due to the limited light penetration beyond the pigmented RPE and the decay of the OCT signal with depth by absorption and scattering, the image at the choroidal level shows a significantly lower resolution [13].

In SD-OCT, the contiguous region of RPE and BM is the outermost highly reflective continuous line (Fig. 12.4). RPE/BM thickness in normal eyes correlates positively with age. The thickness of the RPE/BM complex is significantly greater in dry AMD compared to age-appropriate controls.

The SD-OCT image visualizes four hyperreflective lines within the outer retina in a healthy macula (Fig. 12.4). When interpreting a macular scan, all four lines should be identified, provided the image quality is high enough. Of the four lines of the RPE complex, the innermost fine line is the external limiting membrane (ELM), followed by the ellipsoid zone (inner and outer photoreceptor connecting line) and the outer photoreceptor segments (interdigitation line) and the RPE. Beyond the BM are the choriocapillaris and choroid.

Alterations of the RPE/BM complex in retinal diseases can occur as a result of increased detachment (Fig. 12.5), atrophy, tear or thickening of the RPE.

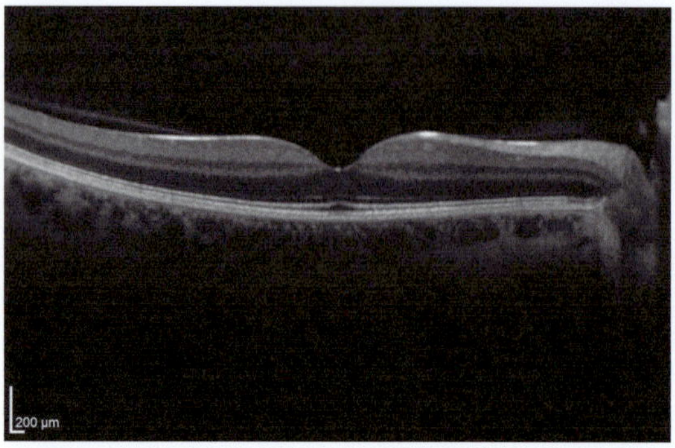

Fig. 12.4 In SD-OCT, four different highly reflective lines can be distinguished in the outer retinal segment. The innermost line is the external limiting membrane (ELM), followed by the inner segments of the cones (connecting line of the inner and outer segment zone), the outer segment line of the cones (interdigitation line) and the outermost segment line of the RPE

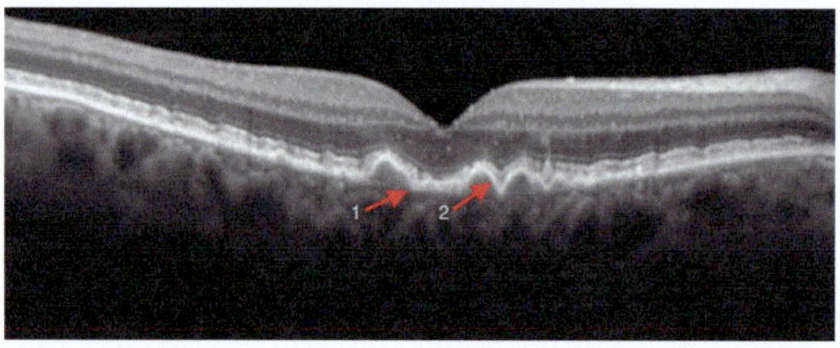

Fig. 12.5 SD-OCT of serous Drusen. The Bruch' membrane (BM) (arrow 1, horizontal fine line) and RPE (arrow 2, highly reflective line of RPE detachment) can be represented as two separate structures

Systematic Verification of RPE Pathologies in SD-OCT

RPE Detachments

The RPE/BM complex in retinal diseases can occur with increased detachment. A pigment epithelial detachment (PED) is an elevation of the RPE from BM with a size of >400 μm width and >75 μm height or >200 μm height. The underlying reflectivity can be divided into homogeneous hypo-reflectivity, hyper-reflectivity and heterogeneous reflectivity. In serous RPE detachment, the RPE is detached and the layer below the RPE is optically empty or only slightly reflective (Fig. 12.6). In an optically empty serous PED, the underlying BM is visible, but not always in crystalline deposits within the detachment cavity (Fig. 12.8).

Serous RPE Detachment (sPED)

In serous RPE detachment, the liquid in the sub-RPE space is optically empty (Fig. 12.6). The separated cavity is surrounded by RPE on one side and BM on the other side. The sPED must be scanned from the macular cube to ensure that the PED is fully serous and no fibrovascular neovascularization can be found.

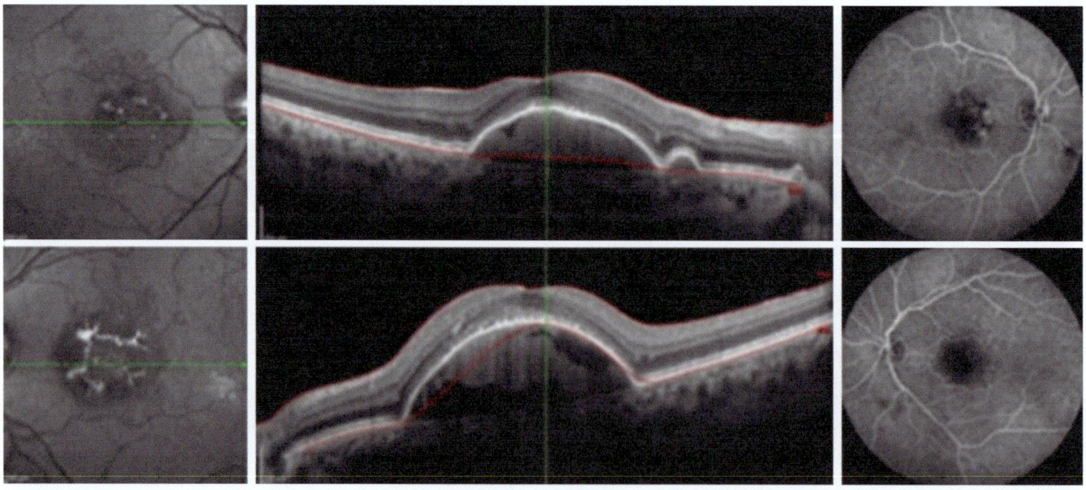

Fig. 12.6 69-year-old patient with VA 0.4, no MMP's (metamorphopsia). Left: Infrared image shows RPE pathologies in butterfly form. Middle (OCT): optically empty area under the RPE (slightly reflective) and attached sensory retina. Right: FLA of the left eye without leakage or staining, of the right eye with staining and no leakage

SD-OCT showed a typical serous PED and slightly constant hyperfluorescence in FLA, but no evidence of choroidal neovascularization (CNV). Treatment was not necessary because no neovascular process was identified in OCT and FLA (no leakage) (Fig. 12.6).

In case of intraretinal cystoid formation and sensory detachment in sPED, a neovascular process must be suspected (Fig. 12.7a, b). In OCT scans, a neovascular highly reflective process or retinal angiomatous proliferation (RAP) lesion must be sought. FLA/OCT-A should be used to identify CNV (type 1 in conjunction with PED). Anti-VEGF treatment has been initiated.

After anti-VEGF treatment (after 3 months), VA (visual acuity) improved to 0.2 and anatomical improvement was achieved. Secondary focal RPE atrophy instead of detachment occurred in OCT after treatment (Fig. 12.7b).

In long-lasting serous PED, the sub-RPE fluid may indicate crystalline deposits (Fig. 12.8). The fluid begins to become turbid after many years of serous RPE detachment.

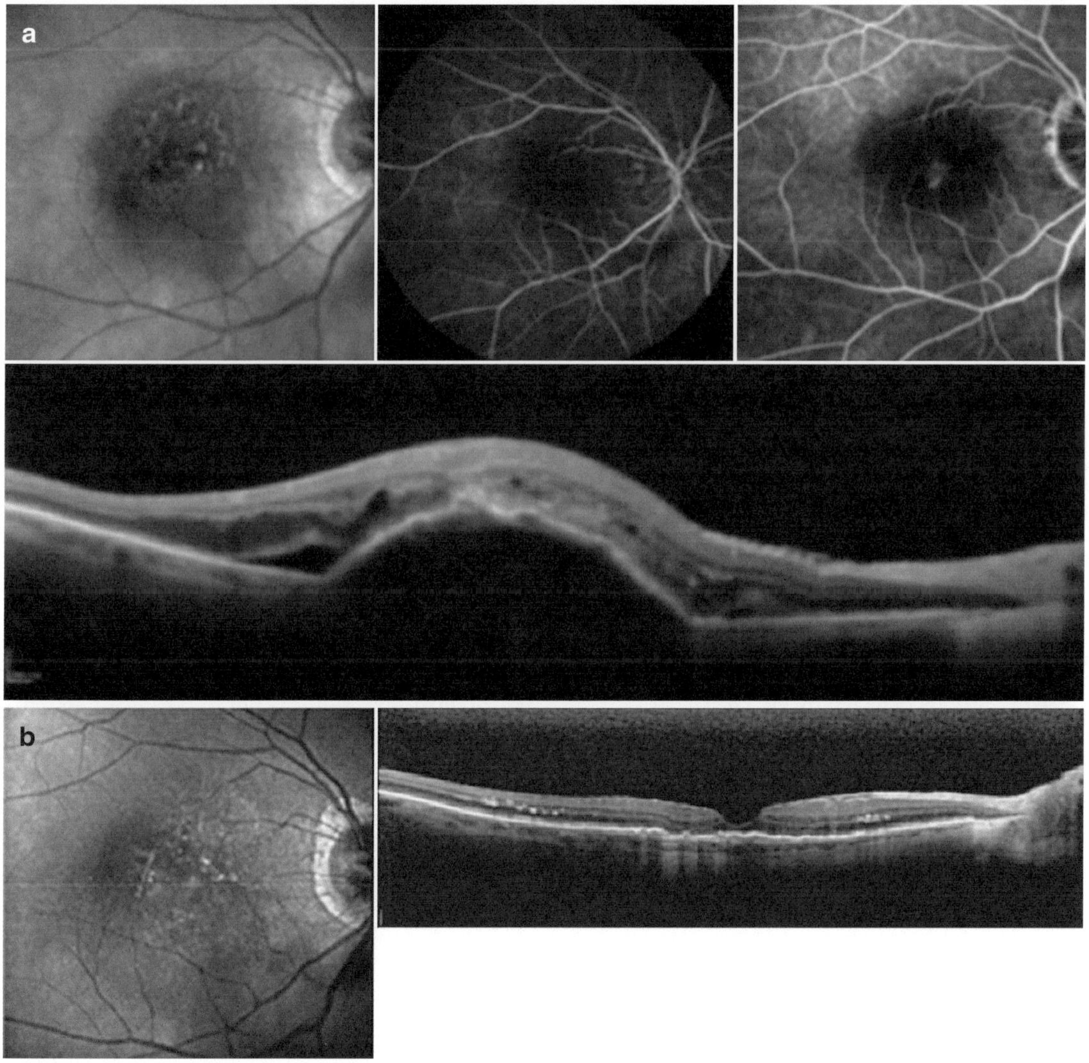

Fig. 12.7 (**a**) 75-year-old patient with VA 0.1. sPED is detected in OCT and sensory detachment and intraretinal cystoid formation. In FLA a leakage in the fovea is detectable and a choroidal neovascularization is suspicious due to the fine leakage. No RAP lesion could be verified in OCT. (**b**) Left: Infrared image after intravitreal treatment, right: OCT shows a subnormal foveal configuration and a focal RPE atrophy with increased light reflection into the choroid

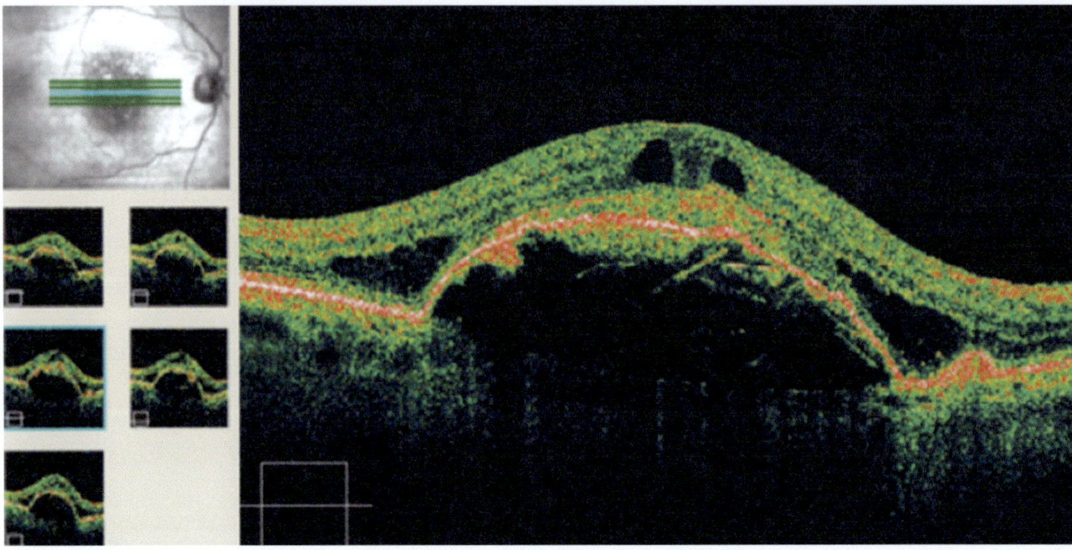

Fig. 12.8 SD-OCT shows crystalline deposits in the sub-RPE cavity as in the long-term RPE detachment. Remarkable is the intraretinal cystoid formation and the sensory detachment, which is rather an intraretinal schisis

Hyperreflective intraretinal and subretinal foci, as seen on SD-OCT, correlated with RPE cells in histology and with funduscopic hyperpigmentation. Any loss or dissociation of RPE leads to hypertransmission of light below the RPE. In histology, the subretinal hyperreflective vitelliform material corresponded to apically expelled RPE organelles and outer segment debris. The occurrence of intraretinal hyperreflective foci was preceded by a thickening of the RPE-BM complex. Over time, the hyperreflective foci of the RPE-BM complex migrate into the retina. Hyperreflective foci in the PED can be quantified and subsequently followed by serial SD-OCT [14]. This RPE foci migration precedes the RPE atrophy detected by the OCT [15].

Fibrovascular RPE Detachment (fPED)

In the event of fibrovascular detachment of the RPE, the space under the RPE is turbid and medium to highly reflective (Fig. 12.9). Depending on the reflectivity of the RPE and the sub-RPE structures, the BM may not be visible. In fPED, always search for RAP lesions or CNV (PNV = pachychoroid CNV) through FLA or OCT-A. In rare cases, ICG is mandatory to detect choroidal polypoidal vasculopathy (PCV) because treatment would be different (anti-VEGF versus photodynamic treatment (PDT)).

Choroidal Polypoidal Vasculopathy (PCV)

In ICG, the PCV is identified by polyps of the choroidal vessels near the optic disc. In OCT the PCV can be visualized by several PED's and medium to highly reflective fibrovascular structures below the RPE. In addition, subretinal hemorrhage often occurs and hard exudates are typical. The hemorrhage often hides the PED finding on the OCT.

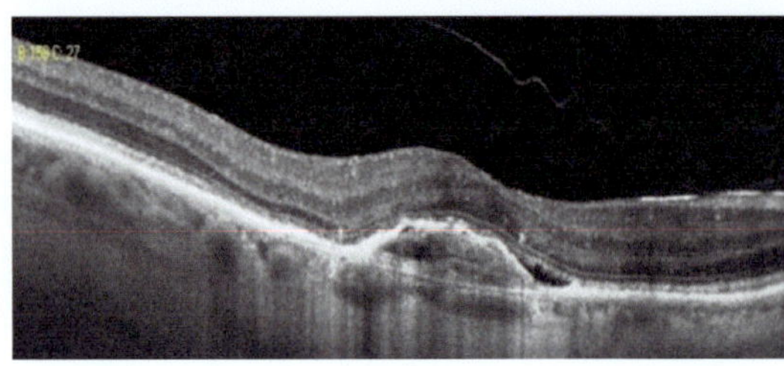

Fig. 12.9 The highly reflective layer of the RPE forms a convex line and the sub-RPE lumen is medium reflective. In addition, there is a sensory detachment laterally to the fovea

In PCV, SD-OCT shows sharp tips and multiple pigment epithelial detachments. This helps in the differentiation from occult CNV's.

The distinction in SD-OCT between PCV and occult CNV shows typical indicators: sharp pigment epithelial detachments, tomographic notch, hyporeflective lumen of the PED, several PED's and hard exudates (funduscopy). These OCT signs occur much more frequently in PCV than in occult CNV. PCV shows lipid and hemorrhage through the polyps and the choroid is typically thickened, changes in RPE are visible and no drusen are visible. SD-OCT detects the vascular lesions of PCV in the sub-RPE space.

This suggests that PCV may be a type 1 CNV variant [15].

The PCV does not respond properly to anti-VEGF treatment. Therefore, it is important to identify PCV in cases of poor response to anti-VEGF and perform ICG in these cases [16]. The treatment differs for occult CNV (type 1) and PCV—therefore, identification is important.

RPE Rip

A possible complication of neovascular AMD (nAMD) may be RPE rip, in which the RPE is torn and leads to a fibrotic scar of the macula (Figs. 12.10 and 12.11b, c). VA decreases as the scar increases. The development process can be

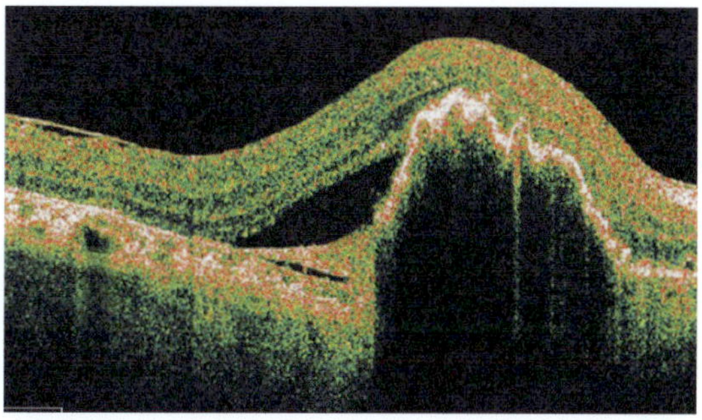

Fig. 12.10 The RPE rip demonstrates an interruption of the RPE layer. The elastic RPE layer shows bundling and a wavy appearance (like a rubber band). A subretinal detachment by the traction of the RPE elevation is typical. The loss of RPE in the RPE rip is associated with inverse shading

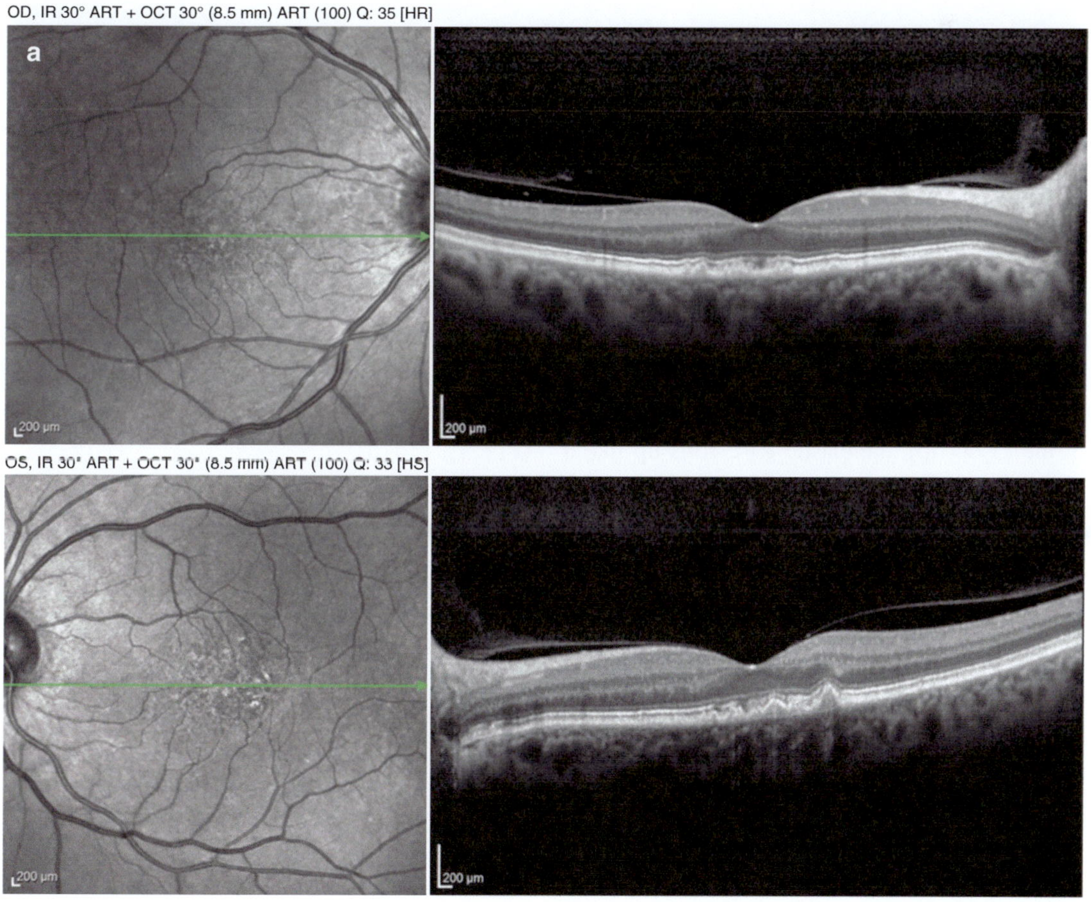

Fig. 12.11 4 years follow-up of a development of RPE rip, from drusen to sPED, RPE rip and subsequent CNV (Type 1). (**a**) SD-OCT shows small miliar, spiky drusen. (**b**) Both eyes developed a sPED, with an RPE rip on the left eye, OCT. (**c**) Increasing scarring and sensory detachment of the rupture side (OS) can be observed in OCT. (**d**) A macular scar in OCT and new intraretinal cystoid formation as an indicator for CNV are found

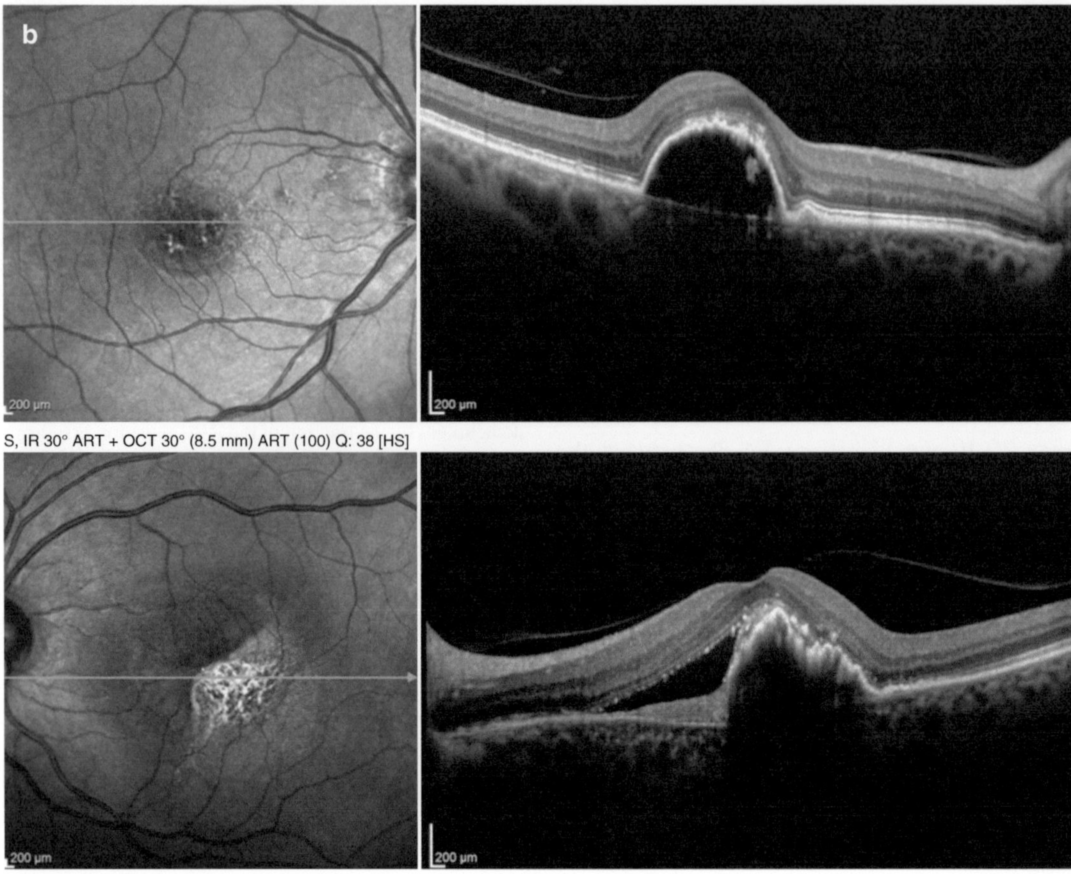

Fig. 12.11 (continued)

observed with modern OCT. In the event of a tear of the PED (rip), the elastic RPE rolls up like a rubber band. The torn part shows atrophy of the RPE with inverse shading of the OCT light beam.

The RPE Rip is most common in an underlying choroidal neovascular process. In the case of an active CNV base, anti-VEGF treatment must be applied and continued. Vascularized PED tears are mainly associated with occult CNV, PCV and RAP lesions.

The follow-up of a patient from 2014 to 2018 with some drusen at the beginning (VA 0.3) and finally an RPE rip and fibrotic scar in 2018 is shown in Fig. 12.11 (VA 0.05) (Fig. 12.11a–d).

Central Serous Chorioretinopathy (CSCR)

Typical OCT findings in CSCR are neurosensory detachment (optically empty subretinal fluid) between the outer retina and the RPE layer and focal serous (s) PED, either as a focus or double detachment (Fig. 12.12a, b). In the acute stage, the focus sPED can often be identified (75%). In rare cases, a double peak sPED is visible. In chronic stages of CSCR RPE, atrophy and loss of photoreceptors

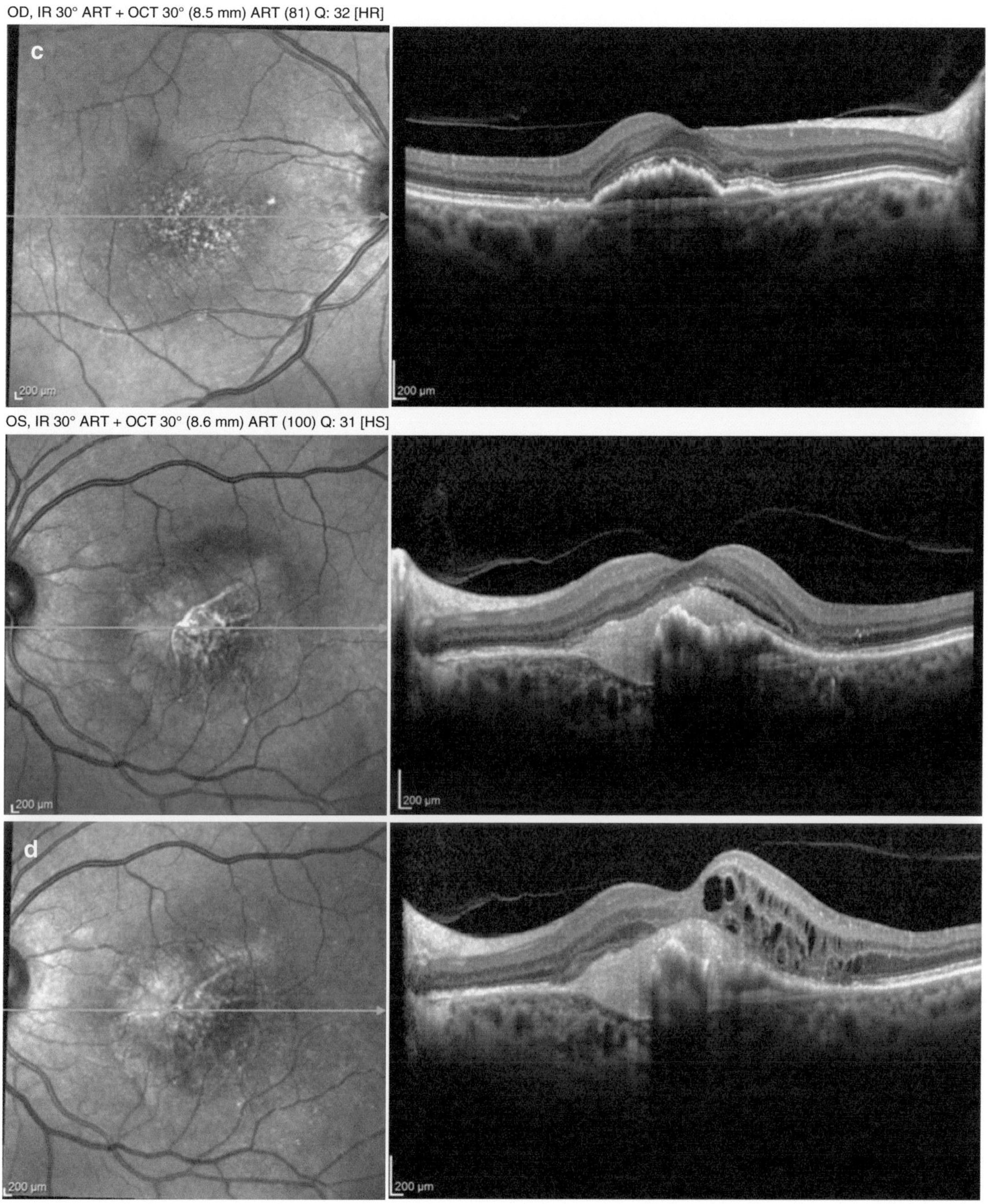

Fig. 12.11 (continued)

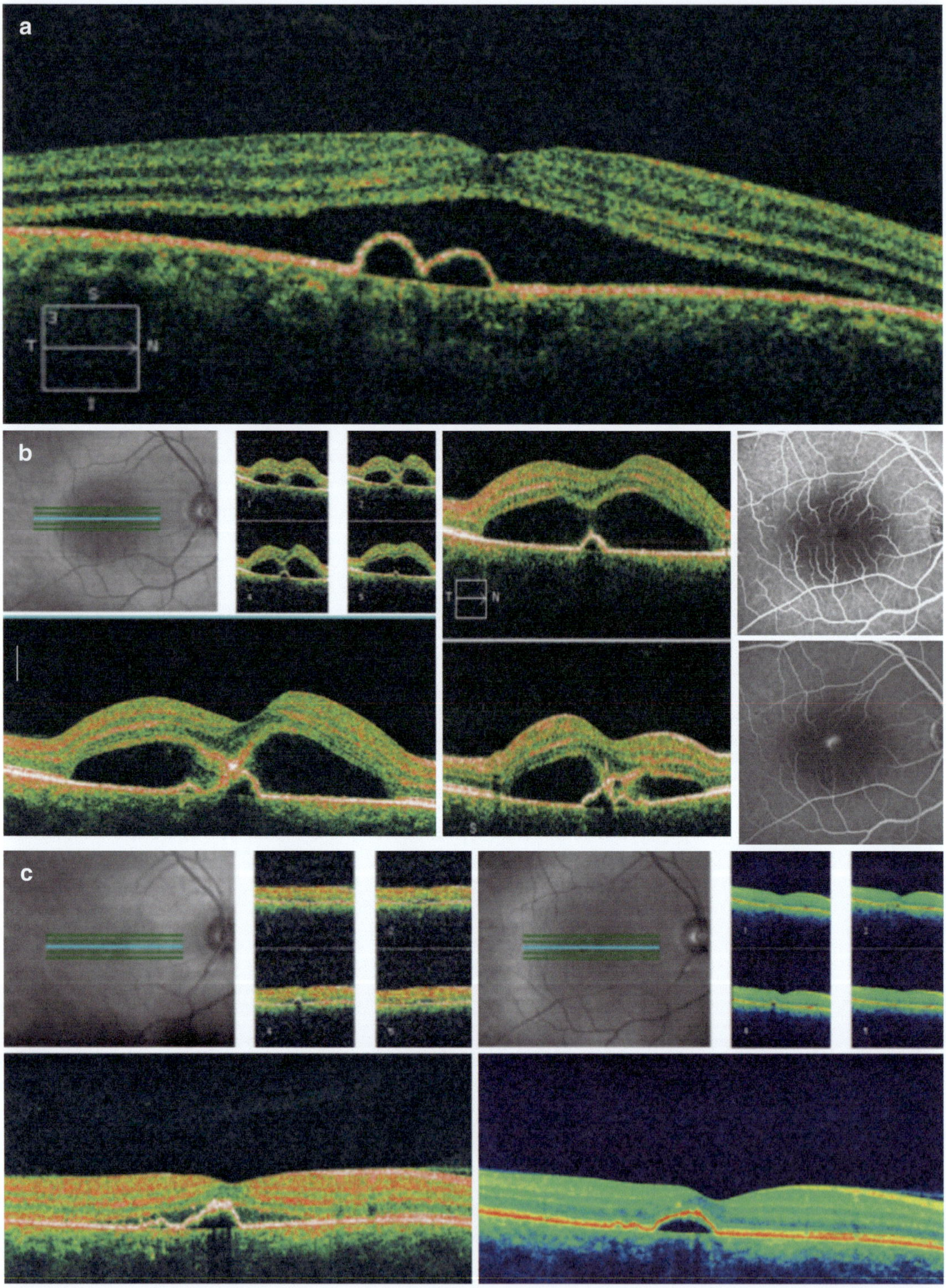

Fig. 12.12 (**a**) OCT in CSCR shows a double peak serous PED and an accompanying sensory retinal detachment. VA is 0.5 OD. Right: FLA shows the typical leakage very close to the fovea (smoke banner phenomenon). (**b**) Left: OCT image shows a sensory detachment and a rare scarring of the retina with the underlying sPED. Right: FLA shows typical subfoveal smoke banner phenomenon, not suitable for laser treatment of sPED (leakage = source point). (**c**) One month later the sensory detachment has resolved, and the VA has improved to 1.0. The sPED remains and may exhibit recurrent CSCR in the future

may occur. CSCR is defined by subretinal fluid and high choroidal permeability on the OCT. The FLA shows a chimney smoke-like pattern and an umbrella leak (Fig. 12.12). The exemplary patient depicted in Fig. 12.12 suffered from visual deterioration in CSCR (VA 0.8). OCT shows sensory detachment and scarring of the sensory retina and the underlying RPE separation in CSCR (rare case). FLA shows sub to juxtafoveal leakage. After treatment, the sensory retina was attached (Fig. 12.12c).

In OCT-A of the superficial and deep retinal plexus, the outer retina and the choriocapillaris showed no altered flow pattern correlating with the leakage point in CSCR [17].

Drusen

Typical signs of early AMD are drusen and atrophy of RPE, in late-stage geographic atrophy and wet AMD. Late AMD exists in dry (85%) and wet (15%) form. In addition to classic late AMD, the lesion shows retinal angiomatous proliferation (RAP) and PCV. Pathological characteristics of AMD are an accumulation of lipofuscin within RPE cells and the appearance of drusen.

The clinical classification of AMD is divided into small drusen (<63 μm), medium drusen (>63 to <125 μm) and large drusen (>125 μm). Small drusen are only droplets and represent normal aging changes. Medium drusen show the early stage of AMD, large drusen the medium AMD including pigmentary changes. Late AMD is defined as neovascular AMD (nAMD) and/or geographic atrophy (GA) [14].

In general, drusen are accumulations of extracellular material and metabolites between BM and RPE (e.g. lipofuscin, cholesterol). The material in SD-OCT has a medium to highly reflective and largely homogeneous form. Drusen can occur as single drusen or in confluent distribution. In addition, the overlying structure may show hyperreflective lesions.

In AMD (dAMD and nAMD), both hard and soft drusen types may occur.

Reticular Drusen (Hard Drusen)

Reticular drusen are granular, irregular and hyperreflexive lesions above the RPE. Hard/reticular drusen show sharp hyperreflexive peaks in OCT compared to flat curved RPE detachments in soft drusen (Figs. 12.5, 12.11a, 12.13, and 12.14) [18, 19].

Soft Drusen

In the early phase, an expansion of the joint structure of BM and RPE in the OCT can be observed. Basal laminar drusen are probably an early form of serous drusen and differ in sub-RPE thickening in SD-OCT (BM can be distinguished from RPE). Soft drusen are identified on OCT by discrete elevations of the RPE layer at the BM level. Soft drusen are typically considered as a collection of optically scattering material (Figs. 12.5 and 12.14) between RPE and BM. In larger drusen or drusenoid PEDs, a greater height of the RPE occurs, often dome-shaped, with hypo- or medium-reflective material separating the RPE from the underlying BM [8, 20].

SD-OCT identifies different types of sub-RPE hyperreflectivity in the regression of calcified drusen.

Type 1 is a multilaminar hyperreflection from the suspected inner part of the BM, type 2 is also a multilaminar hyperreflection from the outer part of the BM and type 3 is a multilaminar fragmented hyperreflection from both parts of the BM. Drusenoid material not removed by macrophages develops calcification (hyperreflection) similar to the arteriosclerosis process. The deposits of lipids and cholesterol, if not removed by macrophages, will likely follow calcification of lipids (hyperreflection in the sub-RPE layer) [21].

Reticular Pseudodrusen

SD-OCT helped to identify so-called reticular pseudodrusen. Reticular pseudodrusen correspond to discrete collections of hyper-reflective material located above the RPE between the RPE and the ellipsoidal zone. Pseudodrusen are hyperreflective granule structures in SD-OCT [8, 20, 22, 23]. The Beaver Dam Eye Study identified reticular drusen as one of the major risk factors for the development of advanced AMD.

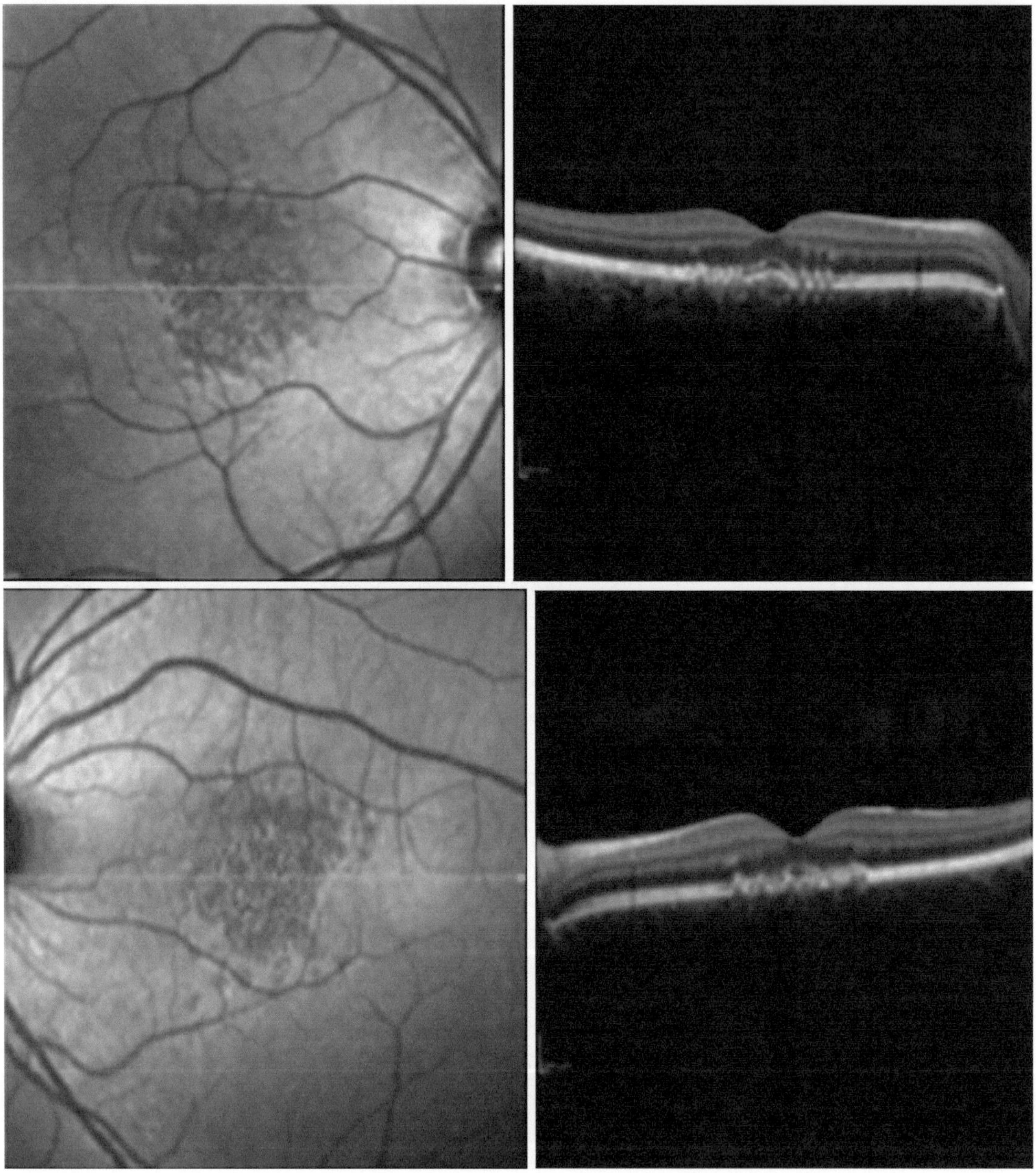

Fig. 12.13 OCT Spectralis demonstrates miliar drusen and VA 1.0 (29-year-old male)

RPE Thickening

RPE Thickening by Neovascularization

Age-Related CNV (nAMD)

The typical finding of OCT in nAMD is fibrovascular RPE thickening and subretinal fluid or cystoid macular edema. Subretinal hemorrhage may also occur. The classification of CNV into classic and occult CNV is based on FLA. But in high-resolution OCT, differentiation can usually also be accomplished.

Classic CNV (type 2) penetrates the RPE/BM complex and is in the subretinal space between

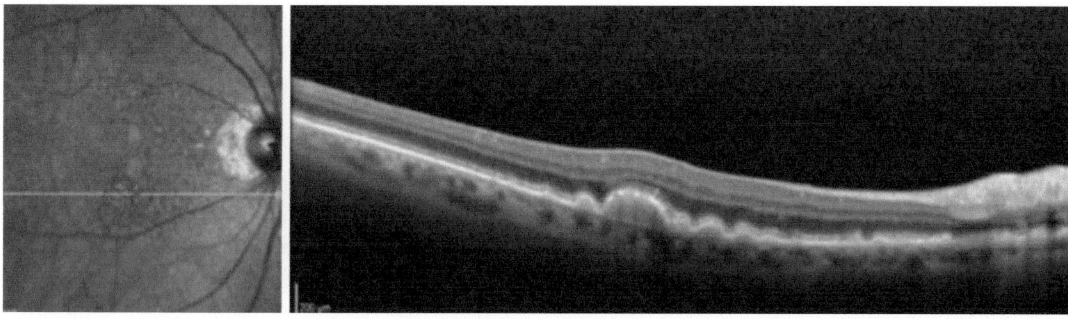

Fig. 12.14 A typical image in serous drusen at early AMD with VA of 1.0. The Spectralis OCT shows a typical curvy RPE separation with a central reflection zone beyond the RPE. The BM is visible as a fine horizontal line beyond the deposition. The drusen show different size and extension

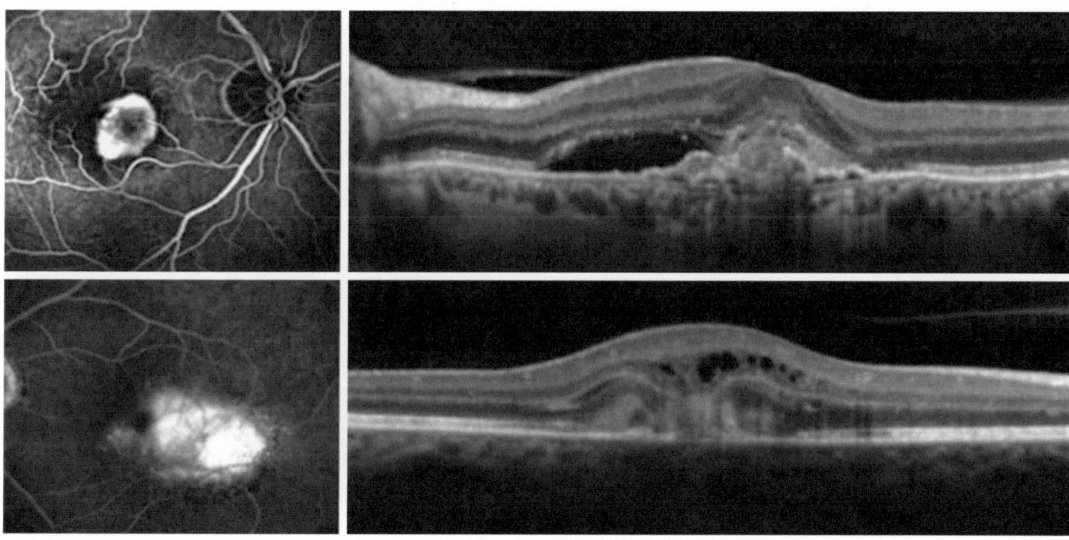

Fig. 12.15 Above: FLA with a typical classic CNV (type 2), sharply defined and above the RPE. OCT (Spectralis) on the right shows the thickening of the RPE/BM layer complex (= neovascular membrane) and subretinal fluid. Below: FLA with occult CNV (type 1), diffuse leakage. OCT shows thickening of the RPE/BM complex and typical intraretinal cystoid formation

the RPE and sensory retina. In FLA, type 2 is well delimited by the visualization of the pathological new subretinal vessels of the macula (Fig. 12.15).

In contrast, the occult CNV (type 1) is the neovascular tissue below the RPE (between RPE and choriocapillaris). In these cases (type 1), the frequency of intraretinal cystoid edema is significantly higher than in classical CNV (type 2). Subretinal fluid is more abundant in classical CNV (Fig. 12.15).

Mixed forms of both types 1 and 2 are common in nAMD. OCT is very important for fluid detection in each retinal and subretinal space and leads to further treatment with anti-VEGF. The indication for the treatment of age-related CNV is based on any fluid within the retina (cystoid spaces or subretinal fluid) regardless of the layer [22, 24, 25].

Type 1 CNV represents the occult CNV (in FLA), which originates from the choriocapillaris. It is often associated with an overlying PED. OCT-A in type 1 CNV shows an entangled network of fine vessels or a round tuft of small-caliber capillaries.

Type 2 CNV corresponds to the classic CNV in FLA (incidence 9–17%). The CNV is located above the RPE in the subretinal space. In the OCT-A, the macula above the RPE presents high flow vessels, which are described as medusa- or glomerulus-shaped patterns.

Type 3 CNV combines type 1 and type 2 patterns. It is previously referred to as RAP lesion or occult chorioretinal anastomosis. Type 3 is predominantly perpendicular to the retinal layers and may extend to the RPE.

OCT-A was compared with multimodal imaging (FLA, ICG, SD-OCT) for the need for treatment in wet AMD. Five results in OCTA were described: (1) form of neovascular lesion, (2) branching patterns (fine or large vessels), (3) anastomoses and vessel loops, (4) peripheral arcade or dense vessel endings, (5) perilesional hypointense halo. Three or more of the criteria represent an active lesion and have been treated with intravitreal injection and two or fewer criteria show an inactive lesion without subsequent treatment. This criterion division corresponds to 95% of the treatment indication by conventional multimodal imaging (FLA, ICG, SD-OCT).

Different types of CNV in exudative AMD can be visualized and differentiated with OCT-A. Type 1 CNV were larger with little differentiation from the surrounding vascular system and were visible on the slab "Mid-Choroid", "CC" and "RPE". In contrast, type 2 CNV showed a sharp demarcation from the surrounding vascular structure reaching to the slab "outer retina" [26]. The use of ICG shows a larger size of CNV compared to different OCT-A devices with different wavelengths, scan patterns and algorithms. Due to different segmented layers for the evaluation of CNV quantitative parameters such as CNV range, vessel density recommends a standardized OCT-A protocol for analysis [27]. OCT-A was generally less successful in detecting CNV compared to ICG. OCT was superior in the detection of CNV type 1 compared to type 2. SD-OCT-A is limited by the detection of blood flow velocity, rather than lesion type [28].

Myopic CNV

Myopic CNV is similar to age-related CNV in OCT. OCT shows similar results in highly myopic CNV. The myopic CNV is typically found as classic CNV (type 2) above the RPE and shows little edema or fluid (very rare intraretinal cysts).

Pachychoroid CNV (PNV)

Pachychoroidal diseases are considered disorders of the RPE and a typical choroidal thickening. Identification of pachychoroidal diseases began in 2013 due to long-wave SS-OCT (EDI enhanced depth imaging) and faster scan acquisition.

Pachychoroidal diseases show an increased choroidal thickness, dilated veins in the Haller layer (pachy veins) and dilution in the Sattler and Choriocapillaris layer.

The choroidal thickness is between 220 and 350 μm, and a thick choroid is defined by a thickness of more than 390 μm.

PNV is typically presented in OCT as CNV with choroidal thickening and missing drusen. Very typical indicators are irregular and very flat PEDs. PNV can be converted to PCV disease.

The spectrum of pachychoroidal diseases includes four different disease groups: Pachychoroidal pigment epitheliopathy (PPE), central serous chorioretinopathy (CSCR), pachychoroidal neovasculopathy (PNV), polypoidal choroidal vasculopathy (PCV). One disease may pass into another. PPE shows small focal RPE detachments, no drusen, and no subretinal fluid and may be a precursor of CSCR. In summary, PPE shows choroidal thickening, thinning in choriocapillaris and changes in RPE [29].

RAP

The RAP lesion described by Yannuzzi 2001 [30] is a specific clinical form of neovascularization in AMD. Neovascularization originates from the outer retinal layer and grows towards RPE (type 3 CNV). RAP-CNV does not respond properly to anti-VEGF treatment.

Hyperreflexive focus on drusen in the outer retinal layer is probably a precursor of the RAP lesion. The identification of precursor signs in SD-OCT is possible by using a B-Scan OCT with high sample density and eye tracking mode. It may take about 21 months to complete progression from precursor to RAP level [31].

RPE Thickening Due to Deposits

Pattern Dystrophy: APMD (Adult Onset Pseudovitelliform Macular Dystrophy)

Pattern dystrophies show a high variety of macular phenomena (butterfly-shaped macular dystrophy, APMD). In funduscopy, a yellow or orange elevation of the fovea in the OCT correlates with a disorder at the RPE level. In pseudovitelliform macular dystrophy (APMD) in adults, moderate to highly reflective material lies beneath the sensory retina and above the RPE [32]. OCT shows a dome-shaped, subretinal, homogeneous hyporeflective layer between the RPE/fracture membrane and the ellipsoid zone of the photoreceptors (Fig. 12.16a, b).

The lesion may also resemble large serous drusen. But APMD occurs with a single foveal yellowish lesion and AMD shows drusen in larger numbers. Discrimination is also possible in the OCT. Serous drusen in OCT show an RPE detachment with an optically empty lumen or a medium reflective filling of the PED (Fig. 12.16a, b). In contrast, APMD shows an increase of a mean reflective convex area above the RPE. This image simulates a CNV in OCT, sometimes also in funduscopy. But unlike CNV, VA is much better and typically OCT shows no subretinal fluid, intraretinal cysts, or hemorrhage.

In about 12% after 6 years, CNV can occur as a rare complication of APMD. In FLA, the drusenoid material leads to staining that can be confused with CNV. The diagnosis is usually obvious, but in difficult cases follow-up of the disease, VA, OCT (fluid accumulation?) and FLA (multimodal imaging) leads to the correct diagnosis.

OCT-A is able to clearly show the presence of CNV, which is hardly visible in the FLA due

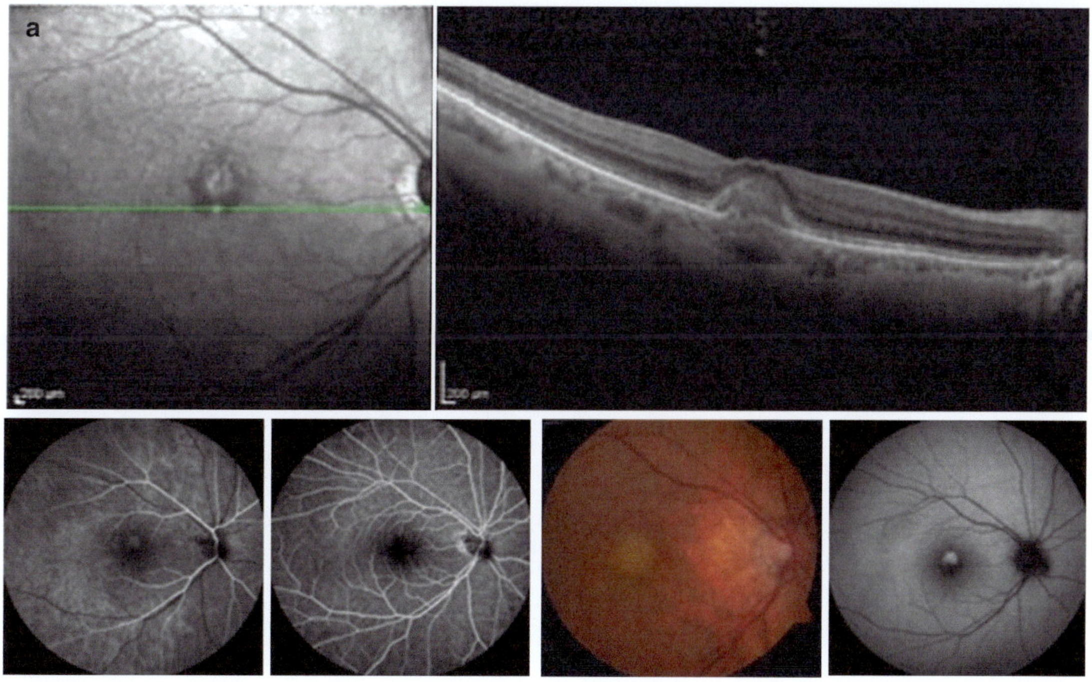

Fig. 12.16 (**a**) VA of both eyes 1.0. OCT shows convex thickening in OD as in CNV, but never accompanied by edema or subretinal fluid. The fundus image shows a typical yellow spot of the macula, also in autofluorescence (AF) a white spot without lipofuscin. The FLA below typically shows no leakage, only slight staining of the lipofuscin deposit. (**b**) SD-OCT shows a convex elevation above RPE-BM without fluid accumulation. The underlying RPE/BM layer is hardly visible under the vitelliform deposit

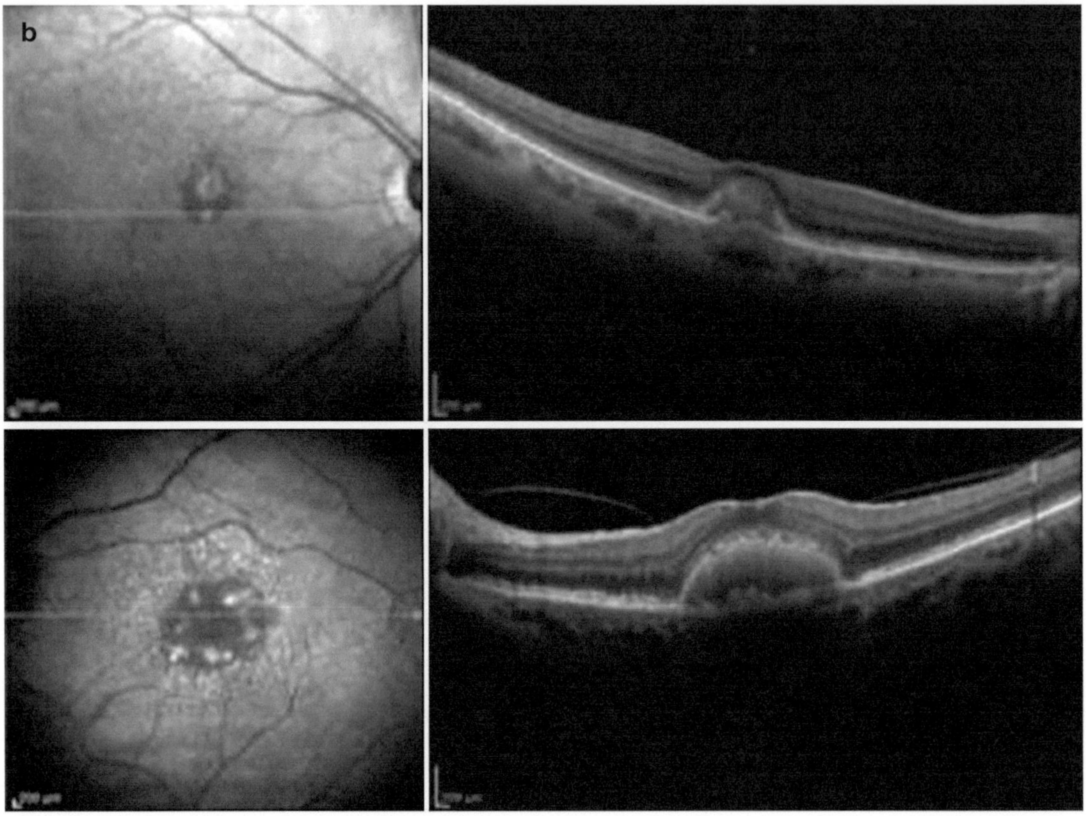

Fig. 12.16 (continued)

to blocking phenomena of vitelliform deposit. Vascular abnormalities in the OCT-A are nonspecific in the superficial and deep capillary plexus. The most important advantage of OCT-A in APMD is the detection of the underlying CNV, which is better detected in OCT-A than in FLA [33].

Best's Disease (Vitelliform Disease)

Best's disease is an autosomal dominant dystrophy of the macula. In vitelliform stage 2 of Best's disease, the subretinal material is homogeneous and hyperreflective. In pseudohypopyon stage 3 there is a homogeneous hyporeflective layer above the hyperreflective layer. This can be misunderstood as subretinal fluid after CNV. The "crumbled egg" stage 4 shows RPE atrophy and hypertrophy (Fig. 12.17). Stage 5, finally, shows a macular scar.

Best's disease very impressively shows that OCT is an image of reflectivity and not histology. The OCT image shows significant distortion of the normal layer structure of the retina.

In OCT, no structure is visible at the photoreceptor and RPE levels, but the VA is 1.0 (Fig. 12.17). Therefore, photoreceptors must be present but are not visible in OCT. The light beam of the OCT is backscattered by the vitelliform deposit and therefore does not reach the photoreceptors and the RPE/BM complex PED. This area does not seem to be absent, but it shows an artifact of the reflectivity image by the OCT.

It is of great interest at which layer vitelliform deposits accumulate. The average thickness of the foveal RPE/BM layer is significantly reduced in Best's disease (all stages) compared to healthy subjects, but not outside the fovea. The vitelliform deposit is most likely located within the interdigitation zone or the RPE/BM complex. It is possible that RPE may continue to form a preserved photoreceptor-RPE complex that provides essential nutrients to the photoreceptors and in turn helps patients maintain better than expected VA for years [34].

Histology shows that the vitelliform deposit between Bruch's membrane and RPE accumulates in the fovea. This material appeared to be derived from degenerating pigment epithelial cells and contained only a few intact lipofuscin granules. Loss of the foveal photoreceptor also occurred above the lesion [35].

The outer retinal layers remains in stage 1, but an interruption can be seen in stage 2–5. The vitelliform material is always found in stage 2 and 3, predominantly in stage 4 and rarely in stage 5. Neurosensory detachment occurred in stages 3 and 4. The more the vitelliform deposit decreased with the progressive development of Best's disease, the more the outer retinal layers were interrupted in the advanced stage [36].

RPE Atrophy

Geographical Atrophy (GA)

The atrophy of RPE is based on two or three criteria in a range of >125 µm: increased signal transmission through the choroid (choroidal

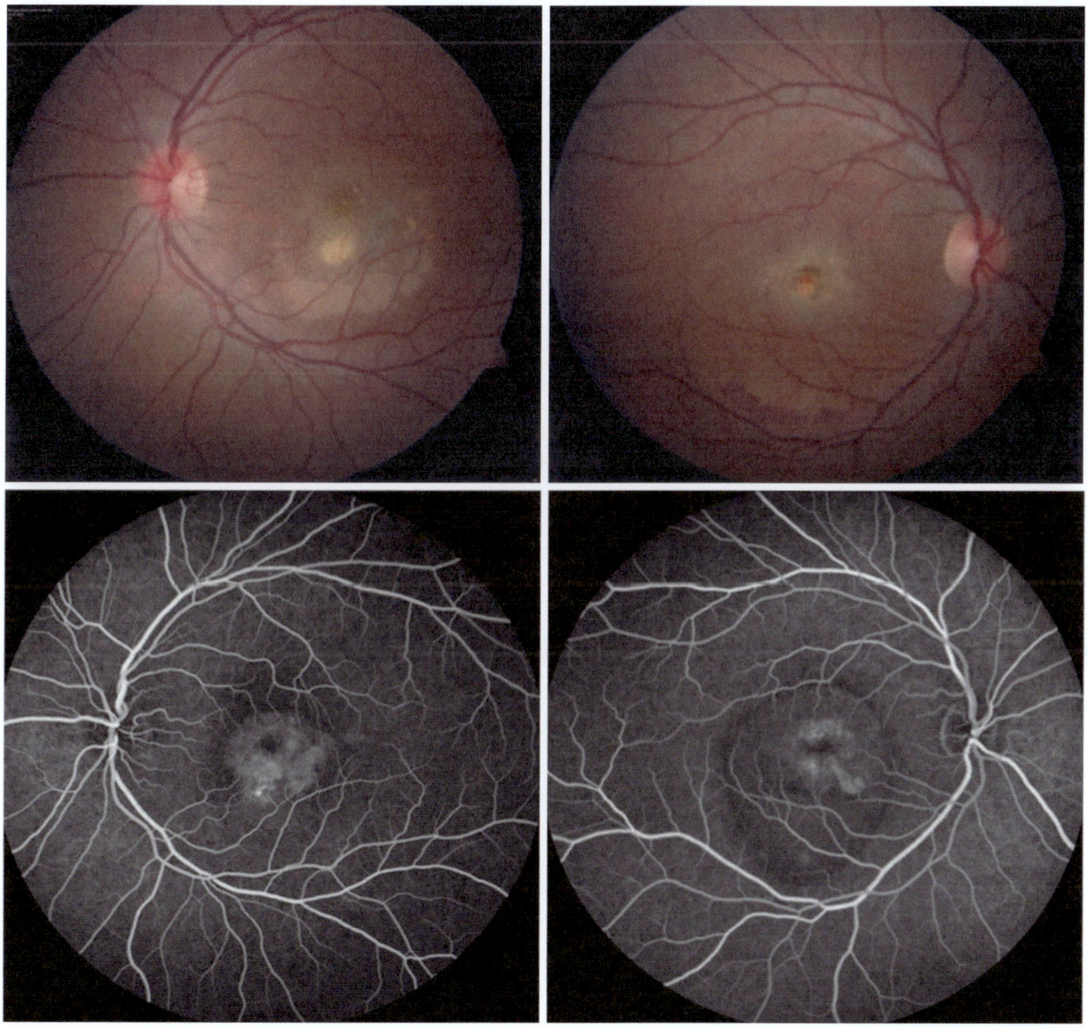

Fig. 12.17 24-year-old male patient, VA 0.8 and 1.0 with Best's disease. The colored fundus image shows typical intermediate morbus Best's (upper line). The FLA of the Best's disease, a patchy, mild hyperfluorescence is visible that corresponds to staining of the vitelliform deposits (center). In SD-OCT, extensive subretinal detachment of the macula over the attached RPE/BM layer (bottom)

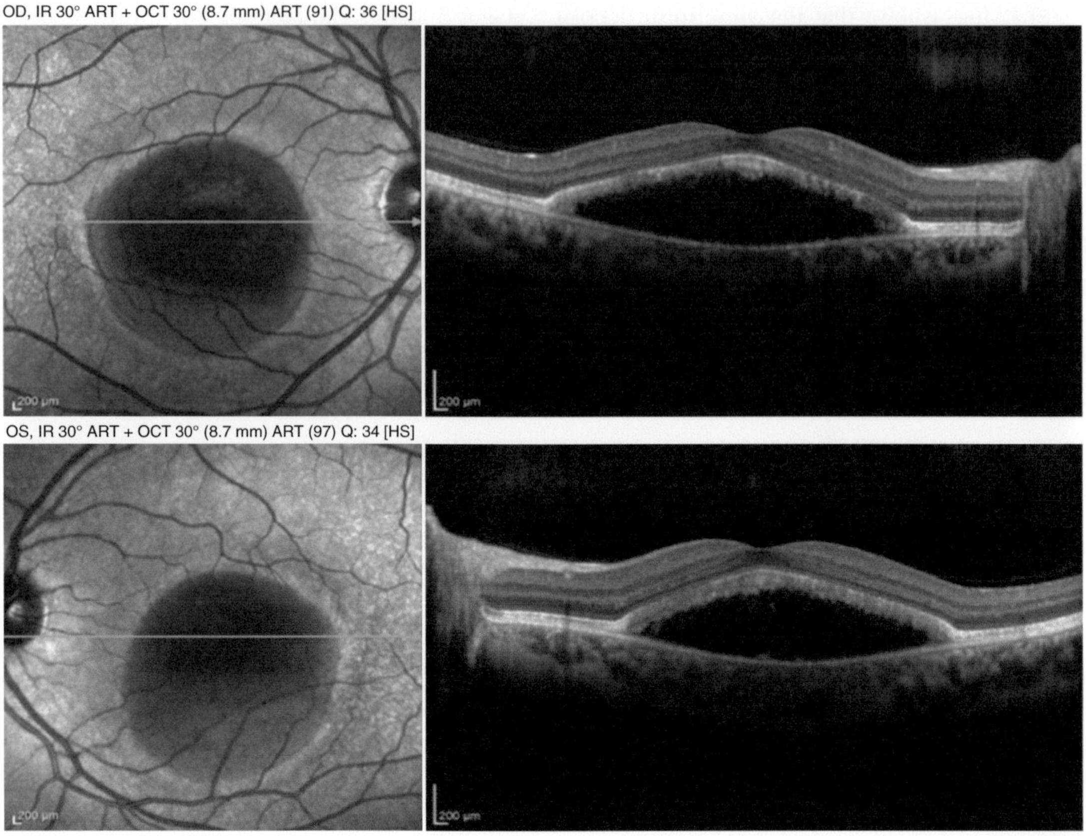

Fig. 12.17 (continued)

hypertransmission), attenuation of the RPE band and loss of the outer retinal layers [19].

GA is a form of dry AMD and occurs with increasing atrophy of the overlying RPE. SD-OCT results in a large-area deficiency of the RPE BM layer with subsequent reverse shadowing in SD-OCT. Due to the absence of the highly reflective RPE layer, the light can penetrate deeper layers (Fig. 12.18).

A broad spectrum of morphological changes in SD-OCT can be found in the GA, both in the surrounding area and in the atrophic region. These changes may represent different disease stages or different molecular heterogeneity [10].

Further longitudinal studies must demonstrate the prognostic effect of these morphological changes. The quantitative indicators for the progression of the disease from early AMD to advanced AMD (within 2 years) were the outer retinal thickness, the drusen area and the hyperreflective focus. Predictive hallmarks for CNV were drusen-centered, while hallmarks for GA were associated with neurosensory retina and age, using artificial intelligence [37].

The magnitude of the RPE visible in OCT and the defects of the photoreceptor in GA lesions differ significantly. These include the outer segments of the photoreceptor that remain in the absence of RPE cells and vice versa. These results are also important for understanding pathogenesis and treatment development [38].

The perfusion of choriocapillaris was significantly reduced adjacent to GA (AMD) measured with OCT-A. Choriocapillaris hypoperfusion was correlated with a loss of the cone photoreceptor. This suggests that reduced choriocapillaris perfusion contributes to the development of GA [39].

Choriocapillaris flow impairment around GA correlates with the annual growth rate of GA

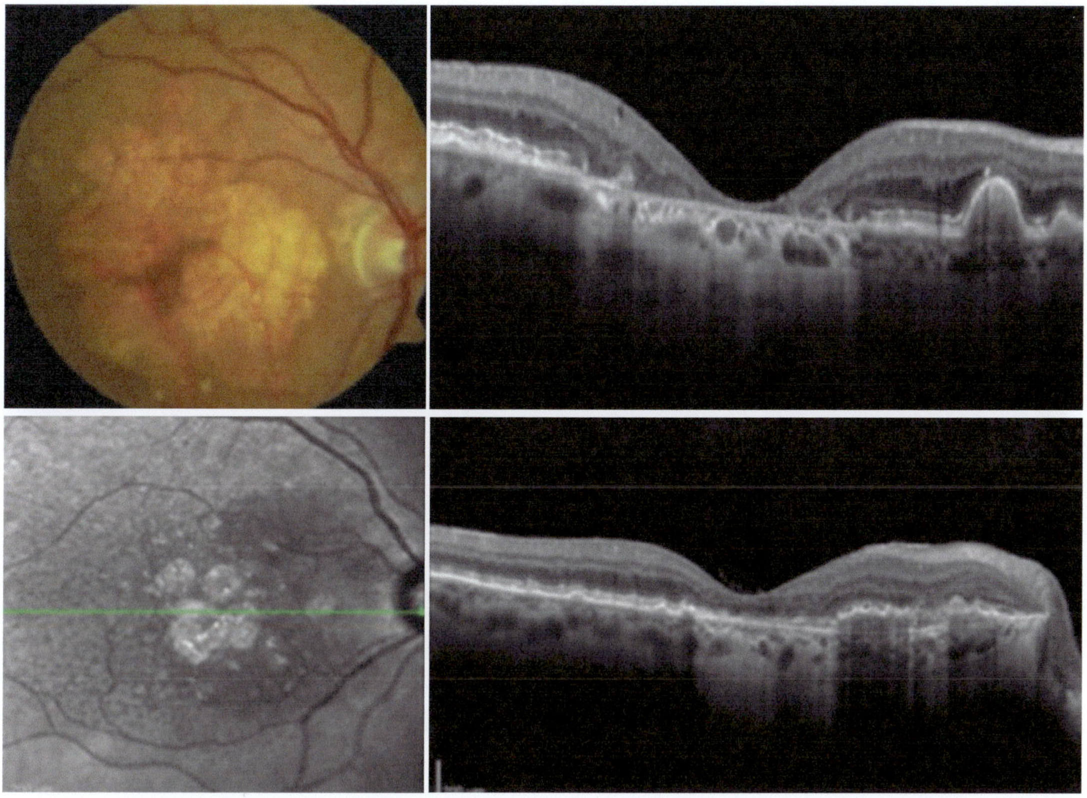

Fig. 12.18 The fundus image shows a typical GA. In OCT, the atrophy of the RPE is subfoveal and additionally large drusen are visible. The OCT identifies typical focal light enhancement as there is no highly reflective RPE

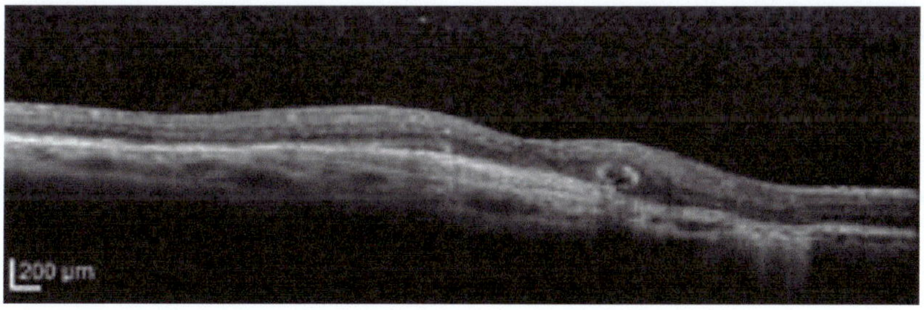

Fig. 12.19 An outer retinal tubulation is identified by OCT over the RPE-BM complex within the outer retinal layers. It is suspected that degenerating photoreceptors are arranged in a circle (circular hyperreflectivity in OCT)

expansion. This shows a useful parameter for prognostic surrogate in patients with GA [40].

A special condition in GA is represented by the outer retinal tubulation (ORT) (Fig. 12.19). It is presumed that degenerating photoreceptors become arranged circular. Individual RPE cells are found in the lumen of the ORT. The ORT must be differentiated from intraretinal cyst formation because unnecessary treatment may possibly be prompted [41].

Stargardt's Disease and Fundus Flavimaculatus

The abnormal deposits in the fundus flavimaculatus can be located on the RPE layer confirmed by OCT. In Stargardt's disease, atrophy of the outer

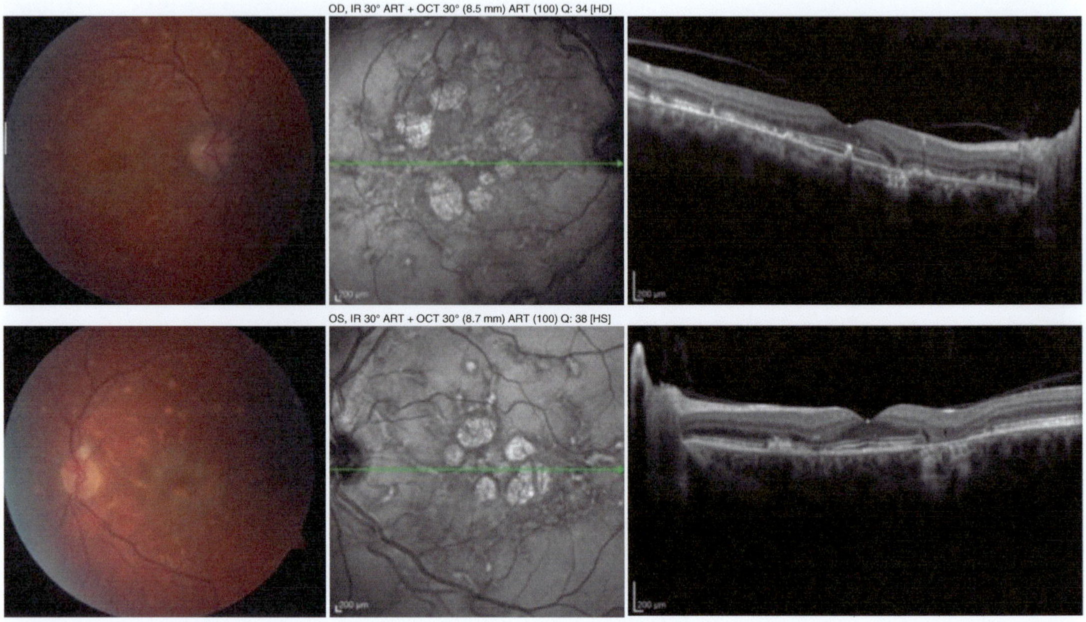

Fig. 12.20 In case of Stargardt's disease with fundus flavimaculatus VA both eyes 1.0. Left: The funduscopic white lesions show focal atrophy of the RPE in OCT. The abnormal deposits in the fundus flavimaculatus can be localized on the RPE layer as focal thickening confirmed by OCT

retinal layers and the RPE can also be observed. Stargardt's disease with fundus flavimaculatus shows focal thickening and atrophy of the RPE simultaneously (Fig. 12.20).

In SD-OCT, the area of ellipsoid zone loss is more reliable than the RPE [42] for monitoring the course of disease in Stargardt's disease.

The choroidal flow signal with OCT-A differs in RPE atrophy in late onset Stargardt's disease and AMD. This choroidal different perfusion may implicate a different pathogenesis of RPE atrophy in both diseases [43].

Choroideremia

A severe loss of RPE in choreoideremic diseases increases the light transmission from OCT to choroid and sclera. The sensory retina appears to lie on the choroid/choriocapillary. Without the highly reflective RPE, deeper penetration into the choroid and sclera is possible.

Choriocapillaris and choroid appear to be almost completely absent (Fig. 12.21). The RPE layer and a very thin choroid lie directly adjacent to the thick sclera. Due to the lack of highly reflective RPE and choroidal vascular supply, the sclera is clearly visible in this situation of choroideremia (Fig. 12.21).

Quantification of the RPE layer and ellipsoid zone on OCT images is highly reproducible and therefore suitable for clinical studies and follow-up [44]. In OCT-A, early vascular abnormalities in the inner retinal layers and choriocapillaris can be observed. In addition, a reduced vascular flow was detectable in preserved macular RPE. OCT-A is useful to detect the vascular situation early in choroideremia [45].

The loss of RPE after inflammation or infectious diseases may lead to the same appearance in OCT, e.g. serpiginous choroiditis, toxoplasmic chorioretinitis, birdshot chorioretinopathy.

Secondary Toxic RPE Damage

Solar/Laser Retinopathy

Looking into the sun or high-energy lasers (such as industrial lasers or non-approved laser pointers) can cause severe retinal damage. The absorption of the laser radiation in visible light (often red 670 nm and green 532 nm) occurs mainly

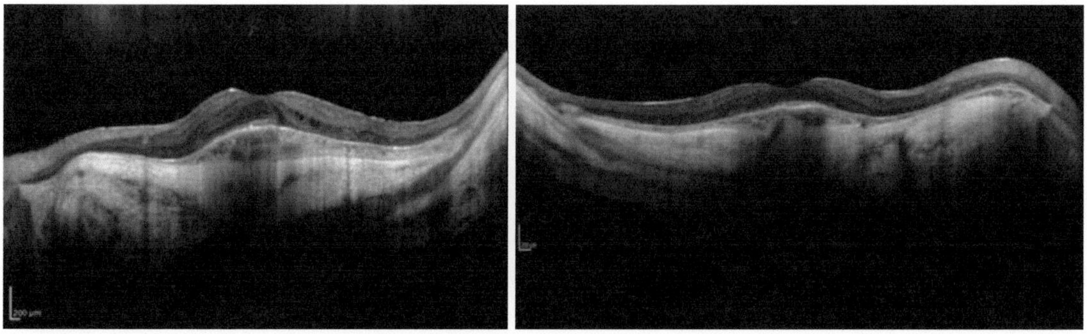

Fig. 12.21 An OCT of choroideremia shows the absence of a highly reflective RPE layer and choriocapillary, but very deep insight into the choroid and sclera

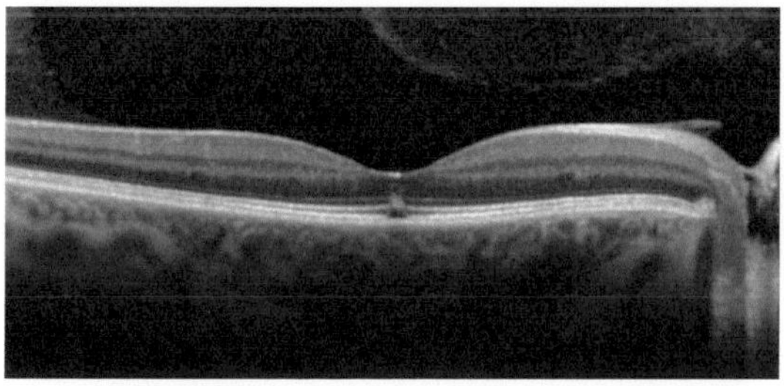

Fig. 12.22 Spectralis OCT image of a 34-year-old woman (VA 0.6) observing a partial solar eclipse without special protective glasses. OCT shows a hyporeflective area subfoveally and a disorder of the photoreceptors

in the outer layers of the retina; the RPE is typically spared (Fig. 12.22). This results in damage that leads to degeneration of the photoreceptors. Sun arc injuries occur in OCT as focal loss of the outer retina and the IS-OS/ellipsoid layer, leaving a small hyporeflective rectangular cavity. Complications of laser exposure include retinal hemorrhage, CNV and chronic macular edema [46, 47]. Histological studies have localized the damage of the outer segments of the foveal photoreceptor and the RPE.

Poppers Maculopathy

Poppers (isopropyl nitrate) are inhaled to give people a brief period of exhilaration. They contain liquid nitrogen chemicals which cause a flush of arterial dilatation. Poppers have recently been used to treat angina pectoris and can affect the macula by causing macular degeneration at an early age at the level of RPE. Poppers maculopathy may occur and presents as vitelliform lesions of the central macula (Fig. 12.23). The pathomechanism is still unclear but may be associated with modulated photoreceptor metabolism due to increased blood NO concentrations and vasodilatation. A vitelliform lesion in OCT of the fovea is shown above the RPE (Fig. 12.23). In SD-OCT, a blurred defect of the outer elements of the photoreceptors can be found. The RPE is slightly affected and appears blurred.

Summary and Future Developments

SD-OCT of the RPE has developed so far that we can now image the retinal microstructure [20]. SD-OCT technology has been successfully implemented in modern OCT systems and enables us to provide high-resolution imaging of the retina in vivo. This has greatly improved our understanding of RPE anatomy and function as well as changes in different pathological units. However, we must bear in mind that OCT is based on reflectivity, so association with histological data must be made carefully. The evaluation of AMD, a disease whose pathogenesis is in the RPE and adjacent structures, has greatly benefited from the introduction of SD-OCT. With the continuing rapid development of new imaging technologies, it is likely that OCT will provide further insights into the pathophysiology and treatment of retinal diseases.

The following developments contribute to the implementation and increasing importance

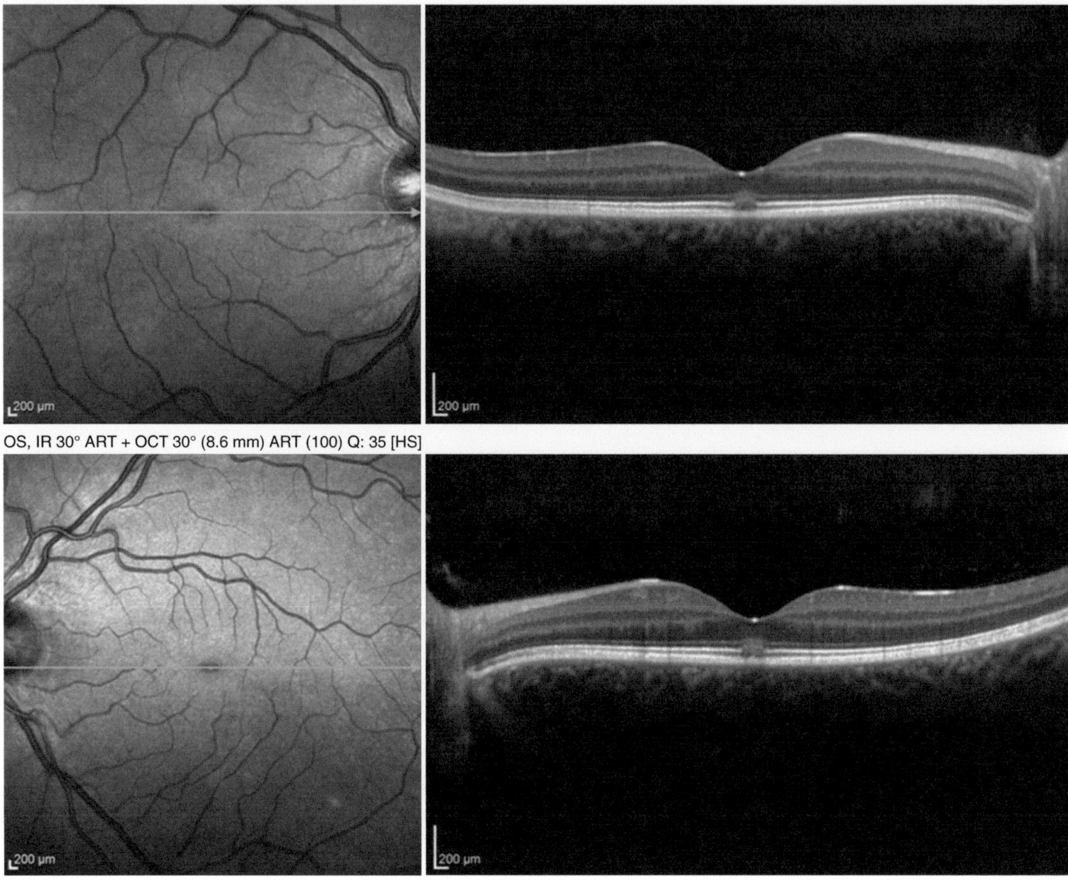

Fig. 12.23 The use of poppers leads to a vitelliform lesion in OCT and a visual deterioration (VA 0.3). The outer retinal layers (photoreceptors) and the RPE layer are affected and blurred

of OCT and OCT-A: Development of higher resolution, faster scan acquisition (software), automated segmentation and OCT angiography. In macular diseases, especially AMD, structural changes can be visualized in a large image analysis and can help in predicting the course of the disease and the prognosis. The development of potential biomarkers is possible. The higher the resolution and the individual layers of the retina can be visualized, the more predictive biomarkers can be developed.

Based on the extensive availability of OCT data, self-learning artificial intelligence (AI) may in the future be able to identify and examine patients and healthy volunteers with macular disease [37]. AI may play an important role for outpatients in the future, although there are limitations in the use of AI only for follow-up [48]. But it may be an option in the future for AI to help study the diseased and healthy population through telemedicine or even an app on the smartphone. The screening values can then lead to consultation with a specialist to confirm a suspected diagnosis.

References

1. Huang D, Swanson E, Lin C, Schuman J, Stinson W, Chang W, et al. Optical coherence tomography. Science. 1991;254:1178–81.
2. Swanson EA, Izatt JA, Hee MR, Huang D, Lin CP, Schuman JS, et al. In vivo retinal imaging by optical coherence tomography. Opt Lett. 1993;18:1864–6.
3. Ash C, Town G, Clement M. Confirmation of spectral jitter: a measured shift in the spectral distribution of intense pulsed light systems using a time-resolved spectrometer during exposure and increased fluence. J Med Eng Technol. 2010;34:97–107.

4. N'soukpoé-Kossi CN, Leblanc RM. Absorption and photoacoustic spectroscopies of lutein and zeaxanthin Langmuir–Blodgett films in connection with the Haidinger's brushes. Can J Chem. 1988;66: 1459–66.
5. Prahl S. Optical absorption of indocyanine green (ICG). 2018. https://omlc.org/spectra/icg/
6. Coscas GJ, Lupidi M, Coscas F, Cagini C, Souied EH. Optical coherence tomography angiography versus traditional multimodal imaging in assessing the activity of exudative age-related macular degeneration: a new diagnostic challenge. Retina. 2015;35:2219–28.
7. Lee JM, Park SC. The argument for swept-source OCT. Ophthalmol Manag. 2016;20:20–2.
8. Karampelas M, Sim DA, Keane PA. Spectral-domain OCT of the RPE. Retin Physician. 2014;11:53–9.
9. Runkle AP, Kaiser PK, Srivastava SK, Schachat AP, Reese JL, Ehlers JP. OCT angiography and ellipsoid zone mapping of macular telangiectasia type 2 from the AVATAR study. Invest Opthalmol Vis Sci. 2017;58:3683.
10. Fleckenstein M, Issa PC, Helb H-M, Schmitz-Valckenberg S, Finger RP, Scholl HPN, et al. High-resolution spectral domain-OCT imaging in geographic atrophy associated with age-related macular degeneration. Invest Opthalmol Vis Sci. 2008;49:4137.
11. Keane PA, Patel PJ, Liakopoulos S, Heussen FM, Sadda SR, Tufail A. Evaluation of age-related macular degeneration with optical coherence tomography. Surv Ophthalmol. 2012;57:389–414.
12. Schmitz-Valckenberg S, Steinberg JS, Fleckenstein M, Visvalingam S, Brinkmann CK, Holz FG. Combined confocal scanning laser ophthalmoscopy and spectral-domain optical coherence tomography imaging of reticular drusen associated with age-related macular degeneration. Ophthalmology. 2010;117:1169–76.
13. Moore DJ, Clover GM. The effect of age on the macromolecular permeability of human Bruch's membrane. Invest Ophthalmol Vis Sci. 2001;42:2970–5.
14. Balaratnasingam C, Messinger JD, Sloan KR, Yannuzzi LA, Freund KB, Curcio CA. Histologic and optical coherence tomographic correlates in drusenoid pigment epithelium detachment in age-related macular degeneration. Ophthalmology. 2017;124: 644–56.
15. Curcio CA, Zanzottera EC, Ach T, Balaratnasingam C, Freund KB. Activated retinal pigment epithelium, an optical coherence tomography biomarker for progression in age-related macular degeneration. Invest Ophthalmol Vis Sci. 2017;58:BIO211–26.
16. De Salvo G, Vaz-Pereira S, Keane PA, Tufail A, Liew G. Sensitivity and specificity of spectral-domain optical coherence tomography in detecting idiopathic polypoidal choroidal vasculopathy. Am J Ophthalmol. 2014;158:1228–1238.e1.
17. Feucht N, Maier M, Lohmann CP, Reznicek L. OCT angiography findings in acute central serous chorioretinopathy. Ophthalmic Surg Lasers Imaging Retina. 2016;47:322–7.
18. Ferris FL, Wilkinson CP, Bird A, Chakravarthy U, Chew E, Csaky K, et al. Clinical classification of age-related macular degeneration. Ophthalmology. 2013;120:844–51.
19. Gattoussi S, Buitendijk GHS, Peto T, Leung I, Schmitz-Valckenberg S, Oishi A, et al. The European Eye Epidemiology spectral-domain optical coherence tomography classification of macular diseases for epidemiological studies. Acta Ophthalmol. 2019;97:364–71.
20. Keane PA, Karampelas M, Sim DA, Sadda SR, Tufail A, Sen HN, et al. Objective measurement of vitreous inflammation using optical coherence tomography. Ophthalmology. 2014;121:1706–14.
21. Querques G, Georges A, Ben Moussa N, Sterkers M, Souied EH. Appearance of regressing drusen on optical coherence tomography in age-related macular degeneration. Ophthalmology. 2014;121:173–9.
22. Klein R, Klein BEK, Tomany SC, Meuer SM, Huang G-H. Ten-year incidence and progression of age-related maculopathy: the Beaver Dam Eye Study. Ophthalmology. 2002;109:1767–79.
23. Sohrab MA, Smith RT, Salehi-Had H, Sadda SR, Fawzi AA. Image registration and multimodal imaging of reticular pseudodrusen. Invest Opthalmol Vis Sci. 2011;52:5743.
24. Regatieri CV, Branchini L, Duker JS. The role of spectral-domain OCT in the diagnosis and management of neovascular age-related macular degeneration. Ophthalmic Surg Lasers Imaging. 2011;42:S56–66.
25. Roberts PK, Baumann B, Schlanitz FG, Sacu S, Bolz M, Pircher M, et al. Retinal pigment epithelial features indicative of neovascular progression in age-related macular degeneration. Br J Ophthalmol. 2017;101:1361–6.
26. Farecki M-L, Gutfleisch M, Faatz H, Rothaus K, Heimes B, Spital G, et al. Characteristics of type 1 and 2 CNV in exudative AMD in OCT-angiography. Graefes Arch Clin Exp Ophthalmol. 2017;255: 913–21.
27. Corvi F, Cozzi M, Barbolini E, Nizza D, Belotti M, Staurenghi G, et al. Comparison between several optical coherence tomography angiography devices and indocyanine green angiography of choroidal neovascularization. Retina. 2019.
28. Told R, Sacu S, Hecht A, Baratsits M, Eibenberger K, Kroh ME, et al. Comparison of SD-optical coherence tomography angiography and indocyanine green angiography in type 1 and 2 neovascular age-related macular degeneration. Invest Opthalmol Vis Sci. 2018;59:2393.
29. Akkaya S. Spectrum of pachychoroid diseases. Int Ophthalmol. 2018;38:2239–46.
30. Yannuzzi LA, Negrão S, Iida T, Carvalho C, Rodriguez-Coleman H, Slakter J, et al. Retinal angiomatous proliferation in age-related macular degeneration. Retina Phila Pa. 2001;21:416–34.
31. Öztaş Z, Menteş J. Retinal angiomatous proliferation: multimodal imaging characteristics and follow-up with eye-tracked spectral domain optical coherence

tomography of precursor lesions. Türk Oftalmol Derg. 2018;48:66–9.
32. Benhamou N, Souied EH, Zolf R, Coscas F, Coscas G, Soubrane G. Adult-onset foveomacular vitelliform dystrophy: a study by optical coherence tomography. Am J Ophthalmol. 2003;135:362–7.
33. Gass JD, Jallow S, Davis B. Adult vitelliform macular detachment occurring in patients with basal laminar drusen. Am J Ophthalmol. 1985;99:445–59.
34. Qian CX, Charran D, Strong CR, Steffens TJ, Jayasundera T, Heckenlively JR. Optical coherence tomography examination of the retinal pigment epithelium in best vitelliform macular dystrophy. Ophthalmology. 2017;124:456–63.
35. O'Gorman S, Flaherty WA, Fishman GA, Berson EL. Histopathologic findings in Best's vitelliform macular dystrophy. Arch Ophthalmol. 1988;106:1261–8.
36. Battaglia Parodi M, Iacono P, Romano F, Bolognesi G, Fasce F, Bandello F. Optical coherence tomography in best vitelliform macular dystrophy. Eur J Ophthalmol. 2017;27:201–4.
37. Schmidt-Erfurth U, Klimscha S, Waldstein SM, Bogunović H. A view of the current and future role of optical coherence tomography in the management of age-related macular degeneration. Eye. 2017;31:26–44.
38. Qu J, Velaga SB, Hariri AH, Nittala MG, Sadda S. Classification and quantitative analysis of geographic atrophy junctional zone using spectral domain optical coherence tomography. Retina. 2018;38:1456–63.
39. Qin J, Rinella N, Zhang Q, Zhou H, Wong J, Deiner M, et al. OCT angiography and cone photoreceptor imaging in geographic atrophy. Invest Opthalmol Vis Sci. 2018;59:5985–92.
40. Nassisi M, Baghdasaryan E, Borrelli E, Ip M, Sadda SR. Choriocapillaris flow impairment surrounding geographic atrophy correlates with disease progression. PLoS One. 2019;14:e0212563.
41. Zweifel SA. Outer retinal tubulation: a novel optical coherence tomography finding. Arch Ophthalmol. 2009;127:1596.
42. Cai CX, Light JG, Handa JT. Quantifying the rate of ellipsoid zone loss in Stargardt disease. Am J Ophthalmol. 2018;186:1–9.
43. Müller PL, Pfau M, Möller PT, Nadal J, Schmid M, Lindner M, et al. Choroidal flow signal in late-onset Stargardt disease and age-related macular degeneration: an OCT-angiography study. Invest Opthalmol Vis Sci. 2018;59:AMD122.
44. Hariri AH, Velaga SB, Girach A, Ip MS, Le PV, Lam BL, et al. Measurement and reproducibility of preserved ellipsoid zone area and preserved retinal pigment epithelium area in eyes with choroideremia. Am J Ophthalmol. 2017;179:110–7.
45. Murro V, Mucciolo DP, Giorgio D, Sodi A, Passerini I, Virgili G, et al. Optical coherence tomography angiography (OCT-A) in young choroideremia (CHM) patients. Ophthalmic Genet. 2019;40(3):201–6.
46. Fujinami K, Yokoi T, Hiraoka M, Nishina S, Azuma N. Choroidal neovascularization in a child following laser pointer-induced macular injury. Jpn J Ophthalmol. 2010;54:631–3.
47. Wyrsch S, Baenninger PB, Schmid MK. Retinal injuries from a handheld laser pointer. N Engl J Med. 2010;363:1089–91.
48. Harkness Eye Institute, Columbia University, New York, United States, Kapoor R, Whigham BT, Al-Aswad LA. Artificial intelligence and optical coherence tomography imaging. Asia-Pac J Ophthalmol [Internet] 2019 [cited 2019 Jun 11]. http://www.apjo.org/Apjo/pdf/id/654.html.

13 RPE Autofluorescence

Stefan Dithmar and Nil Celik

Introduction

Fundus autofluorescence (FAF) imaging is an important noninvasive method in the clinical routine for diagnosis and monitoring of different hereditary and degenerative retinal diseases. The autofluorescent signal is based on naturally occurring fluorophores, which absorb and emit light of particular wavelengths [1]. The most important autofluorescent substance is lipofuscin (LF), which accumulates with age in postmitotic cells, especially in the retinal pigment epithelium (RPE).

FAF imaging in the clinical routine is useful for diagnostics, phenotype-genotype correlation, identification of predictive markers for disease progression and monitoring the disease and the effect of treatment [2]. FAF imaging is not only in vivo but also ex vivo a useful tool to understand pathophysiological mechanisms in the RPE in a cellular and subcellular basis.

RPE Fluorophores

Lipofuscin

Lipofuscin (LF) of the retinal pigment epithelium (RPE) is the major source of fundus autofluorescence (Fig. 13.1). The RPE plays an essential role in the normal function of the neurosensory retina. In particular the permanent phagocytosis and lysosomal catabolism of photoreceptor outer segments (POS) by post mitotic RPE cells are essential for normal photoreceptor function. With advancing age there is a gradually increasing failure of the break-

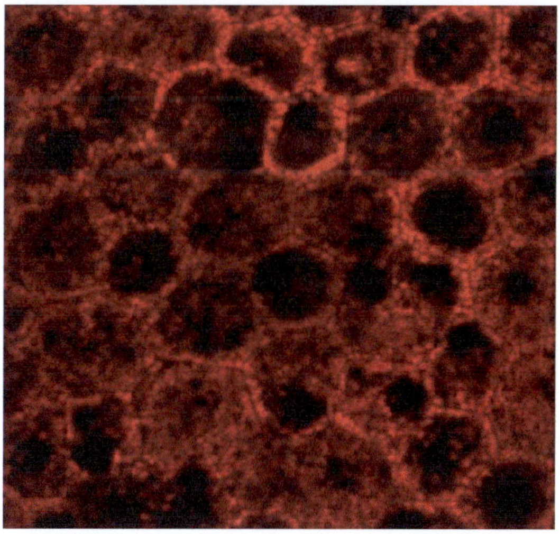

Fig. 13.1 Monolayer of polygonal cells in the RPE: lipofuscin granules are most densely packed closer to the cell membrane

S. Dithmar (✉)
Department of Ophthalmology, HSK Wiesbaden, University of Mainz, Wiesbaden, Germany

N. Celik
Department of Ophthalmology, University Hospital Heidelberg, Heidelberg, Germany

A. K. Klettner, S. Dithmar (eds.), *Retinal Pigment Epithelium in Health and Disease*,
https://doi.org/10.1007/978-3-030-28384-1_13

down of photoreceptor discs, leading to an accumulation of LF in the lysosomal compartment of RPE cells [3–5]. Since the degradation of photoreceptor outer segments is highest in the central retina, the age-related lipofuscin concentration is highest in the corresponding central RPE. LF is supposed to be cell toxic depending on the intracellular concentration of LF granules and can lead to cell death [6]. It is assumed that LF causes RPE atrophy. Clinical studies have shown that regions of elevated FAF are associated with loss of retinal sensitivity. A higher tendency for atrophy progression in areas of intense fundus autofluorescent signal has been shown [7]. Intracellular accumulation of lipofuscin increases the risk of age-related macular degeneration (AMD) [8]. The intracellular concentration of LF granules changes not only due to age, but also in degenerative and hereditary macular dystrophies such as AMD, Best's vitelliform degeneration and Stargardt's disease.

LF consists of mostly lipids and a few proteins [9–11]. It exhibits AF when excited with ultraviolet or blue light. It has an excitation peak at 470 nm and emits yellow-green light with an emission peak at 600 nm (range 500–750 nm) [12]. The main fluorophores are bisretinoids like N-Retinyl-N-retinylidene ethanolamine (A2E), which are metabolic by-products of Vitamin A and the visual cycle [13]. A2E is the first and best characterized fluorophore [14]. In vitro studies indicated that A2E possesses toxic properties, which may inhibit normal cell function via various molecular mechanisms [15–18]. It is discussed that A2E increases the intralysosomal pH level so that lysosomal degradation is inhibited [19]. Furthermore, it has been demonstrated that light exposure of cultured RPE cells induces generation of free radicals [20, 21]. Altogether, several effects of LF are considered to inhibit RPE cell function although the actual pathomechanism has not been detected yet.

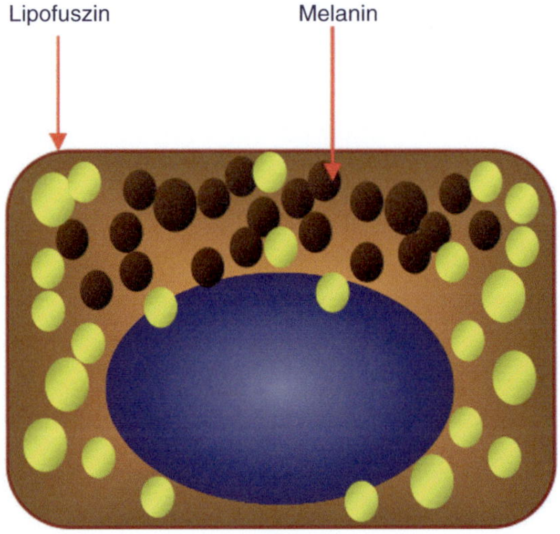

Fig. 13.2 Schematic diagram: typical distribution of lipofuscin (yellow) and melanin (brown) granules. The cell nucleus is found in the basal cytoplasm, while the melanin granules are more densely packed in the central apical zone

Melanin/Melanolipofuscin

Although it is generally accepted that dermal melanin protects the skin from UV light damage, the biological function of RPE melanin is not completely understood. Melanin absorbs excess light that passes through the eye, reducing scattering and improving image resolution (Fig. 13.2). Melanin has been suspected to play a photoprotective role in RPE cells by intercepting reactive oxygen species (ROS). Melanin is the primary fluorophore in near-infrared autofluorescence with a peak excitation at a longer wavelength of 787 nm. Another autofluorescent granule that accumulates in RPE cells and may contribute to the aetiology of AMD is a complex granule exhibiting properties of both melanosomes and lipofuscin granules called melanolipofuscin (MLF). With increasing age, a decrease in melanosomes in the RPE is observed along with an increase in melanolipofuscin (MLF). In contrast to the LF accumulation, MLF accumulation in the RPE has been reported to probably reflect more closely the onset of AMD [22].

Fundus Autofluorescence Imaging Devices In Vivo

In general, the autofluorescent image resolution of the RPE is reduced by structures in front of the retina such as cornea, vitreous body and lens [23, 24]. In order to take these disturbances into account, autofluorescence devices are equipped with correction methods such as applied blocking filters or algorithms for calculating the signal loss [25, 26]. However, the aim of routine clinical examinations is not to quantify the AF signal, but to determine the topographic distribution and temporal change during follow-up examinations.

AF images from different imaging systems or different images cannot be compared. The intensity of the AF signal is represented in pixel gray values, which allows the evaluation of the relative distribution of the AF over the fundus, but not a quantification of the absolute intensities.

Confocal Scanning Laser Ophthalmoscope (cSLO)

The most commonly used device for fundus AF imaging in clinical routine is the confocal scanning laser ophthalmoscope (cSLO), originally developed by Webb et al. [27]. The cSLO is an instrument that projects monochromatic light through a confocal optical system onto the fundus of the eye and detects the reflected light returning from the corresponding focal plane. The confocal property minimizes the scattered light returning from outside the focal plane [28], which increases the image contrast. To further improve contrast, an average series of 5–15 images (up to 100 images) is captured to calculate the mean image. To capture fundus autofluorescence, excitation light with a wavelength of 488 nm is projected onto the fundus and emissions above 500 nm are recorded. Optimum image quality requires the use of a blocking filter to block the short-wave light used for excitation. The maximum illuminance (approx. 2 mW/cm^2) is well below the permissible limits of international standards.

Modified Fundus Photography

Alternatively, modified fundus cameras from several manufacturers are also available on the market [29]. Fundus cameras use a light cone with a longer, red shifted excitation wavelength. This reduces the absorption by the macular pigments and allows the identification of fine central RPE changes [30]. The signal is less strongly reduced by blood and retinal vessels. Absorption through the crystalline lens is also lower. Compared to cSLO, the optic nerve appears more fluorescent in images taken with the fundus camera. Fundus cameras are more resistant to motion artifacts and patients feel less disturbed by the single flash compared to cSLO. However, the images show a lower contrast. Fundus cameras are less expensive than cSLO devices, but require further modifications such as the installation of filters or image processing after acquisition. Another disadvantage is the increased capture of reflected and scattered light. For example, structures outside the retina can erroneously lead to an increased AF signal.

Near-Infrared Fundus Autofluorescence

FAF images are not only available with short-wavelength excitation, but also with near-infrared excitation [31, 32]. Special devices provide excitation of 790 nm and emission over 800 nm. The most interesting target for this modality is the foveal region, where high signals are obtained from the RPE melanin. Also, the choroidal pigment and hyperpigmentations like nevi have a high AF signal in the near-infrared spectra [31].

Normal Fundus Autofluorescence

The normal FAF image is characterized by a central zone of reduced fluorescence intensity caused by absorption by the yellow pigments of the macula (lutein and zeaxanthin) (Fig. 13.3). AF gathers to the perifovea with a maximum at 7–13° and decreases toward the periphery [1, 33]. The perifoveal AF shows an asymmetric distribution with a maximum temporally and superiorly (12° from the fovea) and a lower signal inferiorly and nasally (7–8° from the fovea).

The optic nerve (lack of RPE and lipofuscin) and the retinal vessels (blockage and uptake by the blood) are hypofluorescent. Retinal vessels can appear with fine parallel stripes, which are assumed to be slightly hyperfluorescent due to refraction on the vessel walls.

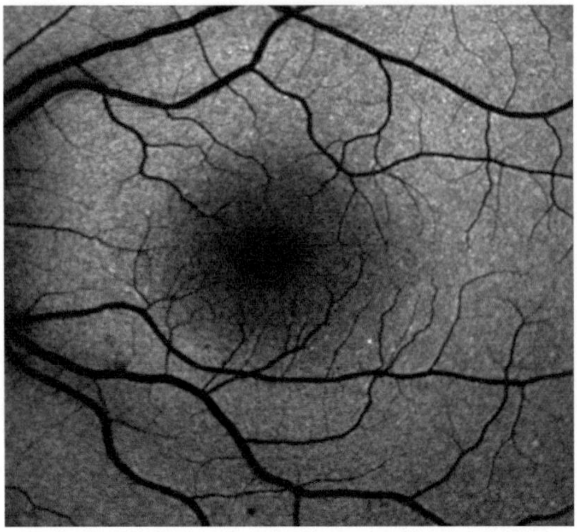

Fig. 13.3 FAF image of the normal RPE. In the central macular region is a reduced level of FAF caused by absorption of the fluorescence by the macular pigments (lutein and zeaxanthin). AF is blocked by retinal blood vessels

The general AF signal intensity is influenced by the clarity of the media. In particular, cataracts are associated with an absorption of blue laser light. Corneal and vitreal opacities are also associated with an impairment of the FAF image quality. For these reasons, quantification of the autofluorescence level at certain retinal sites using the monochromatic method would not be ideal. The use of topographic image data (i.e. the registration of FAF patterns) is more appropriate.

FAF depends on factors such as age and genotype. The distribution of lipofuscin (LF) and thus its autofluorescence almost correlates with the distribution of rods [34].

Not only LF granules possess fluorophores that emit autofluorescence. Fluorophores can be found in practically all tissues, but with different spectral properties and intensities of the emitted light. Fluorophores are present in the choroid and sclera. In the absence of RPE cells, the large choroid vessels are recognizable in autofluorescence mode because the vessel walls are autofluorescent. Normally these signals do not play a role, since the blue excitation light is largely absorbed by the intact layer of the RPE cells.

Pathologic Fundus Autofluorescence

Fundus autofluorescence (FAF) images can disclose the effects of aging and disease at the level of the retinal pigment epithelium. With aging the post mitotic RPE cells accumulate LF granules in the cytoplasm, accompanied by a reduction in the density of the melanin granules. Excessive accumulation of LF (and its characteristic FAF signal) is a marker for multifactorial and degenerative maculopathies, including AMD, idiopathic central serous chorioretinopathy, and purely inherited monogenetic diseases such as Best's vitelliform degeneration and Stargardt's disease [29]. FAF imaging provides a method that can help confirm the diagnosis, differentiate the phenotype, and recognize new prognostic factors, particularly when evaluating AMD. FAF now contributes to our understanding of the pathophysiological role of the RPE as a final common pathway for many retinal and macular diseases. Moreover, it helps with identification of the distribution and density of the macular pigments lutein and zeaxanthin.

Eyes with AMD show a wide spectrum of FAF changes in association with the various stages of disease. In early cases of AMD, there are areas of elevated FAF. These areas do not correspond to visible findings like retinal drusen, however, and they are highly variable (Fig. 13.4). Focal areas of hyperpigmentation are almost always accompanied by elevated FAF (melanolipofuscin), areas of retinal drusen are heterogeneous and can have elevated, reduced, or normal levels of FAF.

Areas of geographic atrophy in the advanced stages of AMD are characterized by a marked reduction in FAF, since in these areas the RPE and its autofluorescent lipofuscin have been destroyed. At the margins of these atrophic areas one finds a variety of FAF patterns (Figs. 13.5, 13.6, and 13.7) [35, 36]. Atrophic areas with diffusely elevated FAF at their margins advance more rapidly than atrophic areas with no or

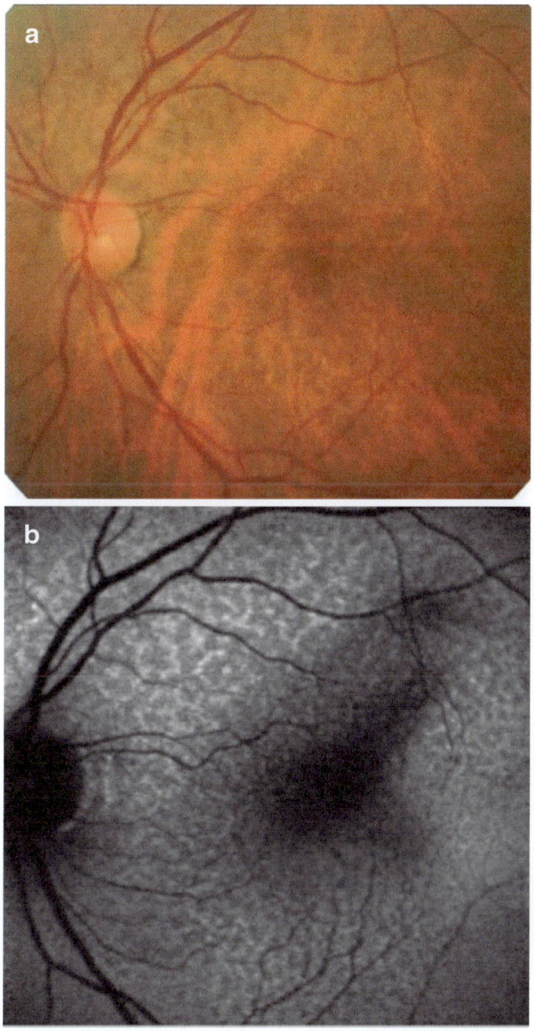

Fig. 13.4 (**a**, **b**) Example of reticulated drusen. Reticulated drusen can be easily identified in FAF images. They can be accompanied by both hyper- and hypointensive autofluorescence regions

only focally elevated FAF. Phenotypic categorization, based on the FAF appearance, allows a prognostic determination of non-exudative AMD in its later stages. In contradistinction to the drusen of AMD, hereditary drusen, which arise at an earlier age, have a generally higher level of autofluorescence (Fig. 13.8). This finding suggests that hereditary drusen have different molecular structures or higher densities of LF granules in the overlying RPE, than do the drusen of AMD. Similarly, pigment epithelial detachments (PED) produce a heterogeneous FAF signal; however, this appears to be determined more by the stage of the PED itself than by the underlying disease process. Elevated FAF intensity could also arise from the fluorophors in the extracellular fluid between the RPE and Bruch's membrane.

Changes in topographic FAF intensity distribution can be found in various retinal diseases and show some characteristic patterns. In Stargardt's disease, for example, one typically finds spots with both increased FAF (LF accumulation) and reduced FAF (already atrophic RPE) in the area of the funduscopically normal looking retina (Fig. 13.9). Best's disease manifests as diffusely elevated levels of FAF with an additional increase of fluorescence intensity in the area of the funduscopically visible yellow deposit that characterizes the vitelliform lesion (Fig. 13.10). This also applies to pattern dystrophies, including adult vitelliform macular dystrophy. FAF findings in cases of retinitis pigmentosa and other photoreceptor dystrophies reflect secondary changes appearing at the level of the retinal pigment epithelium. In some forms, areas with LF accumulation or atrophy zones can be delimited very precisely. A ring with increased autofluorescence at 4–5° eccentricity from the fovea, the so-called "rod ring" (Fig. 13.11), is often found.

Drusen of the optic nerve head are to be differentiated from the drusen of AMD or those of hereditary retinal diseases. Here, the elevated FAF has to do with the calcification of degenerated axonal remnants. A prominently elevated FAF of the optic disc is useful in the differential diagnosis of optic disc elevations of uncertain aetiology (Fig. 13.12).

When interpreting FAF images, it should be taken into account that other structures in the human fundus, e.g. older blood, may exhibit autofluorescent properties in addition to RPE-LF.

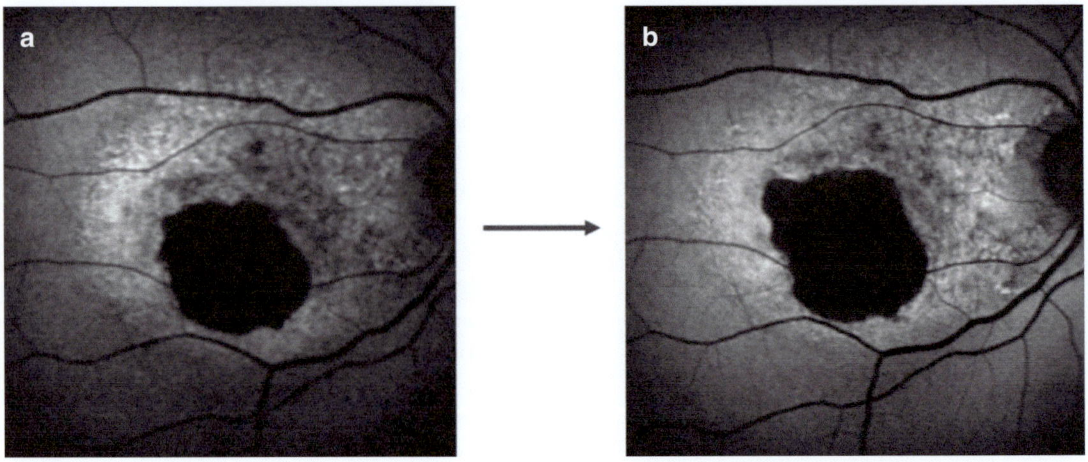

Fig. 13.5 (**a**) Geographic atrophy in a 67-year-old AMD patient: severe reduction of FAF caused by the absence of vital RPE with fluorescent lipofuscin. (**b**) Over a period of 5 years, it can be seen that the extension of the atrophic region occurred at the edges of the lesion where excessive accumulation of LF had previously been localized

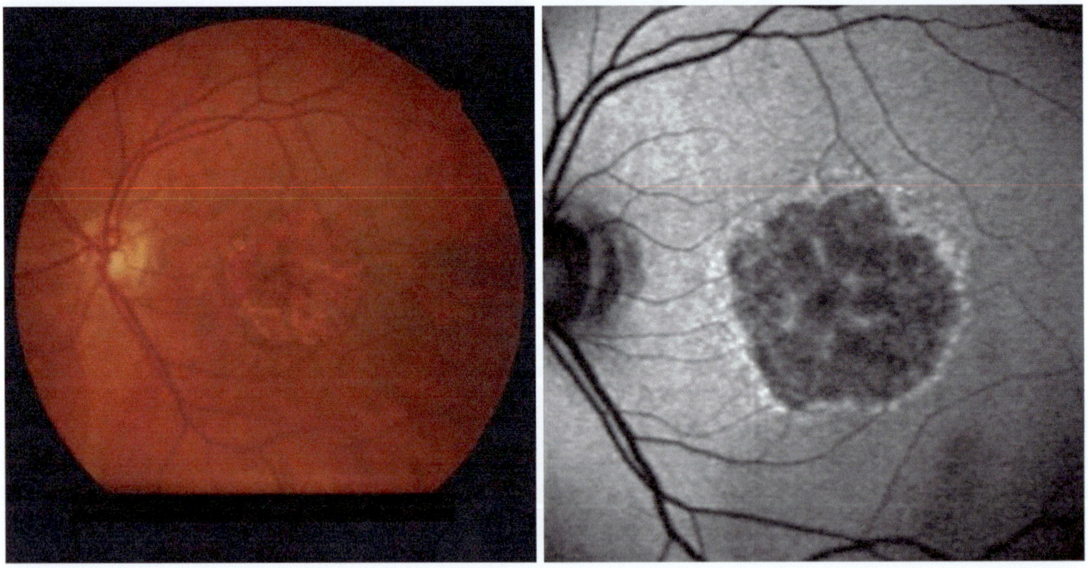

Fig. 13.6 Another example of geographic atrophy in AMD showing a band with an increased FAF signal at the edge of the atrophy zone. These fluorescence patterns at the edge of the atrophy zone can be very different in patients

Autofluorescence Imaging Devices Ex Vivo

Fluorescence Microscopy

Compared to other microscopy methods used in biomedical research, fluorescence microscopy has several advantages in terms of sample preparation as well as the variety of possibilities to extract biologically significant information. A major problem, however, of any standard fluorescence microscopy method compared to non-light-optical microscopy methods remains the intrinsically limited conventional resolution of about 200 nm (widefield microscopy: ~230 nm, confocal microscopy: ~180 nm, two-photon microscopy: ~200 nm) [37–40].

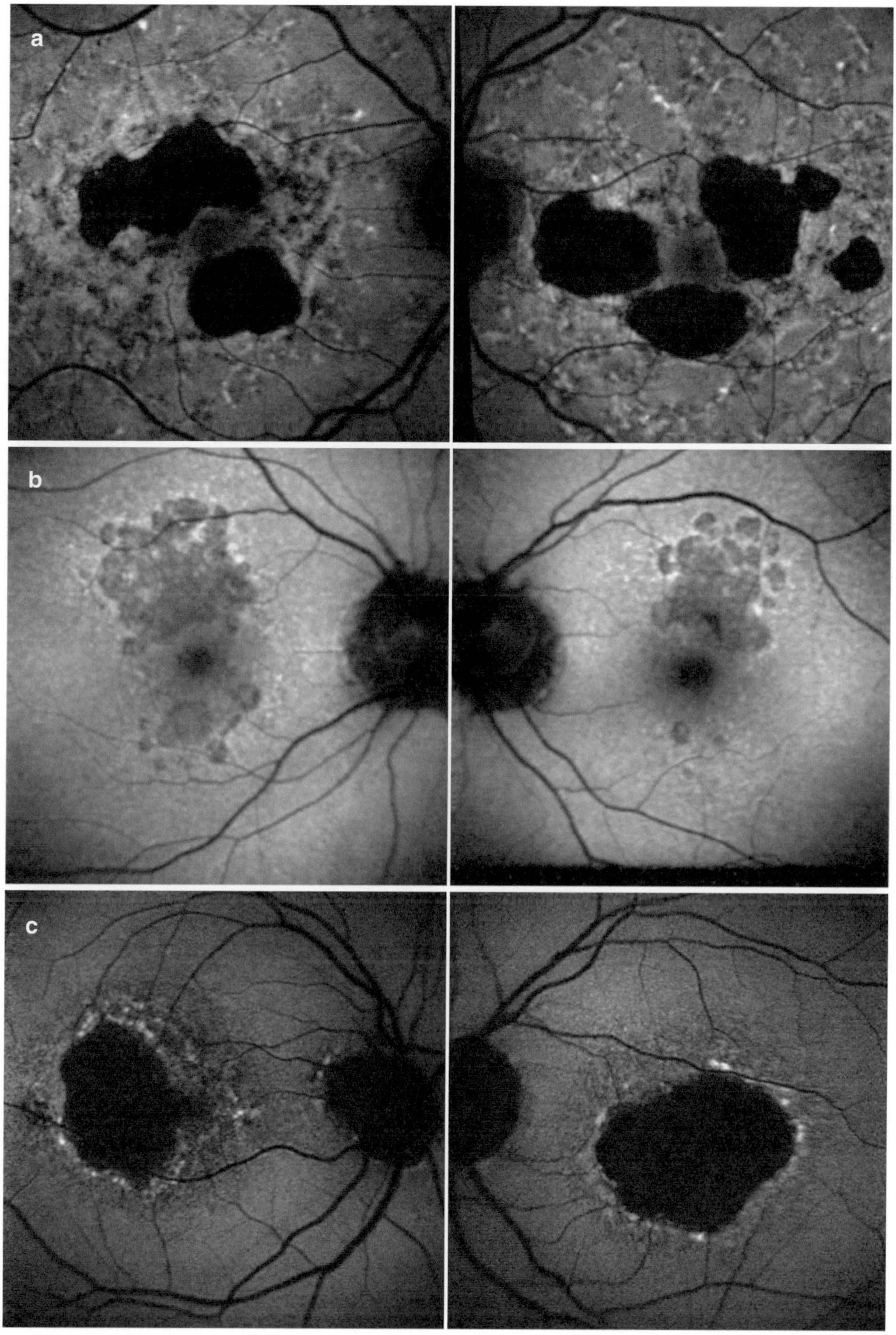

Fig. 13.7 (**a–c**) FAF images in three different patients with geographic atrophy caused by AMD. One can see a pronounced intra-individual left/right symmetry and marked inter-individual variability in the appearance of the atrophic areas and their margins with elevated FAF

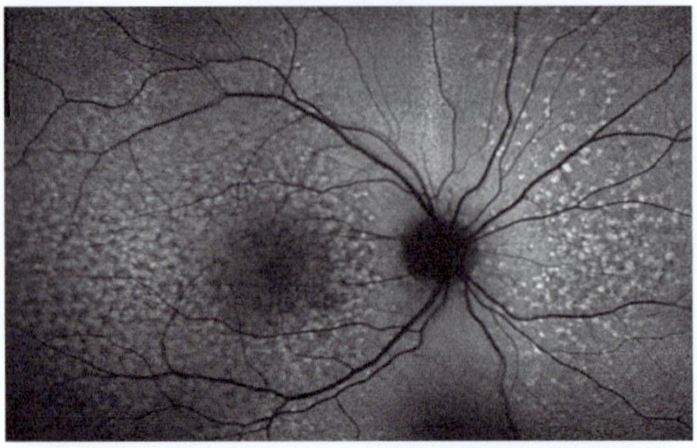

Fig. 13.8 With appropriate image processing software, several adjacent images can be merged into a composite montage. One can see the locations of hereditary drusen. Their points of elevated fluorescence are most densely located in the macula, but are also scattered through retinal areas that are far outside of the macular region

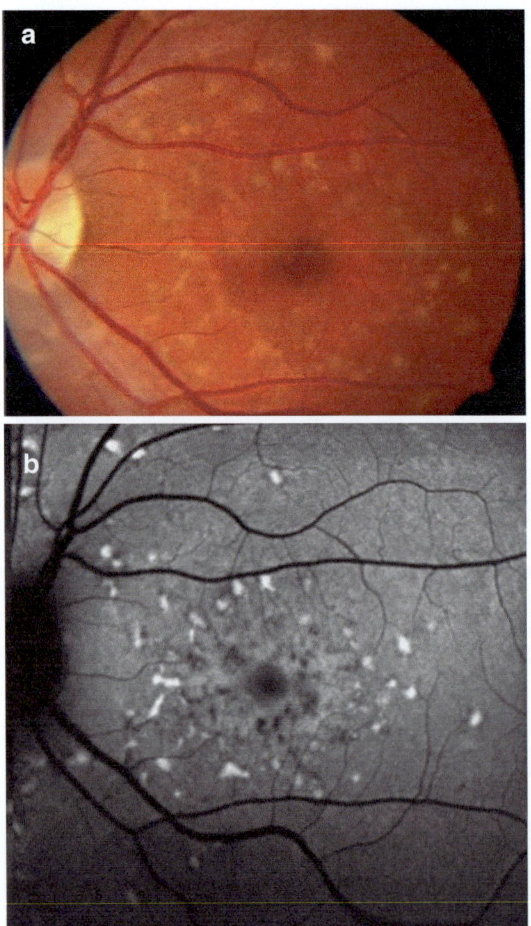

Fig. 13.9 In cases of fundus flavimaculatus or Stargardt's disease, characteristic yellow flecks appear at the level of the RPE (**a**) with increased autofluorescence (**b**) due to an excess accumulation of lipofuscin

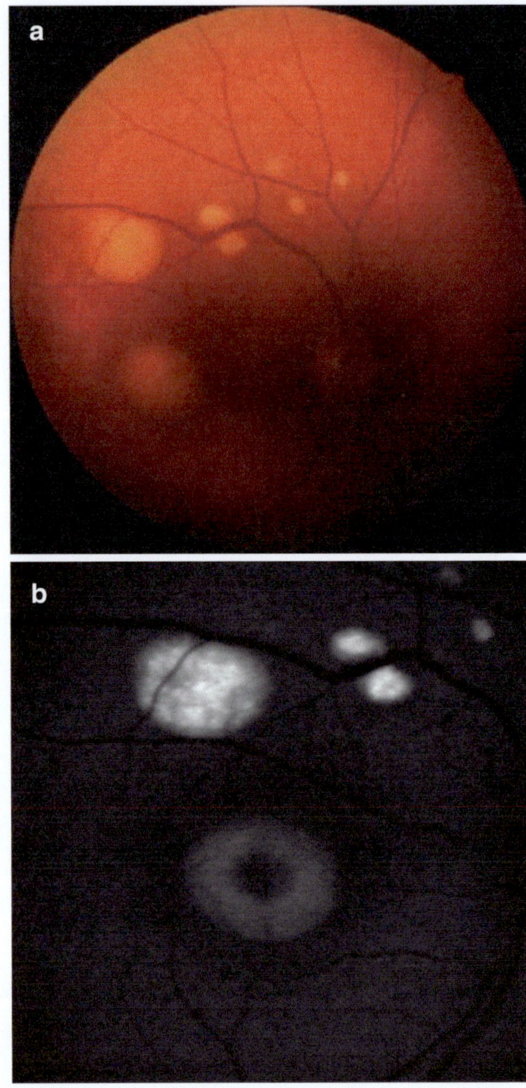

Fig. 13.10 (**a**, **b**) 55-year-old patient with multifocal Best's disease. The yellow (vitelliform) lesions have a strongly elevated autofluorescence due to increased levels of stored lipofuscin

Over the last years different techniques referred to as super resolution fluorescence microscopy have been established to compensate for this deficiency. These techniques (i.e. 4Pi [41], STED [42], SIM/PEM [43] and localization methods [44]) are based on conditions not considered in the original contributions of Abbe [37]. In combination with novel optoelectronical and mathematical tools, these different approaches have allowed the microscope to surpass the conventional resolution limit sub-

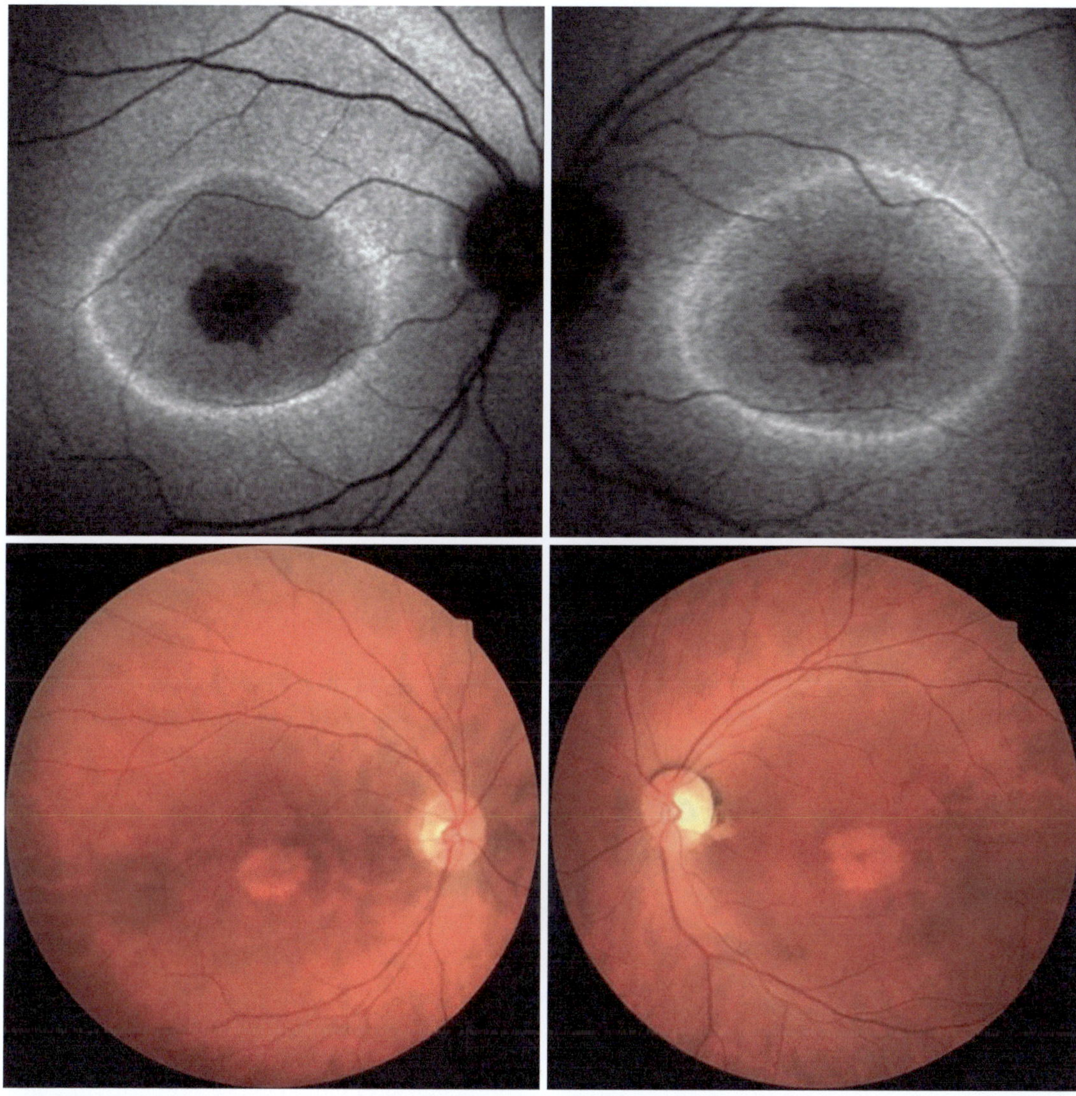

Fig. 13.11 In this 23-year-old patient with an electrophysiologically confirmed cone dystrophy one can see a central zone of atrophy (appearing in the FAF image as dark) surrounded by a ring of elevated FAF called a "rod ring". This phenomenon, whose pathophysiological basis is not well understood, can also appear in patients with other hereditary retinal disorders, including retinitis pigmentosa and Leber's congenital amaurosis

stantially, both in the object plane and in the direction along the optical axis of the microscope system.

Structured Illumination Microscopy

Structured illumination microscopy (SIM) is a relatively new laser-optical fluorescence microscopy technique that offers an improvement in resolution compared to conventional microscopes.

The lateral resolution of a conventional microscope is limited to approximately 200 nm. Structural information of an object below this distance cannot be transferred through the objective lens and into the image plane. The loss of high-resolution information during the imaging process of an object is responsible for the fact that the acquired image is blurred and less distinct compared to the original object.

SIM is capable to shift usually irresolvable object information to resolvable information.

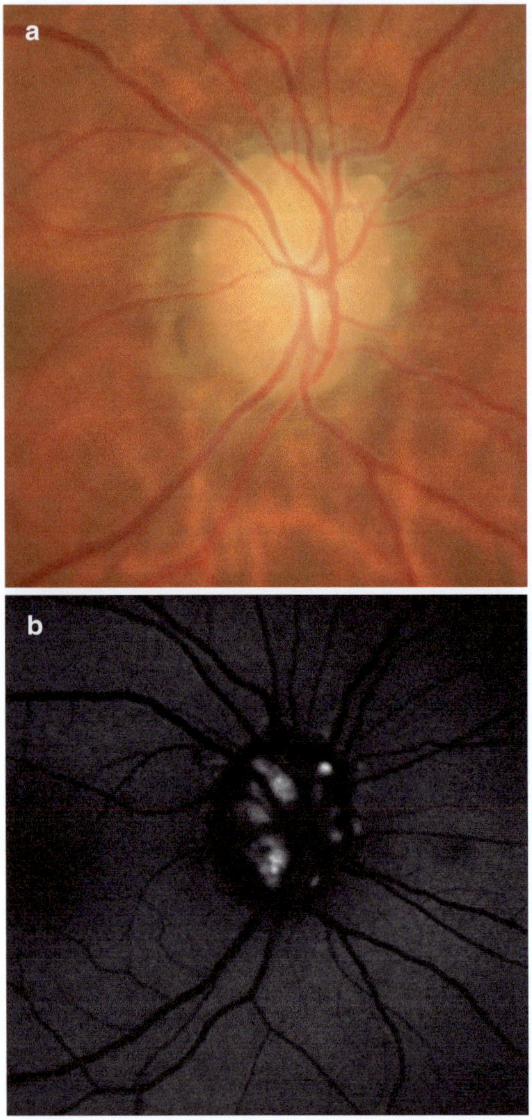

Fig. 13.12 (**a**, **b**) 52-year-old-patient with drusen of the optic nerve. Some drusen show an significantly increased autofluorescence

This is accomplished by an application of a spatially modulated excitation pattern. This shifting process is apparent in everyday life, known as Moiré effect: if two fine gratings are superposed, a coarser, clearly visible grid may appear. If one of the two fine gratings is known, the other superimposed fine grating can be reconstructed. In a similar manner, it is possible to reconstruct the original high-resolution information contained in the acquired SIM data that is generated by a superposition of the excitation pattern with the object's fluorochrome distribution. To accomplish this reconstruction, several images of the object have to be taken with different positions of the illumination pattern. The application of SIM thereby offers a lateral resolution improvement by a factor of 2 in comparison to conventional widefield microscopy and also enables a removal of out of focus information during the reconstruction process to generate optical sections of the object.

SIM has been introduced for high-resolution autofluorescent imaging of RPE cells [45–48].

Intracellular granules like lipofuscin (LF) and melanolipofuscin (MLF) can be visualized and differentiated by SIM (Fig. 13.13). The distinction between LF and MLF granules is especially important since MLF accumulation has been reported to reflect the onset of AMD more closely than LF granules. MLF granules are significantly larger than LF granules, which might be due to fusion of LF granules and melanosomes or autophagocytotic abilities of melanosomes. MLF granules have been reported to be nearly 35% larger than LF granules in flow cytometric analyses [22].

The size of LF granules is related to intracellular location in the ex vivo samples. The closer to Bruch's membrane, the larger they are, suggesting that larger LF granules are transferred towards Bruch's membrane. The basal accumulation of lipofuscin can be explained by the natural apical to basal course of lipofuscin transport through RPE cells [49]. Melanosomes were located significantly more apical than LF and MLF granules.

Examinations of differences of autofluorescence signal intensity related to excitation wavelengths were inconsistent, suggesting that different mixtures of fluorophores within granules can occur. Boulton et al. reported an excitation maximum of extracted LF granules between 360 and 470 nm [50]. Varying probe preparation, proteins surrounding the granules and other factors might contribute to altered excitation behaviour [51]. LF develops within lysosomes from the phagocytosed and metabolized photoreceptor residues. Different

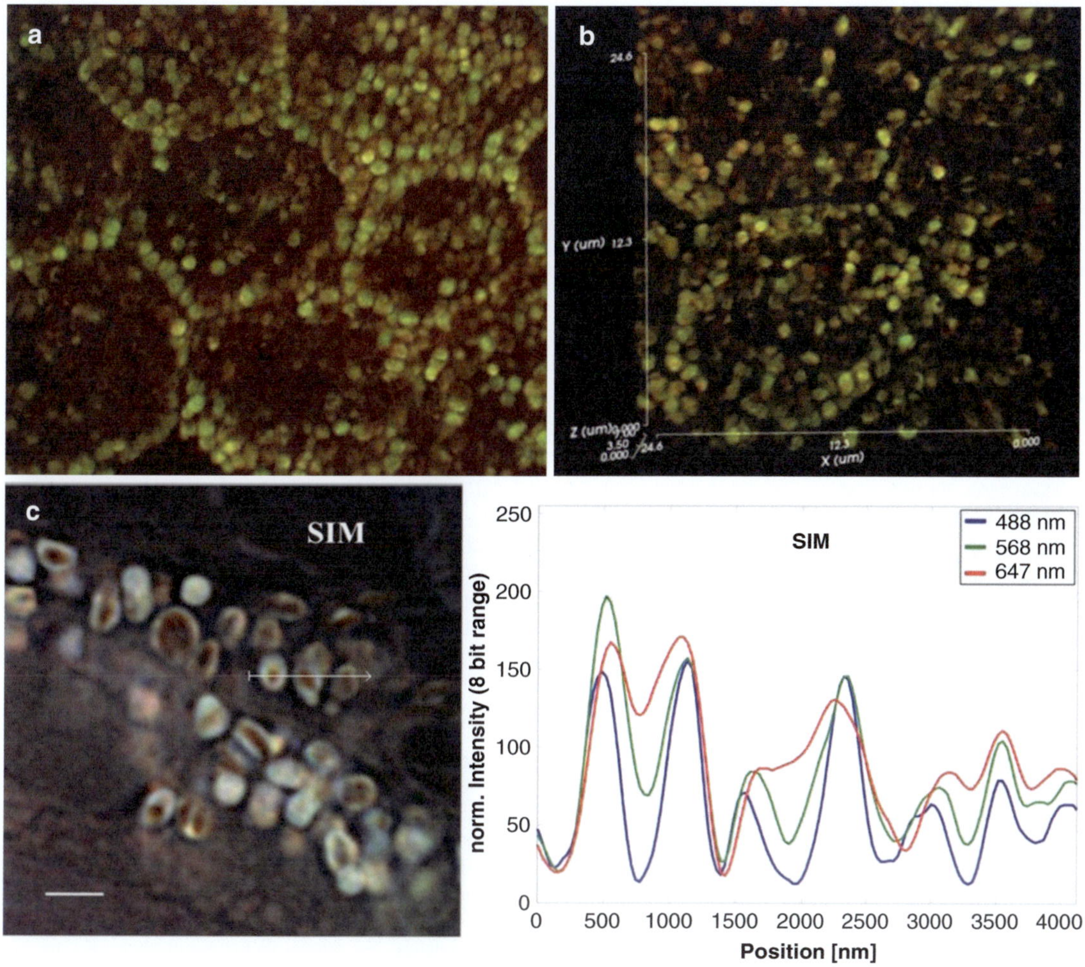

Fig. 13.13 (**a**–**c**) Structured illumination microscopy (SIM) clearly delineates autofluorescent single granules within RPE-cells (ex vivo). (**a**) Hexagonal RPE-cell composite with intracellular autofluorescent granules. (**b**) Single RPE-cells with clearly visible and countable intracellular granules. (**c**) Visible intragranular fluorescence pattern. Emission intensities for different excitation wavelengths along the white arrow have a detailed profile (peaks for lipofuscin rings around central melanin core in melanolipofuscin granules) (scale bar 2 μm)

sizes of LF granules might reflect different stages of LF genesis with small LF granules in early stages. AF properties of LF granules change with growing size showing decreased average emission signals at 647 nm [47]. This indicates an increased presence of fluorophores mainly excitable at 488 and 568 nm in growing or latestage LF granules, or significant loss of fluorophores excitable at 647 nm. No correlation between size and AF was found in MLF granules [47].

Structured illumination microscopy has now also proven to be applicable in vivo. RPE cell cultures can be examined and dynamic intracellular processes can be followed.

The first experiment with a prototype device (Structured Illumination Ophthalmoscope = SIO) recently showed that structured illumination can also be successfully used for fundus examination in humans in a clinical setting (Dithmar et al., unpublished study data).

These developments and the additional implementation of adaptive optics promise completely new insights into RPE autofluorescence phenomena in vivo.

References

1. Delori FC, Dorey CK, Staurenghi G, Arend O, Goger DG, Weiter JJ. In vivo fluorescence of the ocular fundus exhibits retinal pigment epithelium lipofuscin characteristics. Invest Ophthalmol Vis Sci. 1995;36(3):718–29.
2. Schmitz-Valckenberg S, Holz FG, Bird AC, Spaide RF. Fundus autofluorescence imaging: review and perspectives. Retina (Philadelphia, PA). 2008;28(3):385–409.
3. Feeney-Burns L, Hilderbrand ES, Eldridge S. Aging human RPE: morphometric analysis of macular, equatorial, and peripheral cells. Invest Ophthalmol Vis Sci. 1984;25(2):195–200.
4. Weiter JJ, Delori FC, Wing GL, Fitch KA. Retinal pigment epithelial lipofuscin and melanin and choroidal melanin in human eyes. Invest Ophthalmol Vis Sci. 1986;27(2):145–52.
5. Eldred GE, Miller GV, Stark WS, Feeney-Burns L. Lipofuscin: resolution of discrepant fluorescence data. Science (New York, NY). 1982;216(4547): 757–9.
6. Dorey CK, Wu G, Ebenstein D, Garsd A, Weiter JJ. Cell loss in the aging retina. Relationship to lipofuscin accumulation and macular degeneration. Invest Ophthalmol Vis Sci. 1989;30(8):1691–9.
7. Holz FG, Bellmann C, Margaritidis M, Schutt F, Otto TP, Volcker HE. Patterns of increased in vivo fundus autofluorescence in the junctional zone of geographic atrophy of the retinal pigment epithelium associated with age-related macular degeneration. Graefes Arch Clin Exp Ophthalmol. 1999;237(2):145–52.
8. Zhou J, Kim SR, Westlund BS, Sparrow JR. Complement activation by bisretinoid constituents of RPE lipofuscin. Invest Ophthalmol Vis Sci. 2009;50:1392–9.
9. Ng KP, Gugiu B, Renganathan K, Davies MW, Gu X, Crabb JS, Kim SR, Rozanowska MB, Bonilha VL, Rayborn ME, Salomon RG, Sparrow JR, Boulton ME, Hollyfield JG, Crabb JW. Retinal pigment epithelium lipofuscin proteomics. Mol Cell Proteomics. 2008;7(7):1397–405.
10. Feeney L. Lipofuscin and melanin of human retinal pigment epithelium. Fluorescence, enzyme cytochemical, and ultrastructural studies. Invest Ophthalmol Vis Sci. 1978;17(7):583–600.
11. Eldred GM, Miller GV, Stark WS, Feeney-Burns L. Lipofuscin: resolution of discrepant fluorescence data. Science. 1982;216:3.
12. Krebs I, Noemi L, Forrester JV. Fundus autofluorescence. Graefes Arch Clin Exp Ophthalmol. 2011;249(2):309.
13. Parish CA, Hashimoto M, Nakanishi K, Dillon J, Sparrow J. Isolation and one-step preparation of A2E and iso-A2E, fluorophores from human retinal pigment epithelium. Proc Natl Acad Sci U S A. 1998;95(25):14609–13.
14. Feeney-Burns L, Berman ER, Rothman H. Lipofuscin of human retinal pigment epithelium. Am J Ophthalmol. 1980;90(6):783–91.
15. Brunk UT, Wihlmark U, Wrigstad A, Roberg K, Nilsson SE. Accumulation of lipofuscin within retinal pigment epithelial cells results in enhanced sensitivity to photo-oxidation. Gerontology. 1995;41(Suppl 2):201–12.
16. Sparrow JR, Zhou J, Ben-Shabat S, Vollmer H, Itagaki Y, Nakanishi K. Involvement of oxidative mechanisms in blue-light-induced damage to A2E-laden RPE. Invest Ophthalmol Vis Sci. 2002;43(4):1222–7.
17. Schutt F, Davies S, Kopitz J, Holz FG, Boulton ME. Photodamage to human RPE cells by A2-E, a retinoid component of lipofuscin. Invest Ophthalmol Vis Sci. 2000;41(8):2303–8.
18. Bermann M, Schutt F, Holz FG, Kopitz J. Does A2E, a retinoid component of lipofuscin and inhibitor of lysosomal degradative functions, directly affect the activity of lysosomal hydrolases? Exp Eye Res. 2001;72(2):191–5.
19. Holz FG, Schutt F, Kopitz J, Eldred GE, Kruse FE, Volcker HE, Cantz M. Inhibition of lysosomal degradative functions in RPE cells by a retinoid component of lipofuscin. Invest Ophthalmol Vis Sci. 1999;40(3):737–43.
20. Boulton M, Dontsov A, Jarvis-Evans J, Ostrovsky M, Svistunenko D. Lipofuscin is a photoinducible free radical generator. J Photochem Photobiol B. 1993;19(3):201–4.
21. Rozanowska M, Jarvis-Evans J, Korytowski W, Boulton ME, Burke JM, Sarna T. Blue light-induced reactivity of retinal age pigment. In vitro generation of oxygen-reactive species. J Biol Chem. 1995;270(32):18825–30.
22. Warburton S, Davis WE, Southwick K, et al. Proteomic and phototoxic characterization of melanolipofuscin: correlation to disease and model for its origin. Mol Vis. 2007;13:318–29.
23. Sasamoto Y, Gomi F, Sawa M, Sakaguchi H, Tsujikawa M, Nishida K. Effect of cataract in evaluation of macular pigment optical density by autofluorescence spectrometry. Invest Ophthalmol Vis Sci. 2011;52(2):927–32.
24. Sharifzadeh M, Obana A, Gohto Y, Seto T, Gellermann W. Autofluorescence imaging of macular pigment: influence and correction of ocular media opacities. J Biomed Opt. 2014;19(9):96010.
25. Sharifzadeh M, Bernstein PS, Gellermann W. Nonmydriatic fluorescence-based quantitative imaging of human macular pigment distributions. J Opt Soc Am A Opt Image Sci Vis. 2006;23(10):2373–87.
26. van de Kraats J, van Norren D. Optical density of the aging human ocular media in the visible and the UV. J Opt Soc Am A Opt Image Sci Vis. 2007;24(7):1842–57.
27. Webb RH, Hughes GW, Delori FC. Confocal scanning laser ophthalmoscope. Appl Opt. 1987;26(8):1492–9.

28. Sharp PF, Manivannan A, Xu H, Forrester JV. The scanning laser ophthalmoscope—a review of its role in bioscience and medicine. Phys Med Biol. 2004;49(7):1085–96.
29. Yung M, Klufas MA, Sarraf D. Clinical applications of fundus autofluorescence in retinal disease. Int J Retina Vitreous. 2016;2:12.
30. Park SP, Siringo FS, Pensec N, Hong IH, Sparrow J, Barile G, Tsang SH, Chang S. Comparison of fundus autofluorescence between fundus camera and confocal scanning laser ophthalmoscope-based systems. Ophthalmic Surg Lasers Imaging Retina. 2013;44(6):536–43.
31. Weinberger AWA, Lappas A, Kirschkamp T, Mazinani BAE, Huth JK, Mohammadi B, Walter P. Fundus near infrared fluorescence correlates with fundus near infrared reflectance. Invest Ophthalmol Vis Sci. 2006;47(7):3098–108.
32. Keilhauer CN, Delori FC. Near-infrared autofluorescence imaging of the fundus: visualization of ocular melanin. Invest Ophthalmol Vis Sci. 2006;47(8):3556–64.
33. Delori FC, Goger DG, Dorey CK. Age-related accumulation and spatial distribution of lipofuscin in RPE of normal subjects. Invest Ophthalmol Vis Sci. 2001;42(8):1855–66.
34. Curcio CA, Sloan KR, Kalina RE, Hendrickson AE. Human photoreceptor topography. J Comp Neurol. 1990;292(4):497–523.
35. Holz FG, Bellman C, Staudt S, et al. Fundus autofluorescence and development of geographic atrophy in age-related macular degeneration. Invest Ophthalmol Vis Sci. 2001;42:1051–6.
36. Bindewald A, Schmitz-Valkenberg S, Jorzik JJ, Dolar-Szczasny J, Sieber H, Keilhauer C, Weinberger AW, Dithmar S, Pauleikhoff D, Mansmann U, Wolf S, Holz FG. Classification of abnormal fundus autofluorescence patterns in the junctional zone of geographic atrophy in patients with age related macular degeneration. Br J Ophthalmol. 2005;89:874–8.
37. Abbe E. Beitraege zur Theorie des Mikroskops und der mikroskopischen Wahrnehmung. Arch Mikrosk Anat. 1873;9:413–20.
38. Heintzmann R, Ficz G. Breaking the resolution limit in light microscopy. Brief Funct Genomic Proteomic. 2006;5(4):289–301.
39. Bindewald-Wittich A, Han M, Schmitz-Valckenberg S, Snyder SR, Giese GN, Bille JF, Holz FG. Two-photon–excited fluorescence imaging of human RPE cells with a femtosecond Ti:sapphire laser. Invest Ophthalmol Vis Sci. 2006;47(10):4553–7.
40. Han M, Bindewald-Wittich A, Holz FG, Giese G, Niemz MH, Snyder S, Sun H, Yu J, Agopov M, La Schiazza O, Bille JF. Two-photon excited autofluorescence imaging of human retinal pigment epithelial cells. J Biomed Opt. 2006;11(1):010501.
41. Cremer C, Cremer T. Considerations on a laser-scanning-microscope with high resolution and depth of field. Microsc Acta. 1978;81:31–44.
42. Hell SW, Wichmann J. Breaking the diffraction resolution limit by stimulated emission: stimulated-emission-depletion fluorescence microscopy. Opt Lett. 1994;19:780–2.
43. Gustafsson MGL. Surpassing the lateral resolution limit by a factor of two using structured illumination microscopy. J Microsc. 2000;198(2):82–7.
44. Cremer C, von Ketteler A, Lemmer P, Kaufmann R, Weiland Y, Mueller P, Hausmann M, Baddeley D, Amberger R. Far-field fluorescence microscopy of cellular structures at molecular optical resolution. In: Diaspro A, editor. Nanoscopy and multidimensional optical fluorescence microscopy. Boca Raton: Taylor & Francis; 2010.
45. Best G, Amberger R, Baddeley D, Ach T, Dithmar S, Heintzmann R, Cremer C. Structured illumination microscopy of autofluorescent aggregations in human tissue. Micron (Oxford, England: 1993). 2011;42(4):330–5.
46. Ach T, Best G, Ruppenstein M, Amberger R, Cremer C, Dithmar S. High-resolution fluorescence microscopy of retinal pigment epithelium using structured illumination. Ophthalmologe. 2010;107:1037–42.
47. Ach T, Best G, Rossberger S, Heintzmann R, Cremer C, Dithmar S. Autofluorescence imaging of human RPE cell granules using structured illumination microscopy. Br J Ophthalmol. 2012;96(8):1141–4.
48. Rossberger S, Ach T, Best G, Cremer C, Heintzmann R, Dithmar S. High-resolution imaging of autofluorescent particles within drusen using structured illumination microscopy. Br J Ophthalmol. 2013;97(4):518–23.
49. Peters S, Kayatz P, Kociok N, et al. Cellular transport of subretinal material into choroidal and scleral blood vessels: an electron microscopic study. Graefes Arch Clin Exp Ophthalmol. 1999;237:976–83.
50. Boulton M, Docchio F, Dayhaw-Barker P, et al. Age-related changes in the morphology, absorption and fluorescence of melanosomes and lipofuscin granules of the retinal pigment epithelium. Vis Res. 1990;30:1291–303.
51. Schutt F, Ueberle B, Schnolzer M, et al. Proteome analysis of lipofuscin in human retinal pigment epithelial cells. FEBS Lett. 2002;528:217–21.

Part IV

The RPE in Therapy

RPE and Stem Cell Therapy

14

Heli Skottman

Introduction

Retinal pigment epithelium (RPE) is a highly polarized monolayer of cells located between the neural retina and the choroid (see Fig. 14.1). RPE has several vitally important functions as a part of the blood-retinal barrier and in supporting the neural retina: RPE cells provide nutrients for photoreceptors, phagocytose photoreceptor outer segments secrete important molecules including pigment epithelium-derived factor (PEDF) and vascular endothelial growth factor (VEGF), absorb stray light, and control regeneration of visual pigments, ion flow and oxidative damage. For a more extensive review of RPE functions and characteristics, the article by Strauss is highly recommended [1].

Retinal degenerative diseases, such as age-related macular degeneration (AMD), retinitis pigmentosa, and Stargardt macular dystrophy, affect tens of millions of individuals worldwide. For example in AMD, the macula of the eye gradually degenerates, leading to the loss of central vision, and thus hindering tasks such as face recognition, reading, and driving—important cornerstones for individual independence and quality of life. With a steadily increasing life expectancy, the number of people suffering

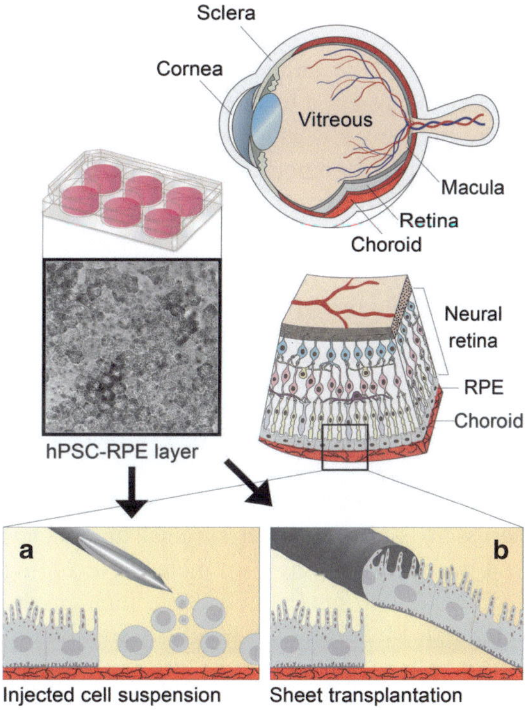

Fig. 14.1 The hPSC-RPE transplantations. The hPSC-RPE cells can be efficiently differentiated and transplanted to the subretinal space between neural retina and choroid. Currently two different transplantation approaches are used (**a**) single-cell suspension injection and (**b**) transplantation of intact RPE cell sheet

from AMD worldwide is predicted to increase to almost 200 million by the year 2020 and to over 280 million by 2040 [2]. There are two types of AMD: dry (atrophic) and wet (neovascular). The

H. Skottman (✉)
Faculty of Medicine and Health Technology, Tampere University, Tampere, Finland
e-mail: heli.skottman@tuni.fi

A. K. Klettner, S. Dithmar (eds.), *Retinal Pigment Epithelium in Health and Disease*,
https://doi.org/10.1007/978-3-030-28384-1_14

dry type accounts for approximately 85–90% of all AMD cases. In its advanced form, known as geographic atrophy (GA), dry AMD leads to RPE degeneration and subsequently photoreceptor death in the macula. The underlying cause of dry AMD remains unknown. Wet AMD is caused by abnormal neovascularization from the choriocapillaris beneath the macula. These new blood vessels tend to bleed, leak fluid, and scar, which damages the photoreceptors. Although there is no cure for AMD, repeated injections of anti-vascular drugs into the eye can slow down the neovascularization and progression of early-stage wet AMD [3–5]. On the other hand, no effective medical or surgical treatment is available for dry AMD, although dietary supplements have been suggested to slow its progression [6]. There is clearly a need to develop a therapy that could preserve or repopulate this important RPE cell layer.

Cell Based Therapy for RPE

One of the most promising future treatments for retinal degeneration is cell replacement therapy [7]. The eye in general is a very attractive target for tissue engineering and cell therapy for several reasons. Firstly, the eye offers easy access to well-developed surgical approaches and non-invasive follow-up methods including high resolution optical coherence tomography (OCT) [7, 8]. Secondly, a relatively small number of cells is sufficient for a cell replacement in the eye as compared to many other organs and tissues. Finally, the eye is generally less prone to immune rejection of transplanted cells, although this advantage may be compromised due to disease pathogenesis such as neovascularization of wet AMD [9, 10].

The single layer of RPE that lies on Bruch's membrane between the photoreceptor outer segments and the choriocapillaris (Fig. 14.1) is a relatively easy target for cell replacement therapy, compared to highly complex neural retina with functional neural connections. Surgical attempts have been made to replace the RPE at the macula, either by moving the macula to the non-diseased periphery or by grafting new RPE under the macula [11]. These are difficult surgeries to perform and can lead to complications such as unplanned retinal detachment, cataract, and double vision [12]. Thus, it is unlikely that these procedures will prove cost effective in combatting the burden of AMD [11]. The earliest attempts of RPE cell transplantation in animal models provided evidence that cell replacement therapy could have potential in treating retinal degeneration. Although the success of these early studies was quite low [13], they encouraged further development of the technology. Later, clinical trials were conducted using fetal [14] or post-mortem adult RPE cells [15–17], as well as retina-RPE complex [18]. Unfortunately, visual acuity of the patients did not improve in the long term. Among these studies, Binder and colleagues were the first to report autologous RPE transplantation for AMD patients with promising outcomes [19]. Taken together, these and other early studies not mentioned here provided proof of concept that RPE cell replacement therapy is possible if a viable source of functional RPE cells is established.

As reviewed by da Cruz and colleagues [20] several cell sources for RPE transplantation have been considered: fetal, autologous, or allogeneic RPE, immortalized RPE cell lines, and stem cells. Among these, the use of fetal tissue is restricted mainly due to poor availability. Autologous RPE cells, on the other hand, may have genetic defects or be functionally impaired due to the disease. Immortalized cell lines likely contain mutations and genetic abnormalities. Thus, the most promising option is either allogeneic RPE cells or RPE cells differentiated from stem cells. Adult human RPE cells isolated from donated eyes can be activated *in vitro* into a stem cell state (RPE stem cells) which are polarized, express RPE markers and have the key physiological properties of native RPE cells making them a candidate for future cell replacement therapy [21, 22]. It is estimated that the macula harbors around 60,000 RPE cells that potentially need replacing. To achieve this, it is necessary to develop technologies to expand RPE stem cells *in vitro*, or to use their paracrine effects to trigger rejuvenation of native RPE *in vivo* [23]. Further preclinical studies are ongoing to develop adult RPE stem cell transplantations towards clinical trials [24]. In addition to the adult RPE stem cells, other stem cell types have been investigated as a source of RPE. Notably, human pluripotent stem cells (hPSC), with their excellent developmental and replicative capacity, can potentially provide an unlimited supply of RPE cells needed to treat the millions of patients suffering from retinal degeneration.

Human embryonic stem cells (hESCs) are usually isolated from surplus embryos of poor quality 4–6 days after *in vitro* fertilization [25]. Due to ethical issues and relatively low availability of these cells, as well as their immunogenic properties, the discovery of the possibility to reprogram human somatic cells to behave like hESCs offered even more exciting opportunities for regenerative medicine [26]. After the discovery of human induced pluripotent stem cells (hiPSC) in 2007, numerous non-integrating and non-viral reprogramming methods have been developed using various cell sources including skin fibroblasts, hair follicles, muscle, peripheral blood lymphocytes and urine [27]. In many respects, hiPSCs resemble hESCs, although epigenetic and genetic abnormalities in the hiPSC lines have been reported [28]. This has raised the issue whether epigenetic marks from the cell source may persist in the reprogrammed hiPSCs. This issue has been under critical evaluation as genomic instability in general is recognized as an important hurdle in the expanding field of stem cell-based therapies. According to the current knowledge, the epigenetic differences observed in some hiPSC lines compared to hESC lines seem to be caused mainly by the reprogramming method and diminish during passaging [29–31]. Further studies are needed to set a threshold for the acceptable level and genomic location of potential epigenetic and genetic changes in the stem cell product manufactured for clinical applications.

Differentiation of RPE from Human Pluripotent Stem Cells

So how can functional RPE cells be obtained from hPSC? During mammalian development, RPE and neural retina both develop from the optic neuroepithelium and share the same progenitors. The neuroepithelium near the anterior part of the neural tube evaginates laterally to form the optic vesicles. Invagination of the distal part of the optic vesicle leads to the formation of the optic cup. By the 6th or 7th week of gestation, the optic cup has differentiated into two epithelial layers. The distal layer then differentiates into the neural retina and the proximal layer develops into the RPE [32]. Since the pioneering work by Sasai and co-workers, hPSC-derived eye organoids mimicking the early retinal developmental steps have been extensively used for modeling eye development *in vitro* [33]. Similarly, *in vitro* differentiation of RPE cells from hPSCs follows the same developmental steps. In [34], Klimanskaya and co-workers were the first to report successful differentiation of RPE cells from hESCs [34]. Many research groups later demonstrated the same also with hiPSCs [35–37]. Since then, numerous research groups have developed methods for obtaining RPE cells from hPSCs, with varying efficiencies. Recent review describe the various differentiation methods in more detail [38], only the general approaches are presented here.

Human PSCs are typically cultured as colonies either on top of a layer of fibroblast feeder cells (mouse embryonic or human foreskin), or without feeder cells (feeder-free) on specific culture substrate in the presence of basic fibroblast growth factor (bFGF) [39–41]. There are two main approaches to initiate RPE differentiation: spontaneous RPE differentiation upon removal of bFGF from the culture medium or directed differentiation using growth factors, inhibitors and/or small molecules. In methods relying on spontaneous differentiation, RPE can be obtained through adherent over growth of hPSC cultures e.g. [34, 42, 43], or by growing embryoid body-like structures in suspension and later plating them down as adherent cultures e.g. [44, 45]. The more directed differentiation approaches attempt to replicate embryonic development by adding specific growth factors, inhibitors, or small molecules at appropriate time points [46–50]. As an example, we have established our own feeder cell-free culture and differentiation method for hPSC-RPE using both of these approaches [51].

Figure 14.2 summarise the differentiation and characterisation approach of RPE cells. In general, depending on the method and cell lines used, pigmented foci usually appear in cultures within 1–4 weeks (see Fig. 14.2a). The pigmented areas are mechanically or enzymatically separated for RPE enrichment. Once separated, pigmented hPSC-RPE cells are seeded on substratum which resembles Bruch's membrane or contains its extracellular matrix (ECM) components such as collagens and laminins [52]. After seeding, hPSC-RPE cells first lose their cobblestone morphology and pigmentation, but regain these characteristics within a few weeks [53] (also highly depending on culture conditions). However, if consecutively passaged, hPSC-RPE cells gradually lose their ability to re-establish RPE features [54]. This is problematic especially if multiple cell doublings are needed to obtain large enough quantities of pure RPE cells. Rho kinase (ROCK) inhibition during passaging may help extend hPSC-RPE passage [55], although it remains to be seen how this affects cell functionality and genetic stability. It is also well acknowledged that hPSC-RPE cells require an additional culture period of several weeks—preferably on permeable cell culture inserts—until they mature to a fully polarized and pigmented monolayer [51, 56, 57]. Furthermore, culture conditions such as the type of substratum and ECM protein coating highly affect hPSC-RPE maturation [52].

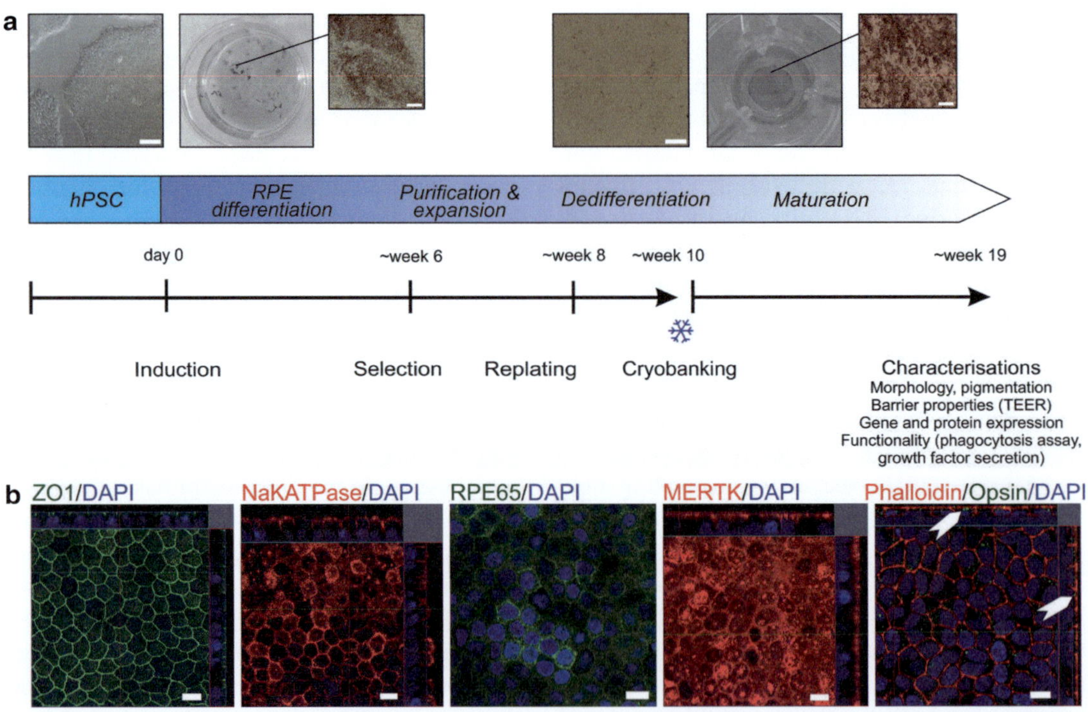

Fig. 14.2 The general hPSC-RPE differentiation and characterisation approach. (**a**) hPSC-RPE differentiation can be divided in induction of differentiation, purification and expantion of pigmented cells, additional replating/passaging and cryopreservation of cells, and finally hPSC-RPE maturation and characterisations. Scale bar 100 µm. (**b**) hPSC-RPE characterized with expression and localization of Zonula Occludens-1 (ZO1), Na+/K+ ATPase, RPE65, MERTK proteins and phagocytosis of photoreceptor outer segments (OPSIN). Scale bar 10 µm

Different hPSC lines may respond very differently to exogenous signals, making it challenging to develop a universal RPE differentiation protocol. It is unlikely that 100% RPE differentiation efficiency will ever be achieved. Thus, further improvements are needed to increase the yield and purity of the RPE cultures in order to obtain sufficient amounts of mature cells with RPE characteristics for safe therapeutic use. Besides establishing more efficient hPSC-RPE differentiation methods, another strategy to improve the purity of RPE populations is to sort cells based on RPE specific marker expression [58]. As safety is a primary consideration for any clinical use of hPSC-RPE and due to the high risk of tumorigenicity, methods to detect any trace of pluripotent cells among the differentiated cells are critically important [59–61]. Another safety concern is the use of animal-derived material such as fetal bovine serum (FBS) and mouse feeder cells. These components are often used in establishment, culture and differentiation of hPSCs, and may transfer non-human pathogens to the patient and cause immune reactions [62, 63]. Finally, cell therapy applications require defined and reproducible conditions in accordance with Good Manufacturing Practice (GMP) during derivation and maintenance of hPSC lines and RPE differentiation [41, 45]. Overall, the variations in differentiation and culture methods influence hPSC-RPE characteristics, which is why critical consideration and planning is needed when aiming for clinical applications. But first, does hPSC-RPE resemble and behave like native human RPE?

Characterization of Stem Cell-Derived RPE Cells

As mentioned earlier, RPE cells have many vitally important characteristics and functions [1]. Thus, it is necessary to verify that hPSC-RPE cells possess these characteristics (See Fig. 14.2b). This is critically important for clinical use, but also for non-clinical applications where hPSC-RPE cells serve as a model of native human RPE. Since the very early studies, putative hPSC-RPE cells were proven to share many characteristics with authentic human RPE: they express RPE specific genes and proteins (e.g. Bestrophin, CRALBP, Na+/K+ATPase, MERTK, Zonula Occludens-1 and Claudin-19), have pigmented cobblestone-like morphology, form tight and highly polarized RPE with high transepithelial electrical resistance (TEER), phagocytose isolated photoreceptor outer segments, and secrete growth factors such as PEDF [34, 35, 45, 64–67]. Moreover, hPSC-RPE cells express many important transporters [68, 69] and aquaporin water channels [56], and possess other physiologically relevant functions [70]. For instance, AMD patient-derived hiPSC-RPE cells have decreased antioxidative defence compared to healthy hiPSC-RPE cells, providing proof of concept that their stress response properties are similar to that of native RPE [71]. RPE cells derived from hiPSCs are in many respects very similar to hESC-RPE cells [51, 72]. Furthermore, a recent comparison of hiPSC lines derived from different somatic cells suggests that hiPSC-RPE functions are more significantly affected by the genetic background of different donors than the epigenetic "memory" associated with the donor tissue [70]. In addition, there is always heterogeneity among hPSC-RPE cultures and cell characteristics and functionality may vary. Thus, it is important to define RPE identity [73, 74] and improve quantitative methods to identify different maturation stages of hPSC-RPE cells. There is ongoing discussion regarding hPSC-RPE characteristics and the various criteria these cells should fulfil in order to be considered authentic RPE cells [73]. For example, Buccholz and co-workers have suggested that the systematic characterization panel of hPSC-RPE should include at least gene and protein analyses, quantitative phagocytosis, TEER measurement, growth factor secretion analysis, retinoid metabolism assay, and functionality in an animal model [35]. To conclude, there is an extensive and ever increasing amount of studies supporting the current knowledge that hPSCs are a promising source of functional RPE cells. The main down-stream applications of these cells are for modelling native RPE for drug testing, for modelling retinal diseases [75], and for RPE cell replacement therapies—the focus of the following subchapters.

Human PSC-RPE Transplantation Studies in Animal Models

The efficacy of hPSC-RPE cell therapy has been extensively studied in different animal models and only some of these are mentioned here as examples. Although large-eyed animal models are preferred especially for the development of subretinal transplantation techniques [76–79], the Royal College of Surgeons (RCS) rat remains a widely used animal model. Its RPE is unable to phagocytose photoreceptor outer segments and therefore photoreceptors degenerate over a period of 3 months after birth [80–82]. The Food and Drug Administration (FDA) recommends the use of this animal model to demonstrate safety and efficacy of hPSC-RPE [74]. The hPSC-RPE transplantation studies follow one of two approaches: injection of a single-cell suspension into the subretinal space, or transplantation of an hPSC-RPE sheet with or without supportive biomaterial matrix (See Fig. 14.1). Both of these approaches have their own pros and cons which are briefly discussed next.

Injection-Based Transplantation

In the first RPE transplantation studies in 2004, primate ESC-derived RPE injected into the subretinal space of RCS rats helped recover retinal function [83]. It was later demonstrated that although single cell suspension injected hPSC-RPE cells survive and improve visual acuity in RCS rats, they rarely form tight epithelia after transplantation and gradually die within 10–15 weeks and cell survival for up to 20–30 weeks seems to be an exception [36, 42, 43, 47, 67, 84]. Besides RCS rats, hPSC-RPE cells have been studied in monkeys and nude rats with a similar outcome [85, 86]. The improvement of visual function has been assessed using electroretinography (ERG) and even using behavioral assays that measure eye or body movements in response to light (optokinetic responses) [36, 47]. The temporary improvements in visual acuity of the RCS rat are thought to be more due to trophic factors [87] secreted by the transplanted cells, or macrophages that might help to phagocytose photoreceptor outer segments [64]. It has been suggested that failure to maintain a long-term improvement may be due to the impaired survival of hPSC-RPE on diseased Bruch's membrane [88–90]. However, injection-based transplantation is fast and technically less challenging than RPE sheet transplantation, which is why it was selected for the first clinical studies in human patients.

RPE Sheet Transplantation

RPE cells are sensitive to local extracellular substrates for anchoring and survival [91], so transplantation of a pre-formed, oriented, polarized monolayer with tight junctions could enhance cell viability and integration into the retina [50, 85]. Moreover, intact RPE monolayers have a higher resistance for oxidative stress and thus could survive better in diseased retina [50]. Finally, the required amount of cells for sheet transplantation is much lower than for subretinal injections [85]. Disadvantages of the transvitreal sheet transplantation are its invasiveness and demands of surgical procedure, although surgical techniques and specialized tools have been developed to ease RPE sheet transplantation into the back of the eye [76, 78].

Retinal degeneration often involves Bruch's membrane—the dynamic, 2–4.7 μm thick, pentalaminar structure which mainly consists of collagens, elastins, laminins, and fibronectin. Its thickness and permeability varies with age, pathological stage, and retinal location [92, 93]. The aged and thickened submacular Bruch's membrane does not support long-term survival and differentiation of transplanted RPE [94, 95]. Consequently, it could be beneficial to transplant hPSC-RPE sheet with a supportive biomaterial scaffold to simultaneously substitute RPE and Bruch's membrane function. In order to best mimic the properties of Bruch's membrane, biomaterial substrates for production and transplantation of hPSC-RPE cells should meet several requirements. First, the scaffold material should support formation of tight hPSC-RPE with proper apical-basal polarization as well as native RPE characteristics. Second, the substrate should be biocompatible, thin enough to fit the subretinal space, with mechanical properties suitable for handling of the cell sheet. Third, and most important, the material needs to enable integration of transplanted cells into the retina. Finally, permeability to fluids and biomolecules is a definite prerequisite for substrates to replace the lost functional role of the damaged Bruch's membrane as a semipermeable barrier [96–99].

Many research groups are focusing on finding an optimal scaffold for RPE transplantation. Decellularized natural scaffolds, such as Bruch's membrane, amniotic membrane, and anterior lens capsule, have been previously suggested as substrates in retinal transplantations [100–102]. These natural scaffolds provide a significant advantage in retaining the complex structure and molecular hierarchy of the ECM while possessing tissue-specific micro- and nanotopography [97, 103]. In addition, natural polymers such as collagen, alginate, and fibroin, provide biocompatible sources of polymers for retinal tissue engineering. Natural polymers also closely mimic the native ECM and possess innate biological activity [97, 104]. Still, biomaterials of natural origin have several disadvantages including poor mechanical properties, batch to batch variation, as well as concerns with immunogenicity, toxic by-products of biodegradation, and pathogen transfer.

Synthetic polymers have multiple attractive characteristics including controlled chemical and physical structure, predictable properties, mechanical durability, high degree of processing flexibility, and high reproducibility in commercial-scale manufacturing processes [97]. The most commonly used synthetic polymers are poly-α-hydroxy-acid-based polymers such as poly(L-lactide) (PLLA), poly(lactide-co-glycolide) (PLGA), poly(ε-caprolactone) (PCL), and combinations of these materials as co-polymers (e.g. PLCL) [97, 105, 106]. Even though synthetic polymers overcome the common drawbacks associated with natural polymers, they tend to be hydrophobic and lack cell binding ligands on the scaffold surface, which results in poor cell attachment without additional surface modifications [106]. Many synthetic biomaterial substrates with distinct architecture have been investigated as potential substrates for RPE [98, 107–109]. Finally, hybrid materials incorporate the beneficial aspects of both biologically active natural polymers and structurally flexible synthetic polymers such as combination of silk fibroin, gelatin and PCL [110]. Hybrid biomaterials show promise as potential Bruch's membrane mimicking substrates for RPE [111, 112].

Most biomaterial studies use either primary RPE cells or immortalized cell lines, and studies of hPSC-RPE cell-biomaterial interactions have only recently gained popularity e.g. [65, 77]. The most disputed property of hPSC-RPE scaffold material is its biostability—are biodegradable scaffolds preferable over biologically inert/non-degradable materials? A biodegradable membrane would provide a temporary support for hPSC-RPE, until the cells remodel and replace it with new ECM layers. A biostable membrane would provide permanent support for the cells and at the same time improve integration of the transplant by providing better permeability, which is likely to be critical for retinal health [65, 113]. For instance, Parylene C (poly(para-xylene)) is a biostable and chemically inert polymer. When combined with Matrigel™ or human vitronectin, Parylene C was shown to support hPSC-RPE growth and functionality both *in vitro* and *in vivo* [114]. Our group has studied the performance of biologically inert polyimide (PI) for hPSC-RPE culture [115] and transplantation [108]. These approaches aim to overcome the disorganized fashion in which RPE cells adhere to Bruch's membrane when injected as a suspension. The plastic polymer is also designed to act as a replacement for the aged and thickened Bruch's membrane, and provides an anchor for the cells while aiding in surgical delivery [11]. It remains an important target for future preclinical and clinical studies to demonstrate whether the best efficacy for hPSC-RPE transplantation is achieved with the less invasive injection method or with the surgically challenging sheet transplantation. Alternatively, perhaps the transplantation method should be chosen based on individual patient and disease status. Finally, further clinical studies will need to demonstrate whether improved retinal function translates into improved cortical representation of images—an outcome which has been observed in humans after transplantation of adult RPE [20].

Clinical Trials with HPSC-RPE Cells

In 2012, 8 years after the first report of successful hESC-RPE differentiation, the first Phase I/II clinical trial using these cells was reported by Schwartz and co-workers, with indication of a good safety profile for patients with Stargardt disease and advanced dry AMD [116]. In the 3-year follow-up study with 18 participants, hESC-RPE cells were administered as a subretinal injection of three dosage cohorts (50,000 cells, 100,000 cells and 150,000 cells). In addition to the safety of the treatment, the authors also demonstrated improved vision in four out of nine AMD patients. Interestingly, only few, if any, pigmented hESC-RPE cells survived in the direct area of GA lesions. Instead, transplanted cells were detected in areas adjacent to the lesions, where they were deposited onto native RPE [117]. A Phase II study with more patients to assess efficacy is expected to report results imminently [23]. Other clinical trials with hPSC-RPE injections are ongoing in several countries including Israel, China, and Korea (for details see recent review [23] and https://clinicaltrials.gov). It remains to be seen if long-term survival and function of subretinally injected cells is achieved.

Unlike hESCs, hiPSCs can be obtained from the patients' own somatic cells, offering the potential for immune-compatibility. To date, one AMD patient has been treated with autologous hiPSC-RPE cells manufactured and transplanted without an artificial scaffold [118]. RPE cells grown on a collagen gel were enzymatically lifted and transplanted as a sheet into the subretinal space of a patient with advanced wet AMD in Japan. It was reported that the patient did not experience any serious side effects and maintained visual acuity 1 year after surgery. The patient did not receive immunosuppressants and showed no signs of rejection. A second patient was recruited to the study, but was put on hold due to genetic mutations in hiPSC-RPE cells. [118, 119] Since then, the approach was modified towards using allogeneic hiPSCs and the clinical trial has resumed [23]

In a clinical trial carried out by The London Project to Cure Blindness in collaboration with Pfizer, two patients with wet AMD were treated with hESC-RPE monolayer immobilized on a polyester membrane [120, 121]. This is the first study demonstrating successful delivery and survival of hESC-RPE patch with a visual acuity gain of two patients treated. Similarly, a clinical trial led by Regenerative Patch Technologies (USA) is aiming to treat GA by transplanting hESC-RPE sheet on parylene C membrane and has very recently published first positive results with 4 out of 5 patients treated [122]. In both of these studies a non-degradable biomaterial with permanent support is used. In contrast, in a clinical trial planned by NEI/NIH, Bharti and co-workers aim to use a biodegradable matrix which will gradually dissolve after successful delivery of the hPSC-RPE cell sheet [38]. Perhaps the final outcomes of these trials will demonstrate what type of biomaterial substrates is better suited for hPSC-RPE delivery—biostable or biodegradable. Overall, it is very encouraging that studies using both cell delivery methods, and both hPSC types, appear to be safe in initial clinical studies.

Future Perspectives for RPE Cell Therapy

Although many clinical trials are ongoing, there are several open questions that need to be addressed and properly answered before safe and effective hPSC based cell therapies are widely available. One of the important and unanswered questions is whether to use hESC or hiPSC for cell replacement therapies. Although considered as functionally equivalent to hESCs, hiPSCs have been shown to harbor subtle differences in gene expression and DNA methylation [123]. Furthermore, there have been reports of point mutations and copy number variation in hiPSCs, which raises possible safety issues [118, 124].

The use of hPSC-RPE in clinical application faces multiple challenges, including manufacturing and characterization of clinical grade cells. The precise list of functional properties absolutely required prior to transplantation, and properties that the cells may or may not acquire once they are correctly integrated into the host tissue, is still missing [73].

Potential tumorigenicity of transplanted cells is a challenge that needs method development and increased understanding to guarantee safety and efficacy of transplanted cells. The pluripotent nature of hPSCs also raises the concern that if any undifferentiated hPSCs were left in the final clinical product, they could increase the risk of tumor or teratoma formation after transplantation. Another challenge is the immune-acceptance of transplanted cells. Although the subretinal space is relatively immune-privileged, damaged blood–retinal barrier, leaky blood vessels, and activated microglia may be present in diseased retina or induced by surgery. This can compromise the immune-privilege and cause cell rejection. Immunogenicity of allogeneic hPSC-RPE cells is therefore an issue [125, 126]. Autologous hiPSC-RPE cells offer minimal risk of cell rejection, but would not be a cost effective strategy on a large scale. Thus, a thorough understanding of the immunogenicity of hPSC-RPE and the optimal immunosuppression regime is essential for future clinical applications. In addition, international cell banking initiatives covering different human leukocyte antigen (HLA) types or universal hPSC lines with standardized cell banking and production methods are needed [127]. Otherwise there is a well-recognized risk that these treatments remain unaffordable for the majority of the patients.

Overall, multifactorial diseases such as AMD need further understanding of the disease pathogenesis, and most likely efficient treatment will require multidisciplinary approaches and personalized medicine. In addition, combination therapy of cell replacement, gene correction, supportive biomaterials and pharmaceuticals may be needed for certain diseases. First, as an example, strategies are being developed to genetically correct hiPSCs prior to differentiation and autologous transplantation [128]. Second, in addition to RPE and photoreceptor degeneration, Bruch's membrane alterations including thickening and accumulation of drusen play an important role in AMD pathogenesis. Thus, further studies are needed to see if artificial scaffolds can replace Bruch's membrane enabling proper RPE cell attachment in the diseased eye, or if novel methods are developed to improve attachment and polarization of injected RPE cells. Third, the critical cell type in early AMD seems to be RPE, while in more advanced cases, it may be necessary to replace neuronal cells either alone or together with RPE cells. Production and transplantation of photoreceptors or their progenitors has shown some promise, but is challenging due to the requirement for functional integration and synaptic contacts with the host neurons [129]. Last but not least, combination of effective medication and new therapeutic agents may be needed together with cell-based therapies to improve their efficacy.

In the end, it would be devastating for the whole field of regenerative medicine if any harm was caused to the patients in ongoing and upcoming clinical trials with hPSC-derived cells. Thus it is important to establish world-wide standards for the proper preclinical and clinical studies to minimize and hopefully avoid poor outcomes [130]. Several clinical trials are in progress around the world and the results will undoubtedly be exciting, but continued research and collaboration are needed to ensure above all safety, and then success of these ground-breaking approaches.

Acknowledgements Heidi Hongisto, Tanja Ilmarinen and Outi Paloheimo are acknowledged for the artwork of Figures.

References

1. Strauss O. The retinal pigment epithelium in visual function. Physiol Rev. 2005;85:845–81. https://doi.org/10.1152/physrev.00021.2004.
2. Wong WL, Su X, Li X, et al. Global prevalence of age-related macular degeneration and disease burden projection for 2020 and 2040: a systematic review and meta-analysis. Lancet Glob Heal. 2014;2:2–e116. https://doi.org/10.1016/S2214-109X(13)70145-1.
3. Heier JS, Brown DM, Chong V, et al. Intravitreal aflibercept (VEGF trap-eye) in wet age-related macular degeneration. Ophthalmology. 2012;119:2537–48. https://doi.org/10.1016/j.ophtha.2012.09.006.
4. Martin DF, Maguire MG, Ying G, et al. Ranibizumab and bevacizumab for neovascular age-related macular degeneration. N Engl J Med. 2011;364:1897–908. https://doi.org/10.1056/NEJMoa1102673.
5. Rosenfeld PJ, Brown DM, Heier JS, et al. Ranibizumab for neovascular age-related macular degeneration. N Engl J Med. 2006;355:1419–31. https://doi.org/10.1056/NEJMoa054481.
6. Group A. Lutein + zeaxanthin and omega-3 fatty acids for age-related macular degeneration: the age-related eye disease study 2 (AREDS2) randomized clinical trial. JAMA J Am Med Assoc. 2013;2:1–11. https://doi.org/10.1001/jama.2013.4997.
7. Zarbin M. Cell-based therapy for degenerative retinal disease. Trends Mol Med. 2016;22:115–34. https://doi.org/10.1016/j.molmed.2015.12.007.
8. Adhi M, Duker JS. Optical coherence tomography—current and future applications. Curr Opin Ophthalmol. 2013;24:213–21. https://doi.org/10.1097/ICU.0b013e32835f8bf8.
9. Stein-Streilein J. Mechanisms of immune privilege in the posterior eye. Int Rev Immunol. 2013;32:42–56. https://doi.org/10.3109/08830185.2012.740535.
10. Zhou R, Caspi RR. Ocular immune privilege. F1000 Biol Rep. 2010;2:pii: 3. https://doi.org/10.3410/B2-3.
11. Ramsden CM, Powner MB, Carr A-JF, et al. Stem cells in retinal regeneration: past, present and future. Development. 2013;140:2576–85. https://doi.org/10.1242/dev.092270.
12. Stanga PE, Kychenthal A, Fitzke FW, et al. Retinal pigment epithelium translocation after choroidal neovascular membrane removal in age-related macular degeneration. Ophthalmology. 2002;109:1492–8.
13. Jha BS, Bharti K. Regenerating retinal pigment epithelial cells to cure blindness: a road towards personalized artificial tissue. Curr Stem Cell Reports. 2015;1:79–91. https://doi.org/10.1007/s40778-015-0014-4.
14. Algvere PV, Berglin L, Gouras P, Sheng Y. Transplantation of fetal retinal pigment epithelium in age-related macular degeneration with subfoveal neovascularization. Graefes Arch Clin Exp Ophthalmol. 1994;232:707–16.
15. Del Priore LV, Kaplan HJ, Tezel TH, et al. Retinal pigment epithelial cell transplantation after subfoveal membranectomy in age-related macular degeneration: clinicopathologic correlation. Am J Ophthalmol. 2001;131:472–80.
16. Peyman GA, Blinder KJ, Paris CL, et al. A technique for retinal pigment epithelium transplantation for age-related macular degeneration secondary to extensive subfoveal scarring. Ophthalmic Surg. 1991;22:102–8.
17. Tezel TH, Del Priore LV, Berger AS, Kaplan HJ. Adult retinal pigment epithelial transplantation in exudative age-related macular degeneration. Am J Ophthalmol. 2007;143:584–95. https://doi.org/10.1016/j.ajo.2006.12.007.
18. Radtke ND, Aramant RB, Petry HM, et al. Vision improvement in retinal degeneration patients by implantation of retina together with retinal pigment epithelium. Am J Ophthalmol. 2008;146:172–82. https://doi.org/10.1016/j.ajo.2008.04.009.
19. Binder S, Stolba U, Krebs I, et al. Transplantation of autologous retinal pigment epithelium in eyes with foveal neovascularization resulting from age-related macular degeneration: a pilot study. Am J Ophthalmol. 2002;133:215–25. https://doi.org/10.1016/S0002-9394(01)01373-3.
20. da Cruz L, Chen FK, Ahmado A, et al. RPE transplantation and its role in retinal disease. Prog Retin Eye Res. 2007;26:598–635. https://doi.org/10.1016/j.preteyeres.2007.07.001.
21. Blenkinsop TA, Saini JS, Maminishkis A, et al. Human adult retinal pigment epithelial stem cell-derived RPE monolayers exhibit key physiological characteristics of native tissue. Investig Ophthalmol Vis Sci. 2015;56:7085–99. https://doi.org/10.1167/iovs.14-16246.
22. Salero E, Blenkinsop TA, Corneo B, et al. Adult human RPE can be activated into a multipotent stem cell that produces mesenchymal derivatives. Cell Stem Cell. 2012;10:88–95. https://doi.org/10.1016/j.stem.2011.11.018.
23. Zhao C, Wang Q, Temple S. Stem cell therapies for retinal diseases: recapitulating development to replace degenerated cells. Development. 2017;144:1368–81. https://doi.org/10.1242/dev.133108.
24. Davis RJ, Blenkinsop TA, Campbell M, et al. Human RPE stem cell-derived RPE preserves photoreceptors in the Royal College of Surgeons rat: method for quantifying the area of photoreceptor sparing. J Ocul Pharmacol Ther. 2016;32:304–9. https://doi.org/10.1089/jop.2015.0162.
25. Skottman H. Derivation and characterization of three new human embryonic stem cell lines in Finland. In Vitro Cell Dev Biol Anim. 2010;46:206–9. https://doi.org/10.1007/s11626-010-9286-2.
26. Takahashi K, Tanabe K, Ohnuki M, et al. Induction of pluripotent stem cells from adult human fibroblasts by defined factors. Cell. 2007;107:861–72. https://doi.org/10.1016/j.cell.2007.11.019.
27. Brandl C, Grassmann F, Riolfi J, Weber B. Tapping stem cells to target AMD: challenges and prospects. J Clin Med. 2015;4:282–303. https://doi.org/10.3390/jcm4020282.

28. Huang K, Shen Y, Xue Z, et al. A panel of CpG methylation sites distinguishes human embryonic stem cells and induced pluripotent stem cells. Stem Cell Reports. 2014;2:36–43. https://doi.org/10.1016/j.stemcr.2013.11.003\rS2213-6711(13)00128-8. [pii]
29. Chin MH, Mason MJ, Xie W, et al. Induced pluripotent stem cells and embryonic stem cells are distinguished by gene expression signatures. Cell Stem Cell. 2009;5:111–23. https://doi.org/10.1016/j.stem.2009.06.008.
30. Nishino K, Toyoda M, Yamazaki-Inoue M, et al. DNA methylation dynamics in human induced pluripotent stem cells over time. PLoS Genet. 2011;7:7. https://doi.org/10.1371/journal.pgen.1002085.
31. Polo JM, Liu S, Figueroa ME, et al. Cell type of origin influences the molecular and functional properties of mouse induced pluripotent stem cells. Nat Biotechnol. 2010;28:848–55. https://doi.org/10.1038/nbt.1667.
32. Fuhrmann S, Zou C, Levine EM. Retinal pigment epithelium development, plasticity, and tissue homeostasis. Exp Eye Res. 2014;123:141–50. https://doi.org/10.1016/j.exer.2013.09.003.
33. Eiraku M, Takata N, Ishibashi H, et al. Self-organizing optic-cup morphogenesis in three-dimensional culture. Nature. 2011;472:51–6. https://doi.org/10.1038/nature09941.
34. Klimanskaya I, Hipp J, Rezai KA, et al. Derivation and comparative assessment of retinal pigment epithelium from human embryonic stem cells using transcriptomics. Cloning Stem Cells. 2004;6:217–45. https://doi.org/10.1089/clo.2004.6.217.
35. Buchholz DE, Hikita ST, Rowland TJ, et al. Derivation of functional retinal pigmented epithelium from induced pluripotent stem cells. Stem Cells. 2009;27:2427–34. https://doi.org/10.1002/stem.189.
36. Carr AJ, Vugler AA, Hikita ST, et al. Protective effects of human iPS-derived retinal pigment epithelium cell transplantation in the retinal dystrophic rat. PLoS One. 2009;4:4. https://doi.org/10.1371/journal.pone.0008152.
37. Hirami Y, Osakada F, Takahashi K, et al. Generation of retinal cells from mouse and human induced pluripotent stem cells. Neurosci Lett. 2009;458:126–31. https://doi.org/10.1016/j.neulet.2009.04.035.
38. Song MJ, Bharti K. Looking into the future: using induced pluripotent stem cells to build two and three dimensional ocular tissue for cell therapy and disease modeling. Brain Res. 2016;1638:2–14. https://doi.org/10.1016/j.brainres.2015.12.011.
39. Crocco MC, Fratnz N, Bos-Mikich A. Substrates and supplements for hESCs: a critical review. J Assist Reprod Genet. 2013;30:315–23. https://doi.org/10.1007/s10815-012-9914-8.
40. Skottman H, Hovatta O. Culture conditions for human embryonic stem cells. Reproduction. 2006;132:691–8.
41. Unger C, Skottman H, Blomberg P, et al. Good manufacturing practice and clinical-grade human embryonic stem cell lines. Hum Mol Genet. 2008;17:R48–53. https://doi.org/10.1093/hmg/ddn079.
42. Lund RD, Wang S, Klimanskaya I, et al. Human embryonic stem cell-derived cells rescue visual function in dystrophic RCS rats. Cloning Stem Cells. 2006;8:189–99. https://doi.org/10.1089/clo.2006.8.189.
43. Vugler A, Carr A-J, Lawrence J, et al. Elucidating the phenomenon of HESC-derived RPE: anatomy of cell genesis, expansion and retinal transplantation. Exp Neurol. 2008;214:347–61. https://doi.org/10.1016/j.expneurol.2008.09.007.
44. Meyer JS, Shearer RL, Capowski EE, et al. Modeling early retinal development with human embryonic and induced pluripotent stem cells. Proc Natl Acad Sci U S A. 2009;106:16698–703. https://doi.org/10.1073/pnas.0905245106.
45. Vaajasaari H, Ilmarinen T, Juuti-Uusitalo K, et al. Toward the defined and xeno-free differentiation of functional human pluripotent stem cell-derived retinal pigment epithelial cells. Mol Vis. 2011;17:558–75.
46. Buchholz DE, Pennington BO, Croze RH, et al. Rapid and efficient directed differentiation of human pluripotent stem cells into retinal pigmented epithelium. Stem Cells Transl Med. 2013;2:384–93. https://doi.org/10.5966/sctm.2012-0163.
47. Idelson M, Alper R, Obolensky A, et al. Directed differentiation of human embryonic stem cells into functional retinal pigment epithelium cells. Cell Stem Cell. 2009;5:396–408. https://doi.org/10.1016/j.stem.2009.07.002.
48. Maruotti J, Sripathi SR, Bharti K, et al. Small-molecule–directed, efficient generation of retinal pigment epithelium from human pluripotent stem cells. Proc Natl Acad Sci. 2015;112:10950–5. https://doi.org/10.1073/pnas.1422818112.
49. Rowland TJ, Blaschke AJ, Buchholz DE, et al. Differentiation of human pluripotent stem cells to retinal pigmented epithelium in defined conditions using purified extracellular matrix proteins. J Tissue Eng Regen Med. 2013;7:642–53. https://doi.org/10.1002/term.1458.
50. Zhu D, Deng X, Spee C, et al. Polarized secretion of PEDF from human embryonic stem cell-derived RPE promotes retinal progenitor cell survival. Investig Ophthalmol Vis Sci. 2011;52:1573–85. https://doi.org/10.1167/iovs.10-6413.
51. Hongisto H, Ilmarinen T, Vattulainen M, et al. Xeno- and feeder-free differentiation of human pluripotent stem cells to two distinct ocular epithelial cell types using simple modifications of one method. Stem Cell Res Ther. 2017;8:291. https://doi.org/10.1186/s13287-017-0738-4.
52. Sorkio A, Hongisto H, Kaarniranta K, et al. Structure and barrier properties of human embryonic stem cell-derived retinal pigment epithelial cells are affected by extracellular matrix protein coating. Tissue Eng Part A. 2014;20:622–34. https://doi.org/10.1089/ten.TEA.2013.0049.
53. Abu Khamidakh AE, Dos Santos FC, Skottman H, et al. Semi-automatic method for Ca2+ imaging data analysis of maturing human embryonic stem cells-derived retinal

pigment epithelium. Ann Biomed Eng. 2016;44:3408–20. https://doi.org/10.1007/s10439-016-1656-9.
54. Singh R, Phillips MJ, Kuai D, et al. Functional analysis of serially expanded human iPS cell-derived RPE cultures. Investig Ophthalmol Vis Sci. 2013;54:6767–78. https://doi.org/10.1167/iovs.13-11943.
55. Croze RH, Thi WJ, Clegg DO. ROCK inhibition promotes attachment, proliferation, and wound closure in human embryonic stem cell-derived retinal pigmented epithelium. Transl Vis Sci Technol. 2016;5(6):7. https://doi.org/10.1167/tvst.5.6.7.
56. Juuti-Uusitalo K, Delporte C, Gregoire F, et al. Aquaporin expression and function in human pluripotent stem cell-derived retinal pigmented epithelial cells. Invest Ophthalmol Vis Sci. 2013;54:3510–9. https://doi.org/10.1167/iovs.13-11800.
57. Juuti-Uusitalo K, Nieminen M, Treumer F, et al. Effects of cytokine activation and oxidative stress on the function of the human embryonic stem cell-derived retinal pigment epithelial cells. Invest Ophthalmol Vis Sci. 2015;56:6265–74. https://doi.org/10.1167/iovs.15-17333.
58. Choudhary P, Whiting PJ. A strategy to ensure safety of stem cell-derived retinal pigment epithelium cells. Stem Cell Res Ther. 2016;7:127. https://doi.org/10.1186/s13287-016-0380-6.
59. Kanemura H, Go MJ, Shikamura M, et al. Tumorigenicity studies of induced pluripotent stem cell (iPSC)-derived retinal pigment epithelium (RPE) for the treatment of age-related macular degeneration. PLoS One. 2014;9:1–11. https://doi.org/10.1371/journal.pone.0085336.
60. Kawamata S, Kanemura H, Sakai N, et al. Design of a tumorigenicity test for induced pluripotent stem cell (iPSC)-derived cell products. J Clin Med. 2015;4:159–71. https://doi.org/10.3390/jcm4010159.
61. Kuroda T, Yasuda S, Kusakawa S, et al. Highly sensitive in vitro methods for detection of residual undifferentiated cells in retinal pigment epithelial cells derived from human iPS cells. PLoS One. 2012;7:1–9. https://doi.org/10.1371/journal.pone.0037342.
62. Martin MJ, Muotri A, Gage F, Varki A. Human embryonic stem cells express an immunogenic nonhuman sialic acid. Nat Med. 2005;11:228–32. https://doi.org/10.1038/nm1181.
63. Sakamoto N, Tsuji K, Muul LM, et al. Bovine apolipoprotein B-100 is a dominant immunogen in therapeutic cell populations cultured in fetal calf serum in mice and humans. Blood. 2007;110:501–8. https://doi.org/10.1182/blood-2007-01-066522.
64. Carr A-J, Vugler A, Lawrence J, et al. Molecular characterization and functional analysis of phagocytosis by human embryonic stem cell-derived RPE cells using a novel human retinal assay. Mol Vis. 2009;15:283–95.
65. Kamao H, Mandai M, Okamoto S, et al. Characterization of human induced pluripotent stem cell-derived retinal pigment epithelium cell sheets aiming for clinical application. Stem Cell Reports. 2014;2:205–18. https://doi.org/10.1016/j.stemcr.2013.12.007.
66. Liao JL, Yu J, Huang K, et al. Molecular signature of primary retinal pigment epithelium and stem-cell-derived RPE cells. Hum Mol Genet. 2010;19:4229–38. https://doi.org/10.1093/hmg/ddq341.
67. Lu B, Malcuit C, Wang S, et al. Long-term safety and function of RPE from human embryonic stem cells in preclinical models of macular degeneration. Stem Cells. 2009;27:2126–35. https://doi.org/10.1002/stem.149.
68. Juuti-Uusitalo K, Vaajasaari H, Ryhänen T, et al. Efflux protein expression in human stem cell-derived retinal pigment epithelial cells. PLoS One. 2012;7:e30089. https://doi.org/10.1371/journal.pone.0030089.
69. Kokkinaki M, Sahibzada N, Golestaneh N. Human induced pluripotent stem-derived retinal pigment epithelium (RPE) cells exhibit ion transport, membrane potential, polarized vascular endothelial growth factor secretion, and gene expression pattern similar to native RPE. Stem Cells. 2011;29:825–35. https://doi.org/10.1002/stem.635.
70. Miyagishima KJ, Wan Q, Corneo B, et al. In pursuit of authenticity: induced pluripotent stem cell-derived retinal pigment epithelium for clinical applications. Stem Cells Transl Med. 2016;5:1562–74. https://doi.org/10.5966/sctm.2016-0037.
71. Chang YC, Chang WC, Hung KH, et al. The generation of induced pluripotent stem cells for macular degeneration as a drug screening platform: identification of curcumin as a protective agent for retinal pigment epithelial cells against oxidative stress. Front Aging Neurosci. 2014;6:191. https://doi.org/10.3389/fnagi.2014.00191.
72. Juuti-Uusitalo K, Delporte C, Grégoire F, et al. Aquaporin expression and function in human pluripotent stem cell–derived retinal pigmented epithelial cells. Invest Opthalmol Vis Sci. 2013;54:3510. https://doi.org/10.1167/iovs.13-11800.
73. Bharti K, Miller SS, Arnheiter H. The new paradigm: retinal pigment epithelium cells generated from embryonic or induced pluripotent stem cells. Pigment Cell Melanoma Res. 2011;24:21–34. https://doi.org/10.1111/j.1755-148X.2010.00772.x.
74. Bharti K, Rao M, Hull SC, et al. Developing cellular therapies for retinal degenerative diseases. Investig Ophthalmol Vis Sci. 2014;55:1191–201. https://doi.org/10.1167/iovs.13-13481.
75. Yvon C, Ramsden CM, Lane A, et al. Using stem cells to model diseases of the outer retina. Comput Struct Biotechnol J. 2015;13:382–9. https://doi.org/10.1016/j.csbj.2015.05.001.
76. Al-Nawaiseh S, Thieltges F, Liu Z, et al. A step by step protocol for subretinal surgery in rabbits. J Vis Exp. 2016;(115):53927. https://doi.org/10.3791/53927.
77. Brant Fernandes RA, Koss MJ, Falabella P, et al. An innovative surgical technique for subretinal transplantation of human embryonic stem cell-derived retinal pigmented epithelium in Yucatan mini pigs: preliminary results. Ophthalmic Surg Lasers Imaging Retina. 2016;47:342–51. https://doi.org/10.3928/23258160-20160324-07.

78. Stanzel BV, Liu Z, Brinken R, et al. Subretinal delivery of ultrathin rigid-elastic cell carriers using a metallic shooter instrument and biodegradable hydrogel encapsulation. Invest Ophthalmol Vis Sci. 2012;53:490–500. https://doi.org/10.1167/iovs.11-8260.
79. Thieltges F, Liu Z, Brinken R, et al. Localized RPE removal with a novel instrument aided by viscoelastics in rabbits. Transl Vis Sci Technol. 2016;5:11. https://doi.org/10.1167/tvst.5.3.11.
80. Dowling JE, Sidman RL. Inherited retinal dystrophy in the rat. J Cell Biol. 1962;14:73–109.
81. Edwards RB, Szamier RB. Defective phagocytosis of isolated rod outer segments by RCS rat retinal pigment epithelium in culture. Science. 1977;197:1001–3.
82. Mullen RJ, LaVail MM. Inherited retinal dystrophy: primary defect in pigment epithelium determined with experimental rat chimeras. Science. 1976;192:799–801.
83. Haruta M, Sasai Y, Kawasaki H, et al. In vitro and in vivo characterization of pigment epithelial cells differentiated from primate embryonic stem cells. Invest Ophthalmol Vis Sci. 2004;45:1020–5.
84. Krohne TU, Westenskow PD, Kurihara T, et al. Generation of retinal pigment epithelial cells from small molecules and OCT4 reprogrammed human induced pluripotent stem cells. Stem Cells Transl Med. 2012;1:96–109. https://doi.org/10.5966/sctm.2011-0057.
85. Diniz B, Thomas P, Thomas B, et al. Subretinal implantation of retinal pigment epithelial cells derived from human embryonic stem cells: improved survival when implanted as a monolayer. Invest Ophthalmol Vis Sci. 2013;54:5087–96. https://doi.org/10.1167/iovs.12-11239.
86. Kamao H, Mandai M, Ohashi W, et al. Evaluation of the surgical device and procedure for extracellular matrix–scaffold–supported human iPSC–derived retinal pigment epithelium cell sheet transplantation. Investig Opthalmol Vis Sci. 2017;58(1):211–20. https://doi.org/10.1167/iovs.16-19778.
87. Shi G, Maminishkis A, Banzon T, et al. Control of chemokine gradients by the retinal pigment epithelium. Invest Ophthalmol Vis Sci. 2008;49:4620–30. https://doi.org/10.1167/iovs.08-1816.
88. Petrus-Reurer S, Bartuma H, Aronsson M, et al. Integration of subretinal suspension transplants of human embryonic stem cell-derived retinal pigment epithelial cells in a large-eyed model of geographic atrophy. Invest Ophthalmol Vis Sci. 2017;58(2):1314–22. https://doi.org/10.1167/iovs.16-20738doi.
89. Sugino IK, Gullapalli VK, Sun Q, et al. Cell-deposited matrix improves retinal pigment epithelium survival on aged submacular human Bruch's membrane. Invest Ophthalmol Vis Sci. 2011;52:1345–58. https://doi.org/10.1167/iovs.10-6112.
90. Sugino IK, Sun Q, Wang J, et al. Comparison of FRPE and human embryonic stem cell-derived RPE behavior on aged human Bruch's membrane. Invest Ophthalmol Vis Sci. 2011;52:4979–97. https://doi.org/10.1167/iovs.10-5386.
91. Tezel TH, Del Priore LV. Reattachment to a substrate prevents apoptosis of human retinal pigment epithelium. Graefes Arch Clin Exp Ophthalmol. 1997;235:41–7.
92. Booij JC, Baas DC, Beisekeeva J, et al. The dynamic nature of Bruch's membrane. Prog Retin Eye Res. 2010;29:1–18. https://doi.org/10.1016/j.preteyeres.2009.08.003.
93. Ramrattan RS, van der Schaft TL, Mooy CM, et al. Morphometric analysis of Bruch's membrane, the choriocapillaris, and the choroid in aging. Invest Ophthalmol Vis Sci. 1994;35:2857–64.
94. Gullapalli VK, Sugino IK, Van Patten Y, et al. Impaired RPE survival on aged submacular human Bruch's membrane. Exp Eye Res. 2005;80:235–48. https://doi.org/10.1016/j.exer.2004.09.006.
95. Sugino IK, Rapista A, Sun Q, et al. A method to enhance cell survival on Bruch's membrane in eyes affected by age and age-related macular degeneration. Invest Ophthalmol Vis Sci. 2011;52:9598–609. https://doi.org/10.1167/iovs.11-8400.
96. Binder S. Scaffolds for retinal pigment epithelium (RPE) replacement therapy. Br J Ophthalmol. 2011;95:441–2. https://doi.org/10.1136/bjo.2009.171926.
97. Hynes SR, Lavik EB. A tissue-engineered approach towards retinal repair: scaffolds for cell transplantation to the subretinal space. Graefes Arch Clin Exp Ophthalmol. 2010;248:763–78. https://doi.org/10.1007/s00417-009-1263-7.
98. Pennington BO, Clegg DO. Pluripotent stem cell-based therapies in combination with substrate for the treatment of age-related macular degeneration. J Ocul Pharmacol Ther. 2016;32:261–71. https://doi.org/10.1089/jop.2015.0153.
99. Sorkio A, Haimi S, Verdoold V, et al. Poly(trimethylene carbonate) as an elastic biodegradable film for human embryonic stem cell-derived retinal pigment epithelial cells. J Tissue Eng Regen Med. 2017;11:3134–44. https://doi.org/10.1002/term.2221.
100. Akrami H, Soheili Z-S, Sadeghizadeh M, et al. Evaluation of RPE65, CRALBP, VEGF, CD68, and tyrosinase gene expression in human retinal pigment epithelial cells cultured on amniotic membrane. Biochem Genet. 2011;49:313–22. https://doi.org/10.1007/s10528-010-9409-1.
101. Kiilgaard JF, Scherfig E, Prause JU, la Cour M. Transplantation of amniotic membrane to the subretinal space in pigs. Stem Cells Int. 2012;2012:716968–5. https://doi.org/10.1155/2012/716968.
102. Nicolini J, Kiilgaard JF, Wiencke AK, et al. The anterior lens capsule used as support material in RPE cell-transplantation. Acta Ophthalmol Scand. 2000;78:527–31.
103. Walters NJ, Gentleman E. Evolving insights in cell-matrix interactions: elucidating how non-soluble properties of the extracellular niche direct stem cell fate. Acta Biomater. 2015;11:3–16. https://doi.org/10.1016/j.actbio.2014.09.038.

104. Rahmany MB, Van Dyke M. Biomimetic approaches to modulate cellular adhesion in biomaterials: a review. Acta Biomater. 2013;9:5431–7. https://doi.org/10.1016/j.actbio.2012.11.019.
105. Lee J, Tae G, Kim YH, et al. The effect of gelatin incorporation into electrospun poly(L-lactide-co-epsilon-caprolactone) fibers on mechanical properties and cytocompatibility. Biomaterials. 2008;29:1872–9. https://doi.org/10.1016/j.biomaterials.2007.12.029.
106. Sorkio A, Porter PJ, Juuti-Uusitalo K, et al. Surface modified biodegradable electrospun membranes as a carrier for human embryonic stem cell-derived retinal pigment epithelial cells. Tissue Eng Part A. 2015;21:2301–14. https://doi.org/10.1089/ten.tea.2014.0640.
107. Calejo MT, Ilmarinen T, Jongprasitkul H, et al. Honeycomb porous films as permeable scaffold materials for human embryonic stem cell-derived retinal pigment epithelium. J Biomed Mater Res A. 2016;104:1646–56. https://doi.org/10.1002/jbm.a.35690.
108. Ilmarinen T, Hiidenmaa H, Kööbi P, et al. Ultrathin polyimide membrane as cell carrier for subretinal transplantation of human embryonic stem cell derived retinal pigment epithelium. PLoS One. 2015;10:e0143669. https://doi.org/10.1371/journal.pone.0143669.
109. Sorkio AE, Vuorimaa-Laukkanen EP, Hakola HM, et al. Biomimetic collagen I and IV double layer Langmuir–Schaefer films as microenvironment for human pluripotent stem cell derived retinal pigment epithelial cells. Biomaterials. 2015;51:257–69. https://doi.org/10.1016/j.biomaterials.2015.02.005.
110. Wang C, Stewart RJ, Kopecek J. Hybrid hydrogels assembled from synthetic polymers and coiled-coil protein domains. Nature. 1999;397:417–20. https://doi.org/10.1038/17092.
111. Warnke PH, Alamein M, Skabo S, et al. Primordium of an artificial Bruch's membrane made of nanofibers for engineering of retinal pigment epithelium cell monolayers. Acta Biomater. 2013;9:9414–22. https://doi.org/10.1016/j.actbio.2013.07.029.
112. Xiang P, Wu K-C, Zhu Y, et al. A novel Bruch's membrane-mimetic electrospun substrate scaffold for human retinal pigment epithelium cells. Biomaterials. 2014;35:9777–88. https://doi.org/10.1016/j.biomaterials.2014.08.040.
113. Stanzel BV, Liu Z, Somboonthanakij S, et al. Human RPE stem cells grown into polarized RPE monolayers on a polyester matrix are maintained after grafting into rabbit subretinal space. Stem Cell Reports. 2014;2:64–77. https://doi.org/10.1016/j.stemcr.2013.11.005.
114. Koss MJ, Falabella P, Stefanini FR, et al. Subretinal implantation of a monolayer of human embryonic stem cell-derived retinal pigment epithelium: a feasibility and safety study in Yucatan minipigs. Graefes Arch Clin Exp Ophthalmol. 2016;254:1553–65. https://doi.org/10.1007/s00417-016-3386-y.
115. Subrizi A, Hiidenmaa H, Ilmarinen T, et al. Generation of hESC-derived retinal pigment epithelium on biopolymer coated polyimide membranes. Biomaterials. 2012;33:8047–54. https://doi.org/10.1016/j.biomaterials.2012.07.033.
116. Schwartz SD, Hubschman J-P, Heilwell G, et al. Embryonic stem cell trials for macular degeneration: a preliminary report. Lancet. 2012;379:713–20. https://doi.org/10.1016/S0140-6736(12)60028-2.
117. Schwartz SD, Regillo CD, Lam BL, et al. Human embryonic stem cell-derived retinal pigment epithelium in patients with age-related macular degeneration and Stargardt's macular dystrophy: follow-up of two open-label phase 1/2 studies. Lancet. 2015;385:509–16. https://doi.org/10.1016/S0140-6736(14)61376-3.
118. Mandai M, Watanabe A, Kurimoto Y, et al. Autologous induced stem-cell–derived retinal cells for macular degeneration. N Engl J Med. 2017;376:1038–46. https://doi.org/10.1056/NEJMoa1608368.
119. Garber K. RIKEN suspends first clinical trial involving induced pluripotent stem cells. Nat Biotechnol. 2015;33:890–1. https://doi.org/10.1038/nbt0915-890.
120. Coffey P. Human embryonic stem cell derived retinal pigment epithelium transplantation in severe exudative age related macular degeneration: so far so visual. In: Annual ARVO 2017 meeting, Baltimore USA; 2017.
121. da Cruz L, Fynes K, Georgiadis O, et al. Phase 1 clinical study of an embryonic stem cell-derived retinal pigment epithelium patch in age-related macular degeneration. Nat Biotechnol. 2018;36:328–37. https://doi.org/10.1038/nbt.4114.
122. Kashani AH, Lebkowski JS, Rahhal FM, et al. A bioengineered retinal pigment epithelial monolayer for advanced, dry age-related macular degeneration. Sci Transl Med. 2018;10:eaao4097. https://doi.org/10.1126/scitranslmed.aao4097.
123. Doi A, Park I-H, Wen B, et al. Differential methylation of tissue- and cancer-specific CpG island shores distinguishes human induced pluripotent stem cells, embryonic stem cells and fibroblasts. Nat Genet. 2009;41:1350–3. https://doi.org/10.1038/ng.471.
124. Howden SE, Gore A, Li Z, et al. Genetic correction and analysis of induced pluripotent stem cells from a patient with gyrate atrophy. Proc Natl Acad Sci U S A. 2011;108:6537–42. https://doi.org/10.1073/pnas.1103388108.
125. Sugita S, Iwasaki Y, Makabe K, et al. Lack of T cell response to iPSC-derived retinal pigment epithelial cells from HLA homozygous donors. Stem Cell Reports. 2016;7:619–34. https://doi.org/10.1016/j.stemcr.2016.08.011.
126. Sugita S, Iwasaki Y, Makabe K, et al. Successful transplantation of retinal pigment epithelial cells from MHC homozygote iPSCs in MHC-matched models. Stem Cell Reports. 2016;7:635–48. https://doi.org/10.1016/j.stemcr.2016.08.010.

127. Gornalusse GG, Hirata RK, Funk SE, et al. HLA-E-expressing pluripotent stem cells escape allogeneic responses and lysis by NK cells. Nat Biotechnol. 2017;35:765–72. https://doi.org/10.1038/nbt.3860.
128. Meyer JS, Howden SE, Wallace KA, et al. Optic vesicle-like structures derived from human pluripotent stem cells facilitate a customized approach to retinal disease treatment. Stem Cells. 2011;29:1206–18. https://doi.org/10.1002/stem.674.
129. Singh MS, Balmer J, Barnard AR, et al. Transplanted photoreceptor precursors transfer proteins to host photoreceptors by a mechanism of cytoplasmic fusion. Nat Commun. 2016;7:13537. https://doi.org/10.1038/ncomms13537.
130. Marks PW, Witten CM, Califf RM. Clarifying stem-cell therapy's benefits and risks. N Engl J Med. 2017;376:1007–9. https://doi.org/10.1056/NEJMp1613723.

RPE and Gene Therapy

15

Knut Stieger and Birgit Lorenz

Introduction

While inherited retinal disorders (IRD) generally lead to neuroretinal degeneration with loss of photoreceptors being the clinically relevant mechanism that leads to severe visual handicaps for the patients, some of the pathologic disease processes originate in the retinal pigment epithelium (RPE). Likewise, age related disorders such as age-related macular degeneration develop with at least parts of the pathologic mechanisms originating from RPE. These observations initiated the development of gene therapeutic approaches targeting the RPE in order to develop cures for these blinding disorders.

Over the past 20 years, tremendous advancements have been made in the development of gene therapeutic strategies for the treatment of inherited retinal dystrophies. More recently, new therapeutic strategies based on the transfer of genetic material into the RPE have been developed to address unmet needs in the handling of age related retinal disorders.

In this chapter, the current knowledge concerning the approach to transfer genetic material into the RPE is delineated together with an overview of the current state of the art in gene therapeutic strategies for RPE based inherited as well as age related retinal disorders. This includes a summary of ongoing clinical trials as well as a description of preclinical ideas that may likely hit the clinical stage in the near future.

Gene Therapeutic Strategies Currently Employed to the RPE

Currently, two different approaches are developed with the ultimate goal to either restore function to a non-functional or absent protein, or knock-down proteins in order to block their function (Fig. 15.1). The former approach is based on gene addition therapy or genome editing, the latter approach solely on genome editing. Gene therapeutic approaches are present at the level of clinical trials in some conditions (Table 15.1), and at the preclinical level for other conditions.

Gene addition therapy is based on the idea to transfer the correct cDNA copy of a gene that is mutated and whose gene product is therefore absent or non-functional, cloned into a eukaryotic expression system into the cells of interest [1]. The transfer is done by means of a viral or non-viral delivery system. The DNA containing the expression cassette is transported intracellularly into the nucleus and transgene expression is started, ultimately leading to restoration of function to the cell. This approach has reached clinical stage for the treatment of RPE65 and

K. Stieger (✉) · B. Lorenz
Department of Ophthalmology, Faculty of Medicine, Justus-Liebig-University Giessen, Giessen, Germany
e-mail: knut.stieger@uniklinikum-giessen.de; birgit.lorenz@uniklinikum-giessen.de

A. K. Klettner, S. Dithmar (eds.), *Retinal Pigment Epithelium in Health and Disease*,
https://doi.org/10.1007/978-3-030-28384-1_15

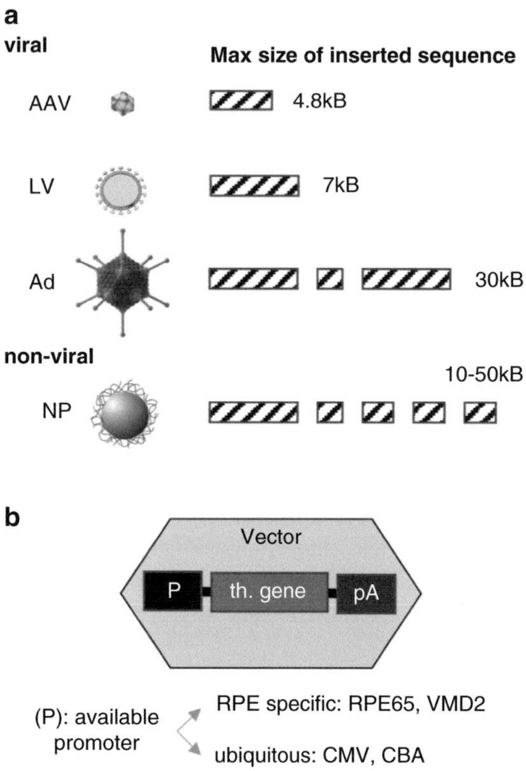

Fig. 15.1 Description of the transfer tools used in RPE based gene therapy. (**a**) Overview of viral and non-viral vectors currently used in RPE based gene therapy and the maximum size of insertable sequence. (**b**) Description of the expression cassette used for gene transfer purposes and overview of currently available promoter sequences. *RPE65* promoter region of the RPE65 gene, *VMD2* promoter region of the human bestrophin 1 gene, *CMV* cytomegalovirus early enhancer promoter, *CBA* chicken beta actin promoter

MERTK deficiency, as well as for the treatment of choroideremia (Table 15.1). For many other inherited retinal dystrophies, preclinical studies are ongoing.

Genome editing is based on the idea to modify the genome at the target site following the induction of a DNA double strand break (DSB). Because such a DSB is very detrimental to the integrity of cells, efficient DNA repair mechanisms exist that close the DSB immediately after its occurrence [2]. DSBs can be induced by highly specific endonucleases, such as the *clustered regulatory interspaced short palindromic repeat—CRISPR associated proteins* (CRISPR-Cas9) system, which has revolutionized molecular biology in the past 5 years but still holds potential risks with regard to eventually negative side effects to the genome integrity. The CRISPR-Cas system is a bacterial immune system against invading phages and different bacteria families use different forms of the Cas proteins, which have specific advantages and disadvantages [3].

Three different repair mechanisms exist: (a) non-homologous end-joining (NHEJ), (b) homology directed repair (HDR), and (c) microhomology mediated endjoining (MMEJ). While the first mechanism functions by directly sticking DNA ends together with small modifications of the DNA ends (insertions, deletion, so-called indel formation), resulting in modification of the genetic information at the target site, the latter two mechanisms employ a template DNA containing the corresponding DNA sequence with long (HDR) or short (MMEJ) homology arms on both sides of the DSB for high fidelity DNA repair without modifications [4]. NHEJ is the predominant repair pathway in dividing and non-dividing cells, HDR and MMEJ normally occur at much lower frequency. Currently, NHEJ as a means to manipulate the genome in RPE cells in both inherited as well as age related retinal disorders is at the early preclinical stage.

Gene Transfer to the RPE

The RPE is a monolayer of neuroectodermal origin situated between the neuroretina and the choriocapillaris of the choroid and forms a functional and morphological entity with the photoreceptors. Therefore, it remains difficult to target these cells separately by any delivery systems and the route of delivery presents a major aspect.

Currently, subretinal deposition of the transfer system is the most efficient way to target RPE cells, while intravitreal delivery systems or suprachoroidal administration are less satisfying. Nonetheless, there are also disadvantages associated with subretinal delivery, as this method is very complex to perform and poses additional stress (sheer stress) to the already compromised retina due to transitory retinal detachment [5]. The retinal microvilli, which surround the

Table 15.1 List of current gene therapy trials for RPE based gene therapeutic applications as by June 2017

Disease	Sponsor	Phase	Vector	NCT	# of patients	Ref
RPE65 Deficiency	Spark Therapeutics	III	AAV2/2.hRPE65v2 (voretigene neparvovec)	00999609	24	[44]
	UCL	I/II	AAV/2/2.hRPE65p.hRPE65 (tgAAG76)	00643747	12	[46]
	MeiraGTx UK II Ltd	I	AAV2/5.OPTIRPE65	02781480	27	[77]
	AGTC	II	AAV2/2.CB.hRPE65	00749957	12	[45]
	UPenn Scheie Eye Institute	I	AAV2/2.CB^{SB}.hRPE65	00481546	15	[43]
	Nantes University Hospital	I	AAV2/4.hRPE65p.hRPE65	01496040	9	
	Hadassah Medical Organisation	I	AAV2/2.CB^{SB}.hRPE65	00821340	10	[78]
MERTK deficiency	Fowzan Alkuraya King Khaled Eye Hospital	I	AAV2/2.VMD2.hMERTK	01482195	6	[61]
Choroideremia	Spark Therapeutics	I,ii	AAV2/2.hCHM	02341807	15	
	NightstaRx	I	AAV2/2.CBA.Rep1	01461213	14	[52]
	Oxford University	II	AAV2/2.CBA.Rep1	02407678	30	
	University Alberta	I/II	AAV2/2.CBA.Rep1	02077361	6	
	University of Miami	II	AAV2/2.CBA.Rep1	02553135	6	
	STZ Eyetrial, Tübingen	II	AAV2/2.CBA.Rep1	02671539	6	

The table includes information regarding sponsor, clinical trial phase, vector administered, the NCT trials.gov number, the number of patients planned to be enrolled and the most recent reference referring to this trial

photoreceptor outer segments and provide the cellular interaction between RPE and photoreceptors, are exposed to mechanical stress during the detachment, and it takes several months for both cell types to get the RPE-photoreceptor interface completely restored. This is one of the reasons why full functional benefit following gene therapeutic intervention associated with subretinal injections should only be expected after up to 6–12 months. Furthermore, subretinal injection leads only to transgene expression within the detached retina, making it impossible to treat the entire retina with one intervention.

Generally, two different delivery systems are available to transfer genetic material into the RPE, viral and non-viral systems (Fig. 15.1a). While viral vectors systems do have the disadvantage of potentially causing immune reactions due to their foreign protein structure, these organisms have developed efficient cell entry systems and mechanisms to promote processing and expression of the transferred genetic material that make these vectors currently the major delivery system. Non-viral systems, such as nanoparticles, still have the limitations of only transferring genetic material into cells without promoting the expression of the transferred material [6].

To better understand the different therapeutic approaches presented in this review, the following paragraphs describe the state of the art in viral and non-viral gene delivery systems, starting with the current gold standard i.e. the adeno-associated virus (AAV) system, followed by two additional virus based systems, lentiviruses and adenoviruses, and a description of nanoparticles that have all been used to target RPE cells.

AAVs

Adeno-associated virus (AAV) is a mammalian single stranded DNA parvovirus. Its genome consists of about 4.7 kB containing two inverted terminal repeats (ITRs) flanking genes for replication (rep) and building the virus capsid (cap) (Fig. 15.1a). AAVs are known to infect non-proliferating and proliferating cells [7]. After infection of the host cell by receptor mediated endocytosis, the virus genome persists as episome in the cell, with few exceptions in dividing cells, where integration is possible in association with the appearance of double strand breaks. In order to generate a recombinant vector, the entire virus sequence except the flanking ITRs is replaced by the expression cassette of choice. Several recombinant AAV (rAAV) serotypes capable to target different cell types have been extensively characterized. While the AAV serotype 2 was employed originally as photoreceptor (PR) and retinal pigment epithelium (RPE) transducing vector for many years, the serotypes 5, 8 and 9 are currently the standard vectors to the retina [8]. More recently, capsid modifications and directed evolution of the capsid have been employed to even further optimize cell tropism in the retina [9]. AAV serotype 4 is the only vector that exclusively targets the RPE and represents therefore an interesting vector for RPE based gene therapy [10].

Though AAVs are promising vehicles for the transfer of genes into the RPE, one main disadvantage is their maximum cargo capacity of 4.7 kB, which is not sufficient to carry cDNAs of many genes with mutations leading to retinal dystrophies or the genetic information for some of the genome modifying nucleases. This may be less problematic for target genes in the RPE, such as RPE65, MERTK or Rep1, but is an issue in genome editing approaches aiming at transferring CRISPR-Cas and template DNA in one vector, or in gene therapeutic approaches targeting genes in photoreceptors [2].

The most widely used CRISPR-Cas variant was discovered in Streptococcus pyogenese (SpCas9) and has a coding sequence size of about 4.2 kB, making it almost too large to be packed as an expression cassette into one AAV together with the necessary guide RNAs, not to speak about the template DNA. To overcome this issue, the CRISPR-Cas system discovered from staphylococcus aureus (SaCas9) has been developed as genome editing tool, because the size is smaller at about 3.2 kB. Nevertheless, a template DNA also does not fit into a vector together with the latter CRISPR system [11, 12].

The problem is currently solved by separation of CRISPR-Cas and guide RNA into one AAV and the template DNA into a second AAV, which would enable genome editing based on HDR in target cells.

Altogether, AAVs are promising vehicles also for genome editing despite their low cargo capacity. They show no immune response when injected in the subretinal space and are able to express genes in non-dividing cells like the RPE.

Lentivirus-Based Vectors

Lentiviruses are retroviruses with an ssRNA genome that is integrated into the DNA of target cells. Because of this random integration, LVs are not as safe as non-integrating vehicles, but able to express transgenes for a very long time, especially in constantly dividing cell populations. To overcome the random integration issue, an integrase deficient lentiviral vector (IDLV) has been developed [13].

The original capsid structure of LVs only allows minor RPE transduction activity following a subretinal injection. In addition, vector purification is limited in the absence of modification to the envelope structure. Interestingly, if the envelope structure is changed by incorporating foreign proteins (ie. pseudotyping of the envelope) such as protein from the vascular stomatitis virus (VSV-G = vesicular stomatitis virus glycoprotein), the vector can be purified much better, and the cellular tropism changes enable a strong transgene expression in RPE cells [14]. Alternatively, envelope pseudotyping with other proteins also enables strong RPE tropism [15].

One big advantage in contrast to AAVs is that LVs can carry large transgenes up to 8 kb [16] (Fig. 15.1a), which may allow to transfer cDNAs of larger target genes or endonucleases and template DNA together in one vector.

Adenovirus Based Vectors

Adenovirus is a large double stranded DNA parvovirus. The size is about 100 nm and therefore about 5 times larger than the AAV, which excludes nuclear entry through the nuclear pores (size of 20 nm) [17]. The capsid is made of hexon proteins and penton base proteins with spikes. There are more than 50 serotypes known that usually cause upper airway infections in humans. The genomic structure is more complex than the AAV genome and consists of early (E) and late (L) genes with respect to their activity in the reproductive cycle. While the first-generation adenovirus vectors were manufactured by replacing small parts of the complex genome, thus leaving lots of viral genes intact, third generation, helper dependent (HD-Ad) vectors have a packaging capacity of more than 30 kB (Fig. 15.1a), which renders them useful for the transfer of large genes or complex genome editing approaches including larger template DNAs [18].

Ad vectors transduce non-dividing cells and the transferred DNA remains episomal, which results only in a transient expression of the transgene of no longer then 3–6 months [19]. Following subretinal injection, Ad serotype 5 (Ad5) has a strong cellular tropism for RPE cells and was used initially in gene therapeutic applications to the RPE. In addition, the serotypes Ad28 and 35 enable transgene expression predominantly in the RPE following subretinal injection [19]. Other serotypes, in particular in combination with changes to the penton base proteins, can change this tropism towards other cells in the retina [15, 20].

Nanoparticles

Nanoparticles (NPs) are made of DNA molecules bound to several different structures such as polymers, liposomes, peptides or complex chemical compounds that are taken up by RPE cells either by phagocytosis or endocytosis and are transported directly into the nucleus [6]. A big advantage of nanoparticles is their capacity to carry up to 14 kB when used as vehicle in the eye [21]. Peptides for ocular delivery (POD) can enter RPE and PR cells *in vivo* after subretinal injection.

In direct comparison to AAVs, NPs, which are composed of polyethylene glycol-substitutes polylysine (CK30PEG) showed levels of transgene expression *in vivo* in mouse retina and RPE that were similar to AAVs, albeit with a lower efficiency per vector genome [21]. Nanoparticles are able to transduce dividing and non-dividing cells due to their transport mechanism [22], the transferred genes remain episomal and show no toxicity in PR and RPE cells. These studies demonstrate the big advantage of NPs in comparison to AAVs, regarding the size of the gene transferred. Because NPs remain episomal, long term transgene expression is limited to few weeks. Recent discoveries of DNA sequences that increase stability of episomal DNA sequences in the nucleus have increased the longevity of transgene expression but it is still not comparable to virus vector mediated transgene expression duration [23]. Since this issue represents the major obstacle for gene addition therapy, in which long term transgene expression is crucial, NP based gene therapeutic approaches have not yet reached clinical stage. However, in genome editing approaches, in which a temporal burst of transgene expression is preferred, NPs may represent the vector of choice in the future.

Taken together, nanoparticles represent a promising technology to transfer genes into the RPE, but the temporarily limited nature of the transgene expression prevents its use for some therapeutic approaches.

Ubiquitous Versus Cell-Type Specific Promoter

Since it remains difficult to target the RPE without touching also photoreceptor cells, in view of safety concerns it may be necessary to limit transgene expression to photoreceptors by specific features included in the expression cassette (Fig. 15.1b). For example, the promoter driving transgene expression can be designed as a cell type specific promoter, thus being only active in the target cell

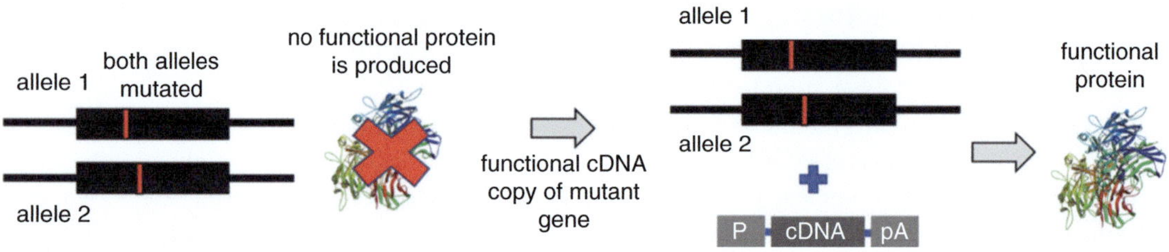

Fig. 15.2 Overview of the gene addition/supplementation therapy approach currently used in RPE based gene therapy. The figure describes the classic gene addition strategy, as it is used in all the current clinical trials. In case of autosomal recessive inheritance, both alleles contain disease causing mutations, which lead to absence of the protein or presence of a non-functional protein. By transfer of an expression cassette containing the correct cDNA of the mutated gene under the control of a promoter (P) and a polyadenylation signal (pA) into the cell using appropriate vector systems, the functional protein can be produced, thus being the basis for potential recovery of function of the cell

and not in any other cell transduced by the vector. For RPE cells, the most abundant promoters used in gene therapeutic studies are the VMD2 promoter (corresponding to the 5′ upstream region of the bestrophin 1 gene) and the RPE65 promoter. In contrast, ubiquitous promoters driving strong transgene expression in the retina and RPE cells include the cytomegalovirus early enhancer and promoter (CMV), the chicken beta actin (CBA) promoter, or the elongation factor 1 alpha short promoter (EFS).

While cell type specific promoters would be the better choice with regard to specificity of transgene expression, concerns remain with regard to potential silencing of transgene expression over time due to other regulatory sequences included in mammalian 5′ upstream regions of genes. However, current observations of declining treatment benefits over time in clinical trials for RPE65 deficiency in humans employing the CMV promoter may also be associated with silencing of the transgene expression cassette, further highlighting this issue in the future design of such therapeutic approaches [24].

Gene Therapy for RPE Based Inherited Retinal Diseases

The very active field of retinal gene addition therapy for RPE based IRDs has advanced the most with several clinical trials ongoing for RPE65 and MERTK deficiency (associated with mutations in *RPE65* or *MERTK*), and choroideremia associated with mutations in *REP1* [25] (Fig. 15.2). Very advanced at the preclinical level are studies aiming at restoring bestrophin 1 expression in the RPE in patients affected with different forms of bestrophinopathies [26]. Furthermore, gene therapeutic applications have been reported for mutations in the LRAT gene and two albinism genes i.e. ocular albinism (OA) 1 gene (now called GPR143) and the tyrosinase gene causing oculocutaneous albinism (OCA) type 1 [27–29]. In this chapter, the focus lies on disease entities, for which the gene therapeutic approaches have been advanced to clinical stage (RPE65, MERTK, choroideremia) or that are just about to enter this stage (bestrophinopathies).

In the last part of the chapter, very recent studies aiming at correcting the genome for MERTK deficiency will also be described.

RPE65 Deficiency

RPE65 encodes for the RPE specific 65 kD protein that has been identified as the isomerohydrolase in the visual cycle, which restores the rhodopsin ligand 11-cis retinal [30]. Lack of RPE65 function results in the absence of 11-cis retinal in rod photoreceptors and thus, complete absence of rod function due to a non-functional phototransduction cascade. Cones seem to have an alternative source for 11-cis retinal, which leads mostly to some preserved cone function at least early in the disease course [31].

Mutations in both alleles of *RPE65* are associated with a spectrum of autosomal recessive retinal dystrophies ranging from Leber congenital amaurosis (LCA) type 2, a very early onset severe retinal dystrophy, to early onset retinal dystrophies (EOSRD, EORD, SEORD) and juvenile retinitis pigmentosa (RP) [32, 33]. Clinical signs include severe (LCA) to moderate (EOSRD, EORD; SEORD) impairment of visual function from birth or with onset in the first months of life, or with onset during the first years of life (ar RP) [34]. The most prominent clinical sign in the majority of patients is profound to absolute night blindness evident from very severe visual handicap at reduced light levels. Nystagmus may be absent, and pupillary reaction to light almost normal, thus differentiating LCA2 from other forms of LCA that are often associated with sluggish to absent pupillary light reflex and a characteristic oculodigital sign. The hallmark sign of RPE65 deficiency is severely reduced or absent fundus autofluorescence (FAF) despite preserved RPE, which is related to the level of residual activity of the isomerohydrolase in the RPE [35]. Lack of RPE65 activity blocks the generation of lipofuscin accumulation in the RPE [36]. At later stages, the absence of FAF may also be caused by atrophic RPE. The range of RPE65 specific phenotypes can be explained by the usually better cone function early in life that ultimately deteriorates leading to complete blindness in many patients from the third decade of life on. The funduscopic aspect early on may be normal and the cone electroretinogram (ERG) recordable yet reduced early on. The subsequent deterioration may be explained by the progressive RPE changes related to increased accumulation of retinyl esters in the RPE cells.

Since the RPE65 protein exerts its function in the RPE, a treatment by gene therapeutic approaches needs to target the RPE, yet the functional improvement is measured at the level of the retina and visual cortex. A variety of animal models have been employed to develop gene addition therapy, and especially the very promising data generated in the naturally occurring dog model [37–39] generated high expectancies for subsequent clinical trials that were started in 2007 [40–42]. To date, clinical data for over 50 patients with RPE65 deficiency demonstrate that improvement in light sensitivity i.e. better performance at lower light levels is the most consistent treatment effect, indicating that rods benefit well from the treatment [43–45] (Table 15.1). However, lack of statistically significant improvement in visual acuity suggests that cone photoreceptors do not profit from the treatment in a similar fashion. Recently reported observations would indicate additional restrictions as to treatment effect: (1) decline of visual function at 3–5 years after initial improvement [24, 46], accompanied (2) by continued thinning of the photoreceptor layer, which likely indicates that the degeneration process of the neurons itself was not halted upon improvement of function [47].

For the treatment of RPE65 deficiency, a medication based on AAV vectors expressing the human RPE65 cDNA under the control of a viral promoter is about to reach approval by the FDA and EMA, as a consequence of the treatment success despite the above-mentioned limitations [48].

Choroideremia

Choroideremia is caused by mutations in the REP1 gene, which encodes the rab escort protein (Rep) 1. This protein is involved in the intracellular trafficking process by facilitating the prenylation of Rab proteins and escorting them to their final destination within the cell. While this protein is expressed in all cells of the body, loss of Rep1 function leads to degeneration of the choroid, RPE and photoreceptors, starting in the periphery with centripetal progression, thus leaving the central retina relatively unaffected until the third to fourth decade or even later [49]. This is related to the presence of a second protein, called Rep2, which can take over the function of Rep1 in all other tissues except retina and RPE. Gene addition in this disease entity aims at restoring Rep1 function to the remaining RPE cells and photoreceptors, thus slowing down of the progression of the disease rather than improving any function per se.

Preclinical data in choroideremia mice and human cells ex vivo employing lentivirus or AAV2 vectors carrying the human CHM cDNA were promising in restoring functional protein levels in RPE cells [50, 51]. These data led to the start of a clinical trial in six patients, demonstrating the safety of the approach [52]. An important aspect in this trial was to evaluate the functional consequences of the temporal detachment of the macular retina from the RPE following the injection. The authors concluded that the observed improvement in visual function in some of the patients and absence of functional loss in the remaining outweigh the risks associated with the treatment. Functional improvement gained in some patients was subsequently reported to be stable for at least 3.5 years, i.e. the duration of this single centre study as published recently [53].

Currently, several clinical trials are ongoing at other sites around the world, including the US, France, and Germany, but no data have been published so far (Table 15.1).

MERTK Deficiency

The receptor *mer tyrosine kinase* (MERTK), which is activated by a multiprotein complex in the presence of discs from the photoreceptor outer segments, recognizes and starts subsequent inclusion of the discs by the RPE membrane for further processing and degradation. When biallelic mutations in the *MERTK* gene abolish its function, this inclusion of the discs by the RPE membrane does not take place, leading to accumulation of debris in the subretinal space, and thus to a loss of the close connection and interaction of these two cell types. The clinical phenotype is that of LCA or EOSRD [54].

The Royal College of Surgeons (RCS) rat, in which phagocytosis of photoreceptor outer segments by RPE cells is impaired due to biallelic mutations in the *mertk* gene [55] was used to study the effects of gene addition employing AAV, lentivirus or adenovirus based vectors, resulting in a reduction of debris formation and increased photoreceptor function, even though the duration of therapeutic effects was only transient [56–58].

Improved AAV vectors containing the human MERTK cDNA under the control of the RPE specific VMD2 promotor showed improved results more recently [59, 60]. A clinical trial was conducted subsequently with six patients that demonstrated the safety of the approach (subretinal injection of AAV vectors) [61]. The patients had visual acuity between 20/50 and 20/3200 before treatment and they received between 1 and 3 injections into the macular area without touching the fovea. Three of the patients reported slight improvement in visual function, which declined subsequently leading to the observation that only one patient hat improved vision at the 2-year post treatment time point. Because of poor fixation and other problems, it was not possible to obtain high definition OCT scans and therefore, reduction of debris or changes of the RPE-photoreceptor interface could not be examined.

Bestrophinopathies

The BEST-1 gene is expressed in the RPE and its gene product, bestrophin 1, is involved in the transport of chlorid ions and the calcium homeostasis within the cells. Loss of function of bestrophin 1 is associated with reduced absorption of fluids from the subretinal space and phagocytosis of photoreceptor outer segments. Mutations in the BEST-1 gene cause either autosomal recessive bestrophinopathy (ARB), autosomal dominant Best vitelliform macular dystrophy (BVMD), or autosomal dominant vitreoretinochoriopathy (VCRP). Depending on the type of disease, clinical features include the presence of circular changes within the macular zone that consist of fluid deposits in a yolk like manner (BVMD), which may lead to increasingly affected central visual acuity. In ARB, patients usually do not have only central visual deficits but rather develop paramacular and peripheral yellowish lesions correlating with increased fundus autofluorescence at the lesion site [62, 63].

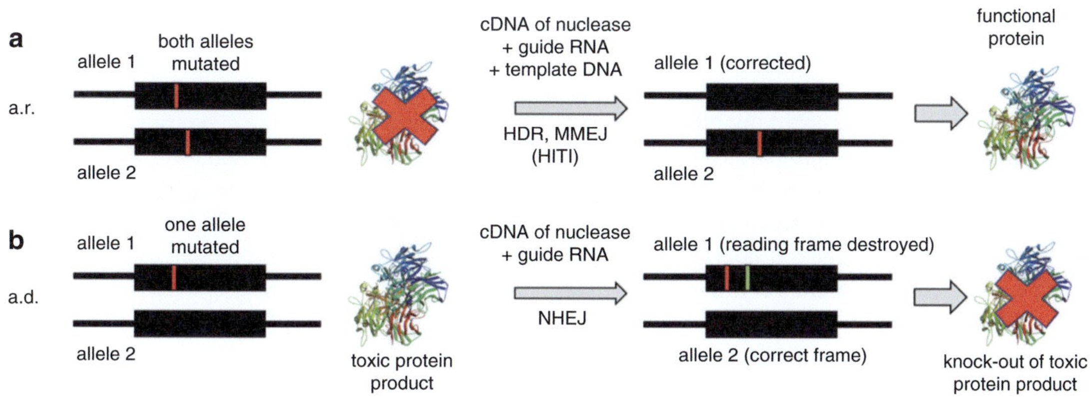

Fig. 15.3 Overview of genome editing approaches. (**a**) In case of inherited disorders with two (autosomal recessive, a.r.) mutated alleles, the transfer of endonucleases, such as CRISPR-Cas, together with the guide RNA and a template DNA, into the nucleus generates double strand breaks (DSB), which are repaired by either homology directed repair (HDR) or microhomology mediated end-joining (MMEJ). Homology independent targeted integration (HITI) of a large DNA sequence was also recently shown. Correction of at least one allele results in the restoration of the correct reading frame and production of the functional protein. (**b**) In case of autosomal dominant (a.d.) disorders with the disease causing mutation (red line) being present only on one allele, therapeutic genome editing is performed by targeted knock-out of the mutant allele. Here, the CRISPR-Cas protein together with the guide RNA but without a template are transferred to the cell and cause a DSB at the target site (green line), which will be repaired by non-homologous end-joining (NHEJ), leading to the destruction of the reading frame and thus to the permanent knock-out of the target allele and subsequent absence of the target protein within the cell

A canine animal model for bestrophin 1 deficiency associated with naturally occurring biallelic mutations develops a retinal disease called canine multifocal retinopathy (CMR), in which multiple circular lesions are visible throughout the retina that are reminiscent of the clinical features observed in human patients [64, 65]. The canine model has been extensively used to study pathogenic mechanisms leading to the typical clinical features in humans, such as the impaired cone associated microvillar ensheathment due to biochemical and structural abnormalities at the RPE-photoreceptor interface [65]. In order to develop a gene therapeutic approach using AAV vectors to transfer the canine Best1 cDNA under the control of the human VMD2 promoter into affected dogs, the promoter and different serotypes of AAV were tested for optimal transgene expression in wildtype dogs and cmr carrier animals [26]. Strong and specific overexpression of bestrophin 1 was observed up to 6 months in animals treated with the AAV serotype 2, which is a promising first step towards the translation of the results to the clinical level.

Genome Editing for MERTK Deficiency

The recent advent of genome editing as therapeutic strategy has opened the field to entirely new concepts on how to treat inherited retinal dystrophies (Fig. 15.3). While still at a very early stage in the development, animal models for IRD are currently used to prove in vitro data or to demonstrate the general feasibility of such an approach, rather than being actual preclinical data meant to be translated to the clinic in short time.

One new approach in genome editing, which was shown to be effective in the RPE in vivo, is the use of NHEJ to introduce missing DNA sequences in disorders that originate from large deletions [66]. Among other model systems, the authors used the RCS rat, in which the pathology is caused by a 1.2 kB deletion in the MERTK gene region including parts of exon 2, and showed partial restoration of full length MERTK expression after genome editing at this locus. Two AAV vectors were subretinally injected expressing CRISPR-Cas9 and two guide RNAs plus the missing DNA sequence of the MERTK gene. The two guide RNAs cut before and after the target site, enabling the cells repair machinery to introduce the missing DNA by NHEJ into the locus. Since this approach functions without large homologous sequences on both sites of the template DNA, the technique was called homology independent targeted integration (HITI). While these experiments represent very interesting data about the capacity of the RPE to repair the genome following the induction of DSBs, the approach is rather not suitable to be used in human patients because the integration at the site is associated with alterations to the genome, which cannot be controlled thus far. In addition, off target toxicity at other sites in the genome cannot be ruled out and more research is needed in order to make this approach ready to go for clinical application.

Gene Therapy for RPE Based Age Related Acquired Retinal Disorders

AMD is an age related, acquired retinal disorder and the leading cause of blindness in the elderly population worldwide. It can be divided into an early phase, in which the chronic activation of the complement system together with a plethora of other factors lead to changes at the RPE-Bruch's Membrane (RPE-BM), leading to the deposit of inflammatory metabolites and lipids in drusen at the Bruch's membrane surface, as well as the atrophy of RPE cells [67, 68]. Geographic RPE atrophy formation leads to subsequent photoreceptor death and blindness. Thickening of the BM and other factors may lead to the rupture of the RPE-BM complex and the subsequent growth of choroidal vessels into the subretinal space, a mechanism termed choroidal neovascularization. This stage of disease is called wet AMD [69].

The two major targets that have been identified for gene therapeutic interventions in AMD are (1) factors involved in complement activation at an earlier stage of the disease, and (2) the major factor for pathologic neovascularisation in the eye in the late form of the disease, the vascular endothelial growth factor (VEGF).

However, not all published strategies target specifically the RPE, but also other cells within the retina and the eye, making the RPE associated changes following the gene transfer difficult to assess. Consequently, in the following chapter, the focus is given to those strategies, which have been explicitly associated with RPE cells.

Targeting the Complement System

During the early stage of AMD progression, chronic activation of the complement system has been associated with changes to the RPE-BM complex. In particular, the observation that polymorphisms in factor H are associated with increased risk for AMD triggered very active research in this field, finally demonstrating that reduced factor H activity is involved in the pathogenesis of AMD [70, 71]. Data from recent clinical trials employing so-called complement therapeutics such as lampalizumab, an antibody against complement factor D, another important factor in the complement cascade, showed treatment benefits in slowing down geographic atrophy formation in patients with dry AMD [72].

Complement factor H physiologically inhibits formation of complement factor 3b on cell surfaces, which is generated continuously through the alternative pathway activation. The assumption that restoration of factor H activity following vector mediated gene transfer of factor H would reduce accumulation of C3b was tested recently in a mouse model of dry AMD. The model was generated by artificially overexpressing C3 in RPE cells by adenovirus vector mediated gene transfer [73]. The mouse exhibits some features similar to those observed in AMD patients, such as increased vascular permeability, endothelial cell proliferation and migration, RPE atrophy, and loss of photoreceptor outer segments. Co-injection of Adenoviral vectors expressing C3 and factor H simultaneously reduced endothelial cell proliferation almost completely and reduced RPE atrophy formation by almost 70%.

Although the model is artificial in its origins, the idea of overexpressing complement factors in the RPE in order to attenuate chronic complement system activation at the RPE-Bruch's Membrane complex seems to be an approach that may likely advance further.

Targeting VEGF

VEGF is expressed, among other cells in the retina, predominantly in the RPE. The RPE–BM complex has a barrier function to keep vessels out of the photoreceptor layer in the retina. If this complex is altered due to chronic insults during the disease progression to the neovascular form of AMD, vessel growth from the choroidea into the retina is possible [74]. This vessel outgrowth into the retina is stimulated by increased VEGF expression due to hypoxic stimuli, which leads to activity changes of endothelial cells and subsequently to the formation of new and error prone vessels. The idea of inhibiting this pathomechanism by blocking the activity of VEGF on the endothelial VEGF receptor through the administration of anti-VEGF molecules to the retina has shown tremendous success over the past 10 years, further corroborating the importance of this factor for the development of the disease [69].

However, important reasons exist that contradict the idea of repeated injections of anti-VEGF molecules, for example the association with increased progression of geographic atrophy [75], which led to the conclusion that alternative approaches are needed to treat these disorders.

One idea would be to knock-out the VEGF allele in RPE cells by use of genome editing in a way to promote NHEJ, which causes indel formation at the target site, thus disrupting the coding sequence and destroying the reading frame. This approach was tested recently by using an AAV vector expressing CRISPR-Cas9 and guide RNAs targeting the VEGF and the Hif1a locus, the latter being an important activator of VEGF expression under hypoxic conditions [76]. As mentioned before, many in vivo experiments for genome editing are proofs of principle rather than definitive treatment approaches, and this is a similar case, although the strategy is appealing. Instead of using SpCas9 or SaCas9 to introduce the DSB, the group used in this study a newly established form from Campylobacter jejuni (CjCas9). The advantage of this Cas protein is the comparatively small size with 2.9 kB, thus enabling the additional inclusion of small template DNAs into one AAV vector. Since a knockout of a target gene is the chosen strategy, no template DNA is necessary and all parts of the system can be transferred with one AAV. The group injected an AAV carrying the CjCas9 under the control of the EFS promoter that allows transgene expression in the RPE and retinal cells. Consequently, indel formation as a result of NHEJ at the target site was found at a frequency of 20–60% in retinal cells and 14–30% in RPE cells, associated with a decreased VEGF level in the cell lysate. When applied to a mouse model for laser induced choroidal neovascularization, mimicking the main pathologic feature in wet AMD, genome editing at the VEGF locus led to decreased lesion sizes by up to 30%.

However, whether a treatment approach based on the targeted destruction of the VEGF locus in RPE cells will ever become a realistic treatment approach in human patients with AMD or other neovascular disorders remains questionable.

Conclusions and Further Outlook

Gene therapeutic approaches targeting the RPE are promising therapeutic strategies for a variety of different disorders. The gene transfer itself is currently the most advanced by using viral vectors and the subretinal route of delivery. Clinical trials are ongoing by means of gene addition therapy for some IRDs and in preparation for others. Genome editing is a tool that needs further characterization in terms of safety and efficacy, but the proof of principle that it can work in the RPE has been shown. Gene therapeutic approaches for dry and wet AMD are still in its infancy but due to the ever-increasing need for alternatives to repeated intraocular protein injections, the chances are high that these strategies will advance to the clinic.

Since the different therapeutic approaches are at different levels of realization, the current questions are manifold. Concerning the clinical trials for gene addition therapy, questions to be solved include the development of highly sensitive and quantifiable methods to describe the therapeutic benefit, which very likely is difficult in each disease treated. Also, optimization of the vector is still an important question, since silencing of transgene expression may be the cause of decreased functional benefit in treated areas more than 3 years after the treatment in patients enrolled in the RPE65 trials.

Concerning genome editing as treatment approach, the complex situation of the DNA repair machinery in post-mitotic cells is almost unknown, and in particular in photoreceptors and RPE cells, nothing is known about the regulatory aspects in the decision making of which pathway will repair the DSB. Until the NHEJ pathway can be controlled or indel formation and off target toxicity can be avoided, this approach is too risky to be used as a treatment approach. Expectations are high for genome editing, particularly with the advent of the CRISPR-Cas technology, but the experiences made in the past with gene therapeutic approaches advancing way too fast into the clinic, leading to fatal events and severe complications should be a strong reminder.

The idea of producing factors in the eye that interfere with the pathogenic pathways in acquired disorders rather than injecting them repeatedly into the vitreous is appealing but needs to be investigated more in detail. Adjustable systems exist that would allow for the external control of transgene expression, allowing to shift expression of these proteins into a therapeutic window.

The future is bright for gene therapeutic applications to the RPE and with the necessary caution and intensive further work several new treatment strategies will likely hit clinical stage, lowering the burden for many patients with diseases of the retina.

References

1. Sengillo JD, Justus S, Cabral T, Tsang SH. Correction of monogenic and common retinal disorders with gene therapy. Genes (Basel). 2017;8(2).
2. Yanik M, Müller B, Song F, Gall J, Wagner F, Wende W, et al. In vivo genome editing as a potential treatment strategy for inherited retinal dystrophies. Prog Retin Eye Res [Internet]. 2017;56:1–18. https://doi.org/10.1016/j.preteyeres.2016.09.001.
3. Cox DBT, Platt RJ, Zhang F. Therapeutic genome editing: prospects and challenges. Nat Med [Internet]. 2015;21(2):121–31. http://www.nature.com/doifinder/10.1038/nm.3793.
4. Maeder ML, Gersbach CA. Genome-editing technologies for gene and cell therapy. Mol Ther [Internet]. 2016;24(3):430–46. http://linkinghub.elsevier.com/retrieve/pii/S1525001616309613.
5. Simunovic MP, Xue K, Jolly JK, MacLaren RE. Structural and functional recovery following limited iatrogenic macular detachment for retinal gene therapy. JAMA Ophthalmol. 2017;135(3):234–41.
6. Adijanto J, Naash MI. Nanoparticle-based technologies for retinal gene therapy. Eur J Pharm Biopharm. 2015;95:353–67.
7. Mak KY, Rajapaksha IG, Angus PW, Herath CB. The adeno-associated virus—a safe and effective vehicle for liver-specific gene therapy of inherited and non-inherited diseases. Curr Gene Ther. 2017;17(1):4–16.
8. Lebherz C, Maguire A, Tang W, Bennett J, Wilson JM. Novel AAV serotypes for improved ocular gene transfer. J Gene Med. 2008;10(4):375–82.
9. Dalkara D, Byrne LC, Klimczak RR, Visel M, Yin L, Merigan WH, et al. In vivo-directed evolution of a new adeno-associated virus for therapeutic outer retinal gene delivery from the vitreous. Sci Transl Med [Internet]. 2013;5(189):189ra76. http://stm.sciencemag.org/cgi/doi/10.1126/scitranslmed.3005708.
10. Weber M. Recombinant adeno-associated virus serotype 4 mediates unique and exclusive long-term transduction of retinal pigmented epithelium in rat, dog, and nonhuman primate after subretinal delivery. Mol Ther [Internet]. 2003 Jun [cited 2012 May 16];7(6):774–81. http://www.nature.com/doifinder/10.1016/S1525-0016(03)00098-4.
11. Gaj T, Gersbach CA, Barbas CF. ZFN, TALEN, and CRISPR/Cas-based methods for genome engineering. Trends Biotechnol [Internet]. 2013;31(7):397–405. https://doi.org/10.1016/j.tibtech.2013.04.004.
12. Ran FA, Cong L, Yan WX, Scott DA, Gootenberg JS, Kriz AJ, et al. In vivo genome editing using Staphylococcus aureus Cas9. Nature. 2015;520(7546):186–91.
13. Philpott NJ, Thrasher AJ. Use of nonintegrating lentiviral vectors for gene therapy. Hum Gene Ther. 2007;18(6):483–9.
14. Duisit G. Five recombinant simian immunodeficiency virus pseudotypes lead to exclusive transduction of retinal pigmented epithelium in rat. Mol Ther [Internet]. 2002 Oct [cited 2012 May 16];6(4):446–54. http://www.nature.com/doifinder/10.1006/mthe.2002.0690.
15. Puppo A, Cesi G, Marrocco E, Piccolo P, Jacca S, Shayakhmetov DM, et al. Retinal transduction profiles by high-capacity viral vectors. Gene Ther. 2014;21(10):855–65.

16. Trapani I, Puppo A, Auricchio A. Vector platforms for gene therapy of inherited retinopathies. Prog Retin Eye Res. 2014;43:108–28.
17. Fougeroux C, Holst PJ. Future prospects for the development of cost-effective adenovirus vaccines. Int J Mol Sci. 2017;18(4).
18. Brunetti-Pierri N, Ng P. Gene therapy with helper-dependent adenoviral vectors: lessons from studies in large animal models. Virus Genes. 2017;53(5):684–91.
19. Ueyama K, Mori K, Shoji T, Omata H, Gehlbach PL, Brough DE, et al. Ocular localization and transduction by adenoviral vectors are serotype-dependent and can be modified by inclusion of rgd fiber modifications. PLoS One. 2014;9(9):e108071.
20. Sweigard JH, Cashman SM, Kumar-Singh R. Adenovirus vectors targeting distinct cell types in the retina. Investig Ophthalmol Vis Sci. 2010;51(4):2219–28.
21. Han Z, Conley SM, Makkia RS, Cooper MJ, Naash MI. DNA nanoparticle-mediated ABCA4 delivery rescues Stargardt dystrophy in mice. J Clin Invest [Internet]. 2012 Sep 4 [cited 2013 Sep 26];122(9):3221–6. http://www.pubmedcentral.nih.gov/articlerender.fcgi?artid=3428101&tool=pmcentrez&rendertype=abstract.
22. Koirala A, Conley SM, Naash MI. A review of therapeutic prospects of non-viral gene therapy in the retinal pigment epithelium. Biomaterials [Internet]. 2013 Sep [cited 2013 Sep 25];34(29):7158–67. http://www.ncbi.nlm.nih.gov/pubmed/23796578.
23. Koirala A, Makkia RS, Conley SM, Cooper MJ, Naash MI. S/MAR-containing DNA nanoparticles promote persistent RPE gene expression and improvement in RPE65-associated LCA. Hum Mol Genet [Internet]. 2013 Apr 15 [cited 2013 Sep 26];22(8):1632–42. http://www.ncbi.nlm.nih.gov/pubmed/23335596.
24. Jacobson SG, Cideciyan AV, Roman AJ, Sumaroka A, Schwartz SB, Heon E, et al. Improvement and decline in vision with gene therapy in childhood blindness. N Engl J Med [Internet]. 2015;372(20):1920–6. http://www.nejm.org/doi/abs/10.1056/NEJMoa1412965%5Cn, http://www.ncbi.nlm.nih.gov/pubmed/25936984.
25. Boye SE, Boye SL, Lewin AS, Hauswirth WW. A comprehensive review of retinal gene therapy. Mol Ther [Internet]. 2013 Mar [cited 2013 Sep 24];21(3):509–19. http://www.ncbi.nlm.nih.gov/pubmed/23358189.
26. Guziewicz KE, Zangerl B, Komaromy AM, Iwabe S, Chiodo VA, Boye SL, et al. Recombinant AAV-mediated BEST1 transfer to the retinal pigment epithelium: analysis of serotype-dependent retinal effects. PLoS One. 2013;8(10):e75666.
27. Surace EM, Domenici L, Cortese K, Cotugno G, Di Vicino U, Venturi C, et al. Amelioration of both functional and morphological abnormalities in the retina of a mouse model of ocular albinism following AAV-mediated gene transfer. Mol Ther [Internet]. 2005 Oct [cited 2012 May 16];12(4):652–8. http://www.ncbi.nlm.nih.gov/pubmed/16023414.
28. Gargiulo A, Bonetti C, Montefusco S, Neglia S, Di Vicino U, Marrocco E, et al. AAV-mediated tyrosinase gene transfer restores melanogenesis and retinal function in a model of oculo-cutaneous albinism type I (OCA1). Mol Ther [Internet]. 2009 Aug [cited 2012 May 16];17(8):1347–54. http://www.pubmedcentral.nih.gov/articlerender.fcgi?artid=2835246&tool=pmcentrez&rendertype=abstract.
29. Batten ML, Imanishi Y, Tu DC, Doan T, Zhu L, Pang J, et al. Pharmacological and rAAV gene therapy rescue of visual functions in a blind mouse model of Leber congenital amaurosis. PLoS Med [Internet]. 2005 Nov [cited 2012 May 16];2(11):e333. http://www.pubmedcentral.nih.gov/articlerender.fcgi?artid=1274279&tool=pmcentrez&rendertype=abstract.
30. Moiseyev G, Chen Y, Takahashi Y, Wu BX, Ma J-X. RPE65 is the isomerohydrolase in the retinoid visual cycle. Proc Natl Acad Sci U S A [Internet]. 2005 Aug 30;102(35):12413–8. http://www.ncbi.nlm.nih.gov/pubmed/16319067.
31. Wang J-S, Kefalov VJ. An alternative pathway mediates the mouse and human cone visual cycle. Curr Biol. 2009;19(19):1665–9.
32. Thompson DA, Gyurus P, Fleischer LL, Bingham EL, McHenry CL, Apfelstedt-Sylla E, et al. Genetics and phenotypes of RPE65 mutations in inherited retinal degeneration. Invest Ophthalmol Vis Sci States. 2000;41(13):4293–9.
33. Lorenz B, Poliakov E, Schambeck M, Friedburg C, Preising MN, Redmond TM. A comprehensive clinical and biochemical functional study of a novel RPE65 hypomorphic mutation. Invest Ophthalmol Vis Sci [Internet]. 2008 Dec [cited 2012 May 16];49(12):5235–42. http://www.ncbi.nlm.nih.gov/pubmed/18599565.
34. Paunescu K, Wabbels B, Preising MN, Lorenz B. Longitudinal and cross-sectional study of patients with early-onset severe retinal dystrophy associated with RPE65 mutations. Graefes Arch Clin Exp Ophthalmol [Internet]. 2005 May [cited 2012 Mar 20];243(5):417–26. http://www.ncbi.nlm.nih.gov/pubmed/15565294.
35. Lorenz B, Wabbels B, Wegscheider E, Hamel CP, Drexler W, Preising MN. Lack of fundus autofluorescence to 488 nanometers from childhood on in patients with early-onset severe retinal dystrophy associated with mutations in RPE65. Ophthalmology [Internet]. 2004 Aug [cited 2012 May 16];111(8):1585–94. http://www.ncbi.nlm.nih.gov/pubmed/15288992.
36. Maiti P, Kong J, Kim SR, Sparrow JR, Allikmets R, Rando RR. Small molecule RPE65 antagonists limit the visual cycle and prevent lipofuscin formation. Biochemistry. 2006;45(3):852–60.
37. Acland GM, Aguirre GD, Ray J, Zhang Q, Aleman TS, Cideciyan AV, et al. Gene therapy restores vision in a canine model of childhood blindness. Nat Genet [Internet]. 2001;28(1):92–5. http://www.ncbi.nlm.nih.gov/pubmed/11326284.
38. Narfstrom K. Functional and structural recovery of the retina after gene therapy in the RPE65 null mutation

dog. Invest Ophthalmol Vis Sci [Internet]. 2003 Apr 1 [cited 2012 May 16];44(4):1663–72. http://www.iovs.org/cgi/doi/10.1167/iovs.02-0595.

39. Le Meur G, Stieger K, Smith AJ, Weber M, Deschamps JY, Nivard D, et al. Restoration of vision in RPE65-deficient Briard dogs using an AAV serotype 4 vector that specifically targets the retinal pigmented epithelium. Gene Ther [Internet]. 2007 Feb [cited 2013 Sep 25];14(4):292–303. http://www.ncbi.nlm.nih.gov/pubmed/17024105.
40. Bainbridge JW, Barker SS, Robbie S, Ophth MRC, Henderson R, et al. Effect of gene therapy on visual function in Leber's congenital amaurosis. N Engl J Med. 2008;358:2231–9.
41. Maguire AM, Simonelli F, Pierce EA, Pugh EN, Mingozzi F, Bennicelli J, et al. Safety and efficacy of gene transfer for Leber's congenital amaurosis. N Engl J Med [Internet]. 2008 May 22 [cited 2013 Sep 26];358(21):2240–8. http://www.pubmedcentral.nih.gov/articlerender.fcgi?artid=2829748&tool=pmcentrez&rendertype=abstract.
42. Hauswirth WW, Aleman TS, Kaushal S, Cideciyan AV, Schwartz SB, Wang L, et al. Treatment of leber congenital amaurosis due to RPE65 mutations by ocular subretinal injection of adeno-associated virus gene vector: short-term results of a phase I trial. Hum Gene Ther [Internet]. 2008 Oct [cited 2013 Sep 26];19(10):979–90. http://www.pubmedcentral.nih.gov/articlerender.fcgi?artid=2940541&tool=pmcentrez&rendertype=abstract.
43. Jacobson SG, Cideciyan A V, Ratnakaram R, Heon E, Schwartz SB, Roman AJ, et al. Gene therapy for leber congenital amaurosis caused by RPE65 mutations: safety and efficacy in 15 children and adults followed up to 3 years. Arch Ophthalmol [Internet]. 2012 Jan [cited 2012 Mar 2];130(1):9–24. http://www.ncbi.nlm.nih.gov/pubmed/21911650.
44. Maguire AM, High KA, Auricchio A, Wright JF, Pierce EA, Testa F, et al. Age-dependent effects of RPE65 gene therapy for Leber's congenital amaurosis: a phase 1 dose-escalation trial. Lancet [Internet]. 2009 Nov 7 [cited 2012 Mar 2];374(9701):1597–605. http://www.ncbi.nlm.nih.gov/pubmed/19854499.
45. Weleber RG, Pennesi ME, Wilson DJ, Kaushal S, Erker LR, Jensen L, et al. Results at 2 years after gene therapy for RPE65-deficient leber congenital amaurosis and severe early-childhood-onset retinal dystrophy. Ophthalmology [Internet]. 2016;123(7):1606–20. https://doi.org/10.1016/j.ophtha.2016.03.003.
46. Bainbridge JWB, Mehat MS, Sundaram V, Robbie SJ, Barker SE, Ripamonti C, et al. Long-term effect of gene therapy on Leber's congenital amaurosis. N Engl J Med [Internet]. 2015;372(20):1887–97. http://www.nejm.org/doi/abs/10.1056/NEJMoa1414221%5Cn, http://www.ncbi.nlm.nih.gov/pubmed/25938638.
47. Cideciyan AV, Jacobson SG, Beltran WA, Sumaroka A, Swider M, Iwabe S, et al. Human retinal gene therapy for Leber congenital amaurosis shows advancing retinal degeneration despite enduring visual improvement. Proc Natl Acad Sci U S A [Internet]. 2013 Feb 5 [cited 2013 Sep 25];110(6):E517–25. http://www.pubmedcentral.nih.gov/articlerender.fcgi?artid=3568385&tool=pmcentrez&rendertype=abstract.
48. Schimmer J, Breazzano S. Investigator outlook: focus on upcoming LCA2 gene therapy phase III results. Hum Gene Ther Clin Dev [Internet]. 2015;26(3):144–9. https://en.wikiversity.org/wiki/Wikiversity_Journal_of_Medicine/Blausen_gallery_2014.
49. Kalatzis V, Hamel CP, IM MD. Choroideremia: towards a therapy. Am J Ophthalmol. 2013;156(3):433–7.e3.
50. Tolmachova T, Tolmachov OE, Barnard AR, de Silva SR, Lipinski DM, Walker NJ, et al. Functional expression of Rab escort protein 1 following AAV2-mediated gene delivery in the retina of choroideremia mice and human cells ex vivo. J Mol Med (Berl) [Internet]. 2013 Jul [cited 2013 Sep 26];91(7):825–37. http://www.pubmedcentral.nih.gov/articlerender.fcgi?artid=3695676&tool=pmcentrez&rendertype=abstract.
51. Tolmachova T, Tolmachov OE, Wavre-Shapton ST, Tracey-White D, Futter CE, Seabra MC. CHM/REP1 cDNA delivery by lentiviral vectors provides functional expression of the transgene in the retinal pigment epithelium of choroideremia mice. J Gene Med. 2012;14(3):158–68.
52. MacLaren RE, Groppe M, Barnard AR, Cottriall CL, Tolmachova T, Seymour L, et al. Retinal gene therapy in patients with choroideremia: initial findings from a phase 1/2 clinical trial. Lancet [Internet]. 2014;383(9923):1129–37. http://www.ncbi.nlm.nih.gov/pubmed/24439297.
53. Edwards TL, Jolly JK, Groppe M, Barnard AR, Cottriall CL, Tolmachova T, et al. Visual acuity after retinal gene therapy for choroideremia. N Engl J Med. 2016;374(20):1996–8.
54. Gal A, Li Y, Thompson DA, Weir J, Orth U, Jacobson SG, et al. Mutations in MERTK, the human orthologue of the RCS rat retinal dystrophy gene, cause retinitis pigmentosa. Nat Genet [Internet]. 2000 Nov [cited 2013 Sep 26];26(3):270–1. http://www.ncbi.nlm.nih.gov/pubmed/11062461.
55. D'Cruz PM, Yasumura D, Weir J, Matthes MT, Abderrahim H, LaVail MM, et al. Mutation of the receptor tyrosine kinase gene Mertk in the retinal dystrophic RCS rat. Hum Mol Genet. 2000;9(4):645–51.
56. Tschernutter M, Schlichtenbrede FC, Howe S, Balaggan KS, Munro PM, Bainbridge JWB, et al. Long-term preservation of retinal function in the RCS rat model of retinitis pigmentosa following lentivirus-mediated gene therapy. Gene Ther [Internet]. 2005 Apr [cited 2013 Sep 26];12(8):694–701. http://www.ncbi.nlm.nih.gov/pubmed/15660111.
57. Vollrath D, Feng W, Duncan JL, Yasumura D, D'Cruz PM, Chappelow A, et al. Correction of the retinal dystrophy phenotype of the RCS rat by viral gene transfer of Mertk. Proc Natl Acad Sci U S A. 2001;98(22):12584–9.
58. Smith AJ, Schlichtenbrede FC, Tschernutter M, Bainbridge JW, Thrasher AJ, Ali RR. AAV-mediated gene transfer slows photoreceptor loss in the RCS rat

model of retinitis pigmentosa. Mol Ther [Internet]. 2003 Aug [cited 2013 Sep 26];8(2):188–95. http://www.ncbi.nlm.nih.gov/pubmed/12907141.

59. Conlon TJ, Deng W-T, Erger K, Cossette T, Pang J, Ryals R, et al. Preclinical potency and safety studies of an AAV2-mediated gene therapy vector for the treatment of MERTK associated retinitis pigmentosa. Hum Gene Ther Clin Dev [Internet]. 2013 Mar [cited 2013 Sep 25];24(1):23–8. http://www.ncbi.nlm.nih.gov/pubmed/23692380.
60. Lavail MM, Yasumura D, Matthes MT, Yang H, Hauswirth WW, Deng W, et al. Retinal degenerative diseases, vol. 854. Basel: Springer; 2016. p. 487–93. https://doi.org/10.1007/978-3-319-17121-0.
61. Ghazi NG, Abboud EB, Nowilaty SR, Alkuraya H, Alhommadi A, Cai H, et al. Treatment of retinitis pigmentosa due to MERTK mutations by ocular subretinal injection of adeno-associated virus gene vector: results of a phase I trial. Hum Genet. 2016;135(3):327–43.
62. Pasquay C, Wang LF, Lorenz B, Preising MN. Bestrophin 1—phenotypes and functional aspects in Bestrophinopathies. Ophthalmic Genet [Internet]. 2015;36(3):193–212. http://informahealthcare.com/doi/abs/10.3109/13816810.2013.863945%5Cn, http://www.tandfonline.com/doi/full/10.3109/13816810.2013.863945#.VeWvy_lVhBc.
63. Johnson AA, Guziewicz KE, Lee CJ, Kalathur RC, Pulido JS, Marmorstein LY, et al. Bestrophin 1 and retinal disease. Prog Retin Eye Res [Internet]. 2016;58:45–69. https://doi.org/10.1016/j.preteyeres.2017.01.006.
64. Guziewicz KE, Zangerl B, Lindauer SJ, Mullins RF, Sandmeyer LS, Grahn BH, et al. Bestrophin gene mutations cause canine multifocal retinopathy: a novel animal model for best disease. Invest Ophthalmol Vis Sci. 2007;48(5):1959–67.
65. Guziewicz KE, Sinha D, Gómez NM, Zorych K, Dutrow EV, Dhingra A, et al. Bestrophinopathy: an RPE-photoreceptor interface disease. Prog Retin Eye Res. 2016;58:70–88.
66. Suzuki K, Tsunekawa Y, Hernandez-Benitez R, Wu J, Zhu J, Kim EJ, et al. In vivo genome editing via CRISPR/Cas9 mediated homology-independent targeted integration. Nature [Internet]. 2016;540(7631):144–9. http://www.nature.com/doifinder/10.1038/nature20565.
67. Adamus G. Can innate and autoimmune reactivity forecast early and advance stages of age-related macular degeneration? Autoimmun Rev. 2017;16(3):231–6.
68. Miller JW. Age-related macular degeneration revisited—piecing the puzzle: the LXIX Edward Jackson Memorial Lecture. Am J Ophthalmol [Internet]. 2013;155(1):1–35. https://doi.org/10.1016/j.ajo.2012.10.018.
69. Miller JW. VEGF: from discovery to therapy: the Champalimaud Award Lecture. Transl Vis Sci Technol [Internet]. 2016;5(2):9. http://www.ncbi.nlm.nih.gov/pubmed/26981331.
70. Langford-Smith A, Keenan TDL, Clark SJ, Bishop PN, Day AJ. The role of complement in age-related macular degeneration: heparan sulphate, a ZIP code for complement factor H? J Innate Immun. 2014;6(4):407–16.
71. Kauppinen A, Paterno JJ, Blasiak J, Salminen A, Kaarniranta K. Inflammation and its role in age-related macular degeneration. Cell Mol Life Sci. 2016;73(9):1765–86.
72. Boyer DS, Schmidt-Erfurth U, van Lookeren Campagne M, Henry EC, Brittain C. The pathophysiology of geographic atrophy secondary to age-related macular degeneration and the complement pathway as a therapeutic target. Retina. 2017;37(5):819–35.
73. Cashman SM, Desai A, Ramo K, Kumar-Singh R. Expression of complement component 3 (C3) from an adenovirus leads to pathology in the murine retina. Investig Ophthalmol Vis Sci. 2011;52(6):3436–45.
74. Gheorghe A, Mahdi L, Musat O. Age-related macular degeneration. Rom J Ophthalmol. 2015;59(2):74–7.
75. Arevalo JF, Lasave AF, Wu L, Acón D, Berrocal MH, Diaz-Llopis M, et al. Intravitreal bevacizumab for choroidal neovascularization in age-related macular degeneration: 5-year results of the Pan-American Collaborative Retina Study Group. Retina. 2016;36(5):859–67.
76. Kim E, Koo T, Park SW, Kim D, Kim K, Cho H-Y, et al. In vivo genome editing with a small Cas9 orthologue derived from Campylobacter jejuni. Nat Commun. 2017;8:14500.
77. Georgiadis A, Duran Y, Ribeiro J, Abelleira-Hervas L, Robbie SJ, Sünkel Laing B, et al. Development of an optimized AAV2/5 gene therapy vector for Leber congenital Amaurosis owing to defects in RPE65. Gene Ther [Internet]. 2016;23(12):857–62. http://www.nature.com/doifinder/10.1038/gt.2016.66.
78. Banin E, Bandah-Rozenfeld D, Obolensky A, Cideciyan AV, Aleman TS, Marks-Ohana D, et al. Molecular anthropology meets genetic medicine to treat blindness in the North African Jewish population: human gene therapy initiated in Israel. Hum Gene Ther [Internet]. 2010;21(12):1749–57. http://www.ncbi.nlm.nih.gov/pubmed/20604683.

RPE and Laser

16

Claus von der Burchard and Johann Roider

Introduction

"Laser" is an acronym for "light amplification by stimulated emission of radiation". A laser device creates a light beam that is distinctly different to other light sources by these characteristics:

1. It usually has a very condensed wavelength spectrum, i.e. the beam is (almost) monochromatic
2. The beam is highly collimated, i.e. the beam only diverges very little
3. The beam usually has a very long coherence length

These physical properties make lasers an ideal tool for delivering light and thereby energy to the eye and especially to the retina. Because of the minimal beam divergence, it can be administered with high precision both in the lab and in eyes. However, to understand the effect of laser application to the retina in general and the retinal pigment epithelium (RPE) in special, it is vital to gain an insight into the physics of laser-tissue interaction.

C. von der Burchard (✉) · J. Roider
Department of Ophthalmology, University Medical Center, University of Kiel, Kiel, Germany
e-mail: claus.vonderburchard@uksh.de; johann.roider@uksh.de

Physics of Laser-Tissue Interaction

Photothermal Effect

The most important principle in laser-RPE interaction is the photothermal effect. This effect prevails mainly when significant laser light is applied for a relatively long period of exposure time, e.g. longer than several milliseconds, typically between 50 and 1000 ms (milliseconds = 10^{-3} s). An additional prerequisite is a chromophore, a light-absorbing structure. The chromophore absorbs photons of a specific wavelength and transforms laser energy into heat. Usually, wavelengths in the visible and near infrared spectrum of light, i.e. about 400–1400 nm, are being used for creating a photothermal effect in the posterior part of the eye. Other, especially shorter wavelengths do not play a role in the posterior part of the eye because they cannot penetrate onto the retina due to water absorption mainly in the cornea.

The by far most important chromophore in the RPE is melanin (Fig. 16.1), which absorbs light throughout the whole visible spectrum of light and near-infrared (with an extinction coefficient decreasing with higher wavelengths). Melanin is densely stacked in melanin granulas, which can be found at the apical side of the RPE cells. It can also be found in the choroid, but overall in lower quantities, less densely stacked, and inhomogeneously distributed. Because of the high overall

A. K. Klettner, S. Dithmar (eds.), *Retinal Pigment Epithelium in Health and Disease*,
https://doi.org/10.1007/978-3-030-28384-1_16

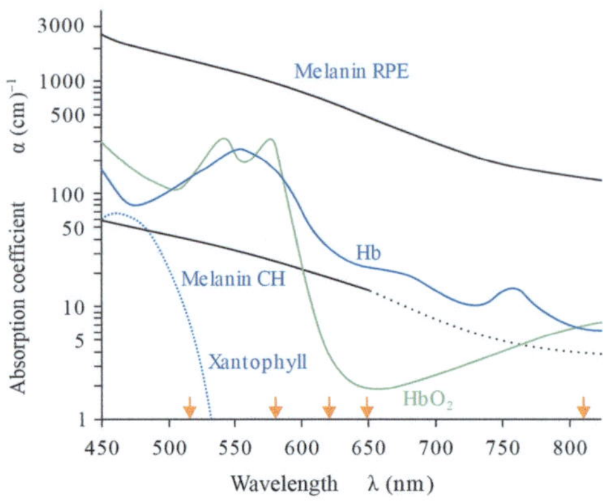

Fig. 16.1 Absorption of retinal chromophores for different wavelengths. (From [1])

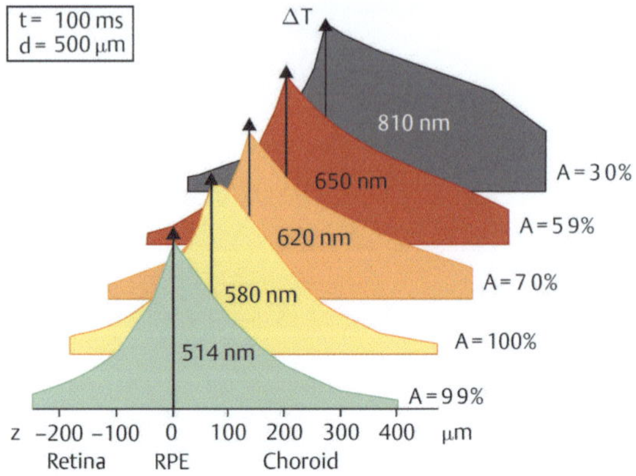

Fig. 16.2 Spacial profile of temperature increase for different laser wavelengths. (From [1])

amount of melanin and its high absorption coefficient, the light absorption of melanin surpasses any other chromophores in the visible spectrum. When considering not only the RPE, but the adjacent retina and choroid, one must also consider the light absorption of blood. The main absorber of blood is hemoglobin, which is higher at lower wavelengths compared to melanin. Another very localized absorber is xanthophyll, which is located in the neural retina only in the foveal region (absorption maximum at around 450 nm). Since nowadays wavelength longer than 514 nm are used for clinically applications, xanthophyll does not play a clinical role anymore. With longer wavelengths, a significant amount of light penetrates to the choroid. This leads to additional heating of the choroid; however, the temperature distribution in the neural retina is similar if exposure times longer than 100 ms are used. Since clinical therapeutic effects are mainly retina or RPE related, the thermal reactions in the choroid are mostly unwanted side effects leading to pain for the patient.

While the translation of light energy into heat initially takes place very localized at the absorbing molecule, the heat will instantly begin to dissipate—to neighboring molecules, organelles and cells. This means that even though the melanin in the RPE (and melanin in the adjacent choroid) is the main photoabsorber, the heat will always spread out in three dimensions both to the surrounding neuroretina and to the choroid and sclera; see Figs. 16.2 and 16.3). The only tactic to decrease spatial spread of heat diffusion is to increase laser power while decreasing exposure time. However, the window for "thermal confinement" is very small: Increase in power leads to high peak temperatures and thereby to a decrease in therapeutic window. When too high powers are used, vaporization can occur and create mechanical damage. Moreover, while the distance of heat diffusion can be slightly reduced, it will not vanish completely [2]. This implicates that with continuous wave lasers, selective RPE treatment is not possible. While this does not affect lab models, the concept of heat conduction is of vital importance in clinical settings: It is actively used in various clinical conditions. For example, in laser retinopexy, a tight scar formation of the RPE and adjacent neuroretina is the desired goal of treatment. At the same time, heat conduction is the main hindrance for laser treatment in the macular region, where irreversible damage of the adjacent photoreceptors is undesirable.

Heat convection, as could theoretically be supposed because of the high blood flow in the choriocapillaris, does not play a role in the usual photocoagulation of under 1 s. It usually prevails with longer exposures of several seconds.

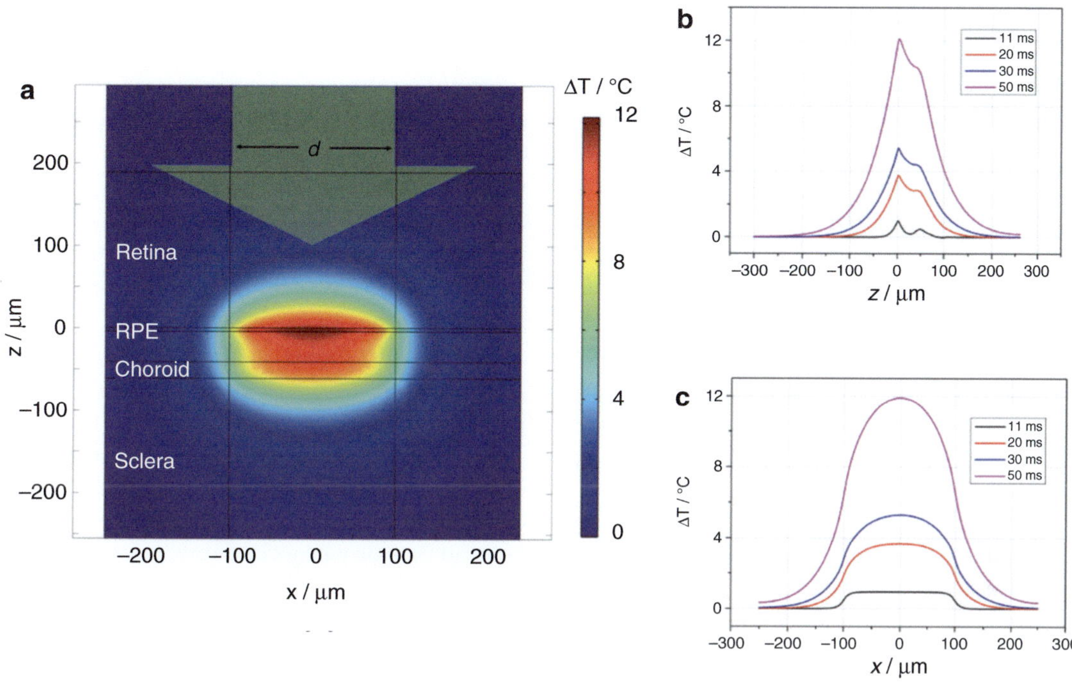

Fig. 16.3 (**a**) Schematic display of temperature changes during a 50 ms, 200 µm irradiation in a rabbit eye. (**b**, **c**) Temperature profiles for different exposure times in the z- and x-axis. (From [3])

Photomechanical Effect

The physical principles of photothermal laser-tissue interactions do not hold up for shorter laser exposure. Photothermal tissue effects can be explained by exposure of proteins to a certain period of temperature elevation. This relationship between exposure time and height of temperature can be described by the Arrhenius law. With shorter pulse durations, this relationship does not hold any more. Other effects are responsible for tissue effects or tissue destruction. These effects usually occur when the exposure time comes to the order of the thermal relaxation time of the absorbing structure. The thermal relaxation time is defined as the time period until a significant amount of heat dissipates out of a target structure. This time is defined slightly different between different authors. For the RPE in total, this time is in the range of a few microseconds (µs = 10^{-6} s), for single melanin granula in the range of about 300–400 nanoseconds (ns = 10^{-9} s). When the laser exposure is in or below the range of the thermal relaxation time, photomechanical effects start to appear. Because of relatively high single pulse energy and low pulse duration, the tissue gets heated to very high temperatures and heating occurs faster than the heat can dissipate out to surrounding organelles. This can lead e.g. to local vaporization, a phenomenon often described as the formation of microbubbles or generation of pressure waves. Microbubbles or pressure waves can cause mechanical damage to surrounding organelles, and according to many theories finally to a disruption of the cell membrane. The result of this treatment is cell death.

Because heat dissipation does not play a role in this mechanical approach, it allows for selective cell destruction. Therefore, lasers based on the photomechanical effect can be used for selective RPE treatment, as will be discussed later.

Photochemical Effect

A third major laser-tissue interaction is the photochemical process, where a long light exposure at a relatively low power does not lead to a significant buildup of heat, but rather induces a photochemical reaction in absorbing molecules. This mechanism prominently plays a role in the cornea (photokeratitis), at the photoreceptors (solar retinopathy and photobiomodulation) and in the choroid/RPE complex (photodynamic therapy). A photochemical effect is defined by an inverse relationship between the energy density of the light (not power density!) and the exposure time.

Photodynamic therapy (PDT) is the most prominent retinal example within the photochemical lasers. PDT works via a photosensitizing drug, e.g. verteporfin, and laser illumination at 690 nm, which is specifically the absorption maximum of the drug. The suspected pathomechanism is that the excited photosensitizing drug creates reactive oxygen intermediates that cause lethal damage to surrounding cells [4]. Dose-dependent cytotoxic influence on endothelial cells causes vascular thrombosis [5, 6]. Via this mechanism, selective destruction of e.g. classic choroidal neovascularization was proposed while healthy retinal tissue is spared [7]. However, these theoretical advantages did only partially hold up because of the simultaneous destruction of the RPE by repeated treatments.

Researchers are currently investigating a concept called photobiomodulation (PBM) for retinal application. In PBM, lights of different wavelengths (590, 670 and 790 nm) were used to stimulate the retina for multiple sessions of a few minutes' duration. The main mechanism of actions seems to be a photochemical effect of the mitochondrial cytochrome c oxidase (COX) [8–10]. By photochemical activation, the enzyme activity is claimed to increase and potentially shift in function. The main focus of PBM are the photoreceptors, but PBM also has been shown to affect RPE cells. Reportedly, PBM treatment increases phagocytosis and decreases VEGF expression [11]. However, extensive research on PBM and the RPE is still missing.

Concepts of RPE Laser Treatment

Clinical laser treatment always consists of a set of different variables that can be altered, mainly consisting out of wavelength, duration of treatment, continuous-wave or pulsed mode, pulse duration, treatment duration, treatment power, and spot size on retina. Theoretically, any slight modification in any of these variables could cause a different laser tissue interaction and a subsequent variable biological response. Therefore, the sheer number of possible combinations make the field of retinal laser treatment confusing at a first glance. To understand retinal laser therapy, it is therefore important to understand the different main concepts into which each distinct combination can then be categorized into.

Classic Continuous-Wave Laser Photocoagulation

The classic application of laser in retinal tissue is tissue destruction by usage of the photothermal effect. Because of heat conduction, destructive RPE photocoagulation will always involve the adjacent choroid and neuroretina. Depending on the treatment goal, a different extent of retinal photocoagulation is intended.

Apart from deliberately applying intense heat for scar formation in retinopexy, the most general intention of laser treatment is to induce some sort of biological response of the RPE and/or neighboring cells that positively affects an ongoing disease. For this purpose, investigations of RPE and laser always must consider the surrounding neuroretina, Bruch's membrane and choroid. While cell culture experiments can ignore these tissues and gain helpful insight into the solitary RPE response to physical phenomena, an experimental setup should always respect the viability of application in tissue.

Dosimetry

Spot size and treatment duration vary depending on the treatment scheme. Clinically, spot sizes between 50 and 500 μm and treatment durations of 20–200 ms are most common.

In order to achieve the intended treatment effect with high precision and reproducibility, one must be able to reproduce the same temperature for the same time span. It is crucial to understand that while laser power and tissue temperature are positively related, multiple factors influence the correlation that can lead to high variabilities intra- and interindividually. Light absorption by the optical media in front of the retina limits the laser power that reaches the retina. The most important examples include cataract, corneal opacities and vitreous hemorrhage. Moreover, retinal pigmentation can vary highly between different individuals and in-between the same individual. Studies have reported that the RPE pigmentation can vary up to factor 3 within the same retina [12].

The easiest solution for this problem for the ophthalmologist is to perform a live observation of the retinal spot during photocoagulation and to adjust laser power for the next spots according to the visual feedback. Photocoagulation leads to a retinal whitening due to changing of the scattering properties of the neural retina, mostly attributed to protein denaturation. This effect becomes barely visible at a tissue temperature of about 65 °C [3] and increases in the extent of whitening with higher temperatures. Also, at the visibility threshold, it takes some time for the whitening to set in. This time-span decreases with increasing laser power; therefore, the time of whitening formation allows for further precision in dosimetry.

While this technique is quite imprecise, it is sufficient for most retinal applications. The most prominent examples of this approach are the following:

- In laser retinopexy, the treatment desires to induce a strong scar-formation between the choroid, the RPE and the neuroretina in order to prevent retinal detachment. In order to achieve a strong scar, high tissue temperatures are required [13, 14], i.e. a solid whitening of the retina
- In panretinal photocoagulation (PRP), treatment rationale is to destroy ischemic neuroretinal cells (details will be discussed later). Again, a distinct retinal whitening is targeted at as a marker of irreversible tissue destruction
- Some applications directly aim to influence vascular structures directly, e.g. ablation of retinal microaneurysms in diabetic retinopathy and other diseases

The above-mentioned examples require distinctly surpassing the visibility threshold. However, it is also important to avoid overpowering. Increasing powers can lead to increasing pain for the patient. Moreover, with increasing power, spot size will increase due to heat dissipation, and ultimately, it can lead to a breakdown of the Bruch membrane with subsequent hemorrhage and possibly formation of choroidal neovascularization. In some animal research models, this effect is used to deliberately create choroidal neovascularization; however, the validity of these models is heavily disputed since these neovascularizations alter significantly from naturally occuring neovascularizations such as in age-related macula degeneration.

In contrast to these above-threshold applications, other treatment modalities focus rather on a biostimulation of the retina than the irreversible tissue destruction. Because the therapeutic range of these modalities lies well-below the funduscopic visibility, more advanced dosimetry schemes must be used. The most well-established procedure is to perform titrating lesions in the peripheral retina to determine the individual visibility threshold and then reduce the power for the treatment lesions by a certain factor, often 0.3–0.5 [15].

However, this approach does not account for the intraindividual pigmentation varieties and therefore is problematic, especially since it is mainly used in the macular region where overtreatment can lead to severe visual impairment. Therefore, smarter and more precise dosimetry solutions are researched; these include dosimetry by optoacoustical feedback [3], optical coherence tomography and others. However, as of today, these modalities are not established in clinical care.

Above-Threshold Laser Treatment

The earliest retinal laser applications were destructive in nature. Diabetic Retinopathy is caused by microvascular damage to the retinal blood perfusion and causes ischemia of the inner retinal layers. Similar ischemia of the inner retinal layers can be found in retinal vein occlusion, although the mechanism is different: Stasis or significant reduction of blood flow leads to insufficient perfusion of the smaller retinal capillaries. In both diseases, hypoxia of the inner retinal layers stimulates the production of pro-angiogenic factors, above all vascular endothelial growth factor (VEGF). Secretion of VEGF in the inner retinal layers and into the adjacent vitreous causes induction of proliferation of retinal blood vessels. While blood vessel proliferation in hypoxic tissue may sound reasonable at a first glance, the unorganized blood vessel growth does not relieve the underlying hypoxia, but instead may lead to uncontrolled epiretinal membrane formation that additionally can cause tractional retinal detachment. Moreover, the new blood vessels are often of fragile nature and thereby lead to vitreous hemorrhage. The idea of laser treatment of ischemic neuroretina is therefore the reduction of VEGF production to stop blood vessel proliferation. Panretinal laser treatment achieves this by a dense treatment of the peripheral retina with high laser powers. This reduces the amount of VEGF producing cells on the one hand, but moreover reduces the number of oxygen-dependent cells in total (the idea being that scar tissue is less energy-dependent than ganglion cells) and thereby leaves more oxygen to the residing cells. Studies have shown an increase in oxygen partial pressure after retinal photocoagulation [16, 17]. It is also suggested that scar formation increases oxygen diffusion from the choroid. Because the areas treated are already regions suffering from hypoxia and thereby are impaired in their function, the sensory defects caused by laser treatment are usually not too severe on the patients; nonetheless, it must be considered that peripheral vision and scotopic vision usually decrease.

Subthreshold Laser Treatment

The concept of large-scale irreversible cell destruction, of course, is problematic for the treatment of the macular region and not viable for the foveal region. Historically, lethal retinal photocoagulation played a role in the management of diabetic macular edema. In the Early Treatment of Diabetic Retinopathy Study (ETDRS), it could be shown that photocoagulation of central microaneurysms (so-called focal grid treatment) could prevent visual acuity loss [18]. However, treatment could also decrease color vision and induce central scotomas. Moreover, as will be discussed below, laser scars can grow over time, so that progressive RPE atrophy can reach the fovea and thereby cause irreversible loss of central vision [19].

The underlying mechanism of macular photocoagulation are still not fully understood. Many researchers believe that changes in cytokine expression are the main underlying principle [20, 21]. Supporting this theory is the fact that milder, less-destructive photocoagulation techniques were shown to lead to similar results as full-strength coagulation. Because of these findings, the original focal grid was clinically replaced by the modified ETDRS technique which require less energy [22]. Treatment goal is not a full-blown retinal coagulation, but only a mild coagulation that still—at least to some extent—affects the photoreceptor layer, but less so the above-lying inner retinal structures.

Continuing the thought of reducing damage, researchers have long sought to find the best cut-off point between being causing as little damage as possible and still being effective for each disease. This led to a variety of different terms and treatment modalities. Therefore, there exists no uniform definition of subthreshold laser treatment. Usually, direct ophthalmoscopic visibility is used as a criterion. However, this does not mean that no alterations can be found in the photoreceptor and other layers, as funduscopy is by far the most crude and one of the least sensitive diagnostic tool for photoreceptor alteration [23].

The term retinal thermostimulation is usually defined as a treatment that only heats the retina by a few degrees without any ultrastructural alterations. The idea is to stimulate a biological response that can positively affect the underlying disease. Well-known examples are Thermostimulation of the Retina (TS-R) [24] or Nondamaging retinal therapy (NRT) [25].

Ultrastructural Workup

Histology

Morphologic changes by laser treatment can be demonstrated by histology even in lesions that are funduscopically invisible [26]. It is noteworthy that these morphological changes can affect the whole retina. In fact, in low intensity lesions around funduscopic threshold, changes of the photoreceptor layer can often be seen earlier than RPE cell damage. Especially, coagulation of the outer segments of the photoreceptors can be found directly after coagulation, but also a discrete pyknosis and condensation of the cell nuclei. RPE cells, on the other hand, often show no histological alterations directly after coagulation, but only a small cellular swelling after 1 month [23, 27].

With higher treatment powers, RPE cell damage becomes more pronounced. Even directly after photocoagulation, absence of a well-organized RPE cell layer can be found. Moreover, within the retina, not only photoreceptors, but also the inner retinal layers (inner nuclear layer and ganglion cell layer) are involved [23]. Histology often shows a pronounced retinal swelling after fixation, which does not exist in-vivo (see Fig. 16.4).

Within the healing process, glia cells replace coagulated tissue. In weak lesions, no strong adhesions are formed in-between the retinal layers and the RPE, which changes with higher treatment powers [13, 14]. This explains the need for high treatment powers in retinopexy.

Optical Coherence Tomography

Optical Coherence Tomography (OCT) allows in-vivo imaging of lesions and is therefore not only much easier to use, but also allows longitudinal insight into lesion development. Therefore, it is not surprising that OCT imaging of laser lesions is more commonly used to characterize laser lesions. However, OCT imaging is different to a histologic work up. Therefore, it is even more important to understand the differences in OCT imaging vs. histology.

Comparative lesion analysis in rabbits has demonstrated several key differences in-between the methods [23] (see Fig. 16.4). Changes in the ellipsoid layer can often be found before funduscopic visibility. When measured, the diameter of the lesions appears wider in OCT than in histology (about 1.5 times). At the same time, involvement of the inner retinal layers can be visualized with less sensitivity than in histology. Especially, during healing processes, the inner layers seem to normalize in OCT imaging, whereas persistent damage can be visualized in histology.

Fluorescence Angiography

In fluorescence angiography, the RPE usually blocks the bright signal of the choriocapillaris

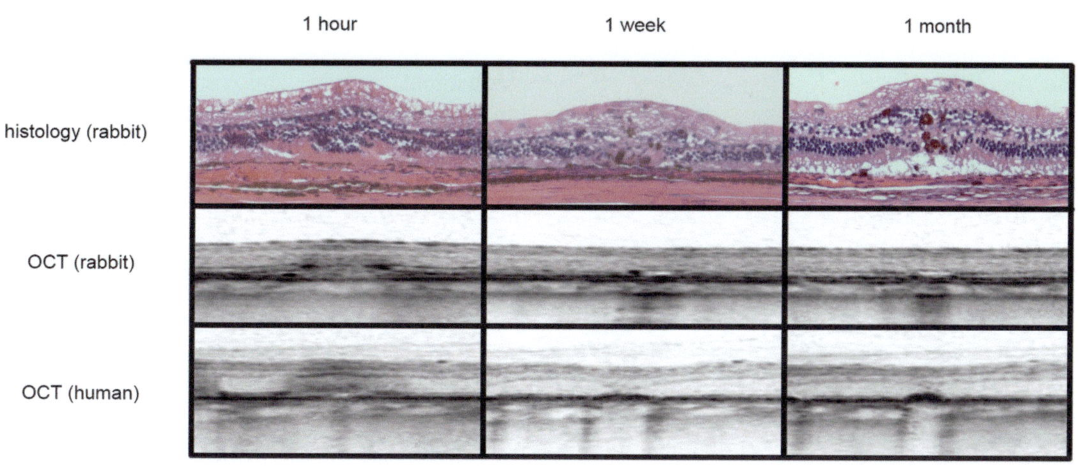

Fig. 16.4 Histology and OCT of an above-threshold lesion (from left to right: after 1 hour, 1 week and 1 month). After 1 hour, disruption of the photoreceptor nuclei and outer segments can be shown. In sequence, glial tissue remodeling with formation of degenerative cysts can be seen. It is noteworthy that the tissue swelling seen in histology does not exist in-vivo, as shown in the OCT. (From [23])

because it absorbs both the exciting as well as the emitting photons. However, when the tight junctions of the RPE break down due to cell damage, fluorescein leakage can be observed, and in case of a cell destruction, a window defect results. This makes fluorescein angiography a highly sensitive means of detecting RPE damage after laser photocoagulation. Angiography is more sensitive in lesion detection; ED-50 threshold was reported at between 50 and 90% of funduscopic threshold [2, 15].

Wound Healing

After photocoagulation, the retinal scar is not necessarily inactive, but can change in morphology for months to years to come. For intense lesions, it is well-known that these lesions can grow over multiple years [28]. The exact mechanisms of this phenomenon are not well-understood, but they must be kept in mind in clinical scenarios, especially when performing coagulations close to the macula.

In contrast, it has been shown that mild photocoagulations can behave quite contrarily. In rats and rabbits, it was reported that mild lesions actually reduce in size over 4 months [26]. The theory is that glial cells that accumulate at the initial scar formation subsequently shrink in size and thereby tear adjacent photoreceptors towards the lesion center. Even more astoundingly, it could be shown that the migrated photoreceptors can make new connections to local inner retinal neurons and thereby restore retinal function [29].

Biological Response

In-vivo experiments have shown that subthreshold lesions can affect protein expression. Studies confirmed up-regulation of heat shock proteins (HSP) even for subthreshold lesions, which are thought to assist cell function repair [30]. In two mice models for age-related macular degeneration (AMD), it could be shown that subthreshold laser application leads to a reduction of the thickness of Bruch's membrane [24], which could be of therapeutic benefit because of better oxygen diffusion from the choroid to the photoreceptors. The exact molecular mechanisms of the effect on Bruch's membrane are not confirmed yet, but HSP expression as well as release of other cell mediators such as matrix metalloproteases are thought to play a major role.

Selective RPE Treatment

Deficiencies in RPE function are considered to play a key role in many diseases, e.g. in chronic serous chorioretinopathy (CSCR), AMD or diabetic macular edema (DME). Numerous organ culture experiments have shown that penetrating RPE lesions lead to RPE regeneration by adjacent cells [32]. Selective RPE destruction is therefore believed to induce RPE rejuvenation and thereby amelioration of cell function and ultimately disease status (Fig. 16.5).

A selective targeting of the RPE cells can be reached by application of the photomechanical effect. The main idea of these treatment regimens is the application of repetitive short pulses with single pulse duration in the range of the thermal relaxation time of the RPE (μs) and a relatively high energy density instead of a subtle single continuous wave radiation. The single pulse energy has to be high enough to create a mechanical tissue RPE effect, but it is not designed to be lethal to the RPE cell with a single shot. Instead, the accumulation of the mechanical damage by repeated microbubble formation is designed to be lethal to RPE cells. Due to thermal confinement, neighboring retinal cells and the Bruch Membrane remain unaffected. This allows for selective pigment epithelium destruction with a high therapeutic window. This treatment modality has been introduced by Roider et al. ([33, 34]) and has been used in treatment of CSCR ([35, 36]), DME ([37]) and other rare clinical pathologies [38].

Selective Retina Therapy (SRT) is using pulses in the microsecond range (usually 1.7 μs), which are theoretically optimized to the

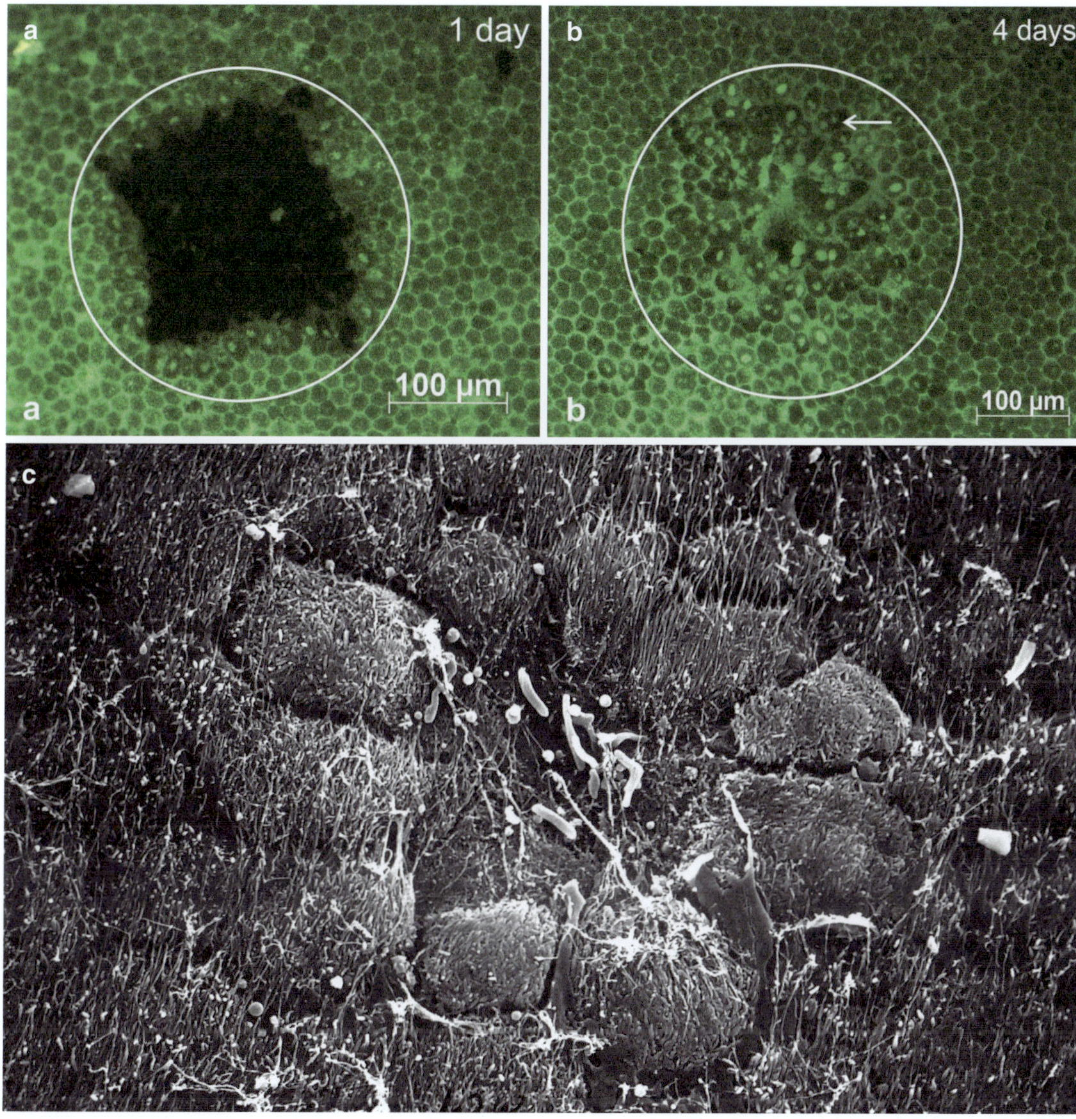

Fig. 16.5 (**a**, **b**) RPE wound healing in organ culture after SRT treatment (from [31]). (**c**) Scanning Electron Microscopy of RPE 1 day after SRT treatment (Photo by Johann Roider)

RPE and have a broad safety margin. Because µs are technically very difficult to generate, Retinal Regeneration Therapy (2RT®) has been introduced, which uses a single laser pulse of 3 nanoseconds, which are technically easy to generate with a frequency double Nd:YAG laser. Both treatment modalities show similar effectiveness in the selective destruction of RPE cells in organ cultures. However, shorter ns pulse durations lead to higher peak temperatures and a decrease of the therapeutic window. A recent multicenter study for treatment of early AMD has reported multiple occurrences of retinal bleedings (7%) after pulsed nanosecond therapy [39] in accordance with the theoretical models of heat dissipation in retinal tissues. No such findings have been reported for pulsed microsecond lasers.

Dosimetry

As with continuous-wave laser application, variations in light absorption and scattering in the optical media and variations in pigment absorption result in the necessity of dosimetry. Lesions in the therapeutic range are funduscopically invisible. In contrast, because of the breakdown of the RPE layer, they demark well in fluorescein angiography. Unfortunately, fluorescein angiography cannot be used for live dosimetry.

However, when over-powered, thermal build-up spreads to the adjacent photoreceptors, resulting in funduscopically visible damage. Titrating lesions in the region of the vascular arcade are again the standard method [39–41]. Similar to subthreshold laser therapy, the power for the treatment lesions is consequently lowered by a certain factor, which makes the procedure imprecise.

Newer techniques include optoacoustic feedback [42] and reflectometry [43] as well as OCT-controlled approaches [44].

Biological Response

Organ cultures have shown that SRT invokes the release of different cell mediators in the phase of the pigment epithelium regeneration. Studies have found an increase of matrix metalloproteases (MMPs) and pigment epithelium derived factor (PEDF). This is thought to positively affect the flux across Bruch's membrane, which plays a key role in AMD pathogenesis [31, 45, 46]. Also, it was found that VEGF levels decreased after treatment [31].

Current Standard Clinical Laser Systems

Historically, the first laser system that became widely accepted for use in ophthalmology was the Argon laser. Argon lasers create a laser beam that consists out of multiple wavelengths; the strongest of which are at 448 and 514 nm. Usually, for uses in ophthalmology, the light is filtered so that it consists out of a monochromatic light at 514 nm (green).

Argon lasers are energy-inefficient and require a gas tube that requires maintenance; therefore, by today they are mostly replaced by frequency-doubled diode Nd:YAG lasers at 532 nm wavelength. Because of the relatively close wavelengths, no significant differences between the laser modalities are to be expected. With the advance of the diode technology, other popular laser systems came to the market. Today additionally laser systems with multiple wavelengths (e.g. yellow at 577 nm) are used and especially for treatment of retinopathy of prematurity (ROP) 810 nm diode lasers are widely found in clinical practice.

References

1. Birngruber R, Weinberg W, Gabel VP. The influence of exposition parameters on the extent of damage in retina coagulation demonstrated by means of a thermal model. In: Jaeger W, (editor). Uveitis. Deutsche Ophthalmologische Gesellschaft Bericht über die 78. Zusammenkunft in Kiel 1980. Wiesbaden: J.F. Bergmann-Verlag; 1981. p. 599–602.
2. Wang J, Quan Y, Dalal R, Palanker D. Comparison of continuous-wave and micropulse modulation in retinal laser therapy. Invest Ophthalmol Vis Sci. 2017;58(11):4722–32. https://doi.org/10.1167/iovs.17-21610.
3. Baade A, von der Burchard C, Lawin M, Koinzer S, Schmarbeck B, Schlott K, Miura Y, Roider J, Birngruber R, Brinkmann R. Power-controlled temperature guided retinal laser therapy. J Biomed Opt. 2017;22(11):1–11. https://doi.org/10.1117/1.JBO.22.11.118001.
4. Schmidt-Erfurth U, Hasan T, Gragoudas E, Michaud N, Flotte TJ, Birngruber R. Vascular targeting in photodynamic occlusion of subretinal vessels. Ophthalmology. 1994;101(12):1953–61.
5. Schlötzer-Schrehardt U, Viestenz A, Naumann GOH, Laqua H, Michels S, Schmidt-Erfurth U. Dose-related structural effects of photodynamic therapy on choroidal and retinal structures of human eyes. Graefes Arch Clin Exp Ophthalmol. 2002;240(9):748–57. https://doi.org/10.1007/s00417-002-0517-4.
6. Schmidt-Erfurth U, Laqua H, Schlötzer-Schrehard U, Viestenz A, Naumann GOH. Histopathological changes following photodynamic therapy in human eyes. Arch Ophthalmol. 2002;120(6):835–44.
7. Photodynamic therapy of subfoveal choroidal neovascularization in age-related macular degeneration with verteporfin: one-year results of 2 randomized clinical trials—TAP report. Treatment of Age-Related Macular Degeneration with Photodynamic Therapy (TAP) Study Group. Arch Ophthalmol. 1999;117(10):1329–45.
8. Begum R, Powner MB, Hudson N, Hogg C, Jeffery G. Treatment with 670 nm light up regulates cytochrome c oxidase expression and reduces inflamma-

tion in an age-related macular degeneration model. PLoS One. 2013;8(2):e57828. https://doi.org/10.1371/journal.pone.0057828.
9. Gkotsi D, Begum R, Salt T, Lascaratos G, Hogg C, Chau K-Y, Schapira AHV, Jeffery G. Recharging mitochondrial batteries in old eyes. Near infra-red increases ATP. Exp Eye Res. 2014;122(May):50–3. https://doi.org/10.1016/j.exer.2014.02.023.
10. Merry GF, Munk MR, Dotson RS, Walker MG, Devenyi RG. Photobiomodulation reduces Drusen volume and improves visual acuity and contrast sensitivity in dry age-related macular degeneration. Acta Ophthalmol. 2017;95(4):e270–7. https://doi.org/10.1111/aos.13354.
11. Fuma S, Murase H, Kuse Y, Tsuruma K, Shimazawa M, Hara H. Photobiomodulation with 670 nm light increased phagocytosis in human retinal pigment epithelial cells. Mol Vis. 2015;21:883–92.
12. Schmidt SY, Peisch RD. Melanin concentration in normal human retinal pigment epithelium. Regional variation and age-related reduction. Invest Ophthalmol Vis Sci. 1986;27(7):1063–7.
13. Wallow IH. Long-term changes in photocoagulation burns. Dev Ophthalmol. 1981;2:318–27.
14. Wallow IH, Tso MO. Failure of formation of chorioretinal adhesions following xenon arc photocoagulation. Mod Probl Ophthalmol. 1974;12(0):189–201.
15. Lavinsky D, Sramek C, Wang J, Huie P, Dalal R, Mandel Y, Palanker D. Subvisible retinal laser therapy: titration algorithm and tissue response. Retina. 2014;34(1):87–97. https://doi.org/10.1097/IAE.0b013e3182993edc.
16. Muqit MMK, Denniss J, Nourrit V, Marcellino GR, Henson DB, Schiessl I, Stanga PE. Spatial and spectral imaging of retinal laser photocoagulation burns. Invest Ophthalmol Vis Sci. 2011;52(2):994–1002. https://doi.org/10.1167/iovs.10-6309.
17. Stefánsson E. Ocular oxygenation and the treatment of diabetic retinopathy. Surv Ophthalmol. 2006;51(4):364–80. https://doi.org/10.1016/j.survophthal.2006.04.005.
18. Early photocoagulation for diabetic retinopathy. ETDRS report number 9. Early Treatment Diabetic Retinopathy Study Research Group. Ophthalmology. 1991;98(5 Suppl):766–85.
19. Schatz H, Madeira D, McDonald HR, Johnson RN. Progressive enlargement of laser scars following grid laser photocoagulation for diffuse diabetic macular edema. Arch Ophthalmol. 1991;109(11):1549–51.
20. Ogata N, Ando A, Uyama M, Matsumura M. Expression of cytokines and transcription factors in photocoagulated human retinal pigment epithelial cells. Graefes Arch Clin Exp Ophthalmol. 2001a;239(2):87–95.
21. Ogata N, Tombran-Tink J, Jo N, Mrazek D, Matsumura M. Upregulation of pigment epithelium-derived factor after laser photocoagulation. Am J Ophthalmol. 2001b;132(3):427–9.
22. Writing Committee for the Diabetic Retinopathy Clinical Research Network, Fong DS, Strauber SF, Aiello LP, Beck RW, Callanan DG, Danis RP, et al. Comparison of the modified early treatment diabetic retinopathy study and mild macular grid laser photocoagulation strategies for diabetic macular edema. Arch Ophthalmol. 2007;125(4):469–80. https://doi.org/10.1001/archopht.125.4.469.
23. Koinzer S, Saeger M, Hesse C, Portz L, Kleemann S, Schlott K, Brinkmann R, Roider J. Correlation with OCT and histology of photocoagulation lesions in patients and rabbits. Acta Ophthalmol. 2013;91(8):e603–11. https://doi.org/10.1111/aos.12188.
24. Tode J, Richert E, Koinzer S, Klettner A, von der Burchard C, Brinkmann R, Lucius R, Roider J. Thermal stimulation of the retina reduces Bruch's membrane thickness in age related macular degeneration mouse models. Transl Vis Sci Technol. 2018;7(3):2. https://doi.org/10.1167/tvst.7.3.2.
25. Lavinsky D, Wang J, Huie P, Dalal R, Lee SJ, Lee DY, Palanker D. Nondamaging retinal laser therapy: rationale and applications to the macula. Invest Ophthalmol Vis Sci. 2016;57(6):2488–500. https://doi.org/10.1167/iovs.15-18981.
26. Paulus YM, Jain A, Gariano RF, Stanzel BV, Marmor M, Blumenkranz MS, Palanker D. Healing of retinal photocoagulation lesions. Invest Ophthalmol Vis Sci. 2008;49(12):5540–5. https://doi.org/10.1167/iovs.08-1928.
27. Marshall J, Mellerio J. Pathological development of retinal laser photocoagulations. Exp Eye Res. 1967;6(4):303–8.
28. Maeshima K, Utsugi-Sutoh N, Otani T, Kishi S. Progressive enlargement of scattered photocoagulation scars in diabetic retinopathy. Retina. 2004;24(4):507–11.
29. Sher A, Jones BW, Huie P, Paulus YM, Lavinsky D, Leung L-SS, Nomoto H, Beier C, Marc RE, Palanker D. Restoration of retinal structure and function after selective photocoagulation. J Neurosci. 2013;33(16):6800–8. https://doi.org/10.1523/JNEUROSCI.1044-12.2013.
30. Sramek C, Mackanos M, Spitler R, Leung L-S, Nomoto H, Contag CH, Palanker D. Non-damaging retinal phototherapy: dynamic range of heat shock protein expression. Invest Ophthalmol Vis Sci. 2011;52(3):1780–7. https://doi.org/10.1167/iovs.10-5917.
31. Richert E, Koinzer S, Tode J, Schlott K, Brinkmann R, Hillenkamp J, Klettner A, Roider J. Release of different cell mediators during retinal pigment epithelium regeneration following selective retina therapy. Invest Ophthalmol Vis Sci. 2018;59(3):1323–31. https://doi.org/10.1167/iovs.17-23163.
32. Del Priore LV, Glaser BM, Quigley HA, Green WR. Response of pig retinal pigment epithelium to laser photocoagulation in organ culture. Arch Ophthalmol. 1989;107(1):119–22. https://doi.org/10.1001/archopht.1989.01070010121039.

33. Roider J, Hillenkamp F, Flotte T, Birngruber R. Microphotocoagulation: selective effects of repetitive short laser pulses. Proc Natl Acad Sci U S A. 1993;90(18):8643–7. https://doi.org/10.1073/pnas.90.18.8643.
34. Roider J, Michaud NA, Flotte TJ, Birngruber R. Response of the retinal pigment epithelium to selective photocoagulation. Arch Ophthalmol. 1992;110(12):1786–92.
35. Klatt C, Saeger M, Oppermann T, Pörksen E, Treumer F, Hillenkamp J, Fritzer E, Brinkmann R, Birngruber R, Roider J. Selective retina therapy for acute central serous chorioretinopathy. Br J Ophthalmol. 2011;95(1):83–8. https://doi.org/10.1136/bjo.2009.178327.
36. Roider J, Brinkmann R, Wirbelauer C, Laqua H, Birngruber R. Subthreshold (retinal pigment epithelium) photocoagulation in macular diseases: a pilot study. Br J Ophthalmol. 2000;84(1):40–7. https://doi.org/10.1136/bjo.84.1.40.
37. Roider J, Liew SHM, Klatt C, Elsner H, Poerksen E, Hillenkamp J, Brinkmann R, Birngruber R. Selective retina therapy (SRT) for clinically significant diabetic macular edema. Graefes Arch Clin Exp Ophthalmol. 2010;248(9):1263–72. https://doi.org/10.1007/s00417-010-1356-3.
38. Koinzer S, Elsner H, Klatt C, Pörksen E, Brinkmann R, Birngruber R, Roider J. Selective retina therapy (SRT) of chronic subfoveal fluid after surgery of rhegmatogenous retinal detachment: three case reports. Graefes Arch Clin Exp Ophthalmol. 2008;246(10):1373–8. https://doi.org/10.1007/s00417-008-0860-1.
39. Guymer RH, Wu Z, Hodgson LAB, Caruso E, Brassington KH, Tindill N, Aung KZ, et al. Subthreshold nanosecond laser intervention in age-related macular degeneration: The LEAD randomized controlled clinical trial. Ophthalmology. 2019;126(6):829–38. https://doi.org/10.1016/j.ophtha.2018.09.015.
40. Brinkmann R, Hüttmann G, Rögener J, Roider J, Birngruber R, Lin CP. Origin of retinal pigment epithelium cell damage by pulsed laser irradiance in the nanosecond to microsecond time regimen. Lasers Surg Med. 2000;27(5):451–64. https://doi.org/10.1002/1096-9101(2000)27:5<451::AID-LSM1006>3.0.CO;2-1.
41. Roider J, Brinkmann R, Wirbelauer C, Laqua H, Birngruber R. Retinal sparing by selective retinal pigment epithelial photocoagulation. Arch Ophthalmol. 1999;117(8):1028–34.
42. Schuele G, Elsner H, Framme C, Roider J, Birngruber R, Brinkmann R. Optoacoustic real-time dosimetry for selective retina treatment. J Biomed Opt. 2005;10(6):064022. https://doi.org/10.1117/1.2136327.
43. Seifert E, Tode J, Pielen A, Theisen-Kunde D, Framme C, Roider J, Miura Y, Birngruber R, Brinkmann R. Selective retina therapy: toward an optically controlled automatic dosing. J Biomed Opt. 2018;23(11):1–12. https://doi.org/10.1117/1.JBO.23.11.115002.
44. Zbinden S, Kucur ŞS, Steiner P, Wolf S, Sznitman R. Automatic assessment of time-resolved OCT images for selective retina therapy. Int J Comput Assist Radiol Surg. 2016;11(6):863–71. https://doi.org/10.1007/s11548-016-1383-6.
45. Ahir A, Guo L, Hussain AA, Marshall J. Expression of metalloproteinases from human retinal pigment epithelial cells and their effects on the hydraulic conductivity of Bruch's membrane. Invest Ophthalmol Vis Sci. 2002;43(2):458–65.
46. Zhang JJ, Sun Y, Hussain AA, Marshall J. Laser-mediated activation of human retinal pigment epithelial cells and concomitant release of matrix metalloproteinases. Invest Ophthalmol Vis Sci. 2012;53(6):2928–37. https://doi.org/10.1167/iovs.11-8585.

Part V

Experimental RPE Models

17 Retinal Pigment Epithelium Cell Culture

Alexa Karina Klettner

Introduction

Retinal pigment epithelium cells (RPE) have been successfully cultivated since the 1920s [1], originally using mainly embryonic chicks as a source for the cells. Since then, the cultivation has been established for many species, following respective trends and technical abilities of the respective times. Species used include (but are not limited to) chicken [1], cat [2], frog (Xenopus laevis) [3], mice [4], rats [5], cow [6], monkey [7], pig [8], and human [9] (Table 17.1). Every model has its advantages and its drawbacks, due to inherent characteristics of the specific species, availability and handling. The preferred species should be chosen according to the investigated research question, availability and expertise of the specific investigator. The following gives a brief (by no means conclusive) overview of some of the used model species and its peculiarities. The cat, for example, was mainly fashionable in the 1980s and is hardly used nowadays [2]. An important feature of the cat is the tapetum lucidum, a reflective layer beneath the RPE, which leads to special adaptations in the RPE, e.g., RPE cells overlaying the tapetum lucidum do not contain melanin. In addition, the Bruch's membrane under the tapetum area is different in its structure and reduced in size [10]. The amphibian Xenopus laevis, on the other hand, is special in the regard that it is able to generate the whole retina, including the RPE [11]. RPE from the mouse is difficult in handling due to size and yield, however, it bears the possibility to culture RPE from genetically modified mice [12]. Porcine RPE is easily available in high amounts from slaughter houses, and its use does not need an ethical approval, as it is considered an active measure for the reduction of animal experimentation. In addition, porcine eyes are easy to handle, as their size correspond well with human eyes [13]. In fact, of all non-primate species, the pig eye resembles the human eye most closely [14] and will be discussed in more detail below. The bovine RPE is also easily obtainable from slaughter houses. However, cows, like cats, have a tapetum lucidum and, as pointed out above, the

Table 17.1 Example of species from which RPE cells have been established with a corresponding example reference

Species	Reference (example)
Chicken	Smith [1]
Cat	Stramm et al. [2]
Frog	Defoe and Easterling [3]
Mice	Gibbs and Williams [4]
Rats	Mayerson et al. [5]
Cow	Heller and Jones [6]
Pig	Chew et al. [8]
Human	Flood et al. [9]

A. K. Klettner (✉)
Department of Ophthalmology, University of Kiel, University Medical Center, Kiel, Schleswig-Holstein, Germany
e-mail: AlexaKarina.Klettner@uksh.de

A. K. Klettner, S. Dithmar (eds.), *Retinal Pigment Epithelium in Health and Disease*,
https://doi.org/10.1007/978-3-030-28384-1_17

RPE covering the tapetum lucidum is not pigmented. Theoretically, the monkey could be considered the best of all animal models for human RPE, and RPE cell culture have been established from these animals [7], however, it is very difficult to obtain for obvious reasons. Finally, human RPE can be considered the best model, however, its availability is limited, and will be discussed below in more detail.

Challenges of RPE Cell Culture

The most important issue considering cell culture is whether the featured cell actually resembles its *in-vivo* counterpart. The question what actually makes up an RPE cell is still debated in the literature. While a signature set of 154 genes has been proposed that are supposed to distinguish RPE cells from other cell types [15], it has been pointed out that an RPE "standard" has be correlated to species and life stage [16]. The RPE *in situ* is a highly differentiated, polarized, pigmented, monolayered epithelial cell that is basally situated on a Bruch's membrane and apically in closec connection with photoreceptor outer segments. In addition, RPE cells are highly "sociable", being in close connection with their neighbor cells, connected via tight junctions and creating the outer blood-retinal-barrier; in addition, they are usually post-mitotic. In this setting, they perform their tasks, such as the recycling of the visual pigment, phagocytosis of photoreceptor outer segments, secrete growth factors, and so on [17].

However, it is inherent to cell culture that in the course of preparation, all that what is typical for an RPE cells is discontinued. An RPE cell to be put in culture needs to be dissociated from the Bruch's membrane (and separated from the photoreceptor outer segments) and dissociated from its neighboring RPE cells, rendering it a single-cell without any connections to a substrate, a tissue or other cells. Inherent to RPE cell culture is a return to a more dedifferentiated state in order to be able to divide and multiply. A trans-differentiation to a mesenchymal phenotype is usual consequence of singling of the RPE [18–20]. Melanin pigmentation is generally lost during the division [9]. The epithelial state has to be regained in culture, but the capability of RPE cells to mature back into it has been described to be limited. Indeed, after each passage of RPE cells, the power of the RPE cells to build up an epithelium is diminished and loss of differentiation during passaging can be seen [21] (Fig. 17.1). Epithelial-mesenchymal transformation is well described in RPE cell culture, and cells of early passage (or population doublings) are needed to achieve acceptable differentiation. The question, however, what can be considered an acceptable differentiation depends on model system used as well as on the research question asked. Generally, differentiation is associated with a pigmented, confluent layer of cobble-stone appearance, for barrier function expression of tight junction proteins and a high transepithelial resistance (TER), and, for polarization, an apical expression of the Na+/K+ ATPase (Table 17.2).

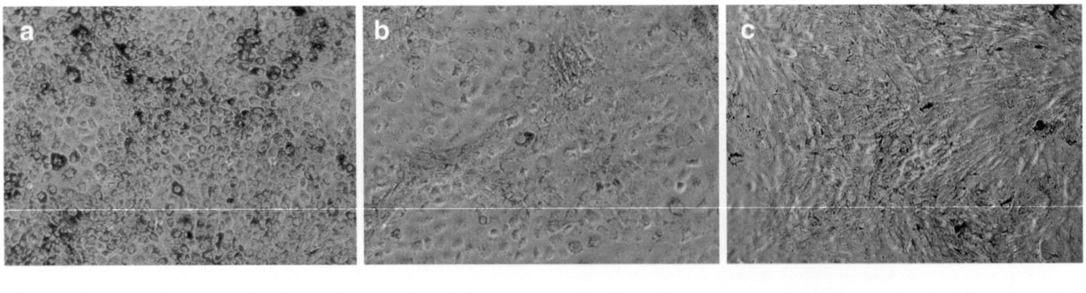

Fig. 17.1 Morphology of primary RPE cells (of porcine origin) at (**a**) passage 0, (**b**) passage 1, (**c**) passage 2. Cobblestone appearance and pigmentation is lost during the course of passaging. Magnification: ×10

Table 17.2 Differentiation marker for cultured RPE cells

Feature	Marker
Morphology	Pigmentation
	Cobble stone appearance
Barrier formation	Tight junction proteins (ZO-1, occludin, claudins)
	Transepithelal resistance
Polarization	Microvilli (apical)
	Na+/K+ ATPase (apical)
	Organelle distribution
	Cytokine secretion
Retinoid cycle	Expression of RPE65
	Expression of 11-cis retinol dehydrogenase
	Expression lecithin retinol acyl transferase
	Expression of CRALBP
Phagocytosis	Uptake of photoreceptor outer segment fragments

Heterogeneity of RPE Cell Culture

To make things even more complicated, RPE cultures have been described to be highly heterogenic [7, 22–24] (Fig. 17.2a, b). Indeed, despite a relatively homogenous appearance, even RPE cells *in situ* have been shown to be heterogenic [25]. Topographical heterogeneity depicts the differences between RPE in the posterior part of the eye (the macula), and the peripheral part of the eye. Posterior RPE differs in its growth potential, lysosomal activities and ion pump potential [25]. Cells in the periphery also have a higher capacity to proliferate compared to the central RPE [26]. It has to be kept in mind when working with primary cells that peripheral cells can outgrow central cells in cell culture [26]. Peripheral and central RPE cells also differ in their expression of cell cycle proteins and of markers of senescence, with the central protein showing elevation of mTOR [26]. Difference can also be found in the nuclei. Apart from measurable differences in nuclei densities [21], RPE cells can present as multi-nuclear cells [27], with multinuclear cells found mainly in the perifovea and periphery [28]. Also, lipofuscin accumulation shows regional differences with the highest concentration found in the perifoveal region [29]. Both multi-nucleation and lipofuscin accumulation reflect the photoreceptor rod/cone topography, implying that RPE heterogeneity at least in these features is connected to the different requirements of photoreceptors in these areas. In addition, RPE cell size is dependent on location, with foveal RPE cells being significantly smaller than those of the perifovea or the periphery [29]. In cell culture, heterogeneity due to location has to be considered, as cells in the center of a culture behave differently from cells in the periphery, showing different migratory behavior and different maturation times. Cells in the periphery may have a delayed formation of tight junctions [30].

Cell Lines

Cell lines are convenient in research, as they have a better availability and are usually less heterogeneity than primary cells, which are generally from genetically divers donors and laborious to prepare. An early immortal RPE cell line to be introduced into the literature was the rat RPE-J line which was created by SV40 infection [31]. Expansion of this cell line occurs at the permissive temperature of 33 °C, while differentiation can be achieved by culture at 40 °C in the presence of retinoic acid. The RPE cell line displays an epithelial morphology, lacks pigmentation, but develops apical microvilli and is capable of phagocytosis [31, 32]. The development of microvilli can be enhanced by the transfection of ezrin [33]. The polarization, however, is not fully developed as the Na+/K+-ATPase can be detected on all surfaces of the cells. Also, vital proteins for the retinoid cycle such as cellular retinaldehyde-binding protein (CRALBP), RPE65, 11-cis-retinol dehydrogenase or lecithin retinol acyl transferase (LRAT), cannot be detected in RPE-J cells [34].

Spontaneously arising cells lines from cultured human RPE have already been described in a pioneering study from the 1970s [35], but have not been broadly utilized. An early immortal human RPE cell line to be described was D407 [36]. A transformed cell line from a 12-year old male donor, this cell line has a

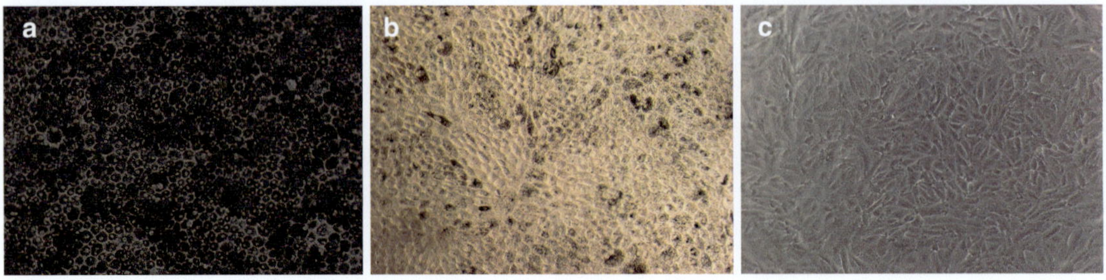

Fig. 17.2 Different levels of pigmentation in RPE cells. Passage 0 primary porcine RPE cells with (**a**) strong and (**b**) light pigmentation. As comparison, a confluent ARPE-19 culture of high passage (**c**) is shown. Magnification ×10

triploid karyotype and submetacentric marker chromosome [36]. Unpigmented, it shows classical cobblestone morphology and exhibits a classical epithelial cytoskeleton, but fails to develop a proper polarization or transepithelial resistance [36, 37]. Proteins of the retinoid cycle are partially expressed, such as CRALBP or RPE65, but not LRAT and are not displaying a functional retinoid metabolism [36, 38, 39]. Vascular endothelial growth factor (VEGF) is secreted by D407 and can be induced by hypoxia [37].

Also, other RPE cell lines are described in the literature, e. g. from mouse RPE, both spontaneously risen [40] or created by transfection with papilloma virus [41], or new human cells lines, both fetal [42] and neonatal [43].

Even though other cell lines have been described and used in RPE research, by far the most common used for experimental studies is the cell line ARPE-19 (for comparison, D407 has currently 87 hits in PubMed, RPE-J has 46 hits and ARPE-19 has 1616 hits). Originally described by Dunn and colleagues [44], it was established from the retinal pigment epithelium of a male, 19-year old donor. The cell line arose spontaneously and was selected for an epithelial phenotype by selective trypsination. The original ARPE-19 cell line was described to express the mRNA of several RPE markers (such as RPE65 or CRALBP) and to be able to differentiate in a polarized mono-cell layer, even though complete polarization was not achieved. The karyotype of the cells was described to be normal, with a deletion in the long arm of chromosome 8 and an addition in the long arm of chromosome 19. The original cell was described to be pigmented, even though pigmentation declined during passage (Fig. 17.2c). The transepithelial resistance was described to be low compared to primary RPE cells [44]. The cells are able to perform phagocytosis of photoreceptor outer segments [32].

Early, it could be seen that the properties of ARPE-19 cells were not uniform but changed during sub-passage and different culture conditions, making comparison of results obtained with ARPE-19 cells of different research group challenging (e.g. [45]). Later passages of ARPE-19 cells were described to have lost their RPE-like morphology, such as cobblestone appearance, and to display strong heterogeneity in culture [45]. In addition, ARPE-19 cell cultures have been shown to contain mortal as well as immortal cells, with immortal cells comprising as much as 73% of the cells of a culture [46]. Also, the karyotype has been changing in the course of the sub-cultivation that happened since Dunn et al. first described the cell line. In addition to translocations, aneuploidies have been detected, e.g. monosomy 16, trisomy 11 or trisomy 18, which appear in heterogenic cell cultures together with cell displaying a normal karyotype. Moreover, different changes can be found in different laboratories, further emphazising the heterogeneity of sub-cultured ARPE-19 cells [47]. It was repeatedly shown that the properties of ARPE-19 cells are highly dependent on culture conditions of the cells (which holds also true, for that matter, for primary RPE cells (e.g. [48])), such as medium choice [45], serum concentration [49], glucose concentrations [50, 51], or substrate offered [52].

The original medium for ARPE-19 cultivation was a mixture of DMEM and F12 [44]. However, later studies suggested the use of other media, such as DMEM without F12 [50] or other medium mixtures [45] which may or may not include additional supplements for more differentiated ARPE-19 cells.

Concerning the substrate to grow the cells on, several have been tested, either resembling native extracellular matrix proteins or substrates as provided by manufacturer's cell culture ware. In a gene analysis comparing the expression profiles of RPE cells, a culture of ARPE-19 cells on plastic proved to be most similar to the native RPE, suggesting that under these conditions, the cells create their own, close-to *in vivo* basement membrane [52]. However, generally, transwell filters are the preferred substrate of ARPE-19 cells as they allow cell polarization (see below).

The gene expression patterns of ARPE-19 cells have been investigated and compared to native RPE or sub-cultured primary RPE, displaying significant different expression profiles [15, 53, 54]. Especially, genes concerning transporter activities, growth factors, extra-cellular matrix remodeling, retinoic acid metabolism, tight junction formation and melanogenesis were reduced compared to native RPE [15]. Of interest, the gene related to phagocytosis, angiogenesis or apoptosis did not show any clear difference in their expression compared to sub-cultured human RPE cells [53]. Not surprisingly, these expression profiles are dependent on culture conditions and can be optimize to more closely resemble native RPE cells by appropriate cultivation protocols [52, 54].

Much effort has been made in order to create well differentiated ARPE-19 cells, with best results being achieved by cultivation of low passage ARPE-19 cells over an extended period of time (2–4 weeks) on transwell filters in low serum [37, 50, 54, 55]. Both pyruvate and glucose have also been discussed as factors for differentiation [50], and other possible factors for differentiation are also found in the literature [56]. Among the characteristics displayed by differentiated ARPE-19 cells are the expression of RPE65 and CRALBP, pigmentation, polarized cell structure, apical microvilli, ability to phagocytose photoreceptor outer segments, assembly of tight junctions, and secretion of VEGF [55]. However, no differentiation protocol has managed to achieve a high transepithelial resistance, which is characteristic for in vivo RPE [16]. TER of ARPE-19 cells has been mostly described to reach about 30–40 Ωcm^2 [37, 44, 45, 57], sometimes reaching up to about 100 Ωcm^2 (e.g. [44, 58]), compared to more than 500 Ω/cm^2 measured for fetal cultured RPE [37, 57, 59] or 200 Ω/cm^2 for native fetal RPE [60]. In addition, ARPE-19 cells do not express the major human claudin (a tight junction protein) claudin-19 [16]. While ARPE-19 monolayers have been used for studies in barrier function (e.g. [58]), ARPE-19 cells, even when well differentiated, are generally not recommend for barrier studies [55, 57].

Primary Cells

Human Fetal RPE Cells

RPE cell cultures obtained from fetal RPE are generally considered to be the most functional RPE cell cultures and present the phenotype of healthy RPE most closely. They are preferably used when highly differentiated RPE cells are needed, as when investigating barrier function [16], retinoid visual cycle [61, 62] or RPE metabolism [63]. RPE cells derived from fetal RPE can overcome some of the obstacles researchers face concerning de-differentiation, loss of pigmentation or low TER, given that the appropriate culture conditions are chosen. Several protocols for fetal human RPE cultures can be found in the literature, differing in substrate, gestation week of the fetal eyes, medium used, or preparation techniques [48, 59, 61, 64, 65]. For example, gestation times of the eyes of the fetuses used varied between 10 and 16 weeks [66], 16–18 weeks [15], 17–22 weeks [67] 18–20 weeks [59] or 21 weeks [48]. Methods include the use of media with various types of supplements, serum-free formulations, calcium-free cell selection, preparation of isolated RPE sheets, or pigmented spheroids [37, 48, 66]. Common to all conditions, however, is a cultivation on a permeable substrate, allowing a polarized differentiation over a time course of several weeks.

An (quite literally) obvious characteristic of RPE cells is its dark pigmentation, which, unfortunately, is usually lost in cell cultures. Similar to other RPE cell cultures, human fetal RPE cells lose their pigment during division, but, in strong contrast to cell lines or adult RPE, they are capable of de novo synthesis of pigment and may regain pigmentation after confluence [57, 59, 65], giving them a classical RPE appearance. In addition, the cells exhibit a strong polarization, as seen in the development of microvilli on the apical side and the correct distribution of organelles [65]. As a widely accepted marker, the Na+/K+-ATPase can be found on the apical surface of differentiated human fetal RPE cells [48, 65].

More important than appearance is function. And indeed, human fetal RPE cells can develop highly differentiated barrier function. Generally, the barrier function is measured in the culture systems as assessed by transepithelial resistance. In strong contrast to RPE cell lines, which TER usually does not exceed 40 Ωcm^2, human fetal RPE cell cultures can develop TER above 400 Ωcm^2 and may reach even 1000 Ωcm^2 or more, which in fact is exceeding its natural tissue TER [16, 37, 57, 60]. In addition, the secretion of the growth factors VEGF and Pigment epithelium derived factor (PEDF) is polarized to the appropriate compartments in human fetal RPE cells [37, 57, 59], in concordance with RPE-choroid explant cultures [68]. The results concerning the amount of VEGF secreted, however, is conflicting with the absolute expression of VEGF in human fetal RPE described to be higher [57] or lower [37] then in ARPE-19. Similar to what is found for cell lines, the differentiation and development of the proper barrier (and other) functions is highly dependent on the medium used and the culture conditions inflicted on the cells [48]. E.g., high glucose has been described to be important for the development of proper barrier function or the expression of RPE65 [48, 65].

The RPE cells are highly important for the visual cycle, the recycling of the 11-cis-retinal. Human fetal RPE cells have been shown to express the proteins needed to fulfil this function, such as RPE65, CRALBP, LRAT and are able to convert all-trans-retinal into all-trans-retinol [57, 61]. Indeed, when studying visual cycle related topics, the ability of the RPE to secrete 11-cis retinal from its apical side has been considered vital and not described in any cell line [61].

While the highly differentiated phenotype of human fetal RPE cells makes them a highly valuable model, it has to be considered, however, that, in addition to ethical concerns about using the tissue of aborted fetuses, they do not represent adult RPE. Adult and fetal RPE differ in their transcriptome [15] and in their profile of trophic factor secretion [67]. Human fetal RPE displayed higher concentrations of VEGF, brain derived growth factor (BDNF), PEDF and lower concentrations of leukemia inhibitory factor (LIF), basic fibroblast growth factor (bFGF) and nerve growth factor (NGF). This correlates with a better ability of fetal RPE cells to support retina survival in an experimental system using porcine retina [67]. As the functional (and nonfunctional) RPE in humans is adult, human fetal RPE cells may be "overachieving", not representing the in vivo situation of the adult situation. This correlates with the life-stage specific definitions of RPE that have been suggested [16].

Adult RPE Cells

Adult Human RPE Cells

An obstacle when using adult human RPE cells is the prolonged post-mortem time before preparation can be conducted, especially when compared to animal donors. The plating efficiency of the cells (the amount of cells actually attaching and dividing) is dependent on the post-mortem time, leading to a reduced yield with increased time [9]. In addition, increased age of the donor is correlated with poor growth characteristics of the cells [9, 35]. Nevertheless, adult human RPE cells can obtain a highly polarized structure and high TER corresponding to *in vivo* measures [69].

Also, they can display a strong and polarized secretion of VEGF, with more VEGF secreted basally than apically [70]. However, complete polarization is still difficult to achieve, with Na+/K+-ATPase found both at the apical and basal membrane, though a stronger expression can be assumed for the apical side [69]. The ability for the retinoid cycle is usually lost in adult human RPE cells, most likely to enzymatic harvesting (trypsination) of the cells [39]. Another problem of adult human RPE may be a general dedifferentiation after long term culture, which is not seen with fetal human RPE [71].

Adult Porcine RPE Cells

Obstacles such as postmortem time and age of donors can be avoided when using porcine adult RPE cells [8, 72, 73]. As outlined above, the porcine eye resembles that of a human, though it has to be kept in mind that it does not contain a macula or fovea. As porcine eyes can be obtained from a slaughter house, the post-mortem time can be controlled and a great variation in donor age avoided. RPE cells obtained from porcine eyes resemble RPE cultures of other species, including a limited capability of cell divisions and dependence on substrate on which they are grown [73]. Also, porcine primary RPE cells display a limited life time in cell culture [73]. Adult porcine RPE cells are capable of phagocytosing photoreceptor outer segments [74–76] and express the visual cycle protein RPE65 [76]. Porcine RPE cells can be polarized in culture and are capable of co-transporting H+ and lactate over the barrier [77], display a TER of about >200 Ω/cm^2 [68, 76, 78] and show an apical expression of the Na+/K+-ATPase when sufficiently cultured [76]. In addition, they show a polarized secretion of VEGF [68, 79]. Thus, porcine adult RPE cells can be considered an alternative to adult human RPE cell culture.

Co-Culture Systems

The major drawback of any cell culture, independent of its origin, is the lack of the three-dimensional interaction with its surrounding cells and tissues. In order to address this, organ specific explant cultures can be generated (see the appropriate chapter of this book). On the cell culture level, three dimensional (3D) cultures or so-called retinas-on-a-chip can add complexity to the *in vitro*-systems. Currently, microfluidic organ-on-a-chip systems are developed which are supposed to mimic organ-specific characteristics on a micro scale, enabling a vasculature-like perfusion. In theory, this system combines various different cell types in a stable and controllable microenvironment, recreating a structure that allows a multiplicity of cell-cell and cell-matrix interaction in a 3D environment [80]. The development of retina-on-a-chip systems for the retinal pigment epithelium is still at the beginning.

The easiest way of 3D culture is the use of retinal pigment epithelium cells and endothelial cells, separated by a porous membrane, as has been done for ARPE-19 and Human Umbilical Vein Endothelial Cells (HUVEC) [81, 82]. However, these cultures may face difficulties, as media components may not be compatible between the cell types and cell death and/or overgrowth of one respective cell type by the other can be observed. In addition, the differentiation of the ARPE-19 cells may be questionable [81]. It should be kept in mind that the use of ARPE-19 cells has its limits as described above. In addition, HUVEC cells are macrovascular while choroidal endothelium consists of microvascular cells which differ in their properties [83, 84]. Other 3D systems use cells closer to the *in vivo* situation, for example human RPE cells and a monkey choroidal endothelial cell line [85]. Using a polycaprolactone (PCL)-gelatin electrospun scaffold, both cell types of the co-culture displayed densely confluent layers, and phagocytic ability as well as cytokine secretion was shown [85]. However, a full assessment of differentiation was not conducted.

One more complex example of a 3D culture of RPE cells describes a microfluidic system using a fibrin-matrix, which also consists of fibroblasts, to represent choroidal vessels [86]. In this system, also ARPE-19 cells as RPE cells and HUVEC were used. The ARPE-19 cells formed a stable monolayer, while the HUVEC cells generated a network of vessel-like structures, which could be used to investigate angiogenic processes in vitro. The RPE cells proved to show stable barrier functions and highly polarized secretion of growth factors VEGF and PEDF, however, the secretion was mostly detected apically, while generally, VEGF is preferable secreted on the basal side [68, 70].

A different approach uses parallel compartments which are interconnected by a grid of microgrooves, which allows contact between the cells, made of a polydimethylsiloxane slab, defining the compartments and a glass chip containing the microgrooves. In addition, electrodes have been added to the glass chip to evaluate the transepithelial resistance [87]. In this system, a co-culture of ARPE-19 cells, a primary human retinal endothelial cells and the neuroblastoma cell line SHSY-5Y was used and differentiation was validated using transepithelial measurements, expression of tight junction proteins and, in case of SHSY-5Y, neuronal markers [87]. Taken together, the development of 3D interacting system of RPE cells and the underlying choroid and the overlying neuronal cells is an exciting new path on the development of more sophisticated cell cultures which needs to be developed further. However, it should be kept in mind that these highly sophisticated models are not suitable for high throughput or high yield experimentation and limited to specific research questions, which require this high complexity of interaction.

Conclusion

The cell culture of the retinal pigment epithelium is a widely used model to study the function of these cells, which has been established from many different species to model for many different research questions. The most appropriate model has to be chosen depending on the research question asked. Caution is advised when using cell lines and it is recommended to verify the differentiation of the cells in the aspect that is going to be studied. Regarding interaction with other cell types and the surrounding tissue, 3D and microfluidic models may offer new and exciting opportunities in the future.

References

1. Smith D. The pigmented epithelium of the embryo chicks eye studied in vivo and in vitro. John Hopkins Hosp Bull. 1920;31:239–46.
2. Stramm LE, Haskins ME, McGovern MM, Aguirre GD. Tissue culture of cat retinal pigment epithelium. Exp Eye Res. 1983;36:91–101.
3. Defoe DM, Easterling KC. Reattachment of retinas to cultured pigment epithelial monolayers from Xenopus laevis. Invest Ophthalmol Vis Sci. 1994;35:2466–76.
4. Gibbs D, Williams DS. Isolation and culture of primary mouse retinal pigmented epithelial cells. Adv Exp Med Biol. 2003;533:347–52.
5. Mayerson PL, Hall MO, Clark V, Abrams T. An improved method for isolation and culture of rat retinal pigment epithelial cells. Invest Ophthalmol Vis Sci. 1985;26:1599–609.
6. Heller J, Jones P. Purification of bovine retinal pigment epithelial cells by dissociation in calcium free buffers and centrifugation in Ficoll density gradients followed by "recovery" in tissue culture. Exp Eye Res. 1980;30:481–7.
7. Matsumoto B, Guérin CJ, Anderson DH. Cytoskeletal redifferentiation of feline, monkey, and human RPE cells in culture. Invest Ophthalmol Vis Sci. 1990;31:879–89.
8. Chew EC, Liew CT, Chew SB, Lee JC, Hou HJ, Yam HF, Ho PC, Ip SM. The growth and behaviour of pig retinal pigment epithelial cells in culture. In Vivo. 1993;7:425–9.
9. Flood MT, Gouras P, Kjeldbye H. Growth characteristics and ultrastructure of human retinal pigment epithelium in vitro. Invest Ophthalmol Vis Sci. 1980;19:1309–20.
10. Braekevelt CR. Retinal epithelial fine structure in the domestic cat (Felis catus). Anat Histol Embryol. 1990;19:58–66.
11. Araki M. Regeneration of the amphibian retina: role of tissue interaction and related signaling molecules on RPE transdifferentiation. Dev Growth Differ. 2007;49:109–20.
12. Koinzer S, Reinecke K, Herdegen T, Roider J, Klettner A. Oxidative stress induces biphasic ERK1/2 activation in the RPE with distinct effects on cell survival at early and late activation. Curr Eye Res. 2015;40:853–7.
13. Sanchez I, Martin R, Ussa F, Fernandez-Bueno I. The parameters of the porcine eyeball. Graefes Arch Clin Exp Ophthalmol. 2011;249:475–82.
14. Middleton S. Porcine ophthalmology. Vet Clin North Am Food Anim Pract. 2010;26:557–72.
15. Strunnikova NV, Maminishkis A, Barb JJ, Wang F, Zhi C, Sergeev Y, Chen W, Edwards AO, Stambolian

D, Abecasis G, Swaroop A, Munson PJ, Miller SS. Transcriptome analysis and molecular signature of human retinal pigment epithelium. Hum Mol Genet. 2010;19:2468–86.
16. Rizzolo LJ. Barrier properties of cultured retinal pigment epithelium. Exp Eye Res. 2014;126:16–26.
17. Strauss O. The retinal pigment epithelium in visual function. Physiol Rev. 2005;85:845–81.
18. Grisanti S, Guidry C. Transdifferentiation of retinal pigment epithelial cells from epithelial to mesenchymal phenotype. Invest Ophthalmol Vis Sci. 1995;36:391–405.
19. Kuriyama F, Ueda Y, Araki M. Complete reconstruction of the retinal laminar structure from a cultured retinal pigment epithelium is triggered by altered tissue interaction and promoted by overlaid extracellular matrices. Dev Neurobiol. 2009;69:950–8.
20. Tamiya S, Liu L, Kaplan HJ. Epithelial-mesenchymal transition and proliferation of retinal pigment epithelial cells initiated upon loss of cell-cell contact. Invest Ophthalmol Vis Sci. 2010;51:2755–63.
21. Sonoi R, Kim MH, Yamada K, Kino-Oka M. Phenotypic heterogeneity of human retinal pigment epithelial cells in passaged cell populations. Biosci Bioeng. 2017;124:227–33.
22. Burke JM. Epithelial phenotype and the RPE: is the answer blowing in the Wnt? Prog Retin Eye Res. 2008;27:579–95.
23. Burke JM, Skumatz CM, Irving PE, McKay BS. Phenotypic heterogeneity of retinal pigment epithelial cells in vitro and in situ. Exp Eye Res. 1996;62:63–73.
24. McKay BS, Irving PE, Skumatz CM, Burke JM. Cell-cell adhesion molecules and the development of an epithelial phenotype in cultured human retinal pigment epithelial cells. Exp Eye Res. 1997;65:661–71.
25. Burke JM, Hjelmeland LM. Mosaicism of the retinal pigment epithelium: seeing the small picture. Mol Interv. 2005;5:241 9.
26. Kokkinopoulos I, Shahabi G, Colman A, Jeffery G. Mature peripheral RPE cells have an intrinsic capacity to proliferate; a potential regulatory mechanism for age-related cell loss. PLoS One. 2011;6:e18921.
27. Ts'o MO, Friedman E. The retinal pigment epithelium. I. Comparative histology. Arch Ophthalmol. 1967;78:641–9.
28. Starnes AC, Huisingh C, McGwin G Jr, Sloan KR, Ablonczy Z, Smith RT, Curcio CA, Ach T. Multinucleate retinal pigment epithelium cells of the human macula exhibit a characteristic and highly specific distribution. Vis Neurosci. 2016;33:e001.
29. Ach T, Huisingh C, McGwin G Jr, Messinger JD, Zhang T, Bentley MJ, Gutierrez DB, Ablonczy Z, Smith RT, Sloan KR, Curcio CA. Quantitative autofluorescence and cell density maps of the human retinal pigment epithelium. Invest Ophthalmol Vis Sci. 2014;55:4832–41.
30. Sonoi R, Kim MH, Kino-Oka M. Facilitation of uniform maturation of human retinal pigment epithelial cells through collective movement in culture. J Biosci Bioeng. 2016;121:220–6.
31. Nabi IR, Mathews AP, Cohen-Gould L, Gundersen D, Rodriguez-Boulan E. Immortalization of polarized rat retinal pigment epithelium. J Cell Sci. 1993;104:37–49.
32. Finnemann SC, Bonilha VL, Marmorstein AD, Rodriguez-Boulan E. Phagocytosis of rod outer segments by retinal pigment epithelial cells requires alpha(v)beta5 integrin for binding but not for internalization. Proc Natl Acad Sci U S A. 1997;94:12932–7.
33. Bonilha VL, Finnemann SC, Rodriguez-Boulan E. Ezrin promotes morphogenesis of apical microvilli and basal infoldings in retinal pigment epithelium. J Cell Biol. 1999;147:1533–48.
34. West KA, Yan L, Miyagi M, Crabb JS, Marmorstein AD, Marmorstein L, Crabb JW. Proteome survey of proliferating and differentiating rat RPE-J cells. Exp Eye Res. 2001;73:479–91.
35. Mannagh J, Arya DV, Irvine AR Jr. Tissue culture of human retinal pigment epithelium. Invest Ophthalmol. 1973;12:52–64.
36. Davis AA, Bernstein PS, Bok D, Turner J, Nachtigal M, Hunt RC. A human retinal pigment epithelial cell line that retains epithelial characteristics after prolonged culture. Invest Ophthalmol Vis Sci. 1995;36:955–64.
37. Geisen P, McColm JR, King BM, Hartnett ME. Characterization of barrier properties and inducible VEGF expression of several types of retinal pigment epithelium in medium-term culture. Curr Eye Res. 2006;31:739–48.
38. Lee H, Chung H, Arnouk H, Lamoke F, Hunt RC, Hrushesky WJ, Wood PA, Lee SH, Jahng WJ. Cleavage of the retinal pigment epithelium-specific protein RPE65 under oxidative stress. Int J Biol Macromol. 2010;47:104–8.
39. von Recum HA, Okano T, Kim SW, Bernstein PS. Maintenance of retinoid metabolism in human retinal pigment epithelium cell culture. Exp Eye Res. 1999;69:97–107.
40. Chen M, Muckersie E, Robertson M, Fraczek M, Forrester JV, Xu H. Characterization of a spontaneous mouse retinal pigment epithelial cell line B6-RPE07. Invest Ophthalmol Vis Sci. 2008;49:3699–706.
41. Catanuto P, Espinosa-Heidmann D, Pereira-Simon S, Sanchez P, Salas P, Hernandez E, Cousins SW, Elliot SJ. Mouse retinal pigmented epithelial cell lines retain their phenotypic characteristics after transfection with human papilloma virus: a new tool to further the study of RPE biology. Exp Eye Res. 2009;88:99–105.
42. Shao Z, Wang H, Zhou X, Guo B, Gao X, Xiao Z, Liu M, Sha J, Jiang C, Luo Y, Liu Z, Li S. Spontaneous generation of a novel foetal human retinal pigment epithelium (RPE) cell line available for investigation on phagocytosis and morphogenesis. Cell Prolif. 2017;50:12386.
43. Najafabadi HS, Soheili ZS, Ganji SM. Behavior of a spontaneously arising human retinal pigment epithelial cell line cultivated on thin alginate film. J Ophthalmic Vis Res. 2015;10:286–94.

44. Dunn KC, Aotaki-Keen AE, Putkey FR, Hjelmeland LM. ARPE-19, a human retinal pigment epithelial cell line with differentiated properties. Exp Eye Res. 1996;62:155–69.
45. Luo Y, Zhuo Y, Fukuhara M, Rizzolo LJ. Effects of culture conditions on heterogeneity and the apical junctional complex of the ARPE-19 cell line. Invest Ophthalmol Vis Sci. 2006;47:3644–55.
46. Kozlowski MR. The ARPE-19 cell line: mortality status and utility in macular degeneration research. Curr Eye Res. 2015;40:501–9.
47. Fasler-Kan E, Aliu N, Wunderlich K, Ketterer S, Ruggiero S, Berger S, Meyer P. The retinal pigment epithelial cell line (ARPE-19) displays mosaic structural chromosomal aberrations. Methods Mol Biol. 2018;1745:305–14.
48. Hu J, Bok D. A cell culture medium that supports the differentiation of human retinal pigment epithelium into functionally polarized monolayers. Mol Vis. 2000;7:14–9.
49. Tian J, Ishibashi K, Honda S, Boylan SA, Hjelmeland LM, Handa JT. The expression of native and cultured human retinal pigment epithelial cells grown in different culture conditions. Br J Ophthalmol. 2005;89:1510–7.
50. Ahmado A, Carr AJ, Vugler AA, Semo M, Gias C, Lawrence JM, Chen LL, Chen FK, Turowski P, da Cruz L, Coffey PJ. Induction of differentiation by pyruvate and DMEM in the human retinal pigment epithelium cell line ARPE-19. Invest Ophthalmol Vis Sci. 2011;52:7148–59.
51. Heimsath EG Jr, Unda R, Vidro E, Muniz A, Villazana-Espinoza ET, Tsin A. ARPE-19 cell growth and cell functions in euglycemic culture media. Curr Eye Res. 2006;31:1073–80.
52. Tian J, Ishibashi K, Handa JT. The expression of native and cultured RPE grown on different matrices. Physiol Genomics. 2004;17:170–82.
53. Cai H, Del Priore LV. Gene expression profile of cultured adult compared to immortalized human RPE. Mol Vis. 2006;12:1–14.
54. Samuel W, Jaworski C, Postnikova OA, Kutty RK, Duncan T, Tan LX, Poliakov E, Lakkaraju A, Redmond TM. Appropriately differentiated ARPE-19 cells regain phenotype and gene expression profiles similar to those of native RPE cells. Mol Vis. 2017;23:60–89.
55. Lynn SA, Keeling E, Dewing JM, Johnston DA, Page A, Cree AJ, Tumbarello DA, Newman TA, Lotery AJ, Ratnayaka JA. A convenient protocol for establishing a human cell culture model of the outer retina. F1000Res. 2018;7:1107.
56. Hazim RA, Volland S, Yen A, Burgess BL, Williams DS. Rapid differentiation of the human RPE cell line, ARPE-19, induced by nicotinamide. Exp Eye Res. 2019;179:18–24.
57. Ablonczy Z, Dahrouj M, Tang PH, Liu Y, Sambamurti K, Marmorstein AD, Crosson CE. Human retinal pigment epithelium cells as functional models for the RPE in vivo. Invest Ophthalmol Vis Sci. 2011;52:8614–20.
58. Mannermaa E, Reinisalo M, Ranta VP, Vellonen KS, Kokki H, Saarikko A, Kaarniranta K, Urtti A. Filter-cultured ARPE-19 cells as outer blood-retinal barrier model. Eur J Pharm Sci. 2010;40:289–96.
59. Maminishkis A, Chen S, Jalickee S, Banzon T, Shi G, Wang FE, Ehalt T, Hammer JA, Miller SS. Confluent monolayers of cultured human fetal retinal pigment epithelium exhibit morphology and physiology of native tissue. Invest Ophthalmol Vis Sci. 2006;47:3612–24.
60. Quinn RH, Miller SS. Ion transport mechanisms in native human retinal pigment epithelium. Invest Ophthalmol Vis Sci. 1992;33:3513–27.
61. Hu J, Bok D. Culture of highly differentiated human retinal pigment epithelium for analysis of the polarized uptake, processing, and secretion of retinoids. Methods Mol Biol. 2010;652:55–73.
62. Hu J, Bok D. The use of cultured human fetal retinal pigment epithelium in studies of the classical retinoid visual cycle and retinoid-based disease processes. Exp Eye Res. 2014;126:46–50.
63. Adijanto J, Philp NJ. Cultured primary human fetal retinal pigment epithelium (hfRPE) as a model for evaluating RPE metabolism. Exp Eye Res. 2014;126:77–84.
64. Song MK, Lui GM. Propagation of fetal human RPE cells: preservation of original culture morphology after serial passage. J Cell Physiol. 1990;143:196–203.
65. Sonoda S, Spee C, Barron E, Ryan SJ, Kannan R, Hinton DR. A protocol for the culture and differentiation of highly polarized human retinal pigment epithelial cells. Nat Protoc. 2009;4:662–73.
66. Gamm DM, Melvan JN, Shearer RL, Pinilla I, Sabat G, Svendsen CN, Wright LS. A novel serum-free method for culturing human prenatal retinal pigment epithelial cells. Invest Ophthalmol Vis Sci. 2008;49:788–99.
67. Kolomeyer AM, Sugino IK, Zarbin MA. Characterization of conditioned media collected from cultured adult versus fetal retinal pigment epithelial cells. Invest Ophthalmol Vis Sci. 2011;52:5973–86.
68. Klettner A, Kaya L, Flach J, Lassen J, Treumer F, Roider J. Basal and apical regulation of VEGF-A and placenta growth factor in the RPE/choroid and primary RPE. Mol Vis. 2015;21:736–48.
69. Hu JG, Gallemore RP, Bok D, Lee AY, Frambach DA. Localization of NaK ATPase on cultured human retinal pigment epithelium. Invest Ophthalmol Vis Sci. 1994;35:3582–8.
70. Blaauwgeers HG, Holtkamp GM, Rutten H, Witmer AN, Koolwijk P, Partanen TA, Alitalo K, Kroon ME, Kijlstra A, van Hinsbergh VW, Schlingemann RO. Polarized vascular endothelial growth factor secretion by human retinal pigment epithelium and localization of vascular endothelial growth factor receptors on the inner choriocapillaris. Evidence for a trophic paracrine relation. Am J Pathol. 1999;155:421–8.
71. Stanzel BV, Blumenkranz MS, Binder S, Marmor MF. Longterm cultures of the aged human RPE do

not maintain epithelial morphology and high transepithelial resistance. Graefes Arch Clin Exp Ophthalmol. 2012;250:313–5.
72. Klettner A, Roider J. Comparison of bevacizumab, ranibizumab, and pegaptanib in vitro: efficiency and possible additional pathways. Invest Ophthalmol Vis Sci. 2008;49:4523–7.
73. Wiencke AK, Kiilgaard JF, Nicolini J, Bundgaard M, Röpke C, La Cour M. Growth of cultured porcine retinal pigment epithelial cells. Acta Ophthalmol Scand. 2003;81:170–6.
74. Feng W, Zheng JJ, Lutz DA, McLaughlin BJ. Loss of RPE phenotype affects phagocytic function. Graefes Arch Clin Exp Ophthalmol. 2003;241:232–40.
75. Klettner A, Möhle F, Lucius R, Roider J. Quantifying FITC-labeled latex beads opsonized with photoreceptor outer segment fragments: an easy and inexpensive method of investigating phagocytosis in retinal pigment epithelium cells. Ophthalmic Res. 2011;46:88–91.
76. Toops KA, Tan LX, Lakkaraju A. A detailed three-step protocol for live imaging of intracellular traffic in polarized primary porcine RPE monolayers. Exp Eye Res. 2014;124:74–85.
77. Hamann S, Kiilgaard JF, la Cour M, Prause JU, Zeuthen T. Cotransport of H+, lactate, and H2O in porcine retinal pigment epithelial cells. Exp Eye Res. 2003;76:493–504.
78. Terasaki H, Shirasawa M, Otsuka H, Yamashita T, Uchino E, Hisatomi T, Sonoda S, Sakamoto T. Different effects of thrombin on VEGF secretion, proliferation, and permeability in polarized and non-polarized retinal pigment epithelial cells. Curr Eye Res. 2015;40:936–45.
79. Shirasawa M, Sonoda S, Terasaki H, Arimura N, Otsuka H, Yamashita T, Uchino E, Hisatomi T, Ishibashi T, Sakamoto T. TNF-α disrupts morphologic and functional barrier properties of polarized retinal pigment epithelium. Exp Eye Res. 2013;110:59–69.
80. Haderspeck JC, Chuchuy J, Kustermann S, Liebau S, Loskill P. Organ-on-a-chip technologies that can transform ophthalmic drug discovery and disease modeling. Expert Opin Drug Discov. 2019;14:47–57.
81. Chen LJ, Ito S, Kai H, Nagamine K, Nagai N, Nishizawa M, Abe T, Kaji H. Microfluidic co-cultures of retinal pigment epithelial cells and vascular endothelial cells to investigate choroidal angiogenesis. Sci Rep. 2017;7:3538.
82. Hamilton RD, Foss AJ, Leach L. Establishment of a human in vitro model of the outer blood-retinal barrier. J Anat. 2007;211:707–16.
83. Lang I, Pabst MA, Hiden U, Blaschitz A, Dohr G, Hahn T, Desoye G. Heterogeneity of microvascular endothelial cells isolated from human term placenta and macrovascular umbilical vein endothelial cells. Eur J Cell Biol. 2003;82:163–73.
84. Shao Z, Friedlander M, Hurst CG, Cui Z, Pei DT, Evans LP, Juan AM, Tahiri H, Duhamel F, Chen J, Sapieha P, Chemtob S, Joyal JS, Smith LE. Choroid sprouting assay: an ex vivo model of microvascular angiogenesis. PLoS One. 2013;8:e69552.
85. Shokoohmand A, Jeon JE, Theodoropoulos C, Baldwin JG, Hutmacher DW, Feigl B. A novel 3D cultured model for studying early changes in age-related macular degeneration. Macromol Biosci. 2017;17:1700221.
86. Chung M, Lee S, Lee BJ, Son K, Jeon NL, Kim JH. Wet-AMD on a chip: modeling outer blood-retinal barrier in vitro. Adv Healthc Mater. 2018;7. https://doi.org/10.1002/adhm.201700028.
87. Yeste J, García-Ramírez M, Illa X, Guimerà A, Hernández C, Simó R, Villa R. A compartmentalized microfluidic chip with crisscross microgrooves and electrophysiological electrodes for modeling the blood-retinal barrier. Lab Chip. 2017;18:95–105.

Retinal Pigment Epithelium Organ Culture

18

Yoko Miura

History of RPE Organ Culture

Studies on the RPE in an explant tissue date back to the 1920s [1–5], long before the cell culture technique was established. Ones of the large interests were then the formation and behavior of the melanosomes in cultures [2, 3] and the self-differentiation of the ocular tissues [5]. Most of these early studies were performed with the explants from embryo chick eye. From the 1950s the culture of the RPE explants from adult human donor eye has been performed and many of the important growth characteristics of RPE cells *in vitro* have been described [6–8]. The development of the improved culture mediums, such as Eagle's medium [9], or Roswell Park Memorial Institute (RPMI) medium [10] in 1950–60s widened the range of experimental possibilities. From 1970s different experiments using RPE explants have been conducted for different purposes. Using a short-term cultivation (at longest for several hours), cellular physiological properties such as active/passive ion transport [11–15] or barrier functions [16] have been studied mainly with RPE-choroid explants in static conditions. On the other hand, RPE morphology [8, 17, 18] was studied from short to long cultivation periods (from hours to weeks), and wound healing of RPE [19–21] and phagocytosis activity of RPE cells [22–24] were studied with the time range from hours to several days under static conditions.

In 2001, by using a new technology of tissue engineering, Framme et al. applied a perfusion culture system [25] for the cultivation of the RPE-choroid tissue explants [26]. Compared to static culture, perfusion culture may provide the tissues with a stable culture environment due to the continuous supply of the nutrients and the removal of wastes. This perfusion system has been widely utilized in the last decade to culture and study RPE explants for different studies, such as a safety testing of the chemical compounds [27, 28], laser-tissue interaction [29, 30], and regulation mechanisms of growth factor secretion [31, 32].

Regarding tissue preservation, maintenance of not only the morphology [29, 30], but also the functionality [30] of RPE in perfusion culture system have been investigated, which revealed the apparent time limit of the cultivation period to investigate the RPE with a good functionality. Recently developed technology may even indicate the metabolic status of the RPE non-invasively by measuring the fluorescence lifetime of the tissue autofluorescence [33, 34]. The fluorescence lifetime of the RPE in the organ culture shows a slow alteration during cultivation, indicating the

Y. Miura (✉)
Institute of Biomedical Optics, University of Lübeck, Lübeck, Germany

Department of Ophthalmology, University of Lübeck, Lübeck, Germany
e-mail: miura@bmo.uni-luebeck.de

A. K. Klettner, S. Dithmar (eds.), *Retinal Pigment Epithelium in Health and Disease*,
https://doi.org/10.1007/978-3-030-28384-1_18

change in the cell metabolic state over time, while the cell viability proven by conventional methods is unchanged. This is motivating researchers to make further attempts to improve metabolic state of the RPE in organ culture as stable as possible so that the tissue can be preserved healthy and thus an experiment with a longer period could be enabled.

Donor of the Eye

The eyes from different vertebrate species, like chick or chick embryo [19–21, 35–38], frog [12, 14], adult newt [39, 40], rabbit [11, 41], pig [17, 26–32, 42–45] or cattle [13, 18, 22–24, 41] have been used as the donor of RPE explants.

Eyes from chick embryo have been utilized more often in earlier days due to the good accessibility. In recent years the studies using chick embryo are mainly focused on the differentiation of the RPE and the retina [20, 36]. The newt eye has an unique characteristics that it can regenerate the entire retina through proliferation and transdifferentiation of RPE cells even in adulthood [46], and thus might serve as an interesting model of the study about treatments for degenerative diseases and RPE regeneration for human eyes [39, 40].

Concerning the genomic homology, the mammalians eyes are considered to serve as a good model for many of human medical studies, e.g. studies for the efficacy and safety of the treatments, or studies for the development of new imaging modalities. Particularly, the domestic pig (*Sus scrofa*) has been shown to have the large similarity in their genome to the human [47] and the eye shows similar anatomy and function as well [48–50]; for example, fully vascularized retina, analogous RPE, no tapetum as compared to cats and dogs, and choroidal vasculature and Bruch's membrane analogous to the human. On the other hand, in the eyes of some lower vertebrates, such as teleost and amphibian eyes, some functions of the RPE have been shown to be apparently different from the ones of the mammalian eyes. For example, their photoreceptors and pigment granules within the RPE undergo positional rearrangements, in response to changes in the light conditions and to circadian rhythms (called "retinomotor movements").

The rabbit eyes are often used for the *in vivo* experiments for the study on laser tissue interaction of the retina [51, 52] due to the similar light absorption characteristics of the retina and the choroid to the human eye [53], or for the study on pharmacokinetics and drug effects [54]. However, the usage of their eyes for cultivation is seldom [11, 41]. Anatomical features of the rabbit eyes have some apparent non-similarities to the human eyes, e.g. the merangiotic (mostly avascular) retina, and a much thinner sclera (0.2–0.25 mm at the equator [50] compared to the pig eyes (0.56–0.86 mm at the equator [49]) and the human eyes (0.53 mm [55]). The scleral thickness may be an influencing factor if the RPE is cultured with the sclera.

Regarding human eyes, enucleated eyes through operations or the eyes from the eye bank have been cultivated and studied by some researchers [6, 8, 56–59]. However, the availability of human eyes is largely different depending on the legal situation. Even though allowed, due to the difficulty of frequent acquisition and in keeping a short post-mortem time, usage of human donor eyes is quite limited in the study with RPE organ culture.

Type of Explant

General Principle for the Preparation of RPE Organ Culture

In RPE organ culture, postmortem time is more critical than in RPE cell culture. Eyes are required to be freshly enucleated and with postmortem time within a few hours, in order to obtain vital RPE cells. Furthermore, the eyes should be kept cool until preparation. Since shedding of rod photoreceptor outer segments and RPE phagocytosis are triggered by a light onset in mammals [60], it is better to keep the eye in a dark condition before and during preparation, if the postmortem phagocytosis activity of the RPE cells is desired to be stabilized before the beginning of experiment [61].

After the extraocular tissues are removed, the eyes need to be immersed shortly in antiseptic solution, than moved into the PBS or culture medium. The eye cup is ready after the removal of the anterior part of the eye, the vitreous and the neural retina. The neural retina may still be left here on the RPE until the later step of the procedure.

In the following paragraphs, different types of culture are introduced; the eye cup, the RPE-choroid-sclera culture, and the RPE-choroid culture.

Eye Cup

RPE cells might be maintained alive for a while in an "eye cup", consisted of the sclera, choroid, Bruch's membrane and RPE [23, 24] (Fig. 18.1a). A few studies have been reported in 1980s that used a bovine eye cup to study RPE's phagocytosis activity [23, 24]. RPE eye cup culture can be defined as the preservation of the RPE in the cup-formed posterior part of the eye, prepared by resecting the sclera in parallel to the corneal limbus at the part of the pars plana to equator position, followed by the removal of the vitreous and the neural retina. The eye cup should be placed in a suitable culture dish and preserved in the enough amount of culture medium. Although culture medium can be provided both inside and outside the eye cup, in most animal eyes the nutrition and fluid transport from the basolateral side of the RPE could be dramatically reduced due to the loss of choroidal blood circulation and low water permeability of the sclera. This effect is assumed to be larger in the eyes with thicker sclera as human and pig eyes [49, 50, 55]. The maximal duration of the preservation of the eye cup in the previous reports was 24 hours. So far, there is no study focusing on the possible duration of RPE preservation in the eye cup organ culture.

Another concern of the RPE eye cup culture is the variety of the size of the explants, due to the individual difference of the eyes, which may cause the inconsistent experimental results due to the inconsistent culture conditions among cultures, such as the medium volume per area and thus eventually the concentration of the metabolic wastes in the culture medium may differ significantly. On this point, the method RPE-choroid-sclera organ culture with the consistent size of the explants as described in Sect. 3.2 is preferred.

RPE-Choroid-Sclera Organ Culture

Compared to the eye cup, the use of resected small explants may have several advantages, such as that they can be cultured in a standard culture dish while being immersed in the culture medium, and that quantitative analysis may be facilitated. In this method, a part of the explant (RPE-choroid-sclera) is resected at a defined size and preserved in culture medium (Fig. 18.1b). As described in Sect. 3.1, the sclera might be the obstacle against the supply of water and nutrition to the RPE cells from their basolateral side. However, considering the ease of preparation and handling of this culture compared to the one without sclera described in Sect. 3.3, it can be also utilized as a model for short-term experiments. It has been utilized in different studies to date for the studies from hours to a few days [11, 17, 24, 41, 56–58, 62, 63]. In recent study, RPE cell viability of the RPE-choroid-sclera explants in a static culture has been confirmed with calcein-AM test at least for 72 hours [64].

RPE-Choroid Organ Culture

In terms of RPE cell preservation the RPE-choroid organ cultures without sclera is considered to be the best way among RPE organ cultures, due to the best supplies of water and nutrition from basolateral sides. It was reported that viable RPE cells of RPE-choroid organ culture can be preserved at least 5 days in a perfusion system (tested with calcein-AM staining), followed by the slow degenerative changes [30]. RPE-choroid organ culture has been used in variety of studies in the last years [26, 30–32, 34, 45, 65]. Since the RPE-choroid sheet needs to be actively removed from the sclera using a scissors and forceps, mechani-

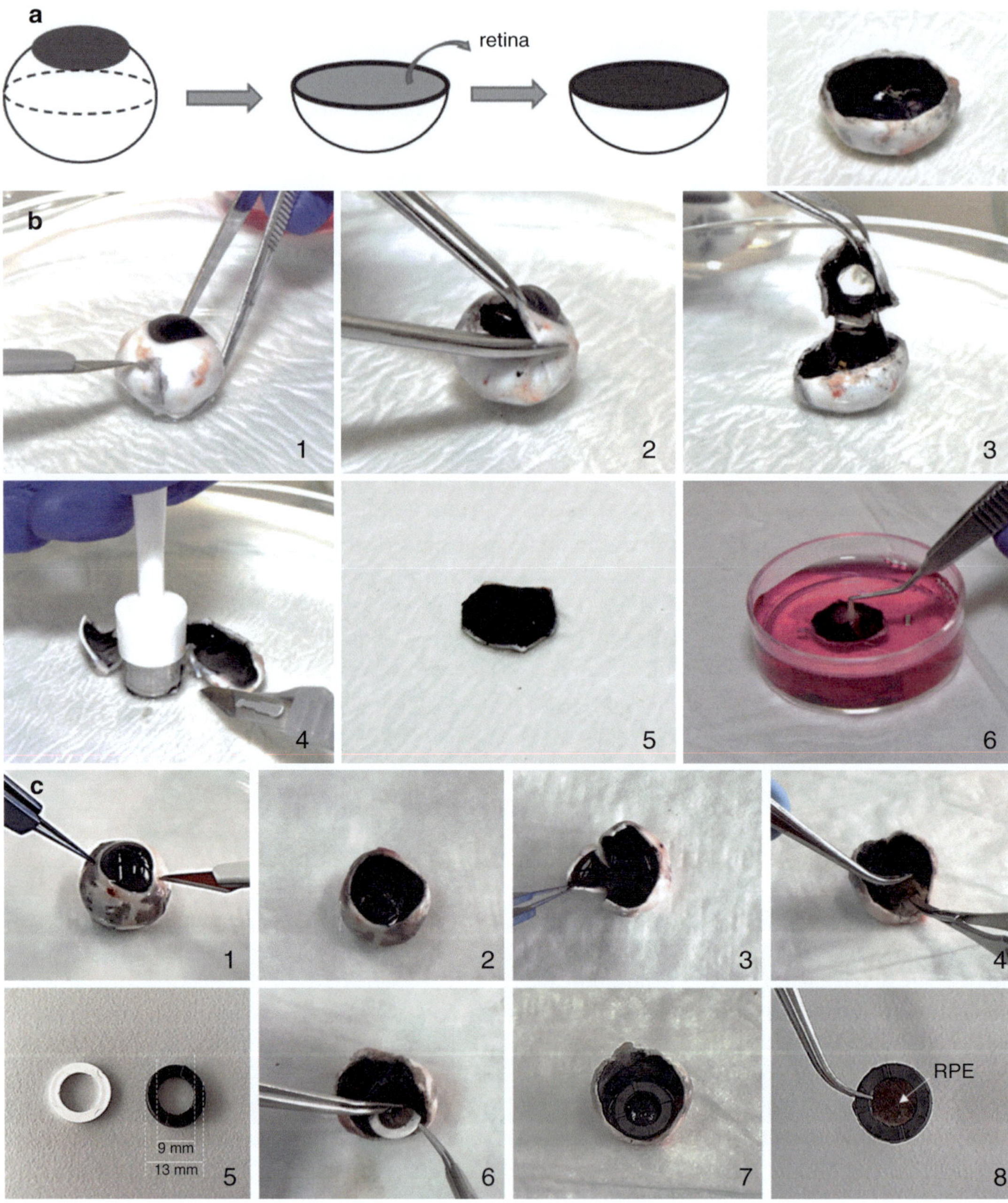

Fig. 18.1 Methods of preparation for different types of RPE explants for organ culture: (**a**) "eye cup" organ culture, (**b**) RPE-choroid-sclera organ culture, and (**c**) RPE-choroid organ culture

cal stress in addition to the stress through the environmental change on tissues has to be taken into consideration. The RPE-choroid sheets with the thickness of just 150–200 μm, which have lost their structural support by the sclera, needs alternative support for cultivation; in previous studies, as a tissue support, either the filters [8, 20, 22] or the special holders [12, 13, 15, 26–32, 44, 45] are mainly used (Fig. 18.1c). The holders have an advantage to keep the explant flat during whole experimental period. The RPE-choroid sheet without holder may lose its flat formation by being waved, rolled, or contracted during cultivation.

Co-Cultivation with Neural Retina

Due to the loss of hydrostatic and osmotic pressure differences, photoreceptor outer segments and RPE lose their adhesion in the postmortem eye [66, 67]. This also means the loss of direct interactions between photoreceptor and RPE, such as phagocytosis of the photoreceptor outer segments by RPE cells after death. The retina in the *ex vivo* condition degenerates faster than the RPE [29]. To date, retinal electric activity, the signals on the electroretinogram (ERG), is preserved at the longest 10 hours in the optimal medium [68]. It suggests that the retinal electric activity disappears already at the first day after preparation, although the morphology is preserved some more days [29]. The attachment does not restore during cultivation.

Kaempf et al. reported that the co-cultivation of the neural retina with RPE-choroid may improve survival of retinal cells compared to cultures of the retina alone, with limited nuclei loss, significant reduction in apoptotic cells in nuclear cell layers, decreased Muller cell hypertrophy, and reduced upregulation of glial fibrillary acid protein, which is upregulated in glial cells following the injury of central nerve system [43]. It may be due to the growth factors secreted by RPE cells for photoreceptor survival, such as pigment epithelium-derived factor (PEDF) [69]. Therefore, it has been considered that the retina-RPE-choroid organ culture might be a good model for the evaluation of interactions between RPE and neural retina, including the signaling molecules or effect of pharmaceuticals on the retina and/or RPE [28]. However, concerning its influence on the RPE, co-culture with the retina might negatively influence the RPE through the metabolites from the degenerating retina. There is, so far, no study has been conducted to clarify the influence of co-cultivated degenerative neural retina on the RPE preservation in an organ culture.

Type of Culture System

Based mainly on the way of medium supply to the explant, the culture method is divided in two ways; static culture and perfusion culture.

Static Culture

In this method, explants including RPE (RPE-choroid, RPE-choroid-sclera, RPE eye cup) with or without supporter (e.g. membrane filter, holders) are preserved in a culture container under static condition, such as in a cell culture dish [20, 23, 24, 42], Lighton tube [8], or Ussing-type chamber [11–14, 35, 44, 45]. They are maintained in a CO_2 incubator (37 °C, 5% CO_2).

The ussing chamber has been developed by Ussing and first applied in the measurement of the Na^+ transport in frog epithelium [70]. Ussing chamber consists of two halves, so that the tissue's apical and basolateral sides are supplied with different culture medium. Studies using Ussing-type chamber with RPE explants contributed greatly to the understanding of the physiological properties of RPE such as ion transports and membrane potentials across the RPE [11–14, 22, 41], or polarized secretion of growth factors or enzymes secreted from RPE cells [44, 45]. In Ussing-type chamber cell biological polarity and transepithelial resistance (TER) can be well preserved. High TER indicates high integrity of RPE tight junctions. Therefore, Ussing-type chamber is useful also for the study of RPE barrier functions. In order to keep the medium temperature around 37 °C, some studies were performed with a modified system with water jacket-surrounded Ussing chamber [11, 13].

Perfusion Culture

Perfusion culture is a culture method in which medium flow is controlled by pumping, and therefore the tissues can be constantly perfused with fresh medium without manual replacement. This method may provide tissues of an environment whose molecular dynamic is closer to under *in vivo* conditions than the static culture. Moreover, perfusion systems may provide a flexible platform to build up different biomimetic environments in various investigations. The general perfusion organ culture techniques were introduced in the 1970s [71, 72], and its application in RPE explants was reported first by Framme et al. in 2002 [26]. They used a system which was originally developed and established by Minuth et al. for the culture of embryonic renal epithelia [25].

Most of the perfusion culture of RPE explants is performed in a closed chamber. The medium should be exposed to the atmosphere, which allows for gas exchange and the partial equilibration of the perfusate O_2/CO_2 levels with the atmosphere. In most studies with RPE explants in perfusion culture system to date have been performed under normal air conditions with silicone rubber tubes having a high oxygen permeability rate [73]. In case aeration is performed and the medium with higher oxygen concentration than in the air is to be provided to the tissues, loss of oxygen from perfusate flowing through the tubing wall during perfusion may be a crucial matter. According to the measurement by Pegg et al., oxygen-aerated medium lost oxygen the most through the silicone rubber tube, compared to other materials as polyvinyl chloride (PVS), polyethylene, or polyamide (Nylon) [74]. Furthermore, silicon rubber had the highest affinity to the fatty acid, which is important for energy and lipid metabolisms of cells [74]. Therefore, the tube material should be selected carefully, taking these points into consideration depending on the purpose of the study.

The perfusion culture system set under the normal air condition has a disadvantage that pH of the culture medium may be changed faster than in the static culture maintained in a 5% CO_2 incubator. In order to minimize the pH increase, buffers such as HEPES (4-(2-hydroxyethyl)-1-piperazineethanesulfonic acid) are usually added in the culture medium. Alternatively aeration of the gas of 5% CO_2 in air and/or pure oxygen might also work for that purpose. Regarding glucose supply, while glucose concentration in the medium decline with time in static culture, it can be maintained at a constant level over time in perfusion culture [75, 76].

Temperature is also an essential parameter for the culture. If the perfusion culture system is maintained outside the incubator, the chamber is to be placed on a warm plate, which keeps the medium temperature around 37 °C. Flow speed of the medium should be controlled by a pump, with which the tissues are not damaged by the hydrodynamic shear stress. For example, the flow speed in the range of 1–2.5 mL/h has been used for the studies using the chamber of 5 mL in volume [26, 27, 30, 32].

Culture Medium

The medium used for RPE organ culture can be principally the same as the medium used for RPE cell culture. In the history of RPE organ culture, RPMI 1640 medium has been used for a long time until the 1980s [8, 22, 24]. In recent studies, Dulbecco's eagles modified medium (DMEM, high glucose) or the mixture of equal part of DMEM (high glucose) and HAM's F12 are often utilized [27, 29–32, 34, 59]. To note is that the glucose concentration of these two mediums are different, where DMEM high glucose contains about 25 mM (4.5 g/L) glucose, whereas DMEM:HMA's F12 contains about 17.5 mM (3.15 g/L). Regarding serum type and concentration, porcine or (fetal) bovine serum with the concentration between 5 and 15% are mostly used.

In perfusion system the medium of inlet is better to be kept in 4 °C and warmed up to 37 °C while it runs through the tubing on the heating plate before supplied to the tissues. A pH stabilizer such as HEPES (4-(2-hydroxyethyl)-1-piperazineethanesulfonic acid) is required for the perfusion culture outside CO_2 incubator, which could be mixed to the culture medium maximally with 25 mM. The pH of the medium may, however, nevertheless increase to some extend compared to the conditions in a CO_2 incubator, if no CO_2-aeration is performed (e.g. Inlet pH 7.29, outlet pH 7.57 [75]).

Preservation and Alteration of the RPE in Organ Culture

Morphological Preservation and Alteration

The RPE in the freshly isolated explants may first retain its native morphology in the culture, such as microvilli, intracellular organelle, and intercellular tight junctions [8, 18] (Fig. 18.2). RPE cells in native tissue are hexagonal in cross-section and averagely approximately 10 μm in height. The apical side of the cell has a number of microvilli and melanosomes, whereas the nucleus is located close to the basal side. According to the short-term structural analysis by McKechnie et al., the explanted RPE first temporarily lacks apical microvilli, but during

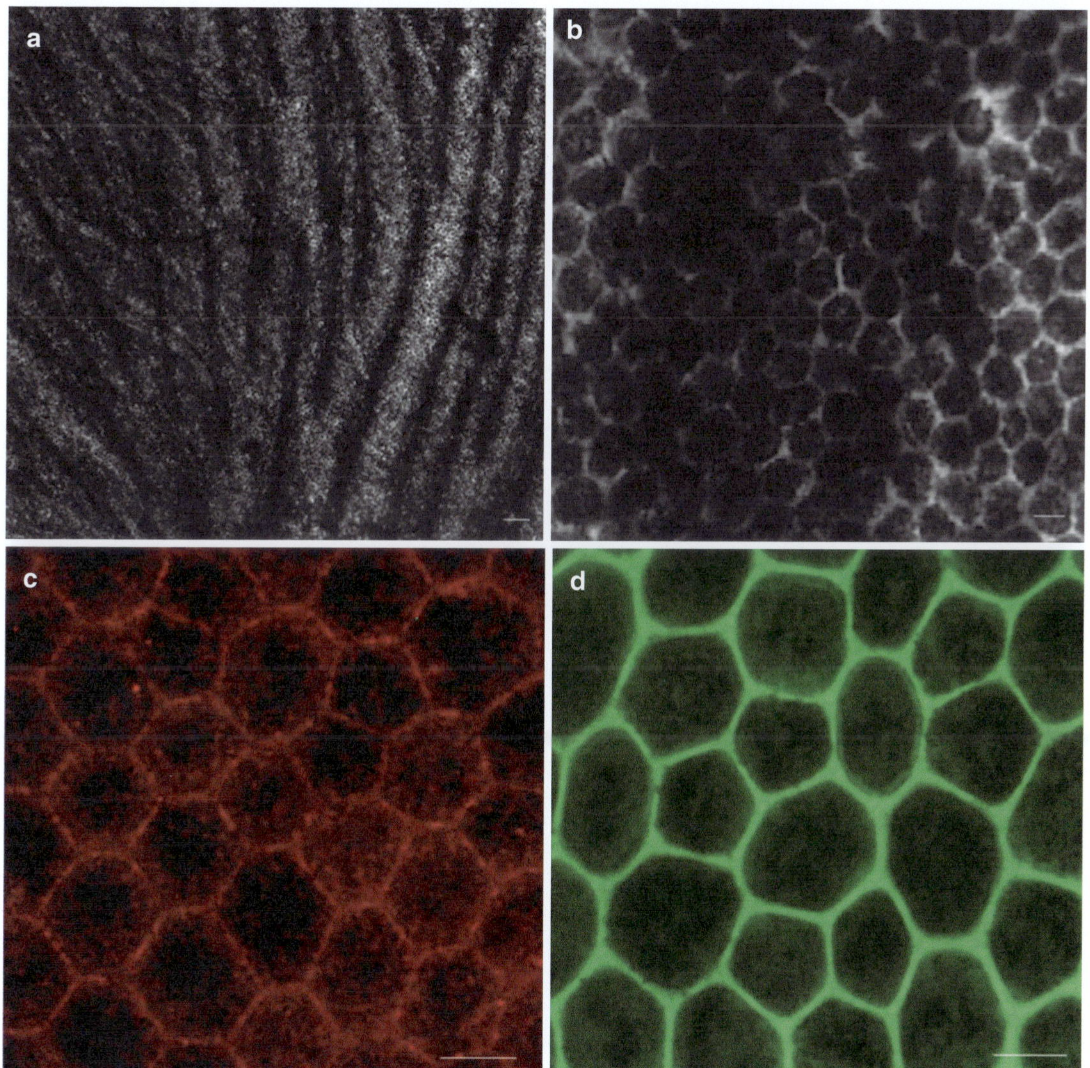

Fig. 18.2 Morphology of the RPE in an RPE-choroid perfusion organ culture after 24 hours of cultivation. (**a**) A bright field image of the RPE with low magnification (Bar = 100 μm), (**b**) A bright field image of the RPE with higher magnification (Bar = 10 μm), (**c**) Immunofluorescence for occludin (Bar = 10 μm), and (**d**) FITC-F-actin staining (Bar = 10 μm). Those highly integrated junctional morphology can be observed at least 5 days of cultivation

the first 3 hours in culture recovery of apical microvilli occurs [18]. Preservation of apical microvilli in the culture for longer term has been also reported [8, 17, 58].

RPE cells in organ culture begin to change in their morphology during cultivation; (1) changes in cell shape, such as rounded, enlarged, flattened, or dome-shaped [8, 17, 30, 58], (2) changes in morphological polarity, such as the apical localization of the melanosomes and the basal localization of the nucleus [30], (3) increase of hypo-pigmented RPE cells [8], (4) decrease of the infoldings of basal plasma membrane [8], (5) shortening of the microvilli [58], (6) changes in junctional integrity and cytoskeleton [30] with irregular alignment of F-actin filament with increasing stress fiber, and the loss of the clear border localization of tight junction proteins (e.g. occludin) [30], and (7) focal nodular proliferation of the RPE [8]. Many of these changes are quite similar to the ones observed in the RPE of aged eyes [51, 77]. Moreover, the dome-shaped change in cell shape resembles to the ones observed consistently in studies of experimental retinal detachments *in vivo* [78–80].

The onset and duration of these degenerative changes of the RPE in organ culture varies among reports [8, 17, 30]. The changes in cell shape (dome-shaped) were observed in most studies at early time points, from several days of cultivation, as the typical initial morphological alterations. However, the time of appearance of further degenerative changes, such as the increase of hypo-pigmented cells, decrease of infoldings of basal plasma membrane, or overt proliferation, are inconsistent; in the study by Tso et al. these changes have been observed at earliest after three days, where the overt changes may begin after 14 days [8], whereas the study by Del Priore showed almost no changes at least for 29 days [17]. The study by Miura et al. showed that the RPE cells in RPE-choroid organ culture in the perfusion system begins to lose their morphological polarity (apical melanosome and basal nucleus) slowly after several days in some cells, partial disruption of junctional integrity after 8 days, but no overt proliferative or degenerative changes were observed over the 8 day's observation period [30]. These differences of the onset of morphological changes may be caused by the culture condition, but might also be largely depending on the sample's initial conditions. Therefore, it is essential to keep the condition of the donor eyes as consistent as possible in the study using RPE explants.

The flattened and less-pigmented RPE cells observed in the long-term studies might be explained as the consequence of the partial cell death and subsequent wound healing. These findings of long-term morphological studies imply that the RPE cells in organ culture do not completely die rapidly, but experience a slow degenerative changes that may take weeks.

Metabolic/Functional Preservation and Alteration

It has been clearly shown that the RPE cells in organ culture have a phagocytosis activities [8, 22–24, 81]. In these studies, phagocytosis activity has been shown in 24–48 hours after tissue preparation, and it is still not well known how much longer the RPE cells in organ culture may have phagocytosis activity. Tso et al. observed abundant endoplasmic reticulum in RPE cells in the organ culture on day 14, suggesting that the cells can be metabolically still active at least until that day [8], which fits well to the morphological changes described in Sect. 6.1 suggesting the degenerative and regenerative changes taking place around that time point.

In order to utilize the RPE organ culture to investigate the healthy RPE, and not degenerating ones, the stable functionality of RPE cells before the onset of overt degenerative change is necessary. One of the essential functions of the RPE is to secrete cytokines to maintain the homeostasis of chorioretinal functions, including growth factors [82]. Among all, vascular endothelial growth factor (VEGF) plays a particularly important role in retinal functions. VEGF is physiologically secreted from the healthy RPE cells, and is crucial not only for the development of the vasculature in the retina and choroid, but also for the development of the neuroretina. VEGF is also known to exert a protective functions for the neuroretina, the RPE, and the choroid [83–86]. Increased stress, e.g. oxidative stress or hypoxia, may lead to the increase of its secretion [31, 87, 88]. A previous study showed that VEGF secretion from RPE of the RPE-choroid explant in a perfusion organ culture was stable until the fifth day of cultivation and started to increase gradually after that. This suggests that the RPE-choroid in perfusion organ culture may be functionally stable for about 5 days before the functional deterioration starts [30]. This interpretation can be supported by the experimental results, showing that the wound made by laser irradiation on the cultured RPE on day 6 could not show normal wound closure, either with incomplete closure or with the closure with overlayed fibroblastic RPE cells, whereas the wound made at the earlier days showed the normal wound closure with a monolayer RPE [30].

Application of RPE Organ Culture in Basic Studies

RPE Wound Healing

The biggest advantage of the RPE wound healing study with RPE explants compared to the study with RPE cell culture is the existence of the Bruch's membrane, the natural substrates of the RPE. An interesting contrast has been demonstrated in previous studies; Integrin antibody 2A10 inhibited cell spreading, migration and proliferation at the wound of the RPE cells grown on fibronectin and on laminin substrates in a cell culture [89], whereas it inhibited cell migration and proliferation, but not cell spreading (increasing of cell size) in an RPE-choroid organ culture [20]. Hergott et al. interpreted these difference that the RPE cells at the wound edge in organ culture have already an adhesion to the Bruch's membrane, on which they spread, whereas the cells in cell culture seemingly need at first to come into contact with the suitable substrates for spreading [20].

Tissue Responses to Laser Irradiation

In clinical practice, retinal laser treatment is conducted with the laser light at the wavelength in the range from green to yellow (around 530–580 nm), which is highly absorbed by the melanosomes in RPE cells [90]. Therefore, RPE cells in organ cultures, which contain numerous melanosomes, are suited for the study on laser-tissue interaction of the RPE. In contrast, RPE cells in cell culture are not suitable for laser studies due to their limited number of melanosomes, because melanosomes are lost during cell division and melanogenesis does not occur actively in RPE cells in cell culture under normal culture conditions [91], thus they reduce melanin content during cultivation. The 532 nm laser radiation has been shown to be absorbed more than 90% by strongly pigmented porcine RPE-choroid explants, whereas only 30–50% in RPE primary cell culture isolated from pigmented porcine eye, and 10–30% in the passaged cultures (Miura, unpublished data). Inhomogeneous pigmentation within a cell culture is also a large disadvantage, as it may cause the inhomogeneous light absorption, leading to the various effects in one culture. As far as the extent of the pigmentation in one RPE explant is homogeneous, the laser effect is depending on the irradiation conditions, such as power, pulse duration, and irradiation time (Fig. 18.3a).

As described above (Sect. 6.2 metabolic characteristics), a laser wound of the RPE made on the sixth day of cultivation in organ culture cannot achieve the normal wound closure [30]. Therefore, the experiments for the normal laser-tissue interaction need to be concluded within the first week of cultivation. The RPE defects of about 200 μm diameter made by a non-thermal laser (selective retina treatment laser) are closed within 4–6 days [30, 92] (Fig. 18.3b).

Phagocytosis Activity

Phagocytosis activity needs high functional polarity of cells. Since engulfment of photoreceptor outer segment by RPE cells occurs only at the apical surface of the cell, it seems obvious

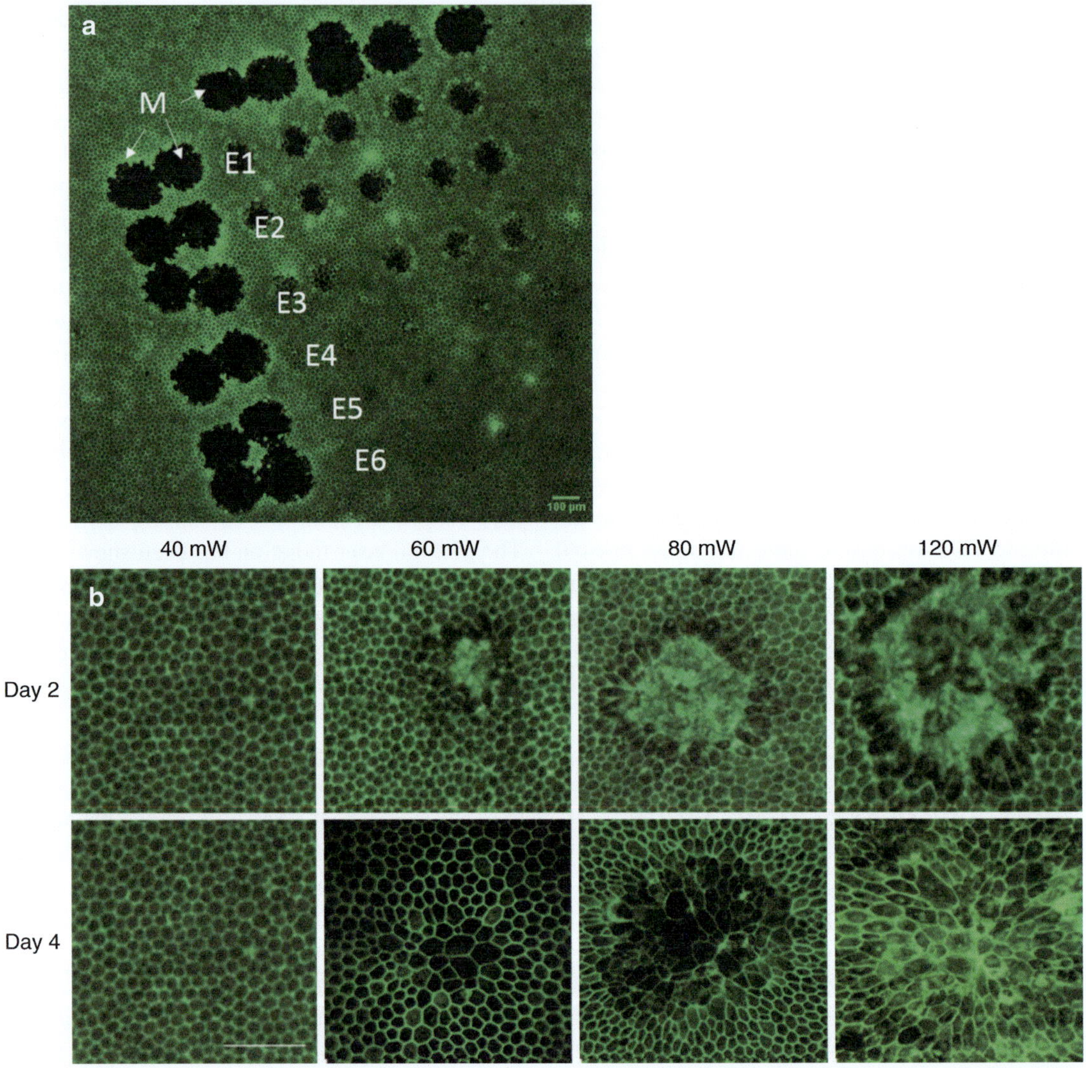

Fig. 18.3 Study of laser-tissue interaction and wound healing of the RPE using RPE organ cultures. (**a**) Calcein-AM cell viability staining directly after laser irradiation with different energy settings. *M* marker (high energy irradiation for the orientation), *E1-E6* decreasing energy settings. Green fluorescence of calcein is positive in living cells, whereas the dead cells are shown as non-fluorescent black region. A decreasing irradiation energy (E1–E6) results in the decrease of dead area (The image was kindly provided by Medical Laser Center Luebeck), (**b**) F-actin fluorescence staining at 2 and 4 days after continuous wave laser irradiation with different power settings. A power-dependent increase of damage size is observed. All wounds are closed after 4 days. (Bar =100 µm)

that organ culture with its higher polarity might be more suitable to understand their phagocytosis activity than cell culture. It has been shown that phagocytosis of latex beads by bovine and human RPE cells in organ culture begins after a latent time period for 4–17 h [22–24, 81]. There seems to be a time-requiring interaction between the cell membrane and latex beads. On the other hand, engulfment of latex beads in human RPE cell culture was observed already after 1–2 hours [93, 94]. Considering these differences in latent time period, there seems to be a significant difference in property of phagocytosis activity between RPE in organ culture and in cell culture.

However, studying the phagocytosis activity with RPE organ culture may have a disadvantage in terms of the microscopic evaluation, where a number of apical melanosomes obstruct the observation of the phagocytized substances, such as latex beads or photoreceptor outer segments in RPE cells. Thus histological study is needed for the morphological evaluation (Fig. 18.4).

Pharmaceutical Research

For short-term tests about toxicity or other biological effects of pharmaceutical agents on RPE cells, the RPE organ culture is considered to be a good model. With the increasing number of new pharmacological applications for retinal diseases, it is considered that the demand of the use of RPE organ culture grows. To date, the safety of indocyanine green (ICG) [28], effect of different anti-VEGF agents [27, 43] or nicotine [31] on RPE cell function have been investigated. However, organ cultures cannot be used for a large scale testing, because it is so far not a high throughput technique.

Transepithelial Transport/Potential

A high functional polarity is required for the transepithelial transport of the ion and fluid. Active transport-generated absorption of fluid across the RPE can be therefore well investigated by the polarized organ culture. For this study, the thick sclera, as the ones of pig or human, are not suitable, and thus RPE-choroid explants are mostly utilized [12, 13, 15, 35], while with the rabbit eyes with thin sclera, Frambach et al. could measure the transepithelial transport and potential using the RPE explant including sclera [41]. As shown in Table 18.1, fresh RPE-choroid organ culture [11–13, 95–97], porcine primary RPE cell culture [98] and human fetal RPE cells (hfRPE) [99] may have their transepithelial resistance (TER) of several hundred $\Omega * cm^2$. The TER of hfRPE

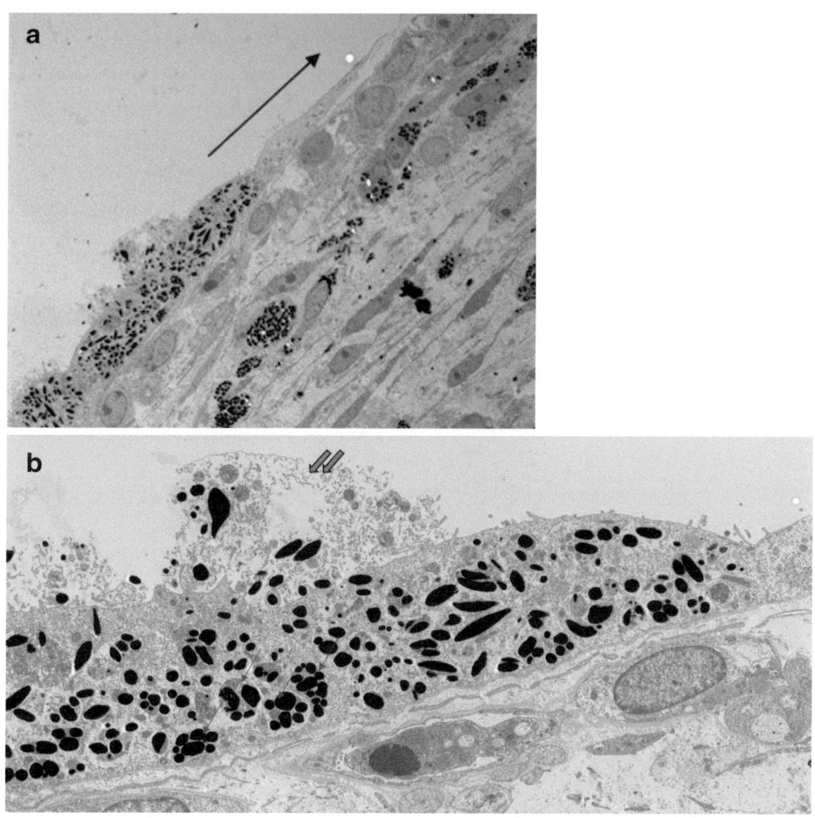

Fig. 18.4 Transmission electron microscopy (TEM) images 48 hours after laser photocoagulation, performed on the first day of cultivation. (**a**) The cells at the leading edge of the wound extend toward the center of the defect (arrow). (**b**) A zoomed image of the cells around the leading edge. It seems that the debris of the dead cells (double arrows) are phagocytized by the surviving RPE cells. Condensed melanosome granules (red arrows) are observed, which are probably the phagocytosed melanosomes originated from the damage RPE cells, suggesting the RPE's active phagocytosis activity in the organ culture

cell culture and primary porcine RPE cell culture can reach much higher, over 1000 Ω∗cm^2, when they are cultivated on the membranes for several weeks. On the other hand, RPE cell culture of human RPE cell lines such as ARPE-19 cells have shown to have significantly lower transepithelial resistance compared to the others, which may be increased maximally around 40 Ω∗cm^2 even after several weeks in cultivation [99] (Table 18.1). For the measurement of those physiological properties, an Ussing-type chamber combined with the equipment for the measurement of potential and resistance is useful. On this point, RPE-choroid explants, which may be utilized directly in the experiment, has an advantage compared to the cell cultures, which need to be cultured for several weeks on the membrane sheet suitable for an experiment with an Ussing-type chamber.

Cytokine Secretion

As described in Sect. 6.2, secretion of cytokines like VEGF from RPE cells, including polarized secretion to apical and basolateral sides, is a crucial indicator of RPE cell function and responses to different stimuli. Therefore, evaluation of cytokine secretion from RPE cells has an important implication for understanding RPE cell behaviors under different conditions. Detection of the polarized secretion of cytokines is also one of the good applications of the RPE-choroid organ culture in an Ussing-type chamber [44, 45]. Klettner et al. showed a differential apical and basal regulation of VEGF-A secretion and primarily choroidal secretion of placenta growth factor (PlGF) [44]. Treumer et al. presented the vectorial release of matrix metalloproteases from RPE cells responding to the laser irradiation, indicating the possible therapeutic mechanism of the selective retina treatment [45]. Perfusion organ culture using a non-Ussing-type chamber can also be used, if the polarity is not an issue, especially in long term and when the influence of certain substances is to be tested [100].

Two-Photon Microscopy and Fluorescence Lifetime Imaging Microscopy

Highly pigmented RPE cells in organ culture is generally difficult to be observed with bright field- as well as fluorescence microscopy due to the strong light absorption by melanosomes. Two-photon microscopy, a non-linear fluorescence microscopy utilizing the laser light with longer wavelength and lower energy than the one photon excitation system (e.g. confocal microscopy), may give different insights about the RPE. A strong light absorption in the melanosomes results in a strong emission of melanin autofluorescence, which presents the RPE cells more clearly [34] (Fig. 18.5a). Study of RPE autofluorescence in two-photon microscopy may provide detailed information about autofluorescence inside/outside RPE cells, insights into the stress-induced autofluorescence [34] (Fig. 18.5b), and the molecular mechanisms at the RPE, such as the visual cycle with retinyl esters [36, 101].

Fluorescence lifetime imaging microscopy (FLIM) is the method to measure and map

Table 18.1 Electrophysiological properties of RPE in explant, human ARPE-19 cell culture, and human fetal RPE cell culture

	RPE-choroid explant[a]	hfRPE cell culture[b]	Primary RPE cell culture[c]	ARPE-19 cell culture[d]
Transmembrane potential (mV)	5.0–12.8	2.6 ± 0.8	No information available	No information available
Transepithelial resistance (TER) (Ω cm^2)	138–350 (fresh)	30 (1w)–1000 (6w)	400 (1w)–1500 (4w)	30 (1w)–43 (5w)

"1w" indicates 1 week after seeding of cells on the membrane
[a]Data from [11, 13, 12, 95–97]
[b]Data from [99, 103]
[c]Data from [98]
[d]Data from [99]

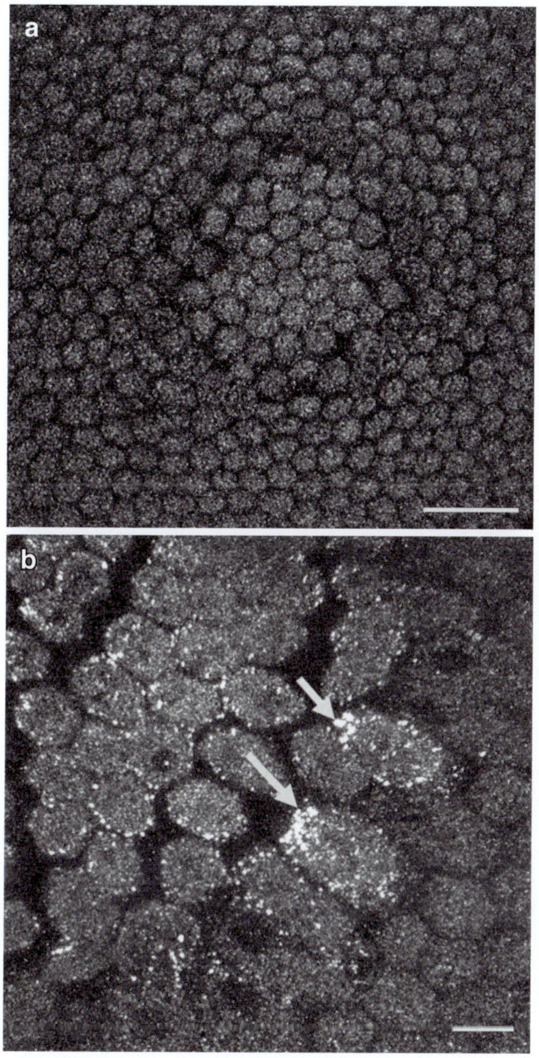

Fig. 18.5 RPE in an organ culture with two-photon microscopy (λex = 730 nm). (**a**) RPE 30 min after thermal laser irradiation (Bar = 50 μM), and (**b**) RPE cells at the rim of coagulation 24 hours after thermal laser irradiation (Bar = 10 μm). Apical melanosomes emit a bright autofluorescence and thus RPE cell shape are well recognized (**a**). Strong stress such as an oxidative stress or heat stress may cause the appearance of bright autofluorescence granular signals (arrows)

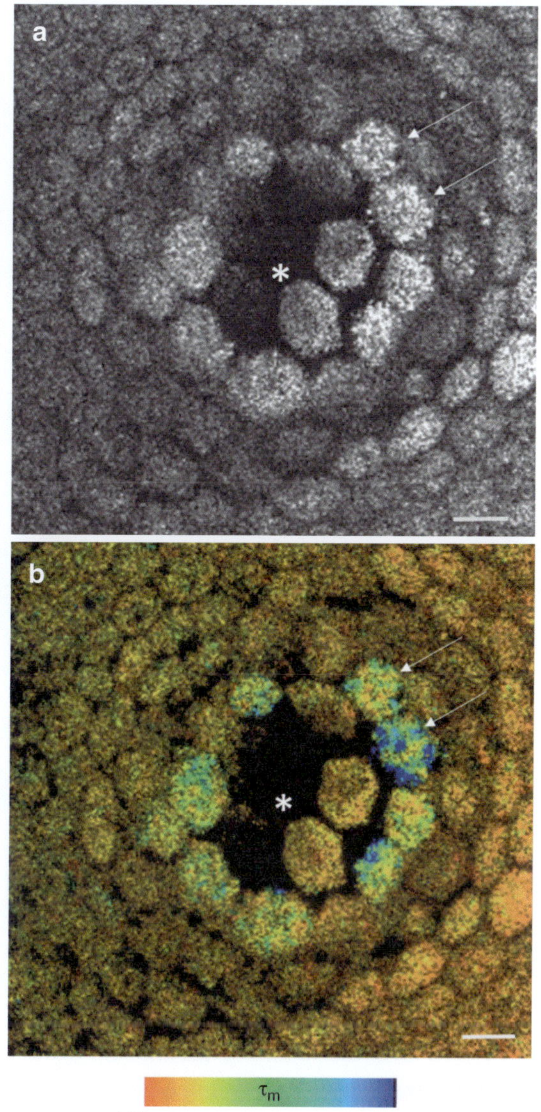

Fig. 18.6 RPE in an organ culture with two-photon excited fluorescence lifetime imaging microscopy (FLIM) 24 hours after thermal laser irradiation (50 mW for 0.1 s. Beam diameter was 300 μm). (**a**) An autofluorescence image with the two-photon microscopy, (**b**) A FLIM image, where the fluorescence lifetime is presented with a pseudo color. The cells around the coagulated region (*) show an increased fluorescence intensity and an prolonged mean fluorescence lifetime (τ_m) (arrows). (Bar = 10 μm)

the fluorescence lifetime of tissues and cells. Measurement of the fluorescence lifetime of the human retina has been enabled in recent years using a fluorescence lifetime imaging ophthalmoscopy (FLIO) [102]. In order to understand the change in fluorescence lifetime of the RPE, usage of the RPE organ culture is necessary, since fluorescence properties of RPE cell culture is completely different from *in vivo* RPE. Oxidative stress around thermal laser irradiation or lipid peroxidation has shown to lead to a significant extension of fluorescence lifetime in the RPE [34] (Fig. 18.6).

Conclusion

With a rapid increase in the number of diagnostic and treatment methods for retinal disease, we face an increasing demand of translational research, in order to understand therapeutic or diagnostic mechanisms, cell responses to different interventions, or to understand unknown aspects of RPE cell functions.

Compared to RPE cell culture, an organ culture from freshly enucleated eyes retains RPE phenotypes closer to *in vivo* tissue, and thus can be beneficial to address specific scientific questions, such as wound healing, secretion of cytokines, laser-tissue interaction, or tissue autofluorescence. There are different forms of cultures; the eye cup culture, the RPE-choroid-sclera culture, and the RPE-choroid culture, and they must be chosen according to the study purpose and required period. The RPE in the culture without sclera seems to be preserved longer than in the one with sclera. The perfusion culture may have an advantage with respect to the *in vivo* mimetic molecular dynamics, and the static culture may have an advantage in the gas atmosphere. The experiments to evaluate RPE functionality is so far recommended to be no longer than 5 days in a perfusion culture due to its degenerative changes, which could be, however, varied through the modifications of culture conditions in the future. In order to broaden the usability of RPE organ culture as an experimental model, it is desired to further optimize the method toward the better tissue preservation.

References

1. Kirby DB. Tissue culture in ophthalmic research. Trans Am Ophthalmol Soc. 1929;27:334–83.
2. Smith DT. Melanin pigment in the pigmented epithelium of the retina of the embryo chick's eyes: studies in vivo and in vitro. Acat Rec. 1920;18:260.
3. Smith DT. The ingestion of melanin pigment granules by tissue cultures. Bull Johns Hopkins Hosp. 1921;22:240.
4. Strangeways TS, Canti RG. Dark-ground illumination of tissue cells cultivated "in vitro". Br Med J. 1926;2(3420):155–7.
5. Strangeways TS, Fell HB. Experimental studies on the differentiation of embryonic tissues growing in vivo and in vitro.—II. The development of the isolated early embryonic eye of the fowl when cultivated in vitro. Proc R Soc B. 1926;100(703):273–83.
6. Albert DM, Tso MO, Rabson AS. In vitro growth of pure cultures of retinal pigment epithelium. Arch Ophthalmol. 1972;88(1):63–9.
7. Barishak YR. In vitro behaviour of the pigmented cells of the retina and uvea of the adult human eye. Acta Ophthalmol. 1960;38:339–46.
8. Tso MO, Albert D, Zimmerman LE. Organ culture of human retinal pigment epithelium and choroid: a model for the study of cytologic behavior of RPE in vitro. Investig Ophthalmol. 1973;12(8):554–66.
9. Eagle H. Amino acid metabolism in mammalian cell cultures. Science. 1959;130(3373):432–7.
10. Moore GE, Gerner RE, Franklin HA. Culture of normal human leukocytes. JAMA. 1967;199(8):519–24.
11. Frambach DA, Valentine JL, Weiter JJ. Initial observations of rabbit retinal pigment epithelium-choroid-sclera preparations. Invest Ophthalmol Vis Sci. 1988;29(5):814–7.
12. Hughes BA, Miller SS, Machen TE. Effects of cyclic AMP on fluid absorption and ion transport across frog retinal pigment epithelium. Measurements in the open-circuit state. J Gen Physiol. 1984;83(6):875–99.
13. Miller SS, Edelman JL. Active ion transport pathways in the bovine retinal pigment epithelium. J Physiol. 1990;424:283–300.
14. Miller SS, Steinberg RH. Passive ionic properties of frog retinal pigment epithelium. J Membr Biol. 1977;36(4):337–72.
15. Steinberg RH, Miller SS, Stern WH. Initial observations on the isolated retinal pigment epithelium-choroid of the cat. Invest Ophthalmol Vis Sci. 1978;17(7):675–8.
16. Steuer H, Jaworski A, Stoll D, Schlosshauer B. In vitro model of the outer blood-retina barrier. Brain Res Brain Res Protoc. 2004;13(1):26–36. https://doi.org/10.1016/j.brainresprot.2003.12.002.
17. Del Priore LV, Glaser BM, Quigley HA, Dorman ME, Green WR. Morphology of pig retinal pigment epithelium maintained in organ culture. Arch Ophthalmol. 1988;106(9):1286–90.
18. McKechnie NM, Keegan WA, Converse CA, Foulds WS. Short-term organ culture of the retinal pigment epithelium in microtitration plates: ultrastructural studies. Graefes Arch Clin Exp Ophthalmol. 1986;224(5):401–6.
19. Hergott GJ, Kalnins VI. Expression of proliferating cell nuclear antigen in migrating retinal pigment epithelial cells during wound healing in organ culture. Exp Cell Res. 1991;195(2):307–14.
20. Hergott GJ, Nagai H, Kalnins VI. Inhibition of retinal pigment epithelial cell migration and proliferation with monoclonal antibodies against the beta 1 integrin subunit during wound healing in organ culture. Invest Ophthalmol Vis Sci. 1993;34(9):2761–8.
21. Hergott GJ, Sandig M, Kalnins VI. Cytoskeletal organization of migrating retinal pigment epithelial cells during wound healing in organ culture. Cell Motil Cytoskeleton. 1989;13(2):83–93. https://doi.org/10.1002/cm.970130203.

22. Feeney L, Mixon RN. An in vitro model of phagocytosis in bovine and human retinal pigment epithelium. Exp Eye Res. 1976;22(5):533–48.
23. Goldhar SW, Basu PK, Ranadive NS. Phagocytosis by retinal pigment epithelium: evaluation of modulating agents with an organ culture model. Can J Ophthalmol. 1984;19(1):33–5.
24. Rosenstock T, Basu R, Basu PK, Ranadive NS. Quantitative assay of phagocytosis by retinal pigment epithelium: an organ culture model. Exp Eye Res. 1980;30(6):719–29.
25. Minuth WW, Stockl G, Kloth S, Dermietzel R. Construction of an apparatus for perfusion cell cultures which enables in vitro experiments under organotypic conditions. Eur J Cell Biol. 1992;57(1):132–7.
26. Framme C, Kobuch K, Eckert E, Monzer J, Roider J. RPE in perfusion tissue culture and its response to laser application. Preliminary report. Ophthalmologica. 2002;216(5):320–8. https://doi.org/66184.
27. Klettner A, Roider J. Comparison of bevacizumab, ranibizumab, and pegaptanib in vitro: efficiency and possible additional pathways. Invest Ophthalmol Vis Sci. 2008;49(10):4523–7. https://doi.org/10.1167/iovs.08-2055.
28. Saikia P, Maisch T, Kobuch K, Jackson TL, Baumler W, Szeimies RM, Gabel VP, Hillenkamp J. Safety testing of indocyanine green in an ex vivo porcine retina model. Invest Ophthalmol Vis Sci. 2006;47(11):4998–5003. https://doi.org/10.1167/iovs.05-1665.
29. Hammer M, Richter S, Kobuch K, Mata N, Schweitzer D. Intrinsic tissue fluorescence in an organotypic perfusion culture of the porcine ocular fundus exposed to blue light and free radicals. Graefes Arch Clin Exp Ophthalmol. 2008;246(7):979–88. https://doi.org/10.1007/s00417-008-0789-4.
30. Miura Y, Klettner A, Noelle B, Hasselbach H, Roider J. Change of morphological and functional characteristics of retinal pigment epithelium cells during cultivation of retinal pigment epithelium-choroid perfusion tissue culture. Ophthalmic Res. 2010;43(3):122–33. https://doi.org/10.1159/000252979.
31. Klettner A. Oxidative stress induced cellular signaling in RPE cells. Front Biosci. 2012;4:392–411.
32. Klettner A, Westhues D, Lassen J, Bartsch S, Roider J. Regulation of constitutive vascular endothelial growth factor secretion in retinal pigment epithelium/choroid organ cultures: p38, nuclear factor kappaB, and the vascular endothelial growth factor receptor-2/phosphatidylinositol 3 kinase pathway. Mol Vis. 2013;19:281–91.
33. Miura Y. Evaluation of mitochondrial function of the retinal tissue with FLIO. In: Paper presented at the FLIM2018, Berlin. 2018.
34. Miura Y, Huettmann G, Orzekowsky-Schroeder R, Steven P, Szaszak M, Koop N, Brinkmann R. Two-photon microscopy and fluorescence lifetime imaging of retinal pigment epithelial cells under oxidative stress. Invest Ophthalmol Vis Sci. 2013;54(5):3366–77. https://doi.org/10.1167/iovs.13-11808.
35. Gallemore RP, Steinberg RH. Effects of DIDS on the chick retinal pigment epithelium. I. Membrane potentials, apparent resistances, and mechanisms. J Neurosci. 1989;9(6):1968–76.
36. Imanishi Y, Sun W, Maeda T, Maeda A, Palczewski K. Retinyl ester homeostasis in the adipose differentiation-related protein-deficient retina. J Biol Chem. 2008;283(36):25091–102. https://doi.org/10.1074/jbc.M802981200.
37. Nagai H, Kalanins VI. An apical tension-sensitive microfilament system in retinal pigment epithelial cells. Exp Cell Res. 1996;223(1):63–71.
38. Sandig M, Kalnins VI. Morphological changes in the zonula adhaerens during embryonic development of chick retinal pigment epithelial cells. Cell Tissue Res. 1990;259(3):455–61.
39. Chiba C, Nakamura K, Unno S, Saito T. Intraocular implantation of DNA-transfected retinal pigment epithelium cells: a new approach for analyzing molecular functions in the newt retinal regeneration. Neurosci Lett. 2004;368(2):171–5. https://doi.org/10.1016/j.neulet.2004.07.009.
40. Yoshikawa T, Mizuno A, Yasumuro H, Inami W, Vergara MN, Del Rio-Tsonis K, Chiba C. MEK-ERK and heparin-susceptible signaling pathways are involved in cell-cycle entry of the wound edge retinal pigment epithelium cells in the adult newt. Pigment Cell Melanoma Res. 2012;25(1):66–82. https://doi.org/10.1111/j.1755-148X.2011.00935.x.
41. Frambach DA, Valentine JL, Weiter JJ. Topical phenylephrine for mydriasis affects rabbit retinal pigment epithelial transport. Invest Ophthalmol Vis Sci. 1989;30(2):343–4.
42. Delpriore LV, Glaser BM, Quigley HA, Green WR. Response of pig retinal-pigment epithelium to laser photocoagulation in organ-culture. Arch Ophthalmol. 1989;107(1):119–22.
43. Kaempf S, Johnen S, Salz AK, Weinberger A, Walter P, Thumann G. Effects of bevacizumab (Avastin) on retinal cells in organotypic culture. Invest Ophthalmol Vis Sci. 2008;49(7):3164–71. https://doi.org/10.1167/iovs.07-1265.
44. Klettner A, Kaya L, Flach J, Lassen J, Treumer F, Roider J. Basal and apical regulation of VEGF-A and placenta growth factor in the RPE/choroid and primary RPE. Mol Vis. 2015;21:736–48.
45. Treumer F, Klettner A, Baltz J, Hussain AA, Miura Y, Brinkmann R, Roider J, Hillenkamp J. Vectorial release of matrix metalloproteinases (MMPs) from porcine RPE-choroid explants following selective retina therapy (SRT): towards slowing the macular ageing process. Exp Eye Res. 2012;97(1):63–72. https://doi.org/10.1016/j.exer.2012.02.011.
46. Chiba C, Hoshino A, Nakamura K, Susaki K, Yamano Y, Kaneko Y, Kuwata O, Maruo F, Saito T. Visual cycle protein RPE65 persists in new retinal cells during retinal regeneration of adult newt. J Comp Neurol. 2006;495(4):391–407. https://doi.org/10.1002/cne.20880.
47. Archibald AL, Bolund L, Churcher C, Fredholm M, Groenen MA, Harlizius B, Lee KT, Milan D, Rogers J, Rothschild MF, Uenishi H, Wang J, Schook LB, Swine Genome Sequencing Consortium. Pig genome sequence—analysis and publication strat-

egy. BMC Genomics. 2010;11:438. https://doi.org/10.1186/1471-2164-11-438.
48. Middleton S. Porcine ophthalmology. Vet Clin North Am Food Anim Pract. 2010;26(3):557–72. https://doi.org/10.1016/j.cvfa.2010.09.002.
49. Olsen TW, Sanderson S, Feng X, Hubbard WC. Porcine sclera: thickness and surface area. Invest Ophthalmol Vis Sci. 2002;43(8):2529–32.
50. Prince JH. Anatomy and histology of the eye and orbit in domestic animals. Springfield: C.C. Thomas; 1960.
51. Koinzer S, Schlott K, Ptaszynski L, Bever M, Kleemann S, Saeger M, Baade A, Caliebe A, Miura Y, Birngruber R, Brinkmann R, Roider J. Temperature-controlled retinal photocoagulation—a step toward automated laser treatment. Invest Ophthalmol Vis Sci. 2012;53(7):3605–14. https://doi.org/10.1167/iovs.11-8588.
52. Sher A, Jones BW, Huie P, Paulus YM, Lavinsky D, Leung LS, Nomoto H, Beier C, Marc RE, Palanker D. Restoration of retinal structure and function after selective photocoagulation. J Neurosci. 2013;33(16):6800–8. https://doi.org/10.1523/JNEUROSCI.1044-12.2013.
53. Spering HG. Laser eye effects. Washington, DC: The National Academies Press; 1968.
54. Myers AC, Lovestam Adrian M, Bruun A, Ghosh F, Andreasson S, Ponjavic V. Retinal function and morphology in rabbit after intravitreal injection of VEGF inhibitors. Curr Eye Res. 2012;37(5):399–407. https://doi.org/10.3109/02713683.2011.611609.
55. Olsen TW, Aaberg SY, Geroski DH, Edelhauser HF. Human sclera: thickness and surface area. Am J Ophthalmol. 1998;125(2):237–41.
56. Flaxel C, Bradle J, Acott T, Samples JR. Retinal pigment epithelium produces matrix metalloproteinases after laser treatment. Retina. 2007;27(5):629–34. https://doi.org/10.1097/01.iae.0000249561.02567.fd.
57. Nicolaissen B, Allen C, Nicolaissen A, Arnesen K. Human retinal-pigment epithelium in long-term explant culture. Acta Ophthalmol. 1986;64(1):1–8.
58. Nicolaissen B Jr, Davanger M, Arnesen K. Surface morphology of explants from the human retinal pigment epithelium in culture. A scanning electron microscopic study. Acta Ophthalmol. 1982;60(6):881–93.
59. Wang H, Ninomiya Y, Sugino IK, Zarbin MA. Retinal pigment epithelium wound healing in human Bruch's membrane explants. Invest Ophthalmol Vis Sci. 2003;44(5):2199–210. https://doi.org/10.1167/iovs.02-0435.
60. LaVail MM. Rod outer segment disk shedding in rat retina: relationship to cyclic lighting. Science. 1976;194(4269):1071–4.
61. Sethna S, Finnemann SC. Analysis of photoreceptor rod outer segment phagocytosis by RPE cells in situ. Methods Mol Biol. 2013;935:245–54. https://doi.org/10.1007/978-1-62703-080-9_17.
62. Ikegami Y, Mitsuda S, Araki M. Neural cell differentiation from retinal pigment epithelial cells of the newt: an organ culture model for the urodele retinal regeneration. J Neurobiol. 2002;50(3):209–20. https://doi.org/10.1002/Neu.10031.
63. Nicolaissen B Jr, Kolstad A, Arnesen K. Reactive changes in the human retinal pigment epithelium in vitro. Acta Ophthalmol. 1981;59(4):476–84.
64. Hutfilz A, Lewke B, Miura Y. Fluorescence lifetime imaging ophthalmoscopy of the retinal pigment epithelium during wound healing after selective retina treatment. In: Buzug TH, Heinz, Klein, Stephan, editors. Student Conference 2018 Lübeck. Infinite Science Publishing; 2018. p. 101–4.
65. Richert E, Koinzer S, Tode J, Schlott K, Brinkmann R, Hillenkamp J, Klettner A, Roider J. Release of different cell mediators during retinal pigment epithelium regeneration following selective retina therapy. Invest Ophthalmol Vis Sci. 2018;59(3):1323–31. https://doi.org/10.1167/iovs.17-23163.
66. Kita M, Marmor MF. Effects on retinal adhesive force in vivo of metabolically active agents in the subretinal space. Invest Ophthalmol Vis Sci. 1992;33(6):1883–7.
67. Marmor MF, Yao XY. The metabolic dependency of retinal adhesion in rabbit and primate. Arch Ophthalmol. 1995;113(2):232–8.
68. Luke M, Weiergraber M, Brand C, Siapich SA, Banat M, Hescheler J, Luke C, Schneider T. The isolated perfused bovine retina—a sensitive tool for pharmacological research on retinal function. Brain Res Brain Res Protoc. 2005;16(1–3):27–36. https://doi.org/10.1016/j.brainresprot.2005.09.001.
69. Jablonski MM, Tombran-Tink J, Mrazek DA, Iannaccone A. Pigment epithelium-derived factor supports normal development of photoreceptor neurons and opsin expression after retinal pigment epithelium removal. J Neurosci. 2000;20(19):7149–57.
70. Ussing HH, Zerahn K. Active transport of sodium as the source of electric current in the short-circuited isolated frog skin. Acta Physiol Scand. 1951;23(2–3):110–27. https://doi.org/10.1111/j.1748-1716.1951.tb00800.x.
71. McAteer JA, Hegre OD. A continuous-flow method of organ culture. In Vitro. 1978;14(9):795–803.
72. Rose GG, Kumegawa M, Nikai H, Bracho M, Cattoni M. The dual-rotary circumfusion system for mark II culture chambers. I. Design, control, and monitoring of the system and the cultures. Microvasc Res. 1970;2(1):24–60.
73. Robb WL. Thin silicone membranes—their permeation properties and some applications. Ann N Y Acad Sci. 1968;146(1):119–37.
74. Pegg DE, Fuller BJ, Foreman J, Green CJ. The choice of plastic tubing for organ perfusion experiments. Cryobiology. 1972;9(6):569–71.
75. Miura Y. Retinal pigment epithelium-choroid organ culture. Expert Rev Ophthalmol. 2011;6(6):669–80. https://doi.org/10.1586/eop.11.70.
76. Sugiura S, Sakai Y, Nakazawa K, Kanamori T. Superior oxygen and glucose supply in perfusion cell cultures compared to static cell cultures demonstrated by simulations using the finite element

method. Biomicrofluidics. 2011;5(2):22202. https://doi.org/10.1063/1.3589910.
77. Bonilha VL. Age and disease-related structural changes in the retinal pigment epithelium. Clin Ophthalmol. 2008;2(2):413–24.
78. Abdal Monaim M, Suleiman JH, Ashraf M. Morphological recovery in the reattached retina of the toad Bufo marinus: a new experimental model of retinal detachment. Arch Med Res. 2005;36(2):107–12. https://doi.org/10.1016/j.arcmed.2004.12.013.
79. Anderson DH, Guerin CJ, Erickson PA, Stern WH, Fisher SK. Morphological recovery in the reattached retina. Invest Ophthalmol Vis Sci. 1986;27(2):168–83.
80. Tsuboi S, Pederson JE, Toris CB. Functional recovery of retinal pigment epithelial damage in experimental retinal detachment. Invest Ophthalmol Vis Sci. 1987;28(11):1788–94.
81. Essner E, Roszka JR, Schreiber JH. Phagocytosis and surface morphology in cultured retinal pigment epithelial cells. Invest Ophthalmol Vis Sci. 1978;17(11):1040–8.
82. Campochiaro PA. Cytokine production by retinal pigmented epithelial cells. Int Rev Cytol. 1993;146:75–82.
83. Byeon SH, Lee SC, Choi SH, Lee HK, Lee JH, Chu YK, Kwon OW. Vascular endothelial growth factor as an autocrine survival factor for retinal pigment epithelial cells under oxidative stress via the VEGF-R2/PI3K/Akt. Invest Ophthalmol Vis Sci. 2010;51(2):1190–7. https://doi.org/10.1167/iovs.09-4144.
84. Klettner A. Physiological functions of VEGF in the retina and its possible implications of prolonged anti-VEGF therapy. Biology, regulation and clinical significance. Hauppauge: Nova Publishing; 2013.
85. Nishijima K, Ng YS, Zhong LC, Bradley J, Schubert W, Jo N, Akita J, Samuelsson SJ, Robinson GS, Adamis AP, Shima DT. Vascular endothelial growth factor-A is a survival factor for retinal neurons and a critical neuroprotectant during the adaptive response to ischemic injury. Am J Pathol. 2007;171(1):53–67. https://doi.org/10.2353/ajpath.2007.061237.
86. Saint-Geniez M, Maldonado AE, D'Amore PA. VEGF expression and receptor activation in the choroid during development and in the adult. Invest Ophthalmol Vis Sci. 2006;47(7):3135–42. https://doi.org/10.1167/iovs.05-1229.
87. Ghiso N, Rohan RM, Amano S, Garland R, Adamis AP. Suppression of hypoxia-associated vascular endothelial growth factor gene expression by nitric oxide via cGMP. Invest Ophthalmol Vis Sci. 1999;40(6):1033–9.
88. Ogata N, Yamanaka R, Yamamoto C, Miyashiro M, Kimoto T, Takahashi K, Maruyama K, Uyama M. Expression of vascular endothelial growth factor and its receptor, KDR, following retinal ischemia-reperfusion injury in the rat. Curr Eye Res. 1998;17(11):1087–96.
89. Chu PG, Grunwald GB. Functional inhibition of retinal pigment epithelial cell-substrate adhesion with a monoclonal antibody against the beta 1 subunit of integrin. Invest Ophthalmol Vis Sci. 1991;32(6):1763–9.
90. Mainster MA. Wavelength selection in macular photocoagulation. Tissue optics, thermal effects, and laser systems. Ophthalmology. 1986;93(7):952–8.
91. Boulton ME. Studying melanin and lipofuscin in RPE cell culture models. Exp Eye Res. 2014;126:61–7. https://doi.org/10.1016/j.exer.2014.01.016.
92. Treumer F, Flohr C, Klettner A, Nolle B, Roider J. [Expression of matrix metalloproteinase-19 in the human cornea. Wound healing in the MMP-19 knock-out mouse model]. Der Ophthalmologe. 2010;107(7):647–53. https://doi.org/10.1007/s00347-009-2045-7.
93. Akeo K, Tanaka Y, Uemura Y, Fujiwara T. Electron-microscopic comparative studies of phagocytic processes between outer segments and latex microspheres in cultured human retinal-pigment epithelial-cells. In Vitro Cell Dev Biol. 1988;24(5):445–50.
94. Zhao MW, Jin ML, He S, Spee C, Ryan SJ, Hinton DR. A distinct integrin-mediated phagocytic pathway for extracellular matrix remodeling by RPE cells. Invest Ophthalmol Vis Sci. 1999;40(11):2713–23.
95. Bialek S, Joseph DP, Miller SS. The delayed basolateral membrane hyperpolarization of the bovine retinal pigment epithelium: mechanism of generation. J Physiol. 1995;484(Pt 1):53–67.
96. Joseph DP, Miller SS. Apical and basal membrane ion transport mechanisms in bovine retinal pigment epithelium. J Physiol. 1991;435:439–63.
97. Quinn RH, Miller SS. Ion transport mechanisms in native human retinal pigment epithelium. Invest Ophthalmol Vis Sci. 1992;33(13):3513–27.
98. Miura Y, Klettner A, Roider J. VEGF antagonists decrease barrier function of retinal pigment epithelium in vitro: possible participation of intracellular glutathione. Invest Ophthalmol Vis Sci. 2010;51(9):4848–55. https://doi.org/10.1167/iovs.09-4699.
99. Ablonczy Z, Dahrouj M, Tang PH, Liu Y, Sambamurti K, Marmorstein AD, Crosson CE. Human retinal pigment epithelium cells as functional models for the RPE in vivo. Invest Ophthalmol Vis Sci. 2011;52(12):8614–20. https://doi.org/10.1167/iovs.11-8021.
100. Klettner A, Recber M, Roider J. Comparison of the efficacy of aflibercept, ranibizumab, and bevacizumab in an RPE/choroid organ culture. Graefes Arch Clin Exp Ophthalmol. 2014;252(10):1593–8. https://doi.org/10.1007/s00417-014-2719-y.
101. Alexander NS, Palczewska G, Palczewski K. Semi-automated discrimination of retinal pigmented epithelial cells in two-photon fluorescence images of mouse retinas. Biomed Opt Express. 2015;6(8):3032–52. https://doi.org/10.1364/BOE.6.003032.
102. Schweitzer D, Schenke S, Hammer M, Schweitzer F, Jentsch S, Birckner E, Becker W, Bergmann A. Towards metabolic mapping of the human retina.

Microsc Res Tech. 2007;70(5):410–9. https://doi.org/10.1002/jemt.20427.
103. Maminishkis A, Chen S, Jalickee S, Banzon T, Shi G, Wang FE, Ehalt T, Hammer JA, Miller SS. Confluent monolayers of cultured human fetal retinal pigment epithelium exhibit morphology and physiology of native tissue. Invest Ophthalmol Vis Sci. 2006;47(8):3612–24. https://doi.org/10.1167/iovs.05-1622.

Animal Models of Diseases of the Retinal Pigment Epithelium

19

Erica L. Fletcher, Ursula Greferath, Philipp Guennel, Mario Huynh, Quan D. Findlay, Andrew I. Jobling, Joanna A. Phipps, Alice A. Brandli, Yao Mei Wang, Samuel A. Mills, Kiana Kakavand, Robb U. DeIongh, and Kirstan A. Vessey

Introduction

Photoreceptor death accounts for approximately 50% of all cases of irreversible vision loss and a significant proportion of these cases are due to conditions that affect the structure and function of the retinal pigment epithelium (RPE). The RPE lies immediately adjacent to photoreceptors and is integral for maintaining normal vision (Fig. 19.1) [1]. Genetic inheritance, environmental factors and age can influence the myriad of functions of the RPE, leading to deleterious effect on photoreceptor function.

A range of mammalian species are affected by inherited mutations, age or systemic medications agents that can influence the structure and function of the RPE. Inherited retinal degeneration caused by mutations encoding proteins important for RPE function affect many dog, cat, pig and primate species, as well as rodents. In addition, with the advent of gene manipulation, a number of new mouse models have emerged, fostering our understanding of retinal degenerations. Age related changes of the RPE are a contributor to age-related macular degeneration (AMD) and many features of this disease are observed in animals. Table 19.1 provides a summary of the rodent and large mammals that display similarities to a range of human conditions and that are described in this chapter.

The aim of this chapter is to provide an overview of how diseases of the RPE manifest in non-laboratory and laboratory animals and how faithfully each animal model recapitulates human disease. In particular, we examine the information gained from studying laboratory and non-laboratory animals that carry mutations in genes encoding proteins important for RPE function, or that are affected by pharmacological agents that affect RPE function.

Overview of the Structure and Function of the RPE

The RPE is a single layer of cells immediately distal to photoreceptors [2] (Fig. 19.1). This single layer of hexagonal shaped cells provides multiple essential functions, which are required for maintenance of normal photoreceptor function, including absorption of excess light, trans-epithelial transport of water, recycling of photoreceptor outer-segments, transport

E. L. Fletcher (✉) · U. Greferath · P. Guennel
M. Huynh · Q. D. Findlay · A. I. Jobling · J. A. Phipps
A. A. Brandli · Y. M. Wang · S. A. Mills
K. Kakavand · R. U. DeIongh · K. A. Vessey
Department of Anatomy and Neuroscience, The University of Melbourne, Melbourne, VIC, Australia
e-mail: elf@unimelb.edu.au

A. K. Klettner, S. Dithmar (eds.), *Retinal Pigment Epithelium in Health and Disease*,
https://doi.org/10.1007/978-3-030-28384-1_19

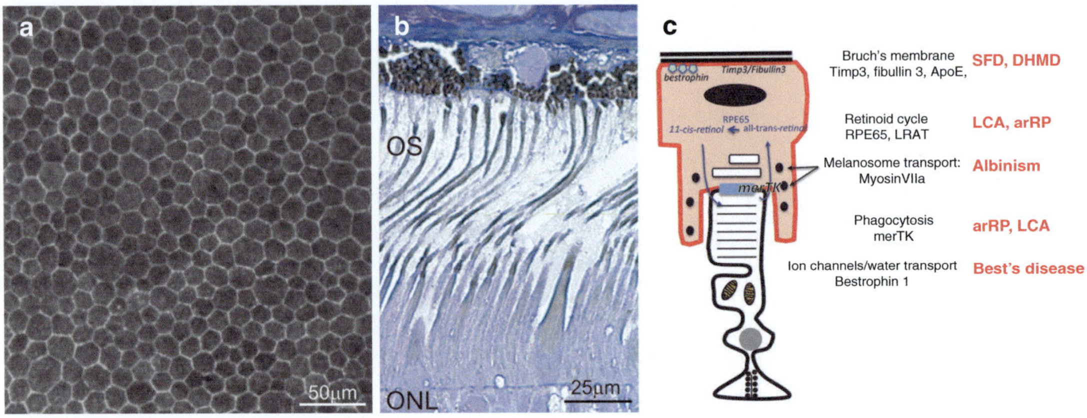

Fig. 19.1 Structure of the retinal pigment epithelium. (**a**) Flatmounted RPE that has been immunolabelled for the actin filament phalloidin. The regular hexagonal pattern of cells is evident. (**b**) Vertical section through the human retina showing the relationship between photoreceptor outer segments and the RPE. Photoreceptor outer segments interdigitate between the apical processes of the RPE. (**c**) Schematic diagram of the RPE showing possible cellular functions modified by inheritance of genetic mutations

Table 19.1 Summary of animal models of RPE disease described in this chapter

RPE function	Gene defect	Animal	Human disease
Phagocytosis of photoreceptor outersegments	*Mertk*	RCS rat, *mer*$^{-/-}$ mouse	Autosomal recessive Retinitis Pigmentosa
Binding of photoreceptor outersgements with RPE microvilli	mi^{vit}	Vitiligo mi^{vit} mouse	Retinal degeneration associated with vitiligo
Ion channel/water transport	*Best1*$^{W93C/W93C}$	*Best1*$^{W93C/W93C}$ knockin mouse	Best vitelliform macular degeneration
Ion channel/water transport	*Best1*	Canine multifocal retinopathy (13 breeds of dog)	Best vitelliform macular degeneration
Extracellular matrix composition of Bruch's membrane—Fibulin 3	Epidermal growth factor-containing fibrillin–like extracellular matrix protein 1	*EFEMP1*^{R345W} mouse	Doyne's Honeycomb retinal dystrophy
Bruch's membrane thickness	*Timp3*	*Timp3*$^{-/-}$, *Timp3*^{Ser156Cys} mice	Sorsby's fundus dystrophy
Lysosomal storage	*CLN6*	*nclf* mouse	Neuronal ceroid lipofuscinoses
Degradation and turnover of spent photoreceptor outersegments	*Abca4*	*Abca4*$^{-/-}$mouse	Stargardt's disease
Degradation and turnover of spent photoreceptor outersegments	*Abca4*	Pitbull terriers	Stargardt's disease
Short chain collagen that is important for adhesion between Bruch's membrane and RPE	Complement 1q Tumor Necrosis Factor 5 gene	*C1QTNF5*^{S163R} knockin mouse	Cone-rod dystrophy
Retinoid recycling	*Lrat*	*Lrat*$^{-/-}$, *Lrat* conditional knockout mice	Leber's congenital amaurosis, Autosomal recessive Retinitis Pigmentosa

Table 19.1 (continued)

RPE function	Gene defect	Animal	Human disease
Retinoid recycling	*Rpe65*	*Rpe65*$^{-/-}$, *rd12*, *Rpe65*^{R91W} mice	Leber's congenital amaurosis, Autosomal recessive Retinitis Pigmentosa
Retinoid recycling	RPE65	Briard sheepdog	Leber's congenital amaurosis, Autosomal recessive Retinitis Pigmentosa
Formation of mature melanosomes	*Oa1*	*Oa1*$^{-/-}$mouse	Ocular albinism
Formation of melanin	Tyrosinase	balb/c mouse, Sprague-Dawley rat	Oculocutaneous albinism
Drusen formation		Aged primates	Early/intermediate AMD
Bruch's membrane thickness	*HTRA1*	*HTRA1*knockin mouse	AMD
Lipid transport	*ApoE*	*ApoE*$^{-/-}$ *ApoEε2*, *ApoEε3*, *ApoEε4* knockin mice	AMD
Lipid transport	*CD36*	*CD36*$^{-/-}$ mouse	AMD
Anti-oxidant mechanisms	*Nrf2*	*Nrf2*$^{-/-}$ mouse	AMD
Anti-oxidant mechanisms	*Sod1*	*Sod1*$^{-/-}$ mouse	AMD
Autophagy	RB1CC1	*Rb1cc1*$^{-/-}$ mouse	AMD

and recycling of retinoids, recycling of ions and finally, secretion of neurotrophic factors. In addition, the RPE dynamically turns over the Bruch's membrane. As shown in Fig. 19.1c, each of these aspects of RPE function can be affected by genetically inherited mutations, toxic substances, or age, and can contribute to major diseases associated with photoreceptor degeneration.

Functions of melanosomes within the RPE: By virtue of the presence of melanin granules within melanosomes of the RPE, excess light is absorbed [3]. It is generally accepted that light absorbed by the RPE prevents the reflection of light that would degrade the visual image. In agreement with this vision-optimization mechanism, melanosomes are located in the apical part of normal RPE cells in close proximity to the microvilli that envelop photoreceptor outer-segments (Fig. 19.1). In addition to their function in light absorption, melanin also plays a role in quenching reactive oxygen species and plays a key role in binding iron. Pigmentation of the RPE involves a several complex processes including the synthesis of melanin from tyrosine via tyrosinase, maturation of melanosomes and finally transport of melanosomes from to peripheral and apical regions of the cell via molecular machinery, including Myosin VIIa [3, 4]. Defects in any of these aspects of melanin biosynthesis or melanosome maturation and transport are associated with albinism, and lead to visual dysfunction of varying severity [5, 6].

Transport of ions, water and nutrients across the RPE: A central function of the RPE is transport of nutrients, waste products, ions and water into and out of the retina [3]. Ion channels and transporters are localized preferentially to the apical or basolateral surfaces of RPE cells. One example of this is Na^+, K^+ATPase which is located on the apical surface and regulates the concentration of sodium and potassium within the subretinal space, causing influx of sodium into RPE cells at the expense of potassium [2, 3]. The sodium gradient that is created by Na^+, K^+ATPase also facilitates the uptake of $HCO3^-$ via Na^+HCO3 and the uptake of potassium and chloride ions via the Na^+-K^+-$2Cl^-$ co-transporter. In combination these systems are important for maintaining intracellular pH and also for maintaining a high sodium concentration in the subretinal space that is critical for maintaining the dark current in rod photoreceptors. In addition to regulation of potassium and sodium, chloride plays an important role in maintaining fluid balance within the RPE and subretinal space. Bestrophin

1, which is localized to the basolateral surface of the RPE, is important for regulating chloride flux in a calcium dependent manner [7, 8].

The RPE is able to transport water and metabolic end products from the subretinal space to the choriocapillaris. Lactate, which is produced predominantly by photoreceptor outer segments, is transported across the RPE via monocarboxylate transporters, notably MCT1 and MCT3 [9, 10]. In the opposite direction, the RPE facilitates transport of glucose from the vasculature to photoreceptors. Glucose transporters, GLUT1 and GLUT3 are highly expressed by the RPE and localized to the basal and apical surfaces [11]. Another nutrient critical for maintaining normal retinal function is retinol which provides the retinoid, 11-cis retinal that is critical for photoreceptor function. Vitamin A (all-trans-retinol) is taken up by the RPE via a receptor mediated process and transported within the RPE via cellular retinol binding protein (CRBP). Once within the RPE, all-trans-retinol undergoes a series of enzymatic isomerizations as part of the retinoid cycle that ultimately leads to the formation of 11-cis retinal that is transported from the RPE to photoreceptors.

Retinoid cycle: The retinoid cycle is a complex recycling system that replenishes 11-cis-retinal, a derivative of Vitamin A that is critical for the conversion of light to a neuronal signal by photoreceptors [2]. Following light exposure, all-trans retinal is transported from photoreceptors to the RPE where it is enzymatically converted back to 11-cis retinal. A number of enzymes important for the isomerization of all-trans retinal to 11-cis retinal are expressed by the RPE including RPE65, lecithin retinol acyltransferase (LRAT), and retinol dehydrogenase (RDH). RPE65 is an isomerase that converts all-trans retinyl esters to 11-cis retinol. LRAT esterifies all-trans retinal to form retinyl esters that form the substrate for RPE65 [12]. Mutations affecting many of these enzymes are associated with photoreceptor dysfunction and death.

Phagocytosis and recycling of photoreceptor outer segments: Photoreceptors are exposed to high amounts of light and thus accumulate photo-damaged proteins and lipids. This is coupled with the generation of photo-oxidative radicals resulting in a high abundance of light-induced toxic substances within photoreceptors. The tips of the photoreceptor outer segments harbour the oldest discs which contain the highest concentration of oxidative radicals, photo-damaged proteins and lipids. Consequently, a major part of photoreceptor renewal process includes the shedding of outer segment tips [13, 14] and the phagocytosis of the shed outer segments by the RPE [2]. Phagocytosis of photoreceptor outer segments involves recognition of outer segments by the RPE, and then processing through a series of phagosomes. The binding of photoreceptor outer segments is dependent on recognition by scavenger receptors, particularly MerTK that is expressed on the apical membrane of the RPE [15]. MerTK is a member of the "TAM" (Tyro3, Axl and Mer) family of scavenger receptors that are widely expressed by cells of the nervous, immune and reproductive system. MerTK is highly expressed by the RPE where is thought to interact with non-muscle myosin allowing the binding and engulfment of photoreceptor outer segments [15]. The integrin component, αVβ5 also plays a role in recognition of photoreceptor outer-segments by the RPE [16]. Mutations affecting MerTK in particular are associated with retinal degeneration.

Secretion of cytokines and growth factors: The RPE is able to produce and secrete various cytokines and growth factors that are required for maintenance of the structural integrity of retina and choriocapillaris including pigment epithelium-derived factor (PEDF), vascular endothelial growth factor (VEGF), Tumour growth factor beta (TGFβ), and a range of fibroblast growth factors [2]. These cytokines and growth factors have a number of roles that include maintaining the immune privileged state within the subretinal space, stabilization of the endothelium of the choriocapillaris [17] and maintenance of neuronal integrity. Release of a number of cytokines is altered with age, potentially altering the environment within the subretinal space and contributing to the development of age related conditions such as age-related macular degeneration [18].

Normal Functions of Bruch's Membrane

The RPE plays an important role in the turnover of Bruch's membrane, a thin (2–4 μm) layer of connective tissue that lies between the RPE and the underlying, choriocapillaris [19]. It is a penta-laminar extracellular matrix composed of primarily elastin and collagen [20]. The importance of Bruch's membrane in retina physiology is the ability to function as both a physical and a biochemical barrier for normal physiological processes and pathological processes such as CNV [19]. Its primary roles include: (1) regulating the diffusion of bio molecules, minerals, antioxidant components, trace elements and serum constituents between the choroid and the RPE [19], (2) providing physical support for RPE cell adhesion, (3) wound healing and (4) acting as a physical barrier that restricts retinal and choroidal cellular migration [19] Given that Bruch's membrane is acellular, transport through it occurs by passive diffusion. Changes to structure or composition of Bruch's membrane can affect diffusion properties, which ultimately affects the function of the RPE and the outer retina.

In summary, the RPE performs a range of functions that are critical for maintaining photoreceptor integrity and function. Retinal degenerations are associated with anomalies that affect virtually every cellular function described above. In the sections below, we outline how animal models with mutations affecting these functions have aided in our understanding of a range of human retinal degenerations.

Modelling Inherited Retinal Diseases Associated with the RPE

Photoreceptor integrity and function is critically dependent on a normal functioning RPE [1]. Consequently, mutations affecting any of the key proteins involved in regulating RPE function are associated with photoreceptor death and ultimately vision loss. As shown in Fig. 19.1, genetic inheritance of a range of mutations affecting RPE function cause retinal degenerations. In this section we summarize how inherited retinal degenerations associated with mutations affecting RPE function influence vision loss in laboratory and non-laboratory animals.

Retinitis Pigmentosa: A Family of Inherited Retinal Degenerations

Retinitis Pigmentosa (RP) refers to a family of inherited retinal degenerations that affects approximately 1:5000 people [21]. It is characterized by gradual loss of rods followed by cones that ultimately leads to complete vision loss. Clinically, RP is associated with deficits in rod photoreceptor function manifesting as a reduction in amplitude the a-wave of the full flash electroretinogram, gradual constriction of the visual field, changes in the retinal fundus including migration of pigment into the retina from the underlying RPE, and attenuation of retinal vasculature. In addition to photoreceptor loss, some forms of RP, called syndromic forms of RP, are associated with degeneration in non-retinal regions of the CNS and/or the body. The commonest syndromic forms of RP include Usher's syndrome and Bardet-Biedl Syndrome. Usher's syndrome is characterized by gradual hearing and vision loss, whilst Bardet-Biedl syndrome is characterized by a range of systemic effects in combination with vision loss. RP is caused by a range of mutations encoding proteins involved in photoreceptor or RPE function. A great deal has been learned about these diseases by understanding the pathogenesis of disease in animals. Moreover, pre-clinical development of therapies including gene therapy, electronic restoration of vision and development of therapeutics has, in many cases, progressed because of positive outcomes in large animal models of disease that have an eye size and structure more similar to humans [22, 23].

Mutations Affecting Phagocytosis of Outer Segments

As noted above, one of the key functions of the RPE is the phagocytosis and recycling of spent outer segment discs. One of the first animal models manifesting photoreceptor degeneration associated with RPE dysfunction was the Royal college of Surgeons rat [24, 25]. The RCS rat develops gradual accumulation of debris within the subretinal space that is accompanied by gradual loss of photoreceptors from postnatal day 18 [25, 26]. As shown in Fig. 19.2, the retinal fundus of RCS rats compared to control rats appears paler possibly as a consequence of the accumulation of debris. In addition, the structure of the retina as viewed using optical coherence tomography (OCT) reveals that a significant proportion of the outer nuclear layer has been replaced by debris. By postnatal day 60, the outer retina shows accumulation of debris that almost entirely replaces the ONL. By this age, few photoreceptors remain, and retinal function is severely compromised [26–28]. The genetic defect that causes retinal degeneration in RCS rat

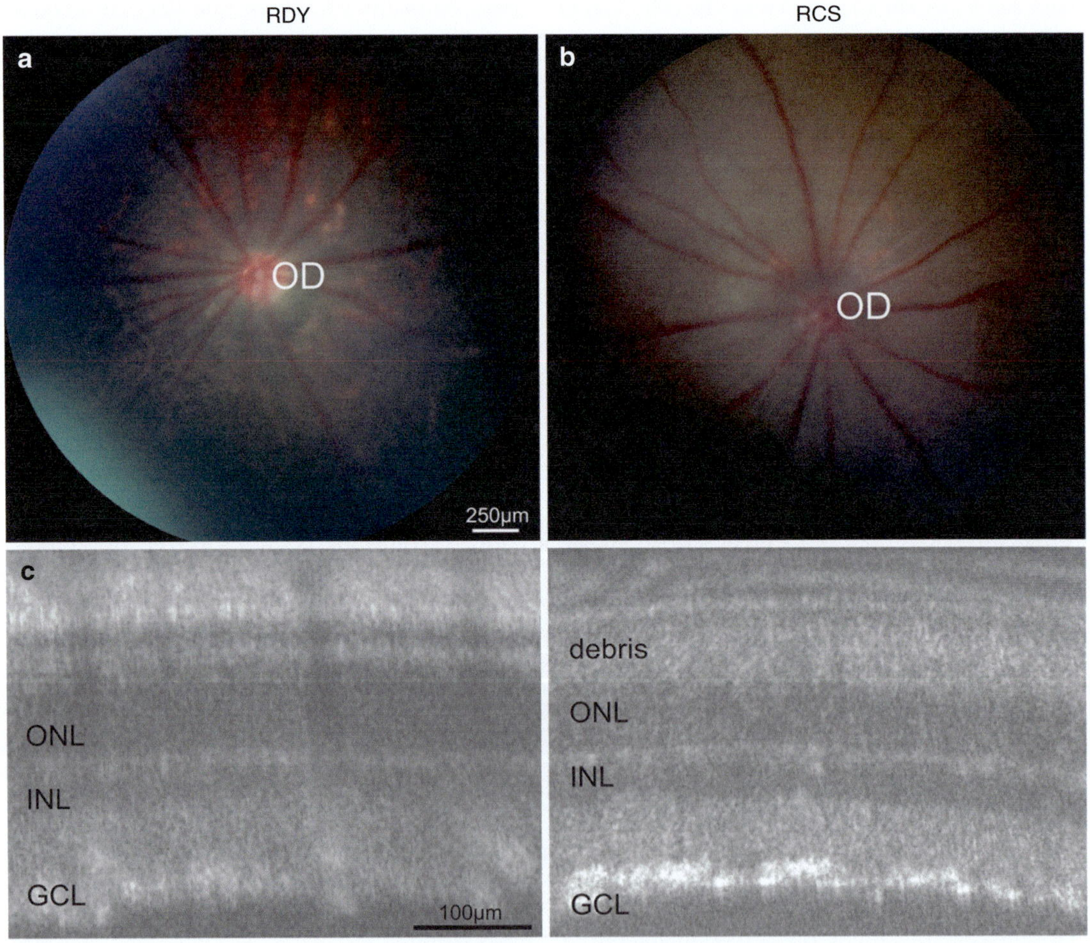

Fig. 19.2 The RCS rat shows defects in phagocytosis by the RPE. (**a**, **b**) Fundus images of a 1 month old RDY (control) and 1 month old RCS rat. The retinal fundus of the RCS rat appears paler possibly because of the accumulation of debris within the subretinal space. (**c**, **d**) Optical coherence tomography of a 1 month old RDY and RCS rat. In contrast to the control (RDY) retina, almost half of the outer retina is replaced by debris. (**e**, **f**) show vertical paraffin sections of the distal retina and RPE stained for haemotoxylin and eosin. The subretinal space shows considerable debris. (**g**, **h**) show vertical sections through the distal retina and RPE immunolabeled for rhodopsin (green) and counter stained for the nuclear marker Hoechst (blue). In contrast to the control RPE, no rhodopsin immunoreactive puncta were observed in the RCS rat RPE suggesting a failure in phagocytosis of photoreceptor outersegments. *RPE* retinal pigment epithelium, *ONL* outer nuclear layer, *INL* inner nuclear layer, *GCL* ganglion cell layer

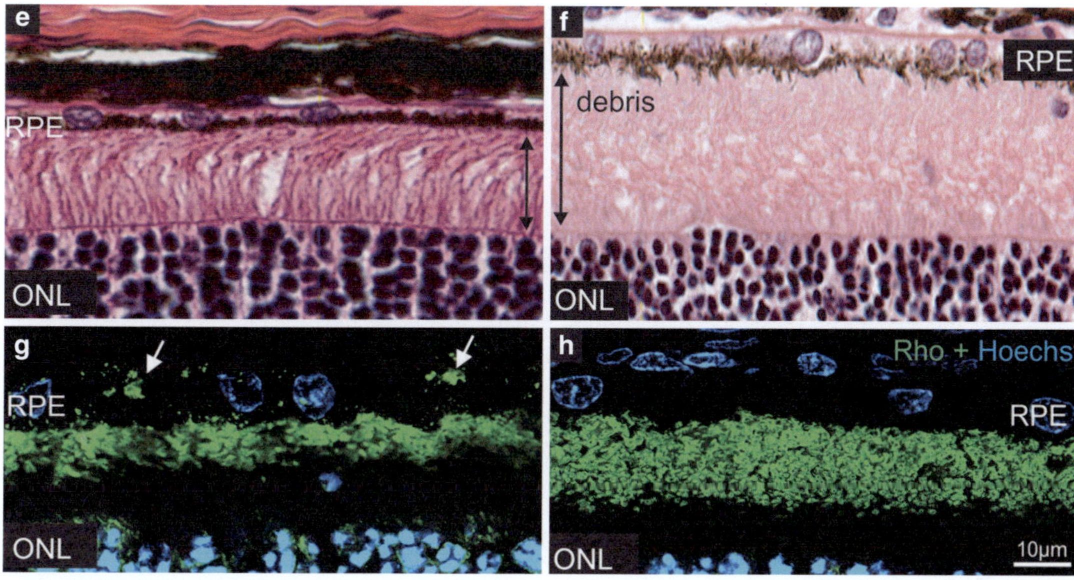

Fig. 19.2 (continued)

and also ~3% of cases of autosomal recessive RP is in *Mertk*, a gene that encodes a transmembrane protein with an extracellular domain important for binding photoreceptor outer segments [29, 30]. This genetic defect leads to the failure of RPE phagocytosis of photoreceptor outer segments, a process crucial for renewal of photoreceptor outer segments. Figure 19.2 shows a vertical section through the RPE of a control and RCS rat. In contrast to the control, no rhodopsin immunoreactive puncta are evident within the RPE of the RCS rat, suggestive of an anomaly in photoreceptor outer segment phagocytosis. Further evidence that RPE dysfunction plays a role in photoreceptor loss in the RCS rat comes from the observation that chimeras formed from the combination of normal and RCS rat embryos display localized retinal degeneration solely in regions where RCS RPE predominates [31]. In addition, gene correction with viral vectors encoding MERTK demonstrate rescue in RCS rats [32] and have been more recently evaluated in a phase I study in humans [33].

Like the RCS rat, accumulation of photoreceptor debris within the subretinal space is a feature of the *mer* knockout mouse and the vitiligo mouse [34, 35]. The vitiligo mi^{vit} mutation causes an anomaly in the relationship between photoreceptor outer segments and the RPE and is associated with gradual photoreceptor loss in homozygous mi^{vit} mice from approximately 2 months of age [36, 37], with complete vision loss within 2 years [35]. There are also marked pigmentary changes within the retinal fundus well before photoreceptor loss and the RPE can appear multilayered, suggestive of abnormal cell proliferation during development [37]. In addition, the RPE microvilli are shortened and closely packed.

Lebers Congenital Amaurosis: Severe Retinal Degenerations Associated with Mutations Affecting the Retinoid Cycle

Leber's congenital amaurosis (LCA) is a severe form of retinal degeneration that leads to irreversible early vision loss often within the first year of life in the absence of any major systemic features [38]. It is accompanied by sensory nystagmus, amaurotic pupils and absence of electrical responses from the retina. It is a rare disease affecting between 1/30,000 and 1/81,000 people. Over 400 mutations in at least 14 genes have been associated with the development of LCA, most of which influence function and integrity of photoreceptors directly (e.g., *GUC2D, AIPL1, CRX*) or the RPE (e.g. *RPE65, LRAT, MERTK*). Mutations in many of the same genes also cause retinitis pigmentosa. Although not well understood, it is possible that the difference in phenotypic severity reflects the importance of the mutant region for protein function or the level of expression. A range of animal models of LCA exist including 13 mouse strains, feline, canine and avian models, most of which carry mutations in genes encoding proteins important for photoreceptor structure and function. However, some rodent and canine species harbour mutations affecting proteins involved in the retinoid cycle, including *Rpe65* and lecithin-retinol acyltransferase *(Lrat)*. Here, we focus on those animal models that are associated with gene mutations affecting RPE dysfunction.

The most widely characterized animal models of LCA are those associated with mutations in *Rpe65* [23]. RPE65 is solely expressed by the RPE and plays a critical role in enzymatic conversion of all-trans retinol to 11-cis retinal. Thus, mutations affecting the expression and function of RPE65 lead to a reduction in the availability of the chromophore, 11-cis retinal, and consequently photoreceptor dysfunction and death [23, 39]. Three mouse models have been identified that carry mutations in *Rpe65*, including the natural mutant *rd12* mouse [40], *Rpe65* null mouse [41] and the *Rpe65*^{R91W} transgenic mouse [42]. *Rpe65* null and *rd12* mice show a slow loss of photoreceptors such that by 12 months of age, only 50% of photoreceptor remain. Moreover, cone photoreceptors are preferentially affected in both these models, with complete loss of short wavelength cones from the inferior retina within 1 month. The loss of cone photoreceptors early in *Rpe65* null mice is consistent with the severe cone photoreceptor loss that has been described in patients with LCA.

Rpe65^{R91W} knock-in mice were generated to express one of the common missense mutations observed in patients with LCA [42]. *Rpe65*^{R91W} mice show partial expression of mutant RPE65 and 10% generation of 11-cis retinal. Despite differences in the level of RPE65 expression compared with *rd12* and *Rpe65* null mice, the phenotype is remarkably similar, showing gradual loss of photoreceptors over a 12-month period.

Like in humans, there are countless genetic mutations that cause retinal degeneration and vision loss in dogs (http://omia.angis.org.au/home) [43]. Loss of vision in dogs is associated with mutations in RPE65. Briard sheepdogs, in particular, can develop an autosomal recessive form of LCA caused by a *RPE65* mutation [44]. These animals are homozygous for a mutation in *RPE65* and develop a slowly progressive retinal degeneration from 1.5 years of age with complete degeneration of photoreceptors in the peripheral retina by 5–7 years of age.

The importance of the retinoid cycle for maintaining photoreceptor integrity is highlighted by severe photoreceptor loss that occurs in response to mutations in another protein important in the retinoid cycle, LRAT. LRAT catalyses the esterification if all-trans retinol to all-trans retinyl esters which forms the substrate that is converted to 11-cis retinol by RPE65. *LRAT* mutations are associated with approximately 1% of all cases of LCA (also referred to as LCA14). Like animals with mutations in RPE65, *LRAT* mutations also lead to a significant reduction in the availability of the chromophore, 11-cis-retinal. *Lrat* knockout mice develop retinal degeneration by two months of age with severe loss of cones occurring prior to rod death. A similar pattern of loss in cones followed by rods was observed in a *Lrat* conditional knockout mouse, where excision of LRAT was achieved selectively in RPE cells by crossing floxed *Lrat* mice with tyrosinase related protein 1(*Tyrp1*)-cre mice [45]. Although the mechanisms by which cones and rods die in *Lrat*-knockout mice remains to be fully understood, there are significant differences in the transport of cone opsin and rhodopsin from the inner segment to the outer segment of photoreceptors. In particular, cone-opsins are mislocalized and accumulate within the inner segment from an early age in *Lrat* knockout mice. The mislocalization of opsin is thought to be critical factor in the subsequent death of cones.

Inherited Macular Degenerations

The macula is a highly specialized region that is preferentially affected in a number of diseases including age-related macular degeneration and inherited macular dystrophies. In humans, there are differences in density of RPE cells and also in the structure of Bruch's membrane in the fovea compared to more peripheral regions that may be a significant factor in the predilection of some conditions to the macula. In addition, the high density of cones in this region of the retina imposes demands on the RPE that are unique to this region of the retina. In studying diseases of the macula, it is important to note that rodents lack a specialized area of the retina of high cone density that has similarities to the human fovea. Thus, mouse models of macula disease are limited to answering questions relating to the role of specific gene pathways in modifying photoreceptor integrity more generally. Specific questions about why the fovea is vulnerable in macula diseases cannot be effectively addressed using rodent models. In contrast, the retinae of large animals including dogs, cats and primates have a specialized area that has similarities to the human macula in that there is a high density of cones in a region located within the temporal retina [46]. Inherited and age-related macular degenerations have been described in some of these larger mammalian species. In the sections below, rodent as well as large animal models of macula disease have been highlighted.

Stargardt's Disease

The commonest form of inherited macular degenerations is Stargardt's disease which is an autosomal recessive disease affecting between 1 in 8,000 and 1 in 10,000 people and that is inherited with a carrier frequency of 1 in 20 [47]. It is characterized by accumulation of lipofuscin within the RPE of the central retinal that leads to RPE dysfunction and death followed by photoreceptor degeneration. ABCA4 is an ATP-binding cassette transporter that is localized to the rim of photoreceptor outer segment disc membranes where it is involved in transport of retinoids from the RPE to photoreceptors [48]. Notably, following isomerization of 11-cis retinal to all-trans retinal by light, all-trans retinal is released into the photoreceptor outer segment and is transported to the disc membrane as a complex with the bisretinoid, N-retinylidene-phosphtidylethanolamine. In the absence of a normal functioning ABCA4 transporter, bisretinoids accumulate within the photoreceptor outer segment and ultimately in the RPE following photoreceptor outer segment phagocytosis. Accumulation of the highly toxic component of lipofuscin, A2E, leads to dysfunction and death of the RPE and subsequently vision loss due to photoreceptor degeneration. Although the gene mutation causal in Stargardt's disease encodes a photoreceptor associated protein, we have included a summary of animal models of this disease because it manifests a profound change in RPE function that has many similarities to other conditions that are directly caused by genes encoding RPE associated proteins.

The pathogenesis of Stargardt's disease has been effectively modelled using the *ABCA4* null mouse. This strain of mouse shows elevated A2E and lipofuscin within the RPE, as well as accumulation of N-retinylidene-phosphtidylethanolamine in photoreceptor outer segments [49, 50]. In addition, A2E induced oxidative stress in the RPE as well as complement activation has been observed in aging *ABCA4* null mice [51]. However, retinal dysfunction and photoreceptor death is slow and only minor changes in dark adaptation have been described even up to 2 years of age [50, 52, 53]. Retinal degeneration associated with an *ABCA4* mutation has been identified in pit bull terriers [54]. Affected animals develop rapid loss of cones followed by rods from between 3 and 6 months of age.

Inherited Macula Degenerations Associated with Bestrophin 1

There are five forms for retinal degeneration associated with mutations in Bestrophin 1 that are broadly referred to as bestrophinopathies [55]. Of the four bestrophins, Bestrophin 1 (Best1) is predominantly expressed by the RPE and is localized to the basolateral surface [56], where it mediates the anion transport, notably chloride, across the RPE cell membrane in a calcium dependent manner [57]. It also regulates intracellular calcium and cell volume [58].

Best vitelliform macular degeneration (BVMD) is the second most common form of inherited macular dystrophy in humans, affecting between 2/10,000 and 1.5/100,000. It is an autosomal dominant condition that is caused by over 200 mutations in Bestrophin 1[55]. It is characterized by excessive accumulation of lipofuscin within the RPE, formation of focal subretinal lesions and subsequently loss of central vision. In addition, there are functional changes in RPE function that are detected by electrooculogram recording and that is considered pathognomonic of the disease. Electrical activity can be elicited from both the RPE and retina in response to a flash of light. For example, the electroretinogram is a series of wavelets of current that are generated by cohorts of neurons in response to a flash of light. The electrooculogram is a much slower currents generated by the RPE. It is thought to arise from depolarization of the basal membrane of the RPE due to increased chloride conductance. In BVMD there is a reduction or absence of the electrooculogram while the ERG remains unaffected.

BVMD progresses through five stages. Stage 1 is characterized by normal vision but with small areas of RPE loss. Stage 2 is characterized by the formation of a well demarcated yellow vitelliform lesion around 2–3 mm in diameter that is centred over the fovea. With time some of the yellow lesion can flatten and resorb, causing a pseudohypopyon indicative of stage 3. During stage 4, the yellow yolk "scrambles" signifying the vitelliruptive stage 3 that is associated with significant vision loss. Finally, during stage 5, there is significant atrophy and choroidal neovascularization. This condition usually presents bilaterally.

Other retinal degenerations associated with mutations in Bestrophin 1 include adult-onset vitelliform macular dystrophy, autosomal recessive bestrophinopathy, autosomal dominant vitreoretinochoroidopathy and retinitis pigmentosa. Adult vitelliform macular dystrophy has many similarities with the milder forms of Best disease with vision preserved in most cases. Autosomal recessive bestrophinopathy is thought to be caused by a "null" mutation in Bestrophin 1 and is associated with a central serous detachment with fibrous subretinal scar most likely caused by choroidal neovascularization. Small yellow vitelliform lesions are also observed.

Best1 knockin mice have been generated that model aspects of human BVMD. Transgenic mice that carry a W93C mutation in the endogenous mouse *Bestrophin* gene have been generated. The W93C mutation was chosen because a large Swedish family with BVMD has been exceptionally well characterized. These mice exhibit many of the signs of human Best disease including accumulation of lipofuscin in the RPE, formation of fluid and debris filled detachments of the retina [59]. Like human BVMD, retinal function in $\mathit{Best1}^{W93C/W93C}$ remains unaffected in the early stages, whereas the electrooculogram is diminished. In addition, large well demarcated detachments of the sensory retina are observed in approximately 40% of heterozygous $\mathit{Best1}^{+/W93C}$ and $\mathit{Best1}^{W93C/W93C}$ mice over 12 months of age that are accompanied by accumulation of lipofuscin in the RPE [59]. Two independently generated Best1 null mice have been generated. In contrast to human BVMD, the electrooculogram is enhanced and there is no change in chloride conductance across the RPE [8, 60]. In addition, there is very little change in retinal integrity, even in mice aged 16–19 months [8].

Canine multifocal retinopathy (cmr1-3) is a naturally occurring autosomal recessive disorder that affects thirteen dog breeds worldwide and that is caused by mutations in bestrophin. These retinopathies show many similarities with human bestrophinopathies [61]. There are three major mutations in the canine Best1 gene that cause disease including a premature stop mutation in exon one (R25X) that was identified in Mastiff breeds [62, 63], a missense mutation (G161D) that affects a rare breed of Coton de Tulear dogs [64] and a frameshift mutation (P463fs) identified in Lapponian Herders [65]. Like their human counterparts, dogs with cmr show a gradual accumulation of lipofuscin within the RPE that is associated with anomalies in cholesterol transport. Importantly, the interaction between photoreceptor outer segments and RPE microvilli is reduced. In particular, the microvilli of RPE cells area retracted, possibly as a developmental consequence of abnormal intracellular calcium regulation. Under normal circumstances, RPE microvilli expand the surface area over which photoreceptors contact the RPE, optimizing photoreceptor outer segment phagocytosis, as well as being a rich source of transporters and ion channels. Separation of photoreceptors from the RPE because of this structural anomaly could be a critical factor in the subsequent detachment of the sensory retina and ultimately the photoreceptor degeneration that occurs [61].

Sorsby Fundus Dystrophy

Bruch's membrane is a five layered basement membrane located between the RPE and choriocapillaris. It contains layers of collagen interspersed with elastin that can vary with age and disease. Being an acellular structure, formation and turnover of Bruch's membrane is dependent on normal function of the RPE. In situations where Bruch's membrane becomes thicker, photoreceptor loss can occur because of deprivation of normal nutrient flow from the vasculature to photoreceptors. Sorsby Fundus Dystrophy (SFD) is a rare autosomal dominant macular degeneration caused by mutations in tissue inhibitor of metalloproteinase 3 (*TIMP3*), an important protein for regulating extracellular matrix turnover [66]. Sorsby fundus dystrophy is characterized by the accumulation of protein and lipid within a thickened Bruch's membrane [67] that is associated with rapid loss of central vision followed by peripheral vision. A transgenic mouse has been created that expresses a similar mutation to those with Sorsby fundus dystrophy, a Ser156Cys substitution in murine *Timp3* [68]. These mice display abnormalities within the RPE from 8 months of age, and an increase in thickness of Bruch's membrane from 30 months. However, they do not develop choroidal neovascularization in contrast to the human condition. More recently, a TIMP3 null mouse has been described [69]. However, Bruch's membrane and the RPE remain largely intact over an 18 month period and vision loss is minimal.

Doynes Honeycomb Retinal Dystrophy

Doynes Honeycomb retinal dystrophy or Malattia Leventinese is a rare autosomal dominantly inherited disease of the macula. Although it can present in early adulthood, it has many similarities with age-related macular degeneration. Small amorphous drusen deposits form between the RPE and Bruch's membrane that gradually enlarge and coalesce with disease duration. Atrophy of the RPE and choroidal neovascularization lead to significant vision loss in the later stages of the disease. A single substitution of Arg345 to Trp (R345W) in the gene *EFEMP1* (epidermal growth factor-containing fibrillin–like extracellular matrix protein 1) is responsible for this disease. EFEMP1 encodes a 493 amino acid protein that is belongs to the fibulin family of extracellular matrix proteins. Although the function of this protein remains to be determined, some fibulin proteins play important roles in the assembly of elastin fibres and EFEMP1 is known to interact with TIMP3.

Two knockin mouse strains have been generated that carry the R345W mutation in the endogenous mouse *EFEMP1* gene [70, 71]. These mice show no significant changes in the retinal fundus, nor in retinal integrity over a 2 year period [70, 71]. However, at the ultrastructural level, there are sub-RPE deposits and changes in Bruch's membrane from as early as 4 months of age. The sub-RPE deposits become more pronounced with increasing age and by 12 months of age Bruch's membrane shows changes in composition and the RPE shows signs of atrophy [70]. Bruch's membrane is thicker in 2 year old mice. Despite these histopathological changes in the RPE and Bruch's membrane, retinal function (as measured by the ERG) is normal and there are no significant changes to retinal structure observed [70, 71]. Moreover, no evidence of advanced disease including choroidal neovascularization has been demonstrated [70, 71]. Overall, these data suggest that the *EFEMP1* knockin mice manifest some of the features of very mild human disease.

Other Rare Inherited Cone-Rod Degeneration That Can Be Modelled in Mice

In addition to the conditions described above, there are a number of other very rare cone-rod dystrophies caused by mutations in genes that encode proteins important in RPE function [72]. Complement 1q Tumor Necrosis Factor 5 gene (C1QTNF5), formerly called CTRP5, encodes a short-chain collagen that is thought to be important for adhesion between the RPE and Bruch's membrane. A single missense mutation in this gene (S163R) is associated with late-onset macular degeneration, an autosomal dominant condition that closely resembles age-related macular degeneration. It is characterized by wide spread deposits between the RPE and Bruch's membrane, gradual atrophy of the RPE and choroidal neovascularization in the advanced stages. These changes are associated with loss of central and peripheral vision.

Two knockin mice have been generated to model late onset macular degeneration, both of which carry the S163R mutation in the *C1QTNF5* gene. In addition, the *rd6* mouse model of retinal degeneration carries a spontaneous mutation in membrane-frizzled-related-protein (*mfrp*). The *MFRP* and *C1QTNF5* genes are located immediately adjacent one another in the human and mouse genome and are expressed as a dicistronic transcript. The two proteins colocalize within the RPE and are functionally linked. Heterozygous $CTRP5^{+/S163R}$ mice show loss of cone and rod mediated function from 10 months of age as well as a progressive increase in the presence of discrete autofluorescent lesions across the retinal fundus. In concert with these findings, there are changes in photoreceptors and the RPE with age. In contrast, Shu et al. [73] have analysed a similarly created $Cq1TNF5+/^{SER163R}$ knockin mouse and found no change in rod or cone mediated function in animals aged up to 2 years, nor any RPE pathology. Whilst it is unclear why these two similar strains of mouse would have such disparate pathology, one possible explanation is that the changes in retinal structure and function described could be a result of the strain carrying a background mutation in CRB1, $Crb1^{rd8/rd8}$ [74]. Indeed, a recent study highlighted the widespread inheritance of this in the background of strains of many mouse lines [74].

Disorders Associated with Anomalies in Melanin/Melanosome Synthesis or Transport

Albinism refers to a group of inherited disorders affecting melanin biosynthesis that affects 1 in 18,000 people [4]. There are two main types of albinism that include oculocutaneous albinism where pigmentation in the eye, skin and hair is affected, and ocular albinism, in which pigmentation defects are restricted to the eye. Pigmentation defects are also characteristic of two rare syndromes called Hermansky-Pudlak syndrome and Chediak Higashi syndrome. Oculocutaneous albinism is an autosomal recessive condition associated with mutations in tyrosinase, P gene, tyrosinase-like protein 1 (TYRP1) and the transporter, SLC45A2. In contrast, ocular albinism mostly affects males in an X-linked fashion and is associated with inheritance of a mutation in OA1 (more recently referred to as GPR143). All forms of albinism are associated with lack of pigmentation in the skin and/or eyes together with anomalies in foveal maturation (foveal hypoplasia) and the optic chiasm. As a consequence of a delayed maturation of the macula, anomalies in fixation, and nystagmus also manifest and vision is often poor [4].

Pigmentation of the RPE involves the formation of melanin within dedicated intracellular organelles, called melanosomes [3]. Formation of melanin is a multistep process initiated by the conversion of tyrosine to 3,4dihydroxyphenylalanine (DOPA) by tyrosinase and then formation of melanin via a cascade of reactions. Melanin is formed within specialized organelles called melanosomes that mature through a series of stages that ultimately forms melanised mature organelles. Mature melanosomes move from the perinuclear region towards the periphery of cells, via transport processes involving microtubules and actin-based motor myosin VIIa. Mutations affecting melanin formation, melanosome maturation, or transport of melanosomes can all lead to defects in pigmentation and albinism [3].

The most important enzyme involved in melanogenesis is tyrosinase, which is expressed in the RPE as well as other pigmented cells within the eye. Mutations in tyrosinase cause a decrease or absence of melanin formation and are associated with human oculocutaneous albinism type 1. There are a number of albino strains of mouse and rat including the balb/c mouse and Sprague-Dawley rat that carry spontaneous mutations in tyrosinase (*tyr*^{c}). Comparisons of retinal structure and function of albino strains of rats compared to pigmented strains have revealed only very modest differences. More recently, detailed analysis of the RPE and retina has been undertaken in albino C57Bl6J-c2J compared to the pigmented congenic C57Bl6 strain [5]. Rod mediated function, as measured by the electroretinogram, is reduced in albino C57Bl6-c2J mice compared to control, and photoreceptor density is reduced in mice aged 7 months or older. In addition, there was an absence of melanin in the RPE and a decrease in melanosome number in albino C57Bl6-c2J. Notably, treatment designed to genetically correct the tyrosinase mutation, with subretinal injection of AAV2-CMV-hTYR, ameliorated the deficits in retinal structure and function [5], suggesting that this mutation was intimately involved in the deficits observed.

Ocular albinism is an X-linked form of the disease that is caused by a mutation in the *OA1* gene, also called *GPR143*. Although skin pigmentation is normal, pigmentation of structures within the eye is absent and patients show nystagmus, foveal hypoplasia and reduced vision. OA1 encodes a G protein receptor that localizes to the membrane of mature melanosomes within the RPE. *OA1 null* mice have been created to further understand the mechanisms of this condition and show many of the hallmark signs of human ocular albinism [75]. Like human ocular albinism, *OA1* null mice develop abnormally large melanosomes in the RPE of *OA1* null mice from birth that increase in number with age [75]. These mice have normal retinal function as measured by the electroretinogram but show abnormal development of the ipsilateral ganglion cell axons that project through the optic chiasm. Along with numerous macromelanosomes within the RPE, a greater proportion of melanosomes were located within the apical part of the RPE in *OA1* null mice compared to control mice and also to a greater extent away from the nucleus. These results suggest that the protein product of *OA1* is important for melanosome maturation as well as peripheral displacement within cells [6].

Modelling Alterations in the RPE with Relevance to AMD

Age-related macular degeneration is the leading cause of irreversible vision loss in those over 60 years of age. It is a multifactorial disease with the early stages affecting 1:7 people over 50 years of age. Of these, many advance to the chronic atrophic form the disease or the acute neovascular form of the disease. The RPE and Bruch's membrane play important roles in the pathogenesis of the disease in its earliest form. The RPE progressively accumulates lipofuscin and ultimately the number of RPE cells decreases. At the ultrastructural level, deposits are observed between the RPE and Bruch's membrane, called basal laminar deposits and basal linear deposits. It has been suggested that the formation of basal linear deposits is indicative of progressing AMD, whereas the formation of basal laminar deposits an indicator of RPE and photoreceptor degeneration.

A central feature of early age-related macular degeneration is an increased thickness of Bruch's membrane as well as drusen formation. Drusen are subretinal deposits composed of a large number of different components including lipid, β-amyloid, and complement proteins. Clinically, patients can progress to one or both forms of advanced AMD [76]. Dry AMD is called geographic atrophy and is characterized by RPE atrophy and subsequent photoreceptor degeneration. It is notable that rod photoreceptors are initially affected, followed by cones. Approximately 10% of patients develop the wet form of AMD which is associated with pathological growth of blood vessels from the choroid into the macula. Although the underlying mechanism for angiogenesis in AMD is complex, it is now well accepted that the angiogenic growth factor, Vascular Endothelial Growth Factor, plays a key role.

Development of animal models of AMD has been challenging for a number of reasons. First, commonly used laboratory animals, such as rats and mice, do not possess a macula, nor live for many years. Moreover, there are no reported cases of the development of an AMD-like condition in large animals such as cats or dogs. There are also significant differences in the structure of the retina, transport of lipid across the RPE and the regulation of the innate immune system in rodents compared to humans. In addition, the influence of multiple genes in combination with environmental effects makes studying the disease even in aging mice difficult. Indeed, there are no animals that recapitulate all aspects of the disease. Below, we summarize how animals (both non-rodent and rodents) can be used to model specific signs associated with AMD.

Early Age-Related Macular Degeneration in Primates

Drusen are an important biomarker for the development of early stage age-related macular degeneration and their size can provide one way for identifying those most at risk of progression to advanced disease [77]. Drusen consist of an abundance of lipid, immune fragments, amyloid and other constituents. The only animals reported to develop drusen with similarities to human disease are simian primates. Indeed, 32% of a cohort of 278 aged female Macaque monkeys showed drusen within the posterior pole and of these only 10% showed 20 or more deposits. Importantly, the composition of the drusen in these animals was similar to those reported in humans, and included approximately 60 different molecular species including vitronectin, amyloid, complement factors and lipid moieties. Ageing primates not only develop drusen with age, but also demonstrate some similarity in genetic risk profile. In particular, HTRA1 (high temperature requirement factor A1) and ARMS2 (age related maculopathy susceptibility 2) have been associated with drusen formation in primates. Despite these similarities, advanced forms of AMD including geographic atrophy and choroidal neovascularization has not been described in primates. In addition, the development of drusen occurs at a comparatively earlier age in primates with about half of all monkeys affected by the equivalent of 20–30 years of age, compared to humans where approximately 50% are affected by 70 years of age.

Although there are many reports of mouse strains developing discrete white lesions across the retinal fundus, careful analysis of these lesions indicates that they do not contain the same breadth of molecular constituents as humans. Although it has been difficult to correlate precisely "drusen-like" lesions with histopathology in mouse strains, some reports suggest that the lesions arise because of an accumulation of retinal immune cells in the subretinal space. Moreover, some mouse strains carry a recessive mutation in $Crb1^{rd8}$, a gene important for photoreceptor polarization. Homozygous expression of this mutation is associated with discrete white lesions across the retina which correspond to the formation of rosettes within the outer retina [78]. Thus, mouse strains that develop discrete "drusen-like" lesions need to be carefully evaluated.

Diseases of the Retina Associated with Accumulation of Lipofuscin in the RPE

Accumulation of lipofuscin in the RPE is an important ageing change that heralds the onset of advanced atrophic AMD. The relationship between lipofuscin and RPE function and death can be investigated using a range of animal models that show accumulation of lipofuscin in these cells including the ABCA4null mouse model of Stargardt's disease described above and models of neuronal ceroid lipofuscinosis (CLN) [79].

Neuronal ceroid lipofuscinoses (CLNs) are a group of inherited lysosomal storage disorders that lead to progressive neurodegeneration

[80]. Globally they affect between 1:12,500 and 1:100,000 and are characterized by progressive cognitive decline, motor dysfunction, irreversible loss of vision and epilepsy that eventually leads to premature death. There are 14 distinct forms of CLNs, showing differences in the age of onset, and gene product, referred to as CLN1–14 [80]. Most are inherited in an autosomal recessive manner but there are some forms of the adult variant that are inherited in an autosomal dominant fashion [80]. A common feature of all forms of CLN is that all tissues show accumulation of autofluorescent storage material at the cellular level. In the posterior eye both the RPE and all cells in the retina show accumulation of lipofuscin that is associated with gradual photoreceptor dysfunction and death.

A range of large non-laboratory animals are affected by ceroid lipofuscinoses including cows, sheep, and dogs [81]. There are at least 13 mouse models of ceroid lipofuscinoses that mirror many of the features of human disease [82]. Mutations in *CLN6* are associated with a variant of late infantile ceroid lipofuscinosis. *CLN6* encodes a 305 amino acid endoplasmic reticulum membrane protein of unknown function. A spontaneous mutation in *CLN6* causes retinal degeneration in *Cln6* null (also called *nclf*) mice. Figure 19.3 shows retinal fundus images of the *Cln6* null mice (*nclf*) and shows small discrete white lesions across the retina and extensive accumulation of autofluorescent material within the RPE. This mouse strain develops many of the features of human disease including neurodegeneration of the cortex and visual system [83]. Notably, photoreceptor loss occurs from 1 month of age at an age when there is marked gliosis and accumulation of lysosomal storage material

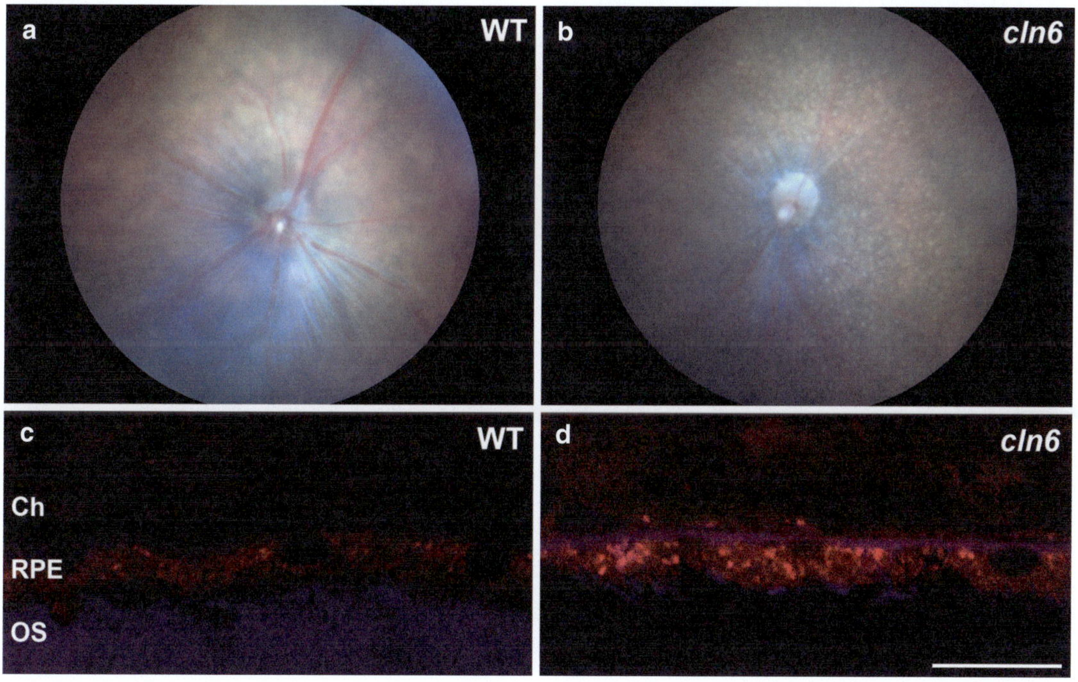

Fig. 19.3 *Cln6* mutant mice show accumulation of lipofucin in the RPE. (**a**, **b**) Images of the retina were collected *in vivo* using a MicronIII fundus camera. Fundus images from 8 month old (**a**) wildtype (WT) and (**b**) *cln6* mutant mice are shown. Many abnormal, hyper-reflective lesions are apparent in the *cln6* mutant fundus. (**c**, **d**) Eyes were collected, processed for histology and transverse retinal cryostat sections were imaged using a confocal microscope. Ultraviolet (blue) and far red (red) excitation wavelengths were used to evaluate auto-fluorescence in the RPE of (**c**) WT and (**d**) *cln6* mutant mice. Increased intensity of auto-fluorescence, indicative of increased lipofucsin deposition, was apparent in the RPE of *cln6* mutant mice. *Ch* choroid, *RPE* retinal pigment epithelium, *OS* outer segments; Scale for **c** and **d**, 20 μm

in both the RPE and all cells of the retina [84]. Moreover, the reduction in visual function occurs prior to anomalies in motor control. Motor performance is tested using the rotarod performance test, whereby animals are placed on a rotating rod and the duration of time that an animal stays on the rod used as an indicator of their balance and coordination. In *Cln6* null mice, motor impairment occurs from 8 months of age, well after loss of visual function [85]. One of the central questions that remains to be explored is why photoreceptors are preferentially affected in ceroid lipofuscinoses, despite widespread cellular accumulation of lipofuscin. With respect to the retina, it is not clear whether an anomaly in RPE function drives photoreceptor loss, or whether lipofuscin interferes with photoreceptor specifically.

Mouse Models Associated with Thickening of Bruch's Membrane

Thickening of Bruch's membrane is a feature of early AMD. This is thought to lead to deprivation of nutrient flow from the choriocapillaris to photoreceptors. There are a range of environmental and genetic factors that can lead to changes in composition of Bruch's membrane and its thickness especially with age. An association between the development and progression of AMD with diet, body mass index, and truncal obesity has been suggested. Dietary factors can affect the integrity of RPE/Bruch membrane in mice. For example, Bruch's membrane is thicker in C57Bl6 mice fed a high fat diet for 6 months compared to mice fed a conventional diet [86]. In addition, a high glycemic index diet is associated with a thicker Bruch's membrane in 16 month old mice compared to similar aged mice fed a low glycemic index diet [87].

Inheritance of a single nucleotide polymorphisms in HTRA1 may elevate risk of developing AMD via mechanisms that involve changes in Bruch's membrane. Notably, a single nucleotide polymorphism in *HTRA1* drives over expression of HTRA1 that ultimately leads to a change in the degradation of extracellular matrix proteoglycans. In agreement with this, transgenic overexpression of *Htra1* in murine RPE cells is associated with disruption and change in composition of Bruch's membrane [88].

Genes involved in lipid transport, including *APOE*, *LIPC*, *CETP* and *ABCA1*, have also been associated with risk of developing advanced AMD. ApoE mediates transport of lipid across cell membranes and is highly expressed by Bruch's membrane. There are two single nucleotide polymorphisms in *APOE* resulting in three different alleles (called ε2, ε3, and ε4). In contrast to the ε4 allele, inheritance of the ε2 allele increases risk of developing AMD [89]. A variety of mice with genetically modified expression of ApoE have been developed including *ApoE*-null mice, and transgenic mice expressing the human ε2, ε3 or ε4 alleles [90–92]. *ApoE*-null mice exhibit raised serum triglycerides and cholesterol and show thickening of Bruch's membrane [90, 93] (Fig. 19.4). ApoE3-Leiden mice which express a dysfunctional form of human ApoE3 develop similar changes in Bruch's membrane to *ApoE*-null mice when fed a high fat diet [91]. Finally, knock-in mice that express the human APOE2, APOE3 or APOE4 proteins under the control of the endogenous mouse *ApoE* promoter develop thickening of Bruchs' membrane and deposits in the basal RPE when fed a high fat diet [92]. Despite the significant changes in Bruch's membrane thickness and composition in these strains of mice, only a small number show progressive disease involving either RPE loss and/or choroidal neovascularization [92].

Anomalies in lipid transport may also explain the changes in Bruch's membrane observed in LDL or CD36 null mice. Low density lipoprotein (LDL) receptor deficient mice are not able to incorporate plasma cholesterol into cells resulting in raised triglyceride levels [94, 95]. These mice show increased thickness of Bruch's membrane when raised on a high fat diet [95]. CD36 is expressed on the basolateral surface of RPE cells and is important for binding of oxidized phospholipids, and perhaps the removal of oxidized lipid from the RPE to the underlying vasculature. *CD36*-null mice develop thickening of Bruch's membrane and subretinal deposits [94].

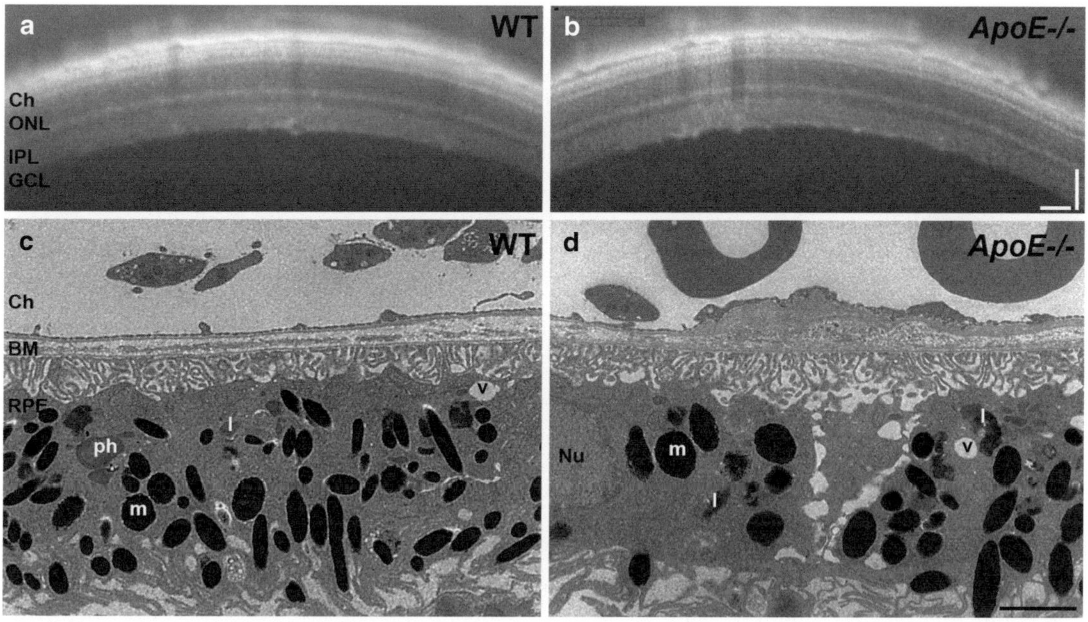

Fig. 19.4 *ApoE*$^{-/-}$ mice show thickening of Bruch's membrane with age. (**a**, **b**) Images of the retinal layer structure in transverse were collected *in vivo* using a Micron III optical coherence tomography (OCT) and fundus camera. OCT images from 13 month old (**a**) wildtype (WT) and (**b**) *ApoE*$^{-/-}$ mice are shown. No changes in retinal layer thickness are apparent in the *ApoE*$^{-/-}$ mice at this time point. (**c**, **d**) Eyes were collected, processed for histology and transverse retinal sections were collected and imaged using a transmission electron microscope. (**c**) In the WT mice, Bruch's membrane (BM) consisted of a thin, five layered structure including the RPE and choroidal basement membranes. The RPE contained many melanosomes (m), small amounts of lipofuscin (l) and occasional phagosomes of outer segments (ph). (**d**) In the *ApoE*$^{-/-}$ mice, Bruch's membrane was thicker and the layered structure less defined. The RPE also contained an apparent increase in lipofuscin content. *Ch* choroid, *BM* Bruch's membrane, *RPE* retinal pigment epithelium, *ONL* outer nuclear layer, *IPL* inner plexiform layer, *GCL* ganglion cell layer, *m* melanosomes, *ph* phagosomes, *Nu* nucleus, *l* lipofuscin, *v* vacuole; Scale for **a** and **b**, vertical 100 μm, horizontal 50 μm; Scale for **c** and **d**, 2 μm

Mouse Models Associated with Oxidative Stress

The retina has the highest oxygen consumption of any tissue of the body, and is therefore prone to oxidative stress [96]. There is increasing evidence that a change in the balance between antioxidant protection and oxidative stress within the RPE can lead to reduced retinal integrity and the development of features of early AMD. The RPE possesses a number of systems that protect it from oxidative stress. These systems are regulated at the transcriptional level via nuclear factor erythroid-2 related factor 2 (Nrf2) that ultimately influences the activity of important anti-oxidant enzymes such as catalase and superoxide dismutase (SOD) or that regulate cellular levels of glutathione and thioredoxin [96]. Factors that reduce expression of Nrf2 or that alter SOD1 or SOD2 activity are associated with oxidative stress and cellular damage within the RPE. Aging as well as smoking, two important risk factors for progression of AMD, are known to reduce Nrf2 mRNA expression in the RPE [97, 98]. Indeed, chronic smoking in C57Bl6 mice has been associated with reduced Nrf2 mRNA expression and RPE degeneration [97]. Nrf2 null mice develop drusen-like lesions within the posterior eye as well as RPE anomalies together with thickening of Bruch's membrane by 12 months of age [99]. Further evidence for an association between oxidative stress and the development of early features of AMD in mice is found in SOD1 null and SOD2 null mice. Like Nrf2 null mice,

SOD1 null mice display an increasing number of drusen-like deposits from nice months of age that are immunoreactive for a number of constituents of drusen including vitronectin and C5 [100]. In addition, thickening of Bruch's membrane, autofluorescence and degeneration of the RPE were also observed [100].

Pharmacological and Transgenic Models Associated with RPE Dysfunction

Chloroquine Toxicity

Hydroxychloroquine is commonly prescribed for the treatment of systemic lupus erythematosus, rheumatoid arthritis, related dermatologic conditions and also as a prophylactic agent to prevent malaria infection [101]. In those treated long term with high doses (generally >5 mg/kg real weight), approximately 7.5% show toxicity that includes RPE dysfunction, depigmentation of the RPE in a ring centred on the fovea (bull's eye maculopathy) and vision loss [102]. The condition is irreversible and thus careful screening is recommended for all patients treated with hydroxychloroquine so as to prevent vision loss [101]. As a consequence of toxicity, hydroxychloroquine is more commonly prescribed than its parent compound chloroquine.

The mechanism(s) by which hydroxychloroquine and chloroquine affect the RPE are not well understood. Several animal models of chloroquine retinopathy have been described which highlight the effect of chloroquine on the RPE. Chronic treatment of primates or cats is associated with RPE loss and subsequent photoreceptor dysfunction [103, 104]. Chloroquine may induce RPE dysfunction and death via mechanisms that influence lysosomal function [105]. Indeed, chloroquine is known to raise the intracellular pH of lysosomes within the RPE [105], causing alkalinization of lysomes. In addition, some studies suggest that binding of the drug to melanin concentrates and/or prolong the effects of the drug.

Modelling RPE Change in Response to Selective Gene Modification

Over the last 30 years studies evaluating the retinal changes that occur in animals that carry mutations encoding proteins in the RPE have greatly expanded our knowledge of disease mechanisms. Our knowledge of the role of the RPE in retinal disease has been enhanced by evaluating animals with spontaneous mutation such as the RCS rat, and then by examining structure-function relationships in "knocking out" or "knocking in" transgenic mouse lines. Much of this information is outlined in the sections above. A limitation of the approaches described so far, is that the genes "knocked-out" are not specific for the RPE only, and are also germ-line mutations that may affect developmental processes. More recently, the Cre-LoxP system has been used to more specifically manipulate gene expression within the RPE in a selective fashion [106]. Cre recombinase is a P1 bacteriophage protein that binds to a 34 bp long target recognition site known as loxP [107]. Through recombination, Cre recombinase has the ability to excise LoxP flanked sequences from the genome. Moreover, using tissue-specific promoters to drive cre recombinase expression provides a means of manipulating gene expression in specific cell types. There are at least four RPE specific Cre lines that have been developed for gene manipulation studies of the RPE, that include the dopachrome tautomerase (Dct)-cre line [108], a tyrosinase related protein line (*Tyrp1*-cre) [109] both of which drive changes in gene expression in a non-inducible fashion. That is, cre expression is present during embryonic development and crossing these mice with floxed mice, results in gene manipulation from an embryonic stage. Two inducible cre lines have also been developed, MCT3-cre and Best1-cre [1, 110]. These mice e use either the tetracycline-inducible system or the estrogen receptor system to control cre expression [1, 110]. Cre recombinase is induced when mice are treated with doxycycline or taxomifen respectively. By crossing *Mct3-CRE*^{ER} with floxed *DTA* mice that express the diphtheria toxin A chain under a ubiquitous promoter, Longbottom and colleagues studies the retinal structural and functional changes that occur in response to selective loss of a proportion of RPE cells [1]. They showed significant loss of photoreceptor structure and function in regions of ablated RPE, highlighting the importance of the RPE for maintaining photoreceptor integrity.

The Cre LoxP system has also been used to study specific cellular processes within the RPE. For example, crossing floxed *Lrat* mice with CMV-cre mice which express cre recombninase in all germ line cells provided a means of selectively ablating Lrat [45]. Using this approach, the importance of Lrat, for maintaining photoreceptor integrity was demonstrated [45]. Using a Cre LoxP system, the importance of autophagy in maintaining RPE integrity has been investigated. Crossing floxed *Rb1cc1*$^{flox/flox}$ mice with Best1-Cre caused the ablation of the RB1CC1 component of the ULK1-ATG13-RB1CC1 autophagy complex, selectively from RPE cells [111]. Ablation of RB1CC1 was associated with a range of anomalies in retinal structure and function [111].

Conclusions

The RPE plays a critical role in maintaining the normal function of photoreceptors. It not only absorbs stray light, but also expressed critical ion channels and transporters that mediate the transport of vital ions and nutrients to and from the underlying vasculature. A range of inherited and age related diseases are caused by mutations and defects in many of the proteins that underpin these functions. A range of large animals as well as laboratory rodents carry similar mutations to those that cause human disease and therefore provide an excellent means for understanding the pathogenesis of these diseases. A great deal has been learned by studying the cellular and functional changes that occur in both small and large animals with mutations affecting the RPE. In addition, these animals provide a method for translating novel treatments to a clinical setting.

Funding

This work was funded by NHMRC ***(#APP1061419)*** to ELF/KAV and an ARC grant LP 150100482 to ELF.

References

1. Longbottom R, Fruttiger M, Douglas RH, Martinez-Barbera JP, Greenwood J, Moss SE. Genetic ablation of retinal pigment epithelial cells reveals the adaptive response of the epithelium and impact on photoreceptors. Proc Natl Acad Sci U S A. 2009;106(44):18728–33.
2. Strauss O. The retinal pigment epithelium in visual function. Physiol Rev. 2005;85(3):845–81.
3. Sparrow JR, Hicks D, Hamel CP. The retinal pigment epithelium in health and disease. Curr Mol Med. 2010;10(9):802–23.
4. Ray K, Chaki M, Sengupta M. Tyrosinase and ocular diseases: some novel thoughts on the molecular basis of oculocutaneous albinism type 1. Prog Retin Eye Res. 2007;26(4):323–58.
5. Gargiulo A, Bonetti C, Montefusco S, Neglia S, Di Vicino U, Marrocco E, Corte MD, Domenici L, Auricchio A, Surace EM. AAV-mediated tyrosinase gene transfer restores melanogenesis and retinal function in a model of oculo-cutaneous albinism type I (OCA1). Mol Ther. 2009;17(8):1347–54.
6. Palmisano I, Bagnato P, Palmigiano A, Innamorati G, Rotondo G, Altimare D, Venturi C, Sviderskaya EV, Piccirillo R, Coppola M, Marigo V, Incerti B, Ballabio A, Surace EM, Tacchetti C, Bennett DC, Schiaffino MV. The ocular albinism type 1 protein, an intracellular G protein-coupled receptor, regulates melanosome transport in pigment cells. Hum Mol Genet. 2008;17(22):3487 501.
7. Johnson AA, Guziewicz KE, Lee CJ, Kalathur RC, Pulido JS, Marmorstein LY, Marmorstein AD. Bestrophin 1 and retinal disease. Prog Retin Eye Res. 2017;58:45–69.
8. Milenkovic A, Brandl C, Milenkovic VM, Jendryke T, Sirianant L, Wanitchakool P, Zimmermann S, Reiff CM, Horling F, Schrewe H, Schreiber R, Kunzelmann K, Wetzel CH, Weber BH. Bestrophin 1 is indispensable for volume regulation in human retinal pigment epithelium cells. Proc Natl Acad Sci U S A. 2015;112(20):E2630–9.
9. Bergersen L, Johannsson E, Veruki ML, Nagelhus EA, Halestrap A, Sejersted OM, Ottersen OP. Cellular and subcellular expression of monocarboxylate transporters in the pigment epithelium and retina of the rat. Neuroscience. 1999;90(1):319–31.
10. Hsu SC, Molday RS. Glucose metabolism in photoreceptor outer segments. Its role in phototransduction and in NADPH-requiring reactions. J Biol Chem. 1994;269(27):17954–9.

11. Ban Y, Rizzolo LJ. Differential regulation of tight junction permeability during development of the retinal pigment epithelium. Am J Physiol Cell Physiol. 2000;279(3):C744–50.
12. Sears AE, Palczewski K. Lecithin:retinol acyltransferase: a key enzyme involved in the retinoid (visual) cycle. Biochemistry. 2016;55(22):3082–91.
13. Young RW. The renewal of photoreceptor cell outer segments. J Cell Biol. 1967;33(1):61–72.
14. Young RW. The renewal of rod and cone outer segments in the rhesus monkey. J Cell Biol. 1971;49(2):303–18.
15. Strick DJ, Feng W, Vollrath D. Mertk drives myosin II redistribution during retinal pigment epithelial phagocytosis. Invest Ophthalmol Vis Sci. 2009;50(5):2427–35.
16. Finnemann SC, Nandrot EF. MerTK activation during RPE phagocytosis in vivo requires alphaVbeta5 integrin. Adv Exp Med Biol. 2006;572:499–503.
17. Barnstable CJ, Tombran-Tink J. Neuroprotective and antiangiogenic actions of PEDF in the eye: molecular targets and therapeutic potential. Prog Retin Eye Res. 2004;23(5):561–77.
18. Calippe B, Augustin S, Beguier F, Charles-Messance H, Poupel L, Conart JB, Hu SJ, Lavalette S, Fauvet A, Rayes J, Levy O, Raoul W, Fitting C, Denefle T, Pickering MC, Harris C, Jorieux S, Sullivan PM, Sahel JA, Karoyan P, Sapieha P, Guillonneau X, Gautier EL, Sennlaub F. Complement factor H inhibits CD47-mediated resolution of inflammation. Immunity. 2017;46(2):261–72.
19. Bhutto I, Lutty G. Understanding age-related macular degeneration (AMD): relationships between the photoreceptor/retinal pigment epithelium/Bruch's membrane/choriocapillaris complex. Mol Aspects Med. 2012;33(4):295–317.
20. Booij JC, Baas DC, Beisekeeva J, Gorgels TG, Bergen AA. The dynamic nature of Bruch's membrane. Prog Retin Eye Res. 2010;29(1):1–18.
21. Hartong DT, Berson EL, Dryja TP. Retinitis pigmentosa. Lancet. 2006;368(9549):1795–809.
22. Aplin FP, Fletcher EL, Luu CD, Vessey KA, Allen PJ, Guymer RH, Shepherd RK, Shivdasani MN. Stimulation of a suprachoroidal retinal prosthesis drives cortical responses in a feline model of retinal degeneration. Invest Ophthalmol Vis Sci. 2016;57(13):5216–29.
23. Cideciyan AV. Leber congenital amaurosis due to RPE65 mutations and its treatment with gene therapy. Prog Retin Eye Res. 2010;29(5):398–427.
24. Bourne MC, Campbell DA, Tansley K. Hereditary degeneration of the rat retina. Br J Ophthalmol. 1938;22(10):613–23.
25. Dowling JE, Sidman RL. Inherited retinal dystrophy in the rat. J Cell Biol. 1962;14:73–109.
26. Fletcher EL, Kalloniatis M. Neurochemical development of the degenerating rat retina. J Comp Neurol. 1997;388(1):1–22.
27. Cuenca N, Pinilla I, Sauve Y, Lund R. Early changes in synaptic connectivity following progressive photoreceptor degeneration in RCS rats. Eur J Neurosci. 2005;22(5):1057–72.
28. Fletcher EL, Kalloniatis M. Neurochemical architecture of the normal and degenerating rat retina. J Comp Neurol. 1996;376(3):343–60.
29. D'Cruz PM, Yasumura D, Weir J, Matthes MT, Abderrahim H, LaVail MM, Vollrath D. Mutation of the receptor tyrosine kinase gene Mertk in the retinal dystrophic RCS rat. Hum Mol Genet. 2000;9(4):645–51.
30. Patel N, Aldahmesh MA, Alkuraya H, Anazi S, Alsharif H, Khan AO, Sunker A, Al-Mohsen S, Abboud EB, Nowilaty SR, Alowain M, Al-Zaidan H, Al-Saud B, Alasmari A, Abdel-Salam GM, Abouelhoda M, Abdulwahab FM, Ibrahim N, Naim E, Al-Younes B, E AlMostafa A, AlIssa A, Hashem M, Buzovetsky O, Xiong Y, Monies D, Altassan N, Shaheen R, Al-Hazzaa SA, Alkuraya FS. Expanding the clinical, allelic, and locus heterogeneity of retinal dystrophies. Genet Med. 2016;18(6):554–62.
31. Mullen RJ, LaVail MM. Inherited retinal dystrophy: primary defect in pigment epithelium determined with experimental rat chimeras. Science. 1976;192(4241):799–801.
32. Vollrath D, Feng W, Duncan JL, Yasumura D, D'Cruz PM, Chappelow A, Matthes MT, Kay MA, LaVail MM. Correction of the retinal dystrophy phenotype of the RCS rat by viral gene transfer of Mertk. Proc Natl Acad Sci U S A. 2001;98(22):12584–9.
33. Ghazi NG, Abboud EB, Nowilaty SR, Alkuraya H, Alhommadi A, Cai H, Hou R, Deng WT, Boye SL, Almaghamsi A, Al Saikhan F, Al-Dhibi H, Birch D, Chung C, Colak D, LaVail MM, Vollrath D, Erger K, Wang W, Conlon T, Zhang K, Hauswirth W, Alkuraya FS. Treatment of retinitis pigmentosa due to MERTK mutations by ocular subretinal injection of adeno-associated virus gene vector: results of a phase I trial. Hum Genet. 2016;135(3):327–43.
34. Duncan JL, LaVail MM, Yasumura D, Matthes MT, Yang H, Trautmann N, Chappelow AV, Feng W, Earp HS, Matsushima GK, Vollrath D. An RCS-like retinal dystrophy phenotype in mer knockout mice. Invest Ophthalmol Vis Sci. 2003;44(2):826–38.
35. Sidman RL, Kosaras B, Tang M. Pigment epithelial and retinal phenotypes in the vitiligo mivit, mutant mouse. Invest Ophthalmol Vis Sci. 1996;37(6):1097–115.
36. Smith SB. C57BL/6J-vit/vit mouse model of retinal degeneration: light microscopic analysis and evaluation of rhodopsin levels. Exp Eye Res. 1992;55(6):903–10.
37. Tang M, Pawlyk BS, Kosaras B, Berson EL, Sidman RL. ERG abnormalities in relation to histopathologic findings in vitiligo mutant mice. Exp Eye Res. 1997;65(2):215–22.
38. den Hollander AI, Roepman R, Koenekoop RK, Cremers FP. Leber congenital amaurosis: genes, proteins and disease mechanisms. Prog Retin Eye Res. 2008;27(4):391–419.
39. Gu SM, Thompson DA, Srikumari CR, Lorenz B, Finckh U, Nicoletti A, Murthy KR, Rathmann

M, Kumaramanickavel G, Denton MJ, Gal A. Mutations in RPE65 cause autosomal recessive childhood-onset severe retinal dystrophy. Nat Genet. 1997;17(2):194–7.
40. Pang JJ, Chang B, Hawes NL, Hurd RE, Davisson MT, Li J, Noorwez SM, Malhotra R, McDowell JH, Kaushal S, Hauswirth WW, Nusinowitz S, Thompson DA, Heckenlively JR. Retinal degeneration 12 (rd12): a new, spontaneously arising mouse model for human Leber congenital amaurosis (LCA). Mol Vis. 2005;11:152–62.
41. Redmond TM, Yu S, Lee E, Bok D, Hamasaki D, Chen N, Goletz P, Ma JX, Crouch RK, Pfeifer K. Rpe65 is necessary for production of 11-cis-vitamin A in the retinal visual cycle. Nat Genet. 1998;20(4):344–51.
42. Samardzija M, von Lintig J, Tanimoto N, Oberhauser V, Thiersch M, Reme CE, Seeliger M, Grimm C, Wenzel A. R91W mutation in Rpe65 leads to milder early-onset retinal dystrophy due to the generation of low levels of 11-cis-retinal. Hum Mol Genet. 2008;17(2):281–92.
43. Nicholas FW, Hobbs M. Mutation discovery for Mendelian traits in non-laboratory animals: a review of achievements up to 2012. Anim Genet. 2014;45(2):157–70.
44. Veske A, Nilsson SE, Narfstrom K, Gal A. Retinal dystrophy of Swedish briard/briard-beagle dogs is due to a 4-bp deletion in RPE65. Genomics. 1999;57(1):57–61.
45. Ruiz A, Ghyselinck NB, Mata N, Nusinowitz S, Lloyd M, Dennefeld C, Chambon P, Bok D. Somatic ablation of the Lrat gene in the mouse retinal pigment epithelium drastically reduces its retinoid storage. Invest Ophthalmol Vis Sci. 2007;48(12):5377–87.
46. Mowat FM, Petersen-Jones SM, Williamson H, Williams DL, Luthert PJ, Ali RR, Bainbridge JW. Topographical characterization of cone photoreceptors and the area centralis of the canine retina. Mol Vis. 2008;14:2518–27.
47. Tanna P, Strauss RW, Fujinami K, Michaelides M. Stargardt disease: clinical features, molecular genetics, animal models and therapeutic options. Br J Ophthalmol. 2017;101(1):25–30.
48. Molday RS, Zhong M, Quazi F. The role of the photoreceptor ABC transporter ABCA4 in lipid transport and Stargardt macular degeneration. Biochim Biophys Acta. 2009;1791(7):573–83.
49. Mata NL, Weng J, Travis GH. Biosynthesis of a major lipofuscin fluorophore in mice and humans with ABCR-mediated retinal and macular degeneration. Proc Natl Acad Sci U S A. 2000;97(13):7154–9.
50. Weng J, Mata NL, Azarian SM, Tzekov RT, Birch DG, Travis GH. Insights into the function of Rim protein in photoreceptors and etiology of Stargardt's disease from the phenotype in abcr knockout mice. Cell. 1999;98(1):13–23.
51. Radu RA, Hu J, Yuan Q, Welch DL, Makshanoff J, Lloyd M, McMullen S, Travis GH, Bok D. Complement system dysregulation and inflammation in the retinal pigment epithelium of a mouse model for Stargardt macular degeneration. J Biol Chem. 2011;286(21):18593–601.
52. Charbel Issa P, Barnard AR, Singh MS, Carter E, Jiang Z, Radu RA, Schraermeyer U, MacLaren RE. Fundus autofluorescence in the Abca4(−/−) mouse model of Stargardt disease—correlation with accumulation of A2E, retinal function, and histology. Invest Ophthalmol Vis Sci. 2013;54(8):5602–12.
53. Mata NL, Tzekov RT, Liu X, Weng J, Birch DG, Travis GH. Delayed dark-adaptation and lipofuscin accumulation in abcr+/− mice: implications for involvement of ABCR in age-related macular degeneration. Invest Ophthalmol Vis Sci. 2001;42(8):1685–90.
54. Kijas JW, Zangerl B, Miller B, Nelson J, Kirkness EF, Aguirre GD, Acland GM. Cloning of the canine ABCA4 gene and evaluation in canine cone-rod dystrophies and progressive retinal atrophies. Mol Vis. 2004;10:223–32.
55. Boon CJ, Klevering BJ, Leroy BP, Hoyng CB, Keunen JE, den Hollander AI. The spectrum of ocular phenotypes caused by mutations in the BEST1 gene. Prog Retin Eye Res. 2009;28(3):187–205.
56. Marmorstein AD, Marmorstein LY, Rayborn M, Wang X, Hollyfield JG, Petrukhin K. Bestrophin, the product of the best vitelliform macular dystrophy gene (VMD2), localizes to the basolateral plasma membrane of the retinal pigment epithelium. Proc Natl Acad Sci U S A. 2000;97(23):12758–63.
57. Rosenthal R, Bakall B, Kinnick T, Peachey N, Wimmers S, Wadelius C, Marmorstein A, Strauss O. Expression of bestrophin-1, the product of the VMD2 gene, modulates voltage-dependent Ca2+ channels in retinal pigment epithelial cells. FASEB J. 2006;20(1):178–80.
58. Marmorstein AD, Cross HE, Peachey NS. Functional roles of bestrophins in ocular epithelia. Prog Retin Eye Res. 2009;28(3):206–26.
59. Zhang Y, Stanton JB, Wu J, Yu K, Hartzell HC, Peachey NS, Marmorstein LY, Marmorstein AD. Suppression of Ca2+ signaling in a mouse model of Best disease. Hum Mol Genet. 2010;19(6):1108–18.
60. Marmorstein LY, Wu J, McLaughlin P, Yocom J, Karl MO, Neussert R, Wimmers S, Stanton JB, Gregg RG, Strauss O, Peachey NS, Marmorstein AD. The light peak of the electroretinogram is dependent on voltage-gated calcium channels and antagonized by bestrophin (best-1). J Gen Physiol. 2006;127(5):577–89.
61. Guziewicz KE, Sinha D, Gomez NM, Zorych K, Dutrow EV, Dhingra A, Mullins RF, Stone EM, Gamm DM, Boesze-Battaglia K, Aguirre GD. Bestrophinopathy: an RPE-photoreceptor interface disease. Prog Retin Eye Res. 2017;58:70–88.
62. Guziewicz KE, Owczarek-Lipska M, Kuffer J, Schelling C, Tontis A, Denis C, Eggen A, Leeb T, Dolf G, Braunschweig MH. The locus for bovine dilated cardiomyopathy maps to chromosome 18. Anim Genet. 2007;38(3):265–9.
63. Guziewicz KE, Slavik J, Lindauer SJ, Aguirre GD, Zangerl B. Molecular consequences of BEST1 gene mutations in canine multifocal retinopathy predict

functional implications for human bestrophinopathies. Invest Ophthalmol Vis Sci. 2011;52(7):4497–505.
64. Guziewicz KE, Aguirre GD, Zangerl B. Modeling the structural consequences of BEST1 missense mutations. Adv Exp Med Biol. 2012;723:611–8.
65. Zangerl B, Wickstrom K, Slavik J, Lindauer SJ, Ahonen S, Schelling C, Lohi H, Guziewicz KE, Aguirre GD. Assessment of canine BEST1 variations identifies new mutations and establishes an independent bestrophinopathy model (cmr3). Mol Vis. 2010;16:2791–804.
66. Weber BH, Vogt G, Wolz W, Ives EJ, Ewing CC. Sorsby's fundus dystrophy is genetically linked to chromosome 22q13-qter. Nat Genet. 1994;7(2):158–61.
67. Hamilton WK, Ewing CC, Ives EJ, Carruthers JD. Sorsby's fundus dystrophy. Ophthalmology. 1989;96(12):1755–62.
68. Weber BH, Lin B, White K, Kohler K, Soboleva G, Herterich S, Seeliger MW, Jaissle GB, Grimm C, Reme C, Wenzel A, Asan E, Schrewe H. A mouse model for Sorsby fundus dystrophy. Invest Ophthalmol Vis Sci. 2002;43(8):2732–40.
69. Janssen A, Hoellenriegel J, Fogarasi M, Schrewe H, Seeliger M, Tamm E, Ohlmann A, May CA, Weber BH, Stohr H. Abnormal vessel formation in the choroid of mice lacking tissue inhibitor of metalloprotease-3. Invest Ophthalmol Vis Sci. 2008;49(7):2812–22.
70. Fu L, Garland D, Yang Z, Shukla D, Rajendran A, Pearson E, Stone EM, Zhang K, Pierce EA. The R345W mutation in EFEMP1 is pathogenic and causes AMD-like deposits in mice. Hum Mol Genet. 2007;16(20):2411–22.
71. Marmorstein LY, McLaughlin PJ, Peachey NS, Sasaki T, Marmorstein AD. Formation and progression of sub-retinal pigment epithelium deposits in Efemp1 mutation knock-in mice: a model for the early pathogenic course of macular degeneration. Hum Mol Genet. 2007;16(20):2423–32.
72. Roosing S, Thiadens AA, Hoyng CB, Klaver CC, den Hollander AI, Cremers FP. Causes and consequences of inherited cone disorders. Prog Retin Eye Res. 2014;42:1–26.
73. Shu X, Luhmann UF, Aleman TS, Barker SE, Lennon A, Tulloch B, Chen M, Xu H, Jacobson SG, Ali R, Wright AF. Characterisation of a C1qtnf5 Ser163Arg knock-in mouse model of late-onset retinal macular degeneration. PLoS One. 2011;6(11):e27433.
74. Mattapallil MJ, Wawrousek EF, Chan CC, Zhao H, Roychoudhury J, Ferguson TA, Caspi RR. The Rd8 mutation of the Crb1 gene is present in vendor lines of C57BL/6N mice and embryonic stem cells, and confounds ocular induced mutant phenotypes. Invest Ophthalmol Vis Sci. 2012;53(6):2921–7.
75. Incerti B, Cortese K, Pizzigoni A, Surace EM, Varani S, Coppola M, Jeffery G, Seeliger M, Jaissle G, Bennett DC, Marigo V, Schiaffino MV, Tacchetti C, Ballabio A. Oa1 knock-out: new insights on the pathogenesis of ocular albinism type 1. Hum Mol Genet. 2000;9(19):2781–8.
76. Coleman HR, Chan CC, Ferris FL 3rd, Chew EY. Age-related macular degeneration. Lancet. 2008;372(9652):1835–45.
77. Ferris FL 3rd, Wilkinson CP, Bird A, Chakravarthy U, Chew E, Csaky K, Sadda SR, Beckman Initiative for Macular Research Classification Committee. Clinical classification of age-related macular degeneration. Ophthalmology. 2013;120(4):844–51.
78. Fletcher EL, Jobling AI, Greferath U, Mills SA, Waugh M, Ho T, de Iongh RU, Phipps JA, Vessey KA. Studying age-related macular degeneration using animal models. Optom Vis Sci. 2014;91(8):878–86.
79. Faller KM, Gutierrez-Quintana R, Mohammed A, Rahim AA, Tuxworth RI, Wager K, Bond M. The neuronal ceroid lipofuscinoses: opportunities from model systems. Biochim Biophys Acta. 2015;1852(10 Pt B):2267–78.
80. Boustany RM. Lysosomal storage diseases—the horizon expands. Nat Rev Neurol. 2013;9(10):583–98.
81. Weber K, Pearce DA. Large animal models for Batten disease: a review. J Child Neurol. 2013;28(9):1123–7.
82. Shacka JJ. Mouse models of neuronal ceroid lipofuscinoses: useful pre-clinical tools to delineate disease pathophysiology and validate therapeutics. Brain Res Bull. 2012;88(1):43–57.
83. Thelen M, Damme M, Schweizer M, Hagel C, Wong AM, Cooper JD, Braulke T, Galliciotti G. Disruption of the autophagy-lysosome pathway is involved in neuropathology of the nclf mouse model of neuronal ceroid lipofuscinosis. PLoS One. 2012;7(4):e35493.
84. Bartsch U, Galliciotti G, Jofre GF, Jankowiak W, Hagel C, Braulke T. Apoptotic photoreceptor loss and altered expression of lysosomal proteins in the nclf mouse model of neuronal ceroid lipofuscinosis. Invest Ophthalmol Vis Sci. 2013;54(10):6952–9.
85. Mirza M, Volz C, Karlstetter M, Langiu M, Somogyi A, Ruonala MO, Tamm ER, Jagle H, Langmann T. Progressive retinal degeneration and glial activation in the CLN6 (nclf) mouse model of neuronal ceroid lipofuscinosis: a beneficial effect of DHA and curcumin supplementation. PLoS One. 2013;8(10):e75963.
86. Dithmar S, Sharara NA, Curcio CA, Le NA, Zhang Y, Brown S, Grossniklaus HE. Murine high-fat diet and laser photochemical model of basal deposits in Bruch membrane. Arch Ophthalmol. 2001;119(11):1643–9.
87. Weikel KA, Fitzgerald P, Shang F, Caceres MA, Bian Q, Handa JT, Stitt AW, Taylor A. Natural history of age-related retinal lesions that precede AMD in mice fed high or low glycemic index diets. Invest Ophthalmol Vis Sci. 2012;53(2):622–32.
88. Vierkotten S, Muether PS, Fauser S. Overexpression of HTRA1 leads to ultrastructural changes in the elastic layer of Bruch's membrane via cleavage of extracellular matrix components. PLoS One. 2011;6(8):e22959.
89. Adams MK, Simpson JA, Richardson AJ, English DR, Aung KZ, Makeyeva GA, Guymer RH, Giles GG, Hopper J, Robman LD, Baird PN. Apolipoprotein E gene associations in age-related macular degeneration: the Melbourne Collaborative Cohort Study. Am J Epidemiol. 2012;175(6):511–8.

90. Dithmar S, Curcio CA, Le NA, Brown S, Grossniklaus HE. Ultrastructural changes in Bruch's membrane of apolipoprotein E-deficient mice. Invest Ophthalmol Vis Sci. 2000;41(8):2035–42.
91. Kliffen M, Lutgens E, Daemen MJ, de Muinck ED, Mooy CM, de Jong PT. The APO(*)E3-Leiden mouse as an animal model for basal laminar deposit. Br J Ophthalmol. 2000;84(12):1415–9.
92. Malek G, Johnson LV, Mace BE, Saloupis P, Schmechel DE, Rickman DW, Toth CA, Sullivan PM, Bowes Rickman C. Apolipoprotein E allele-dependent pathogenesis: a model for age-related retinal degeneration. Proc Natl Acad Sci U S A. 2005;102(33):11900–5.
93. Jobling AI, Guymer RH, Vessey KA, Greferath U, Mills SA, Brassington KH, Luu CD, Aung KZ, Trogrlic L, Plunkett M, Fletcher EL. Nanosecond laser therapy reverses pathologic and molecular changes in age-related macular degeneration without retinal damage. FASEB J. 2015;29(2):696–710.
94. Picard E, Houssier M, Bujold K, Sapieha P, Lubell W, Dorfman A, Racine J, Hardy P, Febbraio M, Lachapelle P, Ong H, Sennlaub F, Chemtob S. CD36 plays an important role in the clearance of oxLDL and associated age-dependent sub-retinal deposits. Aging (Albany NY). 2010;2(12):981–9.
95. Rudolf M, Winkler B, Aherrahou Z, Doehring LC, Kaczmarek P, Schmidt-Erfurth U. Increased expression of vascular endothelial growth factor associated with accumulation of lipids in Bruch's membrane of LDL receptor knockout mice. Br J Ophthalmol. 2005;89(12):1627–30.
96. Datta S, Cano M, Ebrahimi K, Wang L, Handa JT. The impact of oxidative stress and inflammation on RPE degeneration in non-neovascular AMD. Prog Retin Eye Res. 2017;60:201–18.
97. Cano M, Thimmalappula R, Fujihara M, Nagai N, Sporn M, Wang AL, Neufeld AH, Biswal S, Handa JT. Cigarette smoking, oxidative stress, the anti oxidant response through Nrf2 signaling, and age-related macular degeneration. Vision Res. 2010;50(7):652–64.
98. Sachdeva MM, Cano M, Handa JT. Nrf2 signaling is impaired in the aging RPE given an oxidative insult. Exp Eye Res. 2014;119:111–4.
99. Zhao Z, Chen Y, Wang J, Sternberg P, Freeman ML, Grossniklaus HE, Cai J. Age-related retinopathy in NRF2-deficient mice. PLoS One. 2011;6(4):e19456.
100. Imamura Y, Noda S, Hashizume K, Shinoda K, Yamaguchi M, Uchiyama S, Shimizu T, Mizushima Y, Shirasawa T, Tsubota K. Drusen, choroidal neovascularization, and retinal pigment epithelium dysfunction in SOD1-deficient mice: a model of age-related macular degeneration. Proc Natl Acad Sci U S A. 2006;103(30):11282–7.
101. Marmor MF, Kellner U, Lai TY, Melles RB, Mieler WF, American Academy of Ophthalmology. Recommendations on screening for chloroquine and hydroxychloroquine retinopathy (2016 revision). Ophthalmology. 2016;123(6):1386–94.
102. Melles RB, Marmor MF. The risk of toxic retinopathy in patients on long-term hydroxychloroquine therapy. JAMA Ophthalmol. 2014;132(12):1453–60.
103. Meier-Ruge W. Experimental investigation of the morphogenesis of chloroquine retinopathy. Arch Ophthalmol. 1965;73:540–4.
104. Rosenthal AR, Kolb H, Bergsma D, Huxsoll D, Hopkins JL. Chloroquine retinopathy in the rhesus monkey. Invest Ophthalmol Vis Sci. 1978;17(12):1158–75.
105. Guha S, Coffey EE, Lu W, Lim JC, Beckel JM, Laties AM, Boesze-Battaglia K, Mitchell CH. Approaches for detecting lysosomal alkalinization and impaired degradation in fresh and cultured RPE cells: evidence for a role in retinal degenerations. Exp Eye Res. 2014;126:68–76.
106. Nagy A. Cre recombinase: the universal reagent for genome tailoring. Genesis. 2000;26(2):99–109.
107. Metzger D, Chambon P. Site- and time-specific gene targeting in the mouse. Methods. 2001;24(1):71–80.
108. Guyonneau L, Rossier A, Richard C, Hummler E, Beermann F. Expression of Cre recombinase in pigment cells. Pigment Cell Res. 2002;15(4):305–9.
109. Mori M, Metzger D, Garnier JM, Chambon P, Mark M. Site-specific somatic mutagenesis in the retinal pigment epithelium. Invest Ophthalmol Vis Sci. 2002;43(5):1384–8.
110. Iacovelli J, Zhao C, Wolkow N, Veldman P, Gollomp K, Ojha P, Lukinova N, King A, Feiner L, Esumi N, Zack DJ, Pierce EA, Vollrath D, Dunaief JL. Generation of Cre transgenic mice with postnatal RPE-specific ocular expression. Invest Ophthalmol Vis Sci. 2011;52(3):1378–83.
111. Yao J, Jia L, Khan N, Lin C, Mitter SK, Boulton ME, Dunaief JL, Klionsky DJ, Guan JL, Thompson DA, Zacks DN. Deletion of autophagy inducer RB1CC1 results in degeneration of the retinal pigment epithelium. Autophagy. 2015;11(6):939–53.

Index

A. K. Klettner, S. Dithmar (eds.), *Retinal Pigment Epithelium in Health and Disease*,
https://doi.org/10.1007/978-3-030-28384-1

D

E

F

G

MIX
Papier aus verantwortungsvollen Quellen
Paper from responsible sources
FSC® C105338

If you have any concerns about our products,
you can contact us on
ProductSafety@springernature.com

In case Publisher is established outside the EU,
the EU authorized representative is:
Springer Nature Customer Service Center GmbH
Europaplatz 3, 69115 Heidelberg, Germany

Printed by Libri Plureos GmbH
in Hamburg, Germany